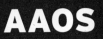

AAOS

Tenth Edition

Emergency

Care and Transportation of the Sick and Injured

Student Workbook

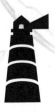

JONES & BARTLETT
LEARNING

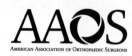

AAOS
AMERICAN ASSOCIATION OF ORTHOPAEDIC SURGEONS

World Headquarters
Jones & Bartlett Learning
5 Wall Street
Burlington, MA 01803
978-443-5000
info@jblearning.com
www.jblearning.com

Jones & Bartlett Learning Canada
6339 Ormindale Way
Mississauga, Ontario L5V 1J2
Canada

Jones & Bartlett Learning International
Barb House, Barb Mews
London W6 7PA
United Kingdom

Substantial discounts on bulk quantities of Jones & Bartlett Learning publications are available to corporations, professional associations, and other qualified organizations. For details and specific discount information, contact the special sales department at Jones & Bartlett Learning via the below contact information or send an email to specialsales@jblearning.com.

Jones & Bartlett Learning books and products are available through most bookstores and online booksellers. To contact Jones & Bartlett Learning directly, call 800-832-0034, fax 978-443-8000, or visit our website, www.jblearning.com.

Production Credits
Chairman of the Board: Clayton Jones
Chief Executive Officer: Ty Field
President: James Homer
SVP, Chief Operating Officer: Don Jones, Jr.
SVP, Chief Technology Officer: Dean Fossella
SVP, Chief Marketing Officer: Alison M. Pendergast
SVP, Chief Financial Officer: Ruth Siporin
Publisher: Kimberly Brophy
Acquisitions Editor, EMS: Christine Emerton
Managing Editor: Carol B. Guerrero
Associate Editor: Amanda Brandt
Associate Editor: Laura Burns
Editorial Assistant: Kara Ebrahim
Reprints & Special Projects Manager: Susan Schultz
Production Assistant: Tina Chen
Director of Marketing: Alisha Weisman

Director of Sales, Public Safety Group: Matthew Maniscalco
VP, Manufacturing and Inventory Control: Therese Connell
Composition: Abella Publishing Services
Text Design: Anne Spencer
Cover Design: Kristin E. Parker
Associate Photo Researcher: Jessica Elias
Cover Image: Cover photographed by Ray Kemp/911 imaging <www.911imaging.com>. Special thanks to Susan Hertzler, Terrance Jackson, Cass Wilson, AllMed, St. Charles County, MO Ambulance District; Photo of EMT patch: © Stephen Coburn/ShutterStock, Inc.
Printing and Binding: Courier Kendallville
Cover Printing: Courier Kendallville

Editorial Credits
Authors: Alan Heckman, BS, NREMTP
Brian Bricker, EMT, CFC

ISBN: 978-1-4496-5023-0

6048

Printed in the United States of America
15 14 13 12   10 9 8 7 6 5

Contents

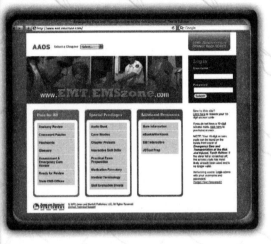

www.EMT.EMSzone.com

ISBN: 978-0-7637-9550-4

The engaging companion website provides a wealth of free resources, including Anatomy Review and Vital Vocabulary. The code printed on the inside front cover of *Emergency Care and Transportation of the Sick and Injured, Tenth Edition* provides students with special user privileges to a more robust gallery of educational resources, including an audio book.

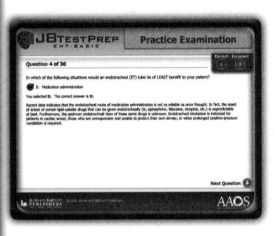

JBTest Prep: EMT-Basic Success

ISBN: 978-0-7637-5783-0

This dynamic program is designed to prepare you to sit for your state or national EMT-Basic certification examination by including the same type of questions you are likely to encounter in a similar electronic environment.

JBTest Prep: EMT-Basic Success provides a series of self-study modules, offering practice examinations and simulated certification examinations using case-based questions and detailed rationales to help you hone your knowledge of the subject matter.

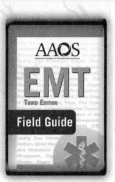

EMT Field Guide, Third Edition

Print ISBN: 978-0-7637-5877-6

iPhone App ISBN: 978-1-4496-0140-9

Fully updated to reflect the new *National EMS Education Standards*, this indispensable resource provides easy access to the vital emergency information needed by BLS personnel. The *Third Edition* of this concise field guide covers patient assessment tools, pediatric guidelines, general pharmacology, and essential information on safe transport. An all-new section on the most common medical emergencies encountered in the field features relevant signs and symptoms and appropriate management steps and makes this a must-have for BLS providers.

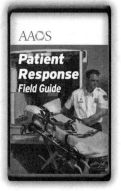

Patient Response Field Guide

Print ISBN: 978-0-7637-6068-7

iPhone App ISBN: 978-0-7637-9925-0

The *Patient Response Field Guide* puts essential assessment and management information into the hands of BLS providers. Key medical and trauma emergencies are presented alphabetically so that they are easily accessible when providers need them most. Each emergency follows a logical structure:

- Pertinent Considerations and Findings—Signs and symptoms, patient history

- Physical Examination—Vital signs, skin condition, assessment guidance

- Treatment—Standard management details for each condition

This indispensible guide includes "Key Question" boxes throughout to remind providers of the questions that may help them rule in or rule out certain conditions.

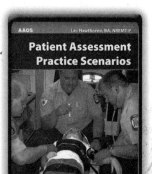

Patient Assessment Practice Scenarios

ISBN: 978-0-7637-7820-0

Patient assessment may be the most challenging subject for EMS students to grasp, and there never seems to be enough time in the classroom for practice. *Patient Assessment Practice Scenarios* allows students to fine-tune their understanding of the patient assessment process. This text includes 150 EMS practice scenarios (75 trauma and 75 medical) that focus on the assessment process as dictated by the National Registry medical assessment and trauma assessment skill sheets.

EMS Systems

General Knowledge

Matching

Match each of the items in the left column to the appropriate definition in the right column.

H	1. ALS	A.	EMS professional trained in ALS interventions
F	2. BLS	B.	A system of internal reviews and audits
M	3. EMT	C.	A system to provide prehospital care to the sick and injured
G	4. AEMT	D.	The physician who authorizes the EMT to perform in the field
A	5. Paramedic	E.	Responsibility of the medical director to ensure that appropriate care is delivered by an EMT
K	6. Medical control	F.	Basic lifesaving interventions, such as CPR
B	7. CQI	G.	EMS professional trained in some ALS interventions
C	8. EMS	H.	Advanced procedures, such as drug administration
L	9. Continuing education	I.	Designated area in which the EMS service is responsible for providing prehospital care
E	10. Quality control	J.	Protects disabled individuals from discrimination
I	11. Primary service area	K.	Physician instruction to EMS team
D	12. Medical director	L.	A required amount of training to maintain skills
J	13. Americans with Disabilities Act	M.	EMS professional trained in BLS interventions

Multiple Choice

Read each item carefully and then select the one best response.

B 1. Control of external bleeding, oxygen administration, and CPR are included in the "scope of practice" of the:

   A. paramedic.

   B. EMT.

   C. AEMT.

   D. EMR.

A 2. Which of the following is NOT true of medical control?

   A. It is determined by the dispatcher.

   B. It may be written or "standing orders."

   C. It may require online radio or phone consultation.

   D. It describes the care authorized by the medical director.

D 3. All of the following are components of continuous quality improvement EXCEPT:

   A. periodic run reviews.

   B. remedial training.

   C. internal reviews and audits.

   D. public seminars and meetings.

_D_   **4.** The major goal of quality improvement is to ensure that:
- **A.** quarterly audits of the EMS system are performed.
- **B.** EMTs have received BLS/CPR training.
- **C.** the public receives the highest standard of care.
- **D.** the proper information is received in the billing department.

_A_   **5.** Federal legislation concerning patient confidentiality is known as:
- **A.** HIPAA.
- **B.** NAACS.
- **C.** EMTALA.
- **D.** FLCPC.

Questions 6–10 are derived from the following scenario: After stocking the ambulance this morning, you and your partner go out for breakfast. While entering the restaurant, you see an older gentleman clutch his chest and collapse to the floor. When you get to him, he has no pulse and is not breathing.

_C_   **6.** Which of the following authorizes you, as an EMT, to provide emergency care to this patient?
- **A.** City council
- **B.** Medical control
- **C.** The medical director
- **D.** The fire chief

_D_   **7.** To treat this patient, you will follow:
- **A.** off-line medical control.
- **B.** online medical control.
- **C.** protocols.
- **D.** all the above.

_D_   **8.** What level of training would allow you to perform an electrocardiogram and advanced life support on this patient?
- **A.** EMR
- **B.** EMT
- **C.** AEMT
- **D.** Paramedic

_A_   **9.** While you checked the patient's airway, breathing, and circulation, your partner considered the benefits of requesting a(n) _____ ambulance to assist with patient care.
- **A.** ALS
- **B.** CQI
- **C.** PSA
- **D.** EMD

_B_   **10.** While you performed CPR on this patient, your partner retrieved the _____, which will deliver an appropriate electrical shock.
- **A.** EMD
- **B.** AED
- **C.** PSA
- **D.** GPS

True/False

If you believe the statement to be more true than false, write the letter "T" in the space provided. If you believe the statement to be more false than true, write the letter "F."

_F_ **1.** EMT personnel are the highest qualified members of the prehospital care team.

_T_ **2.** The EMT scope of practice may include the use of either an automated or manual defibrillator.

_F_ **3.** The purpose of continuous quality improvement (CQI) is to support discipline of personnel.

_T_ **4.** A professional appearance and manner by the EMT will help build a patient's confidence in the EMT's abilities.

_T_ **5.** Essential keys to being a good EMT include compassion and commitment.

_T_ **6.** As a health care professional and an extension of physician care, you are bound by patient confidentiality—even in your own home.

Fill-in-the-Blank

Read each item carefully and then complete the statement by filling in the missing words.

1. _Continuous quality improvement_ is a circular system of continuous internal and external reviews and audits of all aspects of an EMS system.

2. Each EMS system has a physician _medical director_ who authorizes the EMTs in the service to provide medical care in the field.

3. One of the most dramatic recent developments in prehospital emergency care is the use of a(n) _automated external_ defibrillator. _AED_

4. The primary _service_ area is the main area in which an EMS agency operates.

5. A 9-1-1 dispatch center is called a public safety _access point_, or PSAP.

Crossword Puzzle

The following crossword puzzle is an activity provided to reinforce correct spelling and understanding of medical terminology associated with emergency care and the EMT. Use the clues in the column to complete the puzzle.

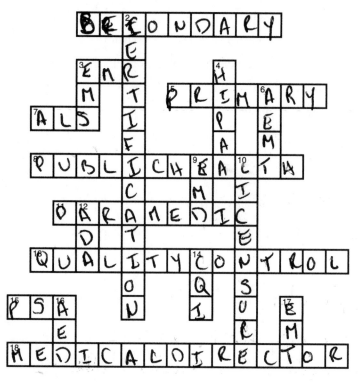

Across

1. Efforts to limit the effects of an injury or illness that you cannot completely prevent are considered _____ prevention.
3. The first trained individual, such as a police officer, fire fighter, lifeguard, or other rescuer, to arrive at the scene of an emergency to provide initial medical assistance
5. Efforts to prevent an injury or illness from ever occurring are known as _____ prevention.
7. Advanced lifesaving procedures
8. Focused on examining the health needs of entire populations with the goal of preventing health problems
11. An individual who has extensive training in advanced life support, including endotracheal intubation, emergency pharmacology, cardiac monitoring, and other advanced assessment and treatment skills
13. The responsibility of the medical director to ensure that the appropriate medical care standards are met by EMTs on each call
15. The designated area in which the EMS service is responsible for the provision of prehospital emergency care and transportation to the hospital
18. The physician who authorizes or delegates to the EMT the authority to provide medical care in the field

Down

1. A process in which a person, an institution, or a program is evaluated and recognized as meeting certain predetermined standards to provide safe and ethical care
2. A multidisciplinary system that represents the combined efforts of several professionals and agencies to provide prehospital emergency care to the sick and injured
4. Federal legislation passed in 1996. Its main effect in EMS is in limiting availability of patients' health care information and penalizing violations of patient privacy.
6. An individual who has training in specific aspects of advanced life support, such as intravenous therapy, and the administration of certain emergency medications
9. A system that assists dispatchers in selecting appropriate units to respond to a particular call for assistance and in providing callers with vital instructions until the arrival of EMS crews
10. The process whereby a state allows individuals to perform a regulated act
12. Comprehensive legislation that is designed to protect individuals with disabilities against discrimination
14. A system of internal and external reviews and audits of all aspects of an EMS system
16. A device that detects treatable life-threatening cardiac arrhythmias (eg, ventricular fibrillation and ventricular tachycardia) and delivers the appropriate electrical shock to the patient
17. An individual who has training in basic life support, including automated external defibrillation, use of a definitive airway adjunct, and assisting patients with certain medications

Critical Thinking

Short Answer

Complete this section with short written answers using the space provided.

1. Describe the EMT's role in the EMS system.

An EMT has the role of providing basic life support (BLS) to a patient on the scene.

2. What role has the US Department of Transportation played in the development of EMS?

DOT has provided EMS with guidelines. It is giving the opportunity for growth in the United States with funding and other management

3. List five roles and/or responsibilities of being an EMT.

① perform evaluation of the scene ② perform patient assesment ③ be on-scene leader ④ ensure and protect patient privacy ⑤ resolve emergency incidents

4. Describe the two basic types of medical direction that help the EMT provide care.

① off-line: standing orders, training, and supervision by the MD
② on-line: direction given over the phone or radio directly from the MD

Ambulance Calls

The following case scenarios provide an opportunity to explore the concerns associated with patient management and to enhance critical-thinking skills. Read each scenario and answer each question to the best of your ability.

1. You are dispatched to a two-car motor vehicle collision (MVC). Upon arrival, you see minimal damage to both vehicles because they were traveling less than 25 mph (40 kph) when the collision occurred. You and your partner interview and examine all the patients and find no apparent injuries. Dispatch contacts you and asks if you need an ALS crew to respond to your location.

Explain how you would respond and why.

Since my partner and I did not note any injuries I would tell
dispatch that an ALS crew was not needed on scene.

2. You and your partner are both EMTs and are dispatched to a private residence for a hanging. You arrive to find a distraught man in the front yard who quickly explains that he found his teenaged daughter in the garage hanging by the neck from an extension cord. You enter the garage and find the patient unresponsive and not breathing but with a weak pulse. Using EMT airway skills, neither of you is able to successfully open the patient's airway enough to provide ventilations.

What should you do?

Since the BLS that my partner and I provided failed to work for this
patient I would called dispatch to request an ALS crew for the
scene.

Workforce Safety and Wellness

General Knowledge

Matching

Match each of the items in the left column to the appropriate definition in the right column.

D	**1.** Cover	**A.** Examples include gloves, gowns, and face shields
A	**2.** PPE	**B.** The process of alarm, reaction, and recovery
C	**3.** OSHA	**C.** Regulatory compliance agency
F	**4.** Posttraumatic stress disorder	**D.** Concealment for protection
B	**5.** General adaptation syndrome	**E.** Capable of causing disease in a susceptible host
E	**6.** Pathogen	**F.** Delayed stress reaction
M	**7.** Transmission	**G.** Encompasses reporting, documentation, and treatment
G	**8.** Postexposure management	**H.** Unwelcome sexual advance
L	**9.** *Emergency Response Guidebook*	**I.** An infection of the liver
I	**10.** Hepatitis	**J.** Contact with blood, body fluids, tissues, or airborne particles
J	**11.** Exposure	**K.** The presence of infectious organisms in or on objects or a patient's body
N	**12.** Infection control	**L.** Resource detailing common hazards and proper responses
H	**13.** Sexual harassment	**M.** The way in which an infectious agent is spread
K	**14.** Contamination	**N.** Procedures to reduce transmission of infection among patients and health care personnel

Multiple Choice

Read each item carefully and then select the one best response.

C   **1.** From the age of 1 to the age of 40, _____ is the leading cause of death.
- **A.** cardiac arrest
- **B.** congenital disease
- **C.** trauma
- **D.** AIDS

C   **2.** The stage of the grieving process where an attempt is made to secure a prize for good behavior or promise to change one's lifestyle is known as:
- **A.** denial.
- **B.** acceptance.
- **C.** bargaining.
- **D.** depression.

A   **3.** The stage of the grieving process that involves refusal to accept diagnosis or care is known as:
- **A.** denial.
- **B.** acceptance.
- **C.** bargaining.
- **D.** depression.

_D_   **4.** The stage of the grieving process that involves an open expression of grief, internalized anger, hopelessness, and/or the desire to die is:
A. denial.
B. acceptance.
C. bargaining.
D. depression.

_B_   **5.** The stage of grieving where the person is ready to die is known as:
A. denial.
B. acceptance.
C. bargaining.
D. depression.

_A_   **6.** When providing support for a grieving person, it is okay to say:
A. "I'm sorry."
B. "Give it time."
C. "I know how you feel."
D. "You have to keep on going."

_D_   **7.** When grieving, family members may express:
A. rage.
B. anger.
C. despair.
D. all of the above.

_C_   **8.** _____ is a response to the anticipation of danger.
A. Rage
B. Anger
C. Anxiety
D. Despair

_B_   **9.** Signs of anxiety include all of the following EXCEPT:
A. diaphoresis.
B. comfort.
C. hyperventilation.
D. tachycardia.

_D_   **10.** Fear may be expressed as:
A. anger.
B. bad dreams.
C. restlessness.
D. all of the above.

_D_   **11.** If you find that you are the target of the patient's anger, make sure that you:
A. are safe.
B. do not take the anger or insults personally.
C. are tolerant and do not become defensive.
D. all of the above.

_D_ **12.** When caring for critically ill or injured patients, _____ will be decreased if you can keep the patient informed at the scene.

    A. confusion

    B. anxiety

    C. feelings of helplessness

    D. all of the above

_D_ **13.** When acknowledging the death of a child, reactions vary, but _____ is/are common.

    A. shock

    B. disbelief

    C. denial

    D. all of the above

_B_ **14.** Negative forms of stress include all of the following EXCEPT:

    A. long hours.

    B. exercise.

    C. shift work.

    D. frustration of losing a patient.

_D_ **15.** Stressors include _____ situations or conditions that may cause a variety of physiologic, physical, and psychological responses.

    A. emotional

    B. physical

    C. environmental

    D. all of the above

_D_ **16.** Prolonged or excessive stress has been proven to be a strong contributor to:

    A. heart disease.

    B. hypertension.

    C. cancer.

    D. all of the above.

_B_ **17.** _____ occur(s) when insignificant stressors accumulate to a larger stress-related problem.

    A. Negative stress

    B. Cumulative stress Pg 46

    C. Psychological stress

    D. Severe stressors

_D_ **18.** Events that can trigger critical incident stress include:

    A. mass-casualty incidents.

    B. serious injury or traumatic death of a child.

    C. death or serious injury of a coworker in the line of duty.

    D. all of the above.

_A_ **19.** The quickest source of energy is _____; however, this supply will last less than a day and is consumed in greater quantities during stress.

    A. glucose (sugar)

    B. carbohydrate

    C. protein

    D. fat

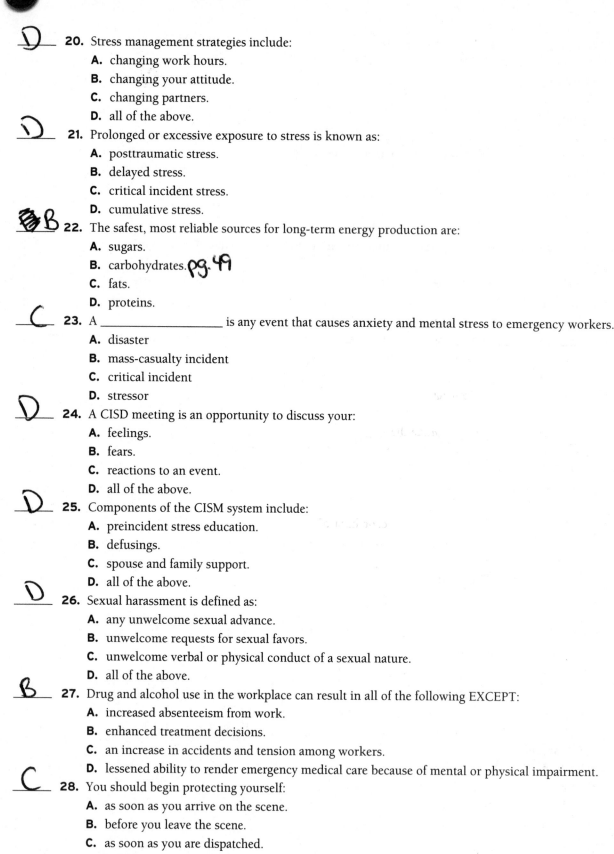

_D_ __ **20.** Stress management strategies include:
   A. changing work hours.
   B. changing your attitude.
   C. changing partners.
   D. all of the above.

_D_ __ **21.** Prolonged or excessive exposure to stress is known as:
   A. posttraumatic stress.
   B. delayed stress.
   C. critical incident stress.
   D. cumulative stress.

_B_ **22.** The safest, most reliable sources for long-term energy production are:
   A. sugars.
   B. carbohydrates. pg. 49
   C. fats.
   D. proteins.

_C_ __ **23.** A _____ is any event that causes anxiety and mental stress to emergency workers.
   A. disaster
   B. mass-casualty incident
   C. critical incident
   D. stressor

_D_ __ **24.** A CISD meeting is an opportunity to discuss your:
   A. feelings.
   B. fears.
   C. reactions to an event.
   D. all of the above.

_D_ __ **25.** Components of the CISM system include:
   A. preincident stress education.
   B. defusings.
   C. spouse and family support.
   D. all of the above.

_D_ __ **26.** Sexual harassment is defined as:
   A. any unwelcome sexual advance.
   B. unwelcome requests for sexual favors.
   C. unwelcome verbal or physical conduct of a sexual nature.
   D. all of the above.

_B_ __ **27.** Drug and alcohol use in the workplace can result in all of the following EXCEPT:
   A. increased absenteeism from work.
   B. enhanced treatment decisions.
   C. an increase in accidents and tension among workers.
   D. lessened ability to render emergency medical care because of mental or physical impairment.

_C_ __ **28.** You should begin protecting yourself:
   A. as soon as you arrive on the scene.
   B. before you leave the scene.
   C. as soon as you are dispatched.
   D. before any patient contact.

_B_ 29. _____ is/are contact with blood, body fluids, tissues, or airborne droplets by direct or indirect contact.

A. Transmission

B. Exposure

C. Handling

D. All of the above

_D_ 30. Modes of transmission for infectious diseases include:

A. blood or fluid splash.

B. surface contamination.

C. needle stick exposure.

D. all of the above.

_A_ 31. The spread of HIV and hepatitis in the health care setting can usually be traced to:

A. careless handling of sharps.

B. improper use of standard precautions.

C. not wearing PPE.

D. sexual interaction with infected persons.

_C_ 32. _____ is equipment that blocks entry of an organism into the body.

A. Vaccination

B. Body substance isolation

C. Personal protective equipment

D. Immunization

_D_ 33. Recommended immunizations include the:

A. MMR vaccine.

B. hepatitis B vaccine.

C. influenza vaccine.

D. all the above.

_D_ 34. Which of the following is an example of a scene hazard?

A. Electricity

B. Vehicle collision

C. Fire

D. All of the above

_B_ 35. You can use a solution of bleach and water at a _____ dilution to clean the unit.

A. 1:1

B. 1:10 pg. 42

C. 1:100

D. 1:1000

_C_ 36. Hazardous materials in vehicles and buildings should be clearly identified using:

A. manifests.

B. MSDS sheets.

C. placards. pg. 63

D. beacons.

_D_ 37. Factors to take into consideration for potential violence include:

A. poor impulse control.

B. substance abuse.

C. depression.

D. all of the above. pg. 71

True/False

If you believe the statement to be more true than false, write the letter "T" in the space provided. If you believe the statement to be more false than true, write the letter "F."

__F__   **1.** Removing the needle from a syringe is the best way to dispose of it safely.

__F__   **2.** Gloves, eye protection, and handwashing are the main components of PPE.

__T__   **3.** Denial is usually the first step in the grieving process.

__F__   **4.** Body fluids are generally not considered infectious substances.

__F__   **5.** Most EMTs never suffer from stress.

__T__   **6.** Physical conditioning and nutrition are two factors the EMT can control in helping to reduce stress.

Fill-in-the-Blank

Read each item carefully and then complete the statement by filling in the missing words.

1. The personal health, safety, and _wellbeing_ of all EMTs are vital to an EMS operation.

2. The struggle to remain calm in the face of horrible circumstances contributes to the _emotional_ _stress_ of the job.

3. The number one cause of all deaths today is _heart_ _disear_.

4. Your safety is the most important consideration at a(n) _hazardous_ materials incident.

5. Proper _handwashing_ is the simplest yet most effective way to control disease transmission.

6. Cover and _concealment_ involve the tactical use of an impenetrable barrier for protection.

7. Almost all dying patients feel some degree of _depressio_ because of internalized anger and other factors.

8. Most _minor_ symptoms may be early signs of severe illness or injury.

Crossword Puzzle

The following crossword puzzle is an activity provided to reinforce correct spelling and understanding of medical terminology associated with emergency care and the EMT. Use the clues in the column to complete the puzzle.

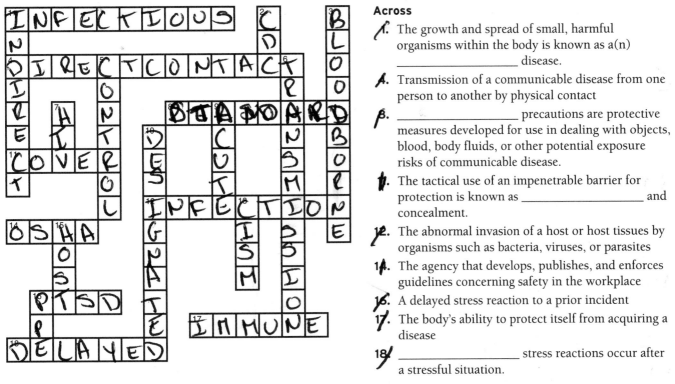

Across

1. The growth and spread of small, harmful organisms within the body is known as a(n) _____ disease.
4. Transmission of a communicable disease from one person to another by physical contact
8. _____ precautions are protective measures developed for use in dealing with objects, blood, body fluids, or other potential exposure risks of communicable disease.
11. The tactical use of an impenetrable barrier for protection is known as _____ and concealment.
12. The abnormal invasion of a host or host tissues by organisms such as bacteria, viruses, or parasites
14. The agency that develops, publishes, and enforces guidelines concerning safety in the workplace
16. A delayed stress reaction to a prior incident
17. The body's ability to protect itself from acquiring a disease
18. _____ stress reactions occur after a stressful situation.

Down

1. Exposure or transmission of disease from one person to another by contact with a contaminated object is called _____ contact.
2. The agency that conducts and supports public health activities and is part of the U.S. Department of Health and Human Services
3. _____ pathogens are pathogenic microorganisms that are present in human blood and can cause disease in humans.
5. Procedures to reduce transmission of infection among patients and health care personnel are known as infection _____.
6. The way in which an infectious disease is spread
7. AIDS is caused by this virus, which damages the cells in the body's immune system
9. _____ stress reactions occur during a stressful situation.
10. The individual in the department who is charged with managing exposures and infection control issues is known as the _____ officer.
13. A process that confronts the responses to critical incidents and defuses them
15. The organism or individual that is attacked by the infecting agent
16. Protective equipment that OSHA requires to be made available to the EMT

Critical Thinking

Multiple Choice

Read each critical-thinking item carefully and then select the best response.

Questions 1–5 are derived from the following scenario: A 12-year-old boy told his grandmother he was going to collect the day's mail, located on the opposite side of the street, for her. As he was returning with the mail, he was struck by a vehicle and was found lying lifeless in the middle of the street.

_C_ **1.** Which of the following would be appropriate to say to the grandmother?
- **A.** "Don't worry. I'm sure he'll be fine."
- **B.** "What were you thinking? You will be reported!"
- **C.** "We're placing him on a backboard to protect his back, and we'll take him to the Columbus Community Hospital. Do you know who his doctor is?"
- **D.** It's best not to spend time talking to the grandmother.

_D_ **2.** As an EMT, you know these types of calls are coming. How can you prepare to meet such stressful situations?
- **A.** Eat a balanced diet.
- **B.** Go for walks or other forms of exercise.
- **C.** Cut down on caffeine and sugars.
- **D.** All of the above.

_B_ **3.** You or your partner may develop _____ after experiencing this call.
- **A.** critical incident stress management
- **B.** posttraumatic stress disorder
- **C.** critical stress debriefing
- **D.** none of the above

_D_ **4.** What signs of stress may you or your partner exhibit?
- **A.** Irritability toward coworkers, family, and friends
- **B.** Loss of interest in work
- **C.** Guilt
- **D.** All of the above

_A_ **5.** When should you begin protecting yourself with standard precautions on this call?
- **A.** As soon as you are dispatched
- **B.** As soon as you arrive
- **C.** After you assess the victim and know what you need
- **D.** After speaking with the grandmother

Short Answer

Complete this section with short written answers using the space provided.

1. Describe the basic concept of standard precautions.

All patients can potentially have an infectious disease that can be transmitted therefore it is most important to protect yourself when in contact with anyone.

2. List the five stages of the grieving process.

①Denial ②Anger ③Bargaining ④Depression ⑤Acceptance

3. List at least five warning signs of stress.

①loss of ~~appetite~~ appetite ②recreational drug/alcohol use ③anxiety
④isolation ⑤loss of work interest

4. List two strategies for managing stress.

~~Exercising~~ ①change work hours
②talk to a professional about feeling stressed

5. Describe the process for proper handwashing.

rinse hands with water, apply soap and water while rubbing
from wrist to finger tips for 20 seconds, dry hands with paper
towel, turn faucet off with same paper towel.

6. List the three layers of clothing recommended for cold weather.

①thin ②thermal middle layer ③outer layer with zippers
for allowing the body to be vented

7. List the four principal determinants of violence.

①past history ②vocal activity ③posture ④physical
activity

8. In what patient care situations should a gown be considered?

When skin will come in contact with secretions, blood,
excretions, contaminated objects, ~~an~~ and body fluids.

Ambulance Calls

The following case scenarios provide an opportunity to explore the concerns associated with patient management and to enhance critical-thinking skills. Read each scenario and answer each question to the best of your ability.

1. In the process of working a motor vehicle collision, your arm is gashed open and you are exposed to the blood of a patient who tells you that he is HIV positive. You have no water supply in which to wash. Your patient is stable, and you are able to control his bleeding with direct pressure.

How would you best manage this situation?

I would continue my patient care until I am able to clean my
wound with alcohol wipes. Then while at the hospital I
will thoroughly wash with soap and water. I will tell my
supervisor right away.

2. You are dispatched to a large apartment complex for a person in respiratory distress. You find the elderly patient living in a dark, messy apartment with many family members, both adults and children, and you know that there have been numerous cases of tuberculosis reported in this particular complex.

With regards to infection control, how would you best manage this situation?

I would wear my personal protective equipment for my hands,
and eyes. Then I would apply the partial rebreather on
the patient. I would advise the facility of the potential

Fill-in-the-Patient Care Report

Read the incident scenario and then complete the following patient care report (PCR).

You and your partner are posted in the parking lot of a convenience store on McBride Avenue just west of Highway 9, cleaning and organizing the back of the ambulance, when emergency tones burst from the radio.

"Truck three, emergency traffic," the dispatcher says.

"Go ahead to three," you respond.

"Truck three, priority one call to 7-9-7-9 Fisher Boulevard for a possible overdose. Show your time of dispatch at oh-nine-twelve."

You copy the assignment, activate the lights and siren, and roll off toward the address, about 14 minutes away.

As you pull up to the address, a towering grey concrete block, housing eight stories of single-room apartments, you are met by a police officer.

"So the mom calls us because she and her daughter were in the middle of a domestic issue," the officer says as he leads you through the lobby and to the elevator. "By the time we got here, the 16-year-old girl had locked herself in the bathroom. I got in there and found her unconscious on the floor with a rig next to her."

"Rig?" your new partner whispers in your ear while you are waiting for the elevator to rumble to the sixth floor.

"Syringe," you say quietly as the officer steps off of the elevator and waves you to an open door.

The clock on the kitchenette microwave reads 9:29 as you enter the small, dimly lit apartment to the sounds of a woman wailing in the bathroom. Two police officers quickly move the distraught mother out of the tiny bathroom so you can get to the unresponsive girl.

"Let's get her out into the living room," you say, using the extremity lift to move the 48-kg (106-lb) patient into the wider floor of the living room. "And watch out for that needle next to her arm; there's no cap on it."

In the living room, you determine that the girl is breathing slowly but adequately and find that she has a slow pulse. You decide to get a full set of vital signs while your partner questions the mother about the girl's history and current drug use. At 0934, the patient's blood pressure is 116/76 mm Hg; her pulse is 46 beats/min; breathing is 8 breaths/min, but with good tidal volume; and she has a pulse oximetry reading of 96%. As you are placing a nonrebreathing mask on the unresponsive girl with 15 L/min of supplemental oxygen, your partner kneels next to you and looks at his notepad.

"She attempted suicide 2 years ago by taking an overdose of aspirin and has been struggling over the past year with a heroin addiction."

"Okay," you say. "Let's get her out to the stretcher and get going."

At 0947, your partner closes you into the back of the ambulance with the patient and climbs into the cab while you obtain a second set of vital signs: blood pressure 114/74 mm Hg, pulse 38 beats/min, respirations 8 breaths/min, and SaO_2 95%. Five minutes later, you arrive at the ambulance bay of the local hospital and quickly move the patient inside. You transfer her care to the emergency department staff after giving a full report to the receiving nurse. After cleaning and preparing the ambulance, you and your partner go back available at 1005.

Fill-in-the-Patient Care Report

EMS Patient Care Report (PCR)				
Date: 9/26/13	Incident No.: 2011-1234	Nature of Call: overdose		Location: 7979 Fisher Blvd
Dispatched: 0912	En Route: 0912	At Scene: 0926	Transport: 0947	At Hospital: 0952	In Service: 1005

Patient Information

Age: 16	Allergies: none
Sex: F	Medications: none
Weight (in kg [lb]): 106 lbs 48 kg 48 kg (106 lbs)	Past Medical History: attempted suicide 2 yrs. ago - again
	Chief Complaint: unresponsive/overdose

Vital Signs

Time: 0934	BP: 116/76	Pulse: 46	Respirations: 8	Sao$_2$: 96%
Time: 0947	BP: 114/74	Pulse: 38	Respirations: 8	Sao$_2$: 95%
Time:	BP:	Pulse:	Respirations:	Sao$_2$:

EMS Treatment

(circle all that apply)

Oxygen @ 6 L/min via (circle one): NC (NRM) Bag-Mask Device	Assisted Ventilation	Airway Adjunct	CPR
Defibrillation	Bleeding Control	Bandaging	Splinting	Other Shock Treatment

Narrative

Skills

Skill Drills

Test your knowledge of this skill by filling in the correct words in the photo captions.

Skill Drill 2-2: Proper Glove Removal Technique

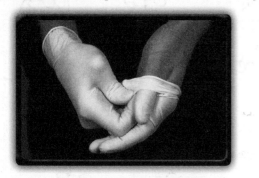

1. Partially remove the first glove by pinching at the ___WRIST___. Be careful to touch only the ___OUTSIDE___ of the glove.

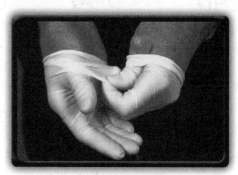

2. Remove the ___SECOND___ glove by pinching the ___EXTERIOR___ with your partially gloved hand.

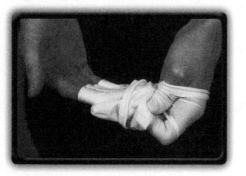

3. Pull the second glove inside-out toward the ___FINGERTIPS___.

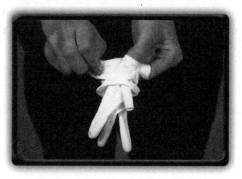

4. Grasp both gloves with your ___FREE___ hand, touching only the clean, ___INTERIOR___ surfaces.

Medical, Legal, and Ethical Issues

General Knowledge

Matching

Match each of the items in the left column to the appropriate definition in the right column.

H **1.** Assault   **A.** Able to make decisions

I **2.** Abandonment   **B.** Specific authorization to provide care expressed by the patient

G **3.** Advance directive   **C.** Confining a person from mental or physical action

E **4.** Battery   **D.** Granted permission

L **5.** Certification   **E.** Touching without consent

A **6.** Competent   **F.** Legal responsibility to provide care

D **7.** Consent   **G.** Written documentation that specifies treatment

F **8.** Duty to act   **H.** Unlawfully placing a patient in fear of bodily harm

B **9.** Expressed consent   **I.** Unilateral termination of care

C **10.** Forcible restraint   **J.** Failure to provide standard of care

M **11.** Implied consent   **K.** Accepted level of care consistent with training

N **12.** Medicolegal   **L.** Process that recognizes that a person has met set standards

J **13.** Negligence   **M.** Legal assumption that treatment was desired

K **14.** Standard of care   **N.** Relating to law or forensic medicine

Multiple Choice

Read each item carefully and then select the one best response.

C **1.** The care that an EMT is able to provide is most commonly defined as a:

  A. duty to act.

  B. competency.

  C. scope of practice.

  D. certification.

A **2.** How the EMT is required to act or behave is called:

  A. the standard of care.

  B. competency.

  C. the scope of practice.

  D. certification.

D **3.** The process by which an individual, an institution, or a program is evaluated and recognized as meeting certain standards is called:

  A. the standard of care.

  B. competency.

  C. the scope of practice.

  D. certification.

___D___ **4.** Negligence is based on the EMT's duty to act, cause, breach of duty, and:

  A. expressed consent.

  B. termination of care.

  C. mode of transport.

  D. real or perceived damages.

___C___ **5.** While treating a patient with a suspected head injury, he becomes verbally abusive and tells you to "leave him alone." If you stop treating him you may be guilty of:

  A. neglect.

  B. battery.

  C. abandonment.

  D. slander.

___B___ **6.** Good Samaritan laws generally are designed to offer protection to persons who render care in good faith. They do not offer protection from:

  A. properly performed CPR.

  B. acts of negligence.

  C. improvising splinting materials.

  D. providing supportive BLS to a DNR patient.

___D___ **7.** Which of the following is generally NOT considered confidential?

  A. Assessment findings

  B. A patient's mental condition

  C. A patient's medical history

  D. The location of the emergency

___D___ **8.** An important safeguard against legal implication is:

  A. responding to every call with lights and siren.

  B. checking ambulance equipment once a month.

  C. transporting every patient to an emergency department.

  D. writing a complete and accurate run report.

___B___ **9.** Your responsibility to provide patient care is called:

  A. scope of practice.

  B. duty to act.

  C. DNR.

  D. standard of care.

___A___ **10.** Presumptive signs of death would not be adequate in cases of sudden death due to:

  A. hypothermia.

  B. acute poisoning.

  C. cardiac arrest.

  D. severe trauma.

___A___ **11.** Definitive or conclusive signs of death that are obvious and clear to even nonmedical persons include all of the following EXCEPT:

  A. profound cyanosis.

  B. dependent lividity.

  C. rigor mortis.

  D. putrefaction.

___D___ **12.** Medical examiners' cases include:

  A. violent death.

  B. suicide.

  C. suspicion of a criminal act.

  D. all of the above.

B **13.** HIPAA is the acronym for the Health Insurance Portability and Accountability Act of 1996. This act:
   A. makes ambulance services accountable for transporting patients in a safe manner.
   B. protects the privacy of health care information and safeguards patient confidentiality.
   C. allows health insurers to transfer an insurance policy to another carrier if a patient does not pay his or her premium.
   D. enables emergency personnel to transfer a patient to a lower level of care when resources are scarce.

True/False

If you believe the statement to be more true than false, write the letter "T" in the space provided. If you believe the statement to be more false than true, write the letter "F."

T **1.** Failure to provide care to a patient once you have been called to the scene is considered negligence.

F **2.** For expressed consent to be valid, the patient must be a minor.

T **3.** If a patient is unconscious and a true emergency exists, the doctrine of implied consent applies.

T **4.** EMTs can legally restrain patients against their will if they pose a threat to themselves or others.

F **5.** DNR orders give you permission not to attempt resuscitation ~~at your discretion.~~

Fill-in-the-Blank

Read each item carefully and then complete the statement by filling in the missing words.

1. The __scope__ of __practice__ outlines the care you are able to provide.

2. The __standard__ of __care__ is the manner in which the EMT must act when treating patients.

3. The legal responsibility to provide care is called the __duty__ __to__ __act__.

4. The determination of __negligence__ is based on duty, breach of duty, damages, and cause.

5. Abandonment is __termination__ of care without transfer to someone of equal or higher training.

6. __Expressed__ consent is given directly by an informed patient, whereas __implied__ consent is assumed in the unconscious patient.

7. Unlawfully placing a person in fear of immediate harm is __assault__, whereas __battery__ is unlawfully touching a person without his or her consent.

8. A(n) __advanced directive__ is a written document that specifies authorized treatment in case a patient becomes unable to make decisions. A written document that authorizes the EMT not to attempt resuscitation efforts is a(n) __DNR order__.

9. Mentally competent patients have the right to __refuse treatment__.

10. Incidents involving child abuse, animal bites, childbirth, and assault have __special reporting__ requirements in many states.

Crossword Puzzle

The following crossword puzzle is an activity provided to reinforce correct spelling and understanding of medical terminology associated with emergency care and the EMT. Use the clues in the column to complete the puzzle.

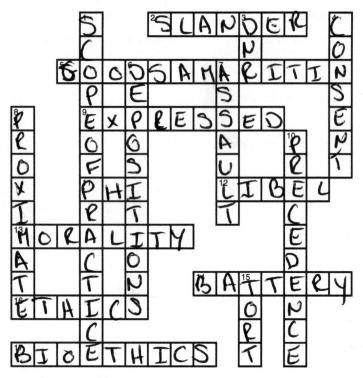

Across

2. False and damaging information about a person that is communicated by the spoken word
5. _____ _____ laws are statutory provisions enacted by many states to protect citizens from liability for errors and omissions in giving good faith emergency medical care.
9. With _____ consent, a patient gives express authorization for provision of care or transport.
11. Any information about health status, provision of health care, or payment for health care that can be linked to an individual
12. False and damaging information about a person that is communicated in writing
13. A code of conduct that can be defined by society, religion, or a person, affecting character, conduct, and conscience
14. Touching a patient or providing emergency care without consent
16. The philosophy of right and wrong, of moral duties, and of ideal professional behavior
17. The study of ethics related to issues that arise in health care

Down

1. Most commonly defined by state law; outlines the care you are able to provide for the patient
3. Written documentation by a physician giving permission to medical personnel not to attempt resuscitation in the event of cardiac arrest is called a(n) _____ order.
4. Permission to render care
6. Oral questions asked of parties and witnesses under oath
7. Unlawfully placing a patient in fear of bodily harm
8. When a person who has a duty abuses it, and causes harm to another individual, the EMT, the agency, and/or the medical director may be sued for negligence. This is called _____ causation.
10. Basing current action on lessons, rules, or guidelines derived from previous similar experiences
15. A wrongful act that gives rise to a civil suit

Critical Thinking

Multiple Choice

Read the scenarios carefully and select the best responses to the questions.

At 2:00 AM, a 17-year-old boy, accompanied by his 19-year-old girlfriend, had driven to the bar to give his father (who had been drinking large amounts of alcohol) a ride home. On the way back, they were involved in a motor vehicle collision. The boy has a large laceration with profuse bleeding on his forehead. His girlfriend is unconscious in the front passenger floor. The father is standing outside the vehicle, appearing heavily intoxicated, and is refusing care.

_B_ **1.** Should the father be allowed to refuse care?

- **A.** Yes. Consent is required before care can be started.
- **B.** No. He is under the influence of drugs/alcohol and is therefore mentally incompetent.
- **C.** Yes, under implied consent.
- **D.** No. You would be guilty of abandonment.

_A_ **2.** Why is it permissible for you to begin treatment on the girlfriend?

- **A.** Consent is implied.
- **B.** Consent has been expressed.
- **C.** Consent was informed.
- **D.** None of the above.

_A_ **3.** As you progress in your care for the patients, the father becomes unconscious. Can you begin/continue care for him now?

- **A.** Yes. Consent is now implied.
- **B.** No. He made his wishes known before he fell unconscious.
- **C.** No. He just needs to sleep it off.
- **D.** Yes. Unconsciousness indicates informed consent.

_C_ **4.** With the son being a minor, what is the best way to gain consent to begin care when his father has an altered mental status or is unconscious?

- **A.** Phone his mother for consent.
- **B.** Call his grandparents for consent.
- **C.** It is a true emergency, so consent is implied.
- **D.** You are covered under the Good Samaritan laws.

You respond to a single-vehicle crash on the highway west of town. Upon arrival you find a 33-year-old man with an open forearm fracture who has self-extricated from his pickup, which is down the roadside embankment. He does not appear to have suffered any other injuries, is fully coherent, and refuses all medical care.

_B_ **5.** In an effort to obtain consent to treat this patient, you should:

- **A.** summon law enforcement and request that the patient be placed into protective custody.
- **B.** clearly explain the consequences of not accepting medical treatment.
- **C.** proceed with treatment; consent is not required because the patient is not being rational.
- **D.** properly document the refusal of care.

_D_ **6.** If you and your partner were out past the end of your scheduled shift and driving the ambulance back to base to go home when you came upon this accident, would you have a legal duty to act?

- **A.** No. If you were not specifically dispatched to the crash, you do not have an obligation to assist.
- **B.** Yes. As a trained and licensed EMT you must assist with every medical emergency that you encounter.
- **C.** No. Because it is past the end of your scheduled shift, you can decide whether you want to stop and help.
- **D.** Yes. As a trained EMT still on-duty for an EMS system, you would have a legal and ethical obligation to stop and assist.

Short Answer

Complete this section with short written answers using the space provided.

1. In many states, certain conditions allow a minor to be treated as an adult for the purpose of consenting to medical treatment. List three of these conditions.

_____

_____

2. When does your responsibility for patient care end?

_____

_____

3. There will be some instances when you will not be able to persuade the patient, guardian, conservator, or parent of a minor child or mentally incompetent patient to proceed with treatment. List five steps you should take to protect all parties involved.

_____

_____

4. List the two rules of thumb that courts consider regarding reports and records.

_____

_____

5. List four steps to take when you are called to a scene involving a potential organ donor.

_____

_____

Ambulance Calls

The following case scenarios provide an opportunity to explore the concerns associated with patient management and to enhance critical-thinking skills. Read each scenario and answer each question to the best of your ability.

1. You are dispatched to a girl complaining of abdominal pain. You arrive to find the 17-year-old girl crying and holding her abdomen. She tells you that she fell down the stairs and that she is pregnant. She is not sure how far along she is, but she is experiencing cramping and spotting. She asks you not to tell anyone and says that if you tell her parents she will refuse transport to the hospital.

What do you do?

_____

_____

_____

2. You are off-duty when you see a child injured while riding his bike. You examine him and find abrasions on both knees, but no other injuries. He needs help getting to his house up the street. He tells you that his mother is not home, but his grandfather is (although he is bedridden). Looking through the window, you see the house is full of clothing, garbage, and papers.

What do you do?

_____

_____

_____

3. It is late in the night when the police summon you to an automobile collision. On arrival, the officer directs you to the back of his patrol car. Sitting on the seat is your patient, snoring loudly with blood covering his face. The officer states that the patient was involved in a drunk-driving accident in which he hit his head on the rearview mirror. The patient initially refused care at the scene. You were called because his wound continues to bleed. Assessment reveals a sleeping 56-year-old man with a deep, gaping wound over the right eye with moderate venous bleeding. During assessment, the patient wakes suddenly and pushes you away. He tells you to leave him alone.

What actions are necessary in the management of this situation?

_____

_____

_____

Fill-in-the-Patient Care Report

Read the incident scenario and then complete the following patient care report (PCR).

It is 2115, and you are just walking out of a grocery store with a small bag of apples when the dispatch tones blare from your portable radio.

"Truck Two," the dispatcher's voice blares from the small speaker. "Emergency call."

You pick up the pace to the ambulance where your partner is fastening his seat belt, answering on the portable as you go. "Dispatch, go for Truck Two."

"Truck Two, I need you to head over to the intersection of Grand and Hopper for a motorcycle versus automobile."

You parrot back the information, jump into the passenger seat, and pull your seat belt into position as your partner activates the lights and siren and pulls out onto the deserted street.

At 7 minutes after dispatch, you arrive at the intersection and see a small blue car with a shattered windshield sitting diagonally in the middle of the intersection. On the opposite side of the road there is a damaged and smoking motorcycle on its side; a person is lying motionless on the pavement nearby.

The driver of the car, who is standing on the side of the road and talking on his cell phone, shouts that he is not injured so you proceed to the woman on the ground. She appears to be approximately 24 years old, is unresponsive to pain, is bleeding from a long forehead laceration, and has inadequate, snoring respirations.

At 9 minutes after dispatch, you have your partner manually immobilize the patient's head and neck while you insert an oropharyngeal airway and begin assisting her respirations with a bag-mask device and 15 L/min of supplemental oxygen.

At 10 minutes after dispatch, a fire truck arrives on scene and one of the fire fighters obtains the patient's vitals while the others prepare the cervical collar and long backboard.

Two minutes later, the fire fighter reports the patient's vitals as: blood pressure, systolic 90, diastolic 54; pulse of 100 beats/min, weak and irregular; respirations of 12 breaths/min with adequate assisted tidal volume; pale, cool, and diaphoretic skin; and a pulse oximetry reading of 94%.

About 5 minutes after obtaining vitals, the patient is appropriately secured to the long backboard and loaded into the ambulance for the short trip to the local university trauma center.

During the 6-minute transport to the trauma center ambulance entrance, you must continue assisting the patient's respirations and cannot repeat the vitals.

It takes a total of 14 minutes to move the patient from your gurney to the bed in the trauma bay, provide a verbal report to the nurse, and prepare the ambulance for your next call.

EMS Patient Care Report (PCR)

Date:	Incident No.:	Nature of Call:		Location:
Dispatched:	En Route:	At Scene:	Transport:	At Hospital:	In Service:

Patient Information

Age:	Allergies:
Sex:	Medications:
Weight (in kg [lb]):	Past Medical History:
	Chief Complaint:

Vital Signs

Time:	BP:	Pulse:	Respirations:	Sao$_2$:
Time:	BP:	Pulse:	Respirations:	Sao$_2$:
Time:	BP:	Pulse:	Respirations:	Sao$_2$:

EMS Treatment
(circle all that apply)

Oxygen @ ___ L/min via (circle one): NC NRM Bag-Mask Device	Assisted Ventilation	Airway Adjunct	CPR
Defibrillation	Bleeding Control	Bandaging	Splinting	Other Shock Treatment

Narrative

Communications and Documentation

General Knowledge

Matching

Match each of the items in the left column to the appropriate definition in the right column.

_____	**1.** Base station	**A.** "Hot line"
_____	**2.** Mobile radio	**B.** A trusting relationship built with your patient
_____	**3.** Portable radio	**C.** Communication through an interconnected series of repeater stations
_____	**4.** Repeater	**D.** Assigned frequency used to carry voice and/or data communications
_____	**5.** Telemetry	**E.** Radio receiver that searches across several frequencies until the message is completed
_____	**6.** UHF	**F.** VHF and UHF channels designated exclusively for EMS use
_____	**7.** VHF	**G.** Vehicle-mounted device that operates at a lower frequency than a base station
_____	**8.** Cellular telephone	**H.** A process in which electronic signals are converted into coded, audible signals
_____	**9.** Dedicated line	**I.** Radio frequencies between 30 and 300 MHz
_____	**10.** MED channels	**J.** Hand-carried or handheld devices that operate at 1 to 5 watts
_____	**11.** Scanner	**K.** Special base station radio that receives messages and signals on one frequency and then automatically retransmits them on a second frequency
_____	**12.** Channel	**L.** Radio frequencies between 300 and 3,000 MHz
_____	**13.** Rapport	**M.** Radio hardware containing a transmitter and receiver that is located in a fixed location

Multiple Choice

Read each item carefully and then select the one best response.

_____ **1.** The base station may be used:

  A. in a single place by an operator speaking into a microphone that is connected directly to the equipment.

  B. remotely through telephone lines.

  C. by radio from a communication center.

  D. all of the above.

_____ **2.** The transmission range of a(n) _____ is more limited than that of mobile or base station radios.

  A. portable radio

  B. 800-MHz radio

  C. cellular phone

  D. UHF radio

_____ **3.** Base stations:

  A. usually have more power than mobile or portable radios.

  B. have higher, more efficient antenna systems.

  C. allow for communication with field units at much greater distances.

  D. all of the above.

_____   **4.** _____ are helpful when you are away from the ambulance and need to communicate with dispatch, another unit, or medical control.

    A. Base stations

    B. Portable radios

    C. Mobile radios

    D. Cellular phones

_____   **5.** Digital signals are also used in some kinds of paging and tone-alerting systems because they transmit _____ and allow for more choices and flexibility.

    A. numerically

    B. faster

    C. alphanumerically

    D. encoded messages

_____   **6.** As with all repeater-based systems, a cellular telephone is useless if the equipment:

    A. fails.

    B. loses power.

    C. is damaged by severe weather or other circumstances.

    D. all of the above.

_____   **7.** Which of the following is FALSE with regard to simplex mode?

    A. When one party transmits, the other must wait to reply.

    B. You must push a button to talk.

    C. It is called a "pair of frequencies."

    D. Radio transmissions can occur in either direction, but not simultaneously in both.

_____   **8.** The principal EMS-related responsibilities of the FCC include:

    A. monitoring radio operations.

    B. establishing limitations for transmitter power output.

    C. allocating specific radio frequencies for use by EMS providers.

    D. all of the above.

_____   **9.** Information given to the responding unit(s) should include all of the following EXCEPT:

    A. the number of patients.

    B. the time the unit will arrive.

    C. the exact location of the incident.

    D. responses by other public safety agencies.

_____   **10.** You must consult with medical control to:

    A. notify the hospital of an incoming patient.

    B. request advice or orders from medical control.

    C. advise the hospital of special situations.

    D. all of the above.

_____   **11.** The patient report commonly includes all of the following EXCEPT:

    A. a list of the patient's medications.

    B. the patient's age and gender.

    C. a brief history of the patient's current problem.

    D. your estimated time of arrival.

_____ **12.** In most areas, medical control is provided by the _____ who work at the receiving hospital.

    A. nurses

    B. physicians

    C. interns

    D. staff

_____ **13.** For _____ reasons, the delivery of sophisticated care, such as assisting patients in taking medications, must be done in association with physicians.

    A. logical

    B. ethical

    C. legal

    D. all of the above

_____ **14.** Standard radio operating procedures are designed to:

    A. reduce the number of misunderstood messages.

    B. keep transmissions brief.

    C. develop effective radio discipline.

    D. all of the above.

_____ **15.** Be sure that you report all patient information in a(n) _____ manner.

    A. objective

    B. accurate

    C. professional

    D. all of the above

_____ **16.** Medical control guides the treatment of patients in the system through all of the following EXCEPT:

    A. hands-on care.

    B. protocols.

    C. direct orders.

    D. postcall review.

_____ **17.** Depending on how the protocols are written, you may need to call medical control for direct orders to:

    A. administer certain treatments.

    B. transport a patient.

    C. request assistance from other agencies.

    D. immobilize a patient.

_____ **18.** When you encounter a patient who is angry, you should be mindful of your:

    A. tone of voice.

    B. attitude.

    C. body language.

    D. all of the above.

_____ **19.** While en route to and from the scene, you should report all of the following to the dispatcher EXCEPT:

    A. any special hazards.

    B. traffic delays.

    C. abandoned vehicles in the median.

    D. road construction.

_____ **20.** Situations that might require special preparation on the part of the hospital include:

    A. HazMat situations.

    B. mass-casualty incidents.

    C. rescues in progress.

    D. all of the above.

_____ **21.** The _____ officially occurs during your oral report at the hospital, not as a result of your radio report en route.

    A. patient report

    B. transfer of care

    C. termination of services

    D. all of the above

_____ **22.** Effective communication between the EMT and health care professionals in the receiving facility is an essential cornerstone of _____ patient care.

    A. efficient

    B. effective

    C. appropriate

    D. all of the above

_____ **23.** Which of the following components MUST be included in the oral report during transfer of care?

    A. The patient's name

    B. Any important history

    C. Vital signs assessed

    D. All of the above

_____ **24.** Your _____ are critically important in gaining the trust of both the patient and family.

    A. gestures

    B. body movements

    C. attitude toward the patient

    D. all of the above

_____ **25.** If the patient is hearing impaired, you should:

    A. stand on the patient's left side.

    B. shout.

    C. speak clearly and distinctly.

    D. use baby talk.

_____ **26.** Functional age relates to the person's:

    A. ability to function in daily activities.

    B. mental state.

    C. activity pattern.

    D. all of the above.

_____ **27.** When caring for a visually impaired patient, you should:

    A. use sign language.

    B. touch the patient only when necessary to render care.

    C. try to avoid sudden movements.

    D. never walk him or her to the ambulance.

_____ **28.** When attempting to communicate with non-English-speaking patients, you should:

    A. use short, simple questions and simple words whenever possible.

    B. always use medical terms.

    C. shout.

    D. position yourself so the patient can read your lips.

_____ **29.** The patient information that is included in the minimum data set includes all of the following EXCEPT:

    A. the chief complaint.

    B. the time that the EMS unit arrived at the scene.

    C. respirations and effort.

    D. skin color and temperature.

_____ **30.** Functions of the patient care report include:

    A. continuity of care.

    B. education.

    C. research.

    D. all of the above.

_____ **31.** A good patient care report documents:

    A. the care that was provided.

    B. the patient's condition on arrival.

    C. any changes.

    D. all of the above.

_____ **32.** When completing the narrative section, be sure to:

    A. describe what you see and what you do.

    B. include only positive findings.

    C. record your conclusions about the incident.

    D. use appropriate radio codes.

_____ **33.** Instances in which you may be required to file special reports with appropriate authorities include:

    A. gunshot wounds.

    B. dog bites.

    C. suspected physical, sexual, or substance abuse.

    D. all of the above.

True/False

If you believe the statement to be more true than false, write the letter "T" in the space provided. If you believe the statement to be more false than true, write the letter "F."

_____ **1.** The two-way radio is at least two units: a transmitter and a receiver.

_____ **2.** Base stations typically have more power and much higher and more efficient antenna systems than mobile or portable radios.

_____ **3.** Ethnocentrism occurs when you consider your own cultural values to be equal to those of others.

_____ **4.** The transmission range of a mobile radio is more limited than that of a portable radio.

_____ **5.** A dedicated line, a special telephone line used for specific point-to-point communications, is always open or under the control of the individuals at each end.

_____ **6.** The written report is a vital part of providing emergency medical care and ensuring the continuity of patient care.

_____ **7.** EMS systems that use repeaters are unable to get good signals from portable radios.

_____ **8.** Small changes in your location will not significantly affect the quality of your transmission.

_____ **9.** Your reporting responsibilities end when you arrive at the hospital.

_____ **10.** Patients deserve to know that you can provide medical care and that you are concerned about their well-being.

Fill-in-the-Blank

Read each item carefully and then complete the statement by filling in the missing words.

1. Written communications, in the form of a(n) _____ _____ _____,

provide you with an opportunity to communicate the patient's story to others who may participate in the patient's care

in the future.

2. A two-way radio consists of two units: a(n) _____ and a(n) _____.

3. A(n) _____ _____, also known as a "hot line", is always open or under the control of

the individuals at each end.

4. With _____, electronic signals are converted into coded, audible signals.

5. Low-power portable radios that communicate through a series of interconnected repeater stations called "cells" are

known as _____ _____.

6. _____ are commonly used in EMS operations to alert on- and off-duty personnel.

7. When the first call to 9-1-1 comes in, the dispatcher must try to judge its relative _____ to begin the appropriate EMS response using emergency medical dispatch protocols.

8. The principal reason for radio communication is to facilitate communication between you and _____ _____.

9. You could be successfully sued for _____ if you describe a patient in a way that injures his or her reputation.

10. Regardless of your system's design, your link to _____ _____ is vital to maintain the high quality of care that your patient requires and deserves.

11. To ensure complete understanding, once you receive an order from medical control, you must _____ the order back, word for word, and then receive confirmation.

12. By their very nature, _____ _____ do not require direct communication with medical control.

13. Maintaining _____ _____ with your patient builds trust and lets the patient know that he or she is your first priority.

14. Children can easily see through lies or deception, so you must always be _____ with them.

15. If the patient does not speak any English, find a family member or friend to act as a(n) _____.

16. The national EMS community has identified a(n) _____ _____ _____ that should enable communication and comparison of EMS runs among agencies, regions, and states.

17. _____ adult patients have the right to refuse treatment.

Crossword Puzzle

The following crossword puzzle is an activity provided to reinforce correct spelling and understanding of medical terminology associated with emergency care and the EMT. Use the clues in the column to complete the puzzle.

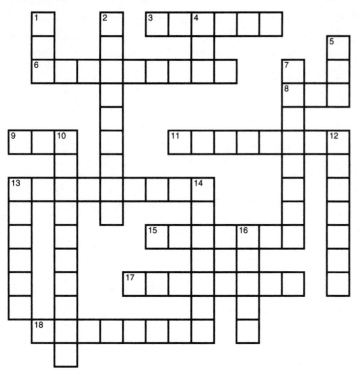

Across

3. The ability to transmit and receive simultaneously

6. A process in which electronic signals are converted into coded, audible signals

8. Radio frequencies between 300 and 3,000 MHz

9. The federal agency that has jurisdiction over interstate and international telephone and telegraph services and satellite communications

11. A special base station radio that receives messages and signals on one frequency and then automatically retransmits them on a second frequency

13. The study of space between people and its effects on communication

15. An assigned frequency or frequencies that are used to carry voice and/or data communications

17. Telecommunication systems that allow a computer to maximize utilization of a group of frequencies

18. A low-power portable radio that communicates through an interconnected series of repeater stations called "cells" is known as a(n) _____ telephone.

Down

1. Small computer terminals inside ambulances that directly receive data from the dispatch center

2. Questions for which the patient must provide detail to give an answer are called _____ questions.

4. The legal document used to record all patient care activities

5. Radio frequencies between 30 and 300 MHz

7. _____ imposition is when one person imposes his or her beliefs, values, and practices on another because he or she believes his or her ideals are superior.

10. _____ questions can be answered in short or single-word responses.

12. A trusting relationship that you build with your patient

13. The use of a radio signal and a voice or digital message that is transmitted to "beepers" or desktop monitor radios

14. A radio receiver that searches across several frequencies until the message is completed

16. Anything that dampens or obscures the true meaning of a message

Critical Thinking

Multiple Choice

Read each critical-thinking item carefully and then select the one best response.

Questions 1–5 are derived from the following scenario: You have just finished an ambulance run where a 45-year-old man had run his SUV into a utility pole. The driver was found slumped over the steering wheel, unconscious. A large electrical wire was lying across the hood of the vehicle. After securing scene safety, you were able to approach the patient and complete a primary assessment, in which you found a 6″ (15.4-cm) laceration across his forehead. The patient regained responsiveness, was alert and oriented, and refused care.

_____ **1.** Should an EMT document this call, even though the patient refused care?

    A. No. You only need to document when you have actually provided care.

    B. No. This was not a billable run.

    C. Yes. It is best signed by the patient as "refusal of care."

    D. Both A and B.

_____ **2.** Which of the following would it be important to document?

    A. That the scene needed to be made safe

    B. That ensuring scene safety delayed care

    C. That you completed a primary assessment

    D. All of the above

_____ **3.** While writing the report, you made an error. How should this be corrected?

    A. Draw a single line through it.

    B. Erase the mistake.

    C. Cover up the mistake with correction fluid.

    D. All of the above.

_____ **4.** What are the consequences of falsifying a report?

    A. It may result in the suspension and/or revocation of your license.

    B. It gives other health care providers a false impression of assessment/findings.

    C. It results in poor patient care.

    D. All of the above.

_____ **5.** If the patient refuses to sign the refusal form:

    A. Sign it yourself and state: "Patient refused to sign."

    B. You cannot let the man leave the scene until he either goes with you or signs the form.

    C. Have a credible witness sign the form testifying that he or she witnessed the patient's refusal of care.

    D. If the patient refuses care, you don't have to document it.

Short Answer

Complete this section with short written answers using the space provided.

1. List the five principal FCC responsibilities related to EMS.

_____

_____

2. Identify what the abbreviation HIPAA stands for and define it.

_____

_____

3. List the six functions of a patient care report.

_____

_____

4. Describe the two types of written report forms generally in use in EMS systems.

_____

_____

Ambulance Calls

The following case scenarios provide an opportunity to explore the concerns associated with patient management and to enhance critical-thinking skills. Read each scenario and answer each question to the best of your ability.

1. You are in the dispatch office filling in for the EMS dispatcher who needed to use the restroom. The phone rings and you answer it to hear a hysterical woman screaming about a child falling into an old well. The only information she is providing is that he is 5 years old and is not making any noise. The address is on the computer display.

How would you best manage this situation, and what additional help would you call for?

_____

_____

_____

2. You respond to an "unknown medical problem" in an area commonly populated by Hispanic Americans. You arrive to find several individuals speaking to a middle-aged man. They seem to be concerned about him and motion you toward the patient. You attempt to gain information about the situation, but your patient does not speak English and you do not speak Spanish. The patient has no outward appearance of any problems.

How would you best manage this situation?

_____

_____

_____

3. You are dispatched to the parking lot of a grocery store for a "confused child." You arrive to find a young boy who is developmentally disabled. He cannot communicate who he is or where he lives. He is frightened but appears otherwise unharmed.

How would you best manage this situation?

_____

_____

_____

Fill-in-the-Patient Care Report

Read the incident scenario and then complete the following patient care report (PCR).

You watch the digital clock on the dashboard change to 5:11 PM and flip through the stack of PCRs that you have accumulated during the past 10 hours of your busy shift, ensuring that they are all complete. Ten minutes later, the dispatcher contacts you on the radio and requests that you and your partner respond to 18553 Old Redwood Highway for a dirt bike accident.

Six minutes later your partner pulls off the main road and into a sprawling, green field dotted with motocross riders in multicolored pads and helmets. One small group of riders off in the distance begins jumping up and down, waving their arms. The ambulance moves slowly across the smooth, solid ground and a minute later you arrive at the group's location. You see a rider lying on the ground with blood covering his lower left leg.

"He ripped his foot off," a teenaged girl with long blonde hair shouts as you step out of the truck. "Please help him quick!"

You kneel next to the 19-year-old injured man as your partner gets the equipment from the back of the ambulance. The young man is pounding his fist on the ground and yelling in pain, holding his injured leg tightly with one gloved hand. The foot of his left leg is hanging limply, almost completely severed from the ankle and bleeding profusely.

You immediately apply pressure to the end of the patient's leg with a trauma dressing as three fire fighters arrive. You direct two of the fire fighters to remove the patient's helmet while you immobilize his spine. Your partner and the third fire fighter prepare the cervical collar and backboard.

Once the patient is completely immobilized on the backboard and your partner has initiated high-flow oxygen therapy with a nonrebreathing mask, you bandage the dressings in place (after noting that the bleeding has almost completely stopped) and direct the loading of the 73-kg (161-lb) patient into the ambulance. You make a mental note that you had been on scene for only 8 minutes.

You obtain a complete set of vital signs just as your partner is pulling out of the grass and back onto the road. You find the following: blood pressure is 104/66 mm Hg; heart rate is 102 beats/min; respirations are 18 breaths/min and unlabored; skin is pale, cool, and moist; and oxygen saturation is 97%. You immediately raise the foot of the backboard about 10″ (25 cm) and cover the patient with a blanket to preserve his body temperature.

After contacting the receiving trauma center with a verbal report and ETA, you repeat the vital signs about 5 minutes after the first set. You find his blood pressure is at 110/72 mm Hg, heart rate is 90 beats/min, respirations are 14 breaths/min and still unlabored, color is returning to his skin, and the pulse oximeter is showing 99%. Just as you finish obtaining the vitals, your partner opens the back doors and you deliver the patient to the waiting team in the trauma bay.

Twenty minutes later, after providing an appropriate report to the charge nurse, turning over care of the patient, and properly cleaning and disinfecting the ambulance, you call yourselves back in service and head back to the post.

Fill-in-the-Patient Care Report

EMS Patient Care Report (PCR)					
Date:	**Incident No.:**	**Nature of Call:**		**Location:**	
Dispatched:	**En Route:**	**At Scene:**	**Transport:**	**At Hospital:**	**In Service:**

Patient Information	
Age: **Sex:** **Weight (in kg [lb]):**	**Allergies:** **Medications:** **Past Medical History:** **Chief Complaint:**

Vital Signs				
Time:	**BP:**	**Pulse:**	**Respirations:**	**Sao$_2$:**
Time:	**BP:**	**Pulse:**	**Respirations:**	**Sao$_2$:**
Time:	**BP:**	**Pulse:**	**Respirations:**	**Sao$_2$:**

EMS Treatment				
(circle all that apply)				
Oxygen @ ___ L/min via (circle one): NC NRM Bag-Mask Device	**Assisted Ventilation**	**Airway Adjunct**		**CPR**
Defibrillation	**Bleeding Control**	**Bandaging**	**Splinting**	**Other Shock Treatment**

Narrative

The Human Body

General Knowledge

Matching

Match each of the items in the left column to the appropriate definition in the right column.

_____ **1.** Anterior

_____ **2.** Capillary

_____ **3.** Anatomic position

_____ **4.** Superior

_____ **5.** Midline

_____ **6.** Carotid

_____ **7.** Medial

_____ **8.** Inferior

_____ **9.** Femoral

_____ **10.** Proximal

_____ **11.** Brachial

_____ **12.** Distal

_____ **13.** Flexion

_____ **14.** Radial

_____ **15.** Posterior

A. Closer to the midline

B. Farther from the midline

C. Farther from the head; lower

D. Standing, facing forward, palms facing forward

E. Imaginary vertical line descending from the middle of the forehead to the floor

F. Front surface of the body

G. Closer to the head; higher

H. Bending of a joint

I. Back or dorsal surface of the body

J. Closer to the midline

K. Connects arterioles to venules

L. Major artery that supplies blood to the head and brain

M. Major artery that supplies blood to the lower extremities

N. Major artery of the lower arm

O. Major artery of the upper arm

For each of the bones listed in the left column, indicate whether it is an upper extremity bone (A) or a lower extremity bone (B).

_____ **16.** Talus

_____ **17.** Patella

_____ **18.** Clavicle

_____ **19.** Fibula

_____ **20.** Calcaneus

_____ **21.** Ulna

_____ **22.** Humerus

A. Upper extremity bone

B. Lower extremity bone

For each of the muscle characteristics described in the left column, select the type of muscle from the right column.

_____ **23.** Attaches to the bone

_____ **24.** Found in the walls of the gastrointestinal tract

_____ **25.** Carries out much of the automatic work of the body

_____ **26.** Forms the major muscle mass of the body

_____ **27.** Under the direct control of the brain

_____ **28.** Found only in the heart

_____ **29.** Responds only to primitive stimulus

_____ **30.** Can tolerate blood supply interruption for only a very short period

_____ **31.** Responsible for all bodily movement

_____ **32.** Has its own blood supply and electrical system

A. Skeletal

B. Smooth

C. Cardiac

For each of the parts of the nervous system in the left column, select the phrase in the right column with which it is associated.

_____ **33.** Spinal cord

_____ **34.** Central nervous system

_____ **35.** Sensory nerves

_____ **36.** Motor nerves

_____ **37.** Brain

_____ **38.** Peripheral nervous system

A. Exits the brain through an opening at the base of the skull

B. Transmit electrical impulses to the muscles, causing them to contract

C. Brain and spinal cord

D. Links the central nervous system to various organs in the body

E. Carry sensations of taste and touch to the brain

F. Controlling organ of the body

Multiple Choice

Read each item carefully and then select the one best response.

_____ **1.** The topographic term used to describe the location of an injury that is toward the midline center of the body is:

    A. lateral.

    B. medial.

    C. midaxillary.

    D. midclavicular.

_____ **2.** Topographically, the term *distal* means:

    A. near the trunk.

    B. associated with a point of reference.

    C. near the free end of the extremity.

    D. toward the center of the body.

_____ **3.** The leaf-shaped flap of tissue that prevents food and liquid from entering the trachea is called the:

    A. uvula.

    B. epiglottis.

    C. laryngopharynx.

    D. cricothyroid membrane.

_____ **4.** Which of the following systems is responsible for releasing chemicals that regulate body activities?

    A. Nervous

    B. Endocrine

    C. Cardiovascular

    D. Skeletal

_____ **5.** Which of the following vessels does NOT carry blood to the heart?

    A. Inferior vena cava

    B. Superior vena cava

    C. Pulmonary vein

    D. Pulmonary artery

_____ **6.** The _____ is connected to the intestine by the bile ducts.

    A. stomach

    B. spleen

    C. appendix

    D. liver

_____ **7.** Which of the following is NOT a function of the urinary system?

    A. Fluid control

    B. Hormone regulation

    C. pH balancing

    D. Waste filtration

True/False

If you believe the statement to be more true than false, write the letter "T" in the space provided. If you believe the statement to be more false than true, write the letter "F."

_____ **1.** The aorta is the major artery that supplies the groin and lower extremities with blood.

_____ **2.** The knee is a ball-and-socket joint.

_____ **3.** The phalanges are the bones of the fingers and toes.

_____ **4.** The right atrium receives blood from the pulmonary veins.

_____ **5.** There are 12 ribs that attach to the sternum.

_____ **6.** Exhaled air contains 21% oxygen.

_____ **7.** The spleen is a muscle that is commonly injured in abdominal blunt-trauma injuries.

Fill-in-the-Blank

Read each item carefully and then complete the statement by filling in the missing words.

1. There is/are _____ cervical vertebrae.

2. The movable bone in the skull is the _____.

3. There is a total of _____ lobes in the right and left lungs.

4. _____ pairs of ribs attach posteriorly to the thoracic vertebrae.

5. The spinal column has _____ vertebrae.

6. The ankle bone is known as the _____.

7. The cerebrum, which is the largest part of the brain, is composed of four lobes: _____, _____, _____, and _____.

8. The _____ space is the space between the cells.

9. The movement of air between the lungs and the environment is called _____.

10. How much air is being effectively moved during ventilation and how much blood is gaining access to the alveoli is called the _____ ratio.

Labeling

Label the following diagrams with the correct terms.

1. Directional Terms

A. _____

B. _____

C. _____

D. _____

E. _____

F. _____

G. _____

H. _____

I. _____

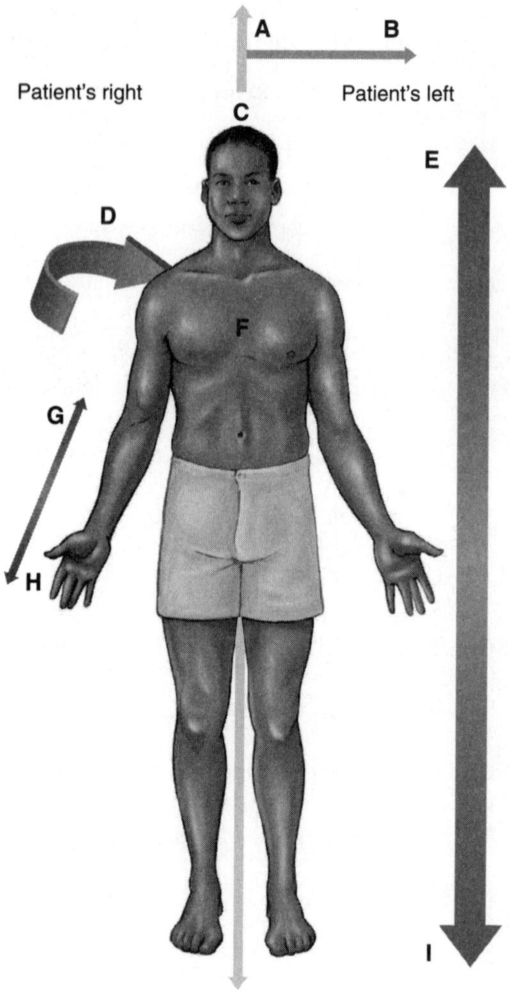

A   B

Patient's right   Patient's left

C

E

D

F

G

H

I

2. Anatomic Positions

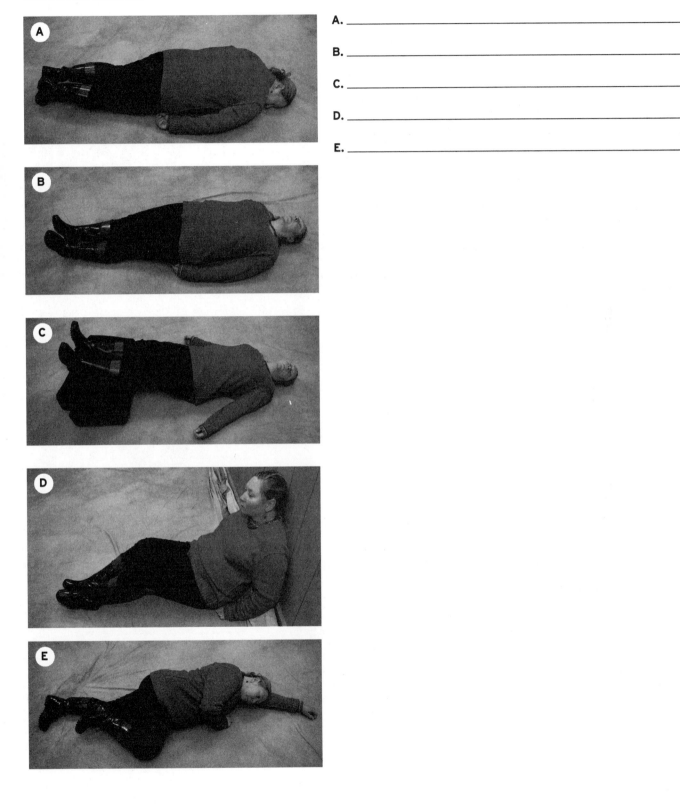

A. _____

B. _____

C. _____

D. _____

E. _____

3. The Skull

A. _____

B. _____

C. _____

D. _____

E. _____

F. _____

G. _____

H. _____

I. _____

J. _____

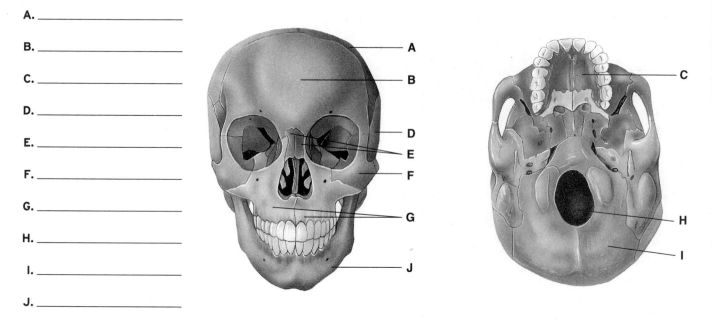

4. The Spinal Column

A. _____

B. _____

C. _____

D. _____

E. _____

F. _____

G. _____

H. _____

I. _____

J. _____

K. _____

L. _____

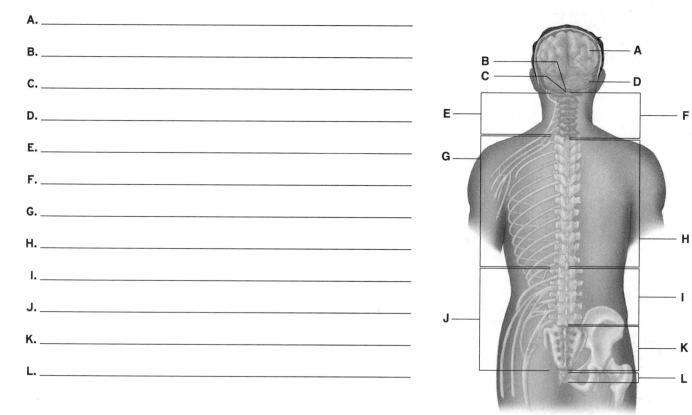

5. The Thorax

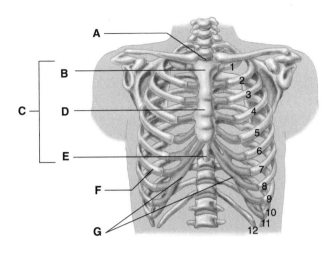

A. _____

B. _____

C. _____

D. _____

E. _____

F. _____

G. _____

6. The Shoulder Girdle

A. _____

B. _____

C. _____

D. _____

E. _____

F. _____

G. _____

7. The Wrist and Hand

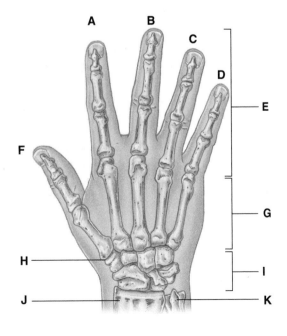

A. _____

B. _____

C. _____

D. _____

E. _____

F. _____

G. _____

H. _____

I. _____

J. _____

K. _____

8. The Pelvis

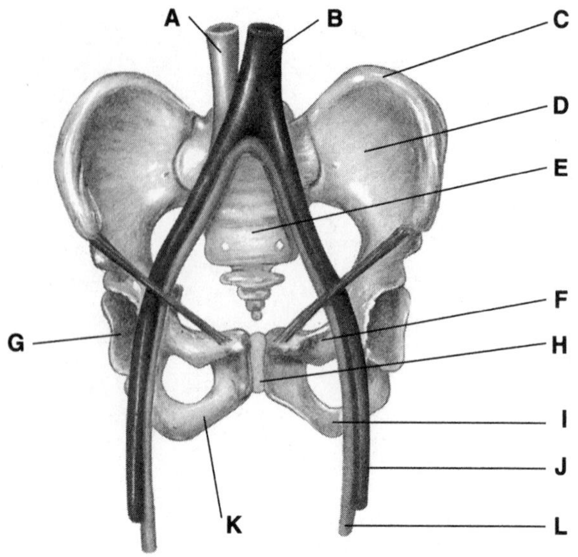

A. _____

B. _____

C. _____

D. _____

E. _____

F. _____

G. _____

H. _____

I. _____

J. _____

K. _____

L. _____

9. The Lower Extremity

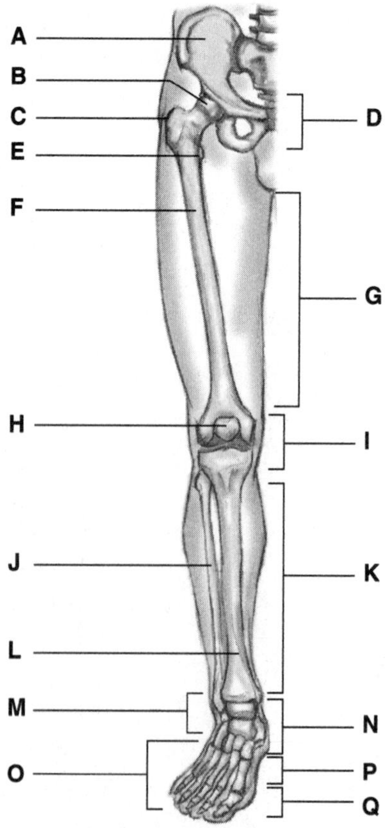

A. _____

B. _____

C. _____

D. _____

E. _____

F. _____

G. _____

H. _____

I. _____

J. _____

K. _____

L. _____

M. _____

N. _____

O. _____

P. _____

Q. _____

10. The Foot

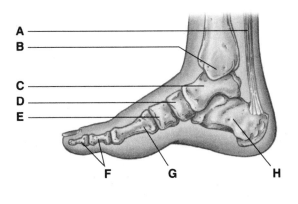

A. _____

B. _____

C. _____

D. _____

E. _____

F. _____

G. _____

H. _____

11. The Respiratory System

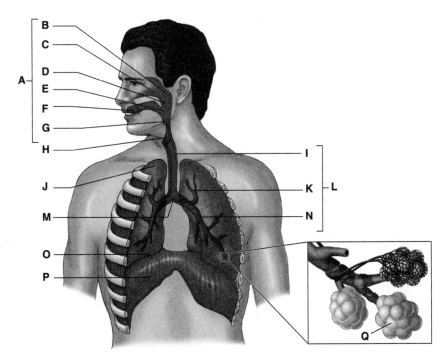

A. _____

B. _____

C. _____

D. _____

E. _____

F. _____

G. _____

H. _____

I. _____

J. _____

K. _____

L. _____

M. _____

N. _____

O. _____

P. _____

Q. _____

12. The Circulatory System

A. _____

B. _____

C. _____

D. _____

E. _____

F. _____

G. _____

H. _____

I. _____

J. _____

K. _____

L. _____

M. _____

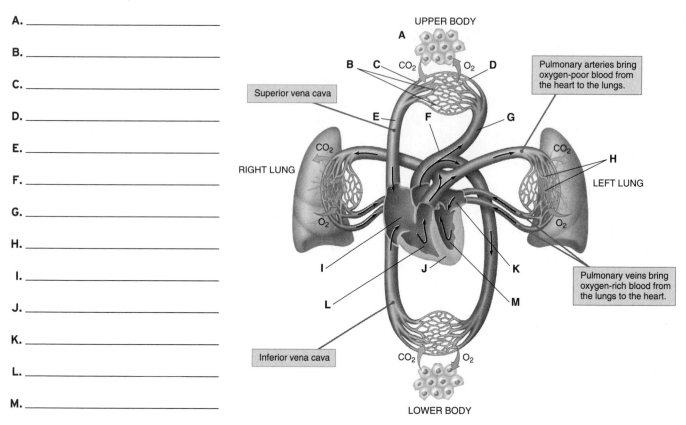

UPPER BODY

A

B C CO_2 O_2 D

Superior vena cava

Pulmonary arteries bring oxygen-poor blood from the heart to the lungs.

E F G

RIGHT LUNG

CO_2

CO_2

LEFT LUNG

H

O_2

O_2

I J K

L M

Inferior vena cava

Pulmonary veins bring oxygen-rich blood from the lungs to the heart.

CO_2 O_2

LOWER BODY

13. Central and Peripheral Pulses

A. _____

B. _____

C. _____

D. _____

E. _____

F. _____

G. _____

H. _____

I. _____

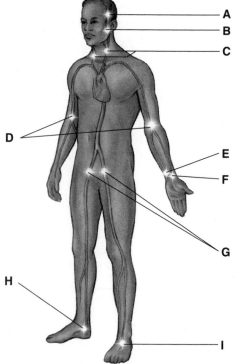

A

B

C

D

E

F

G

H

I

14. The Brain

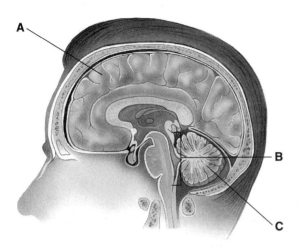

A. _____

B. _____

C. _____

15. Anatomy of the Skin

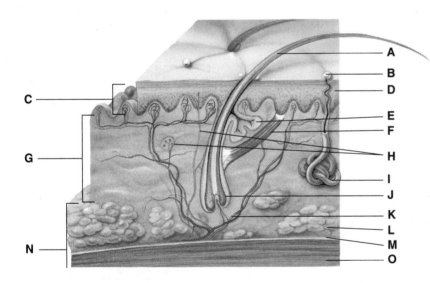

A. _____

B. _____

C. _____

D. _____

E. _____

F. _____

G. _____

H. _____

I. _____

J. _____

K. _____

L. _____

M. _____

N. _____

O. _____

16. The Male Reproductive System

A. _____

B. _____

C. _____

D. _____

E. _____

F. _____

G. _____

H. _____

I. _____

J. _____

K. _____

L. _____

M. _____

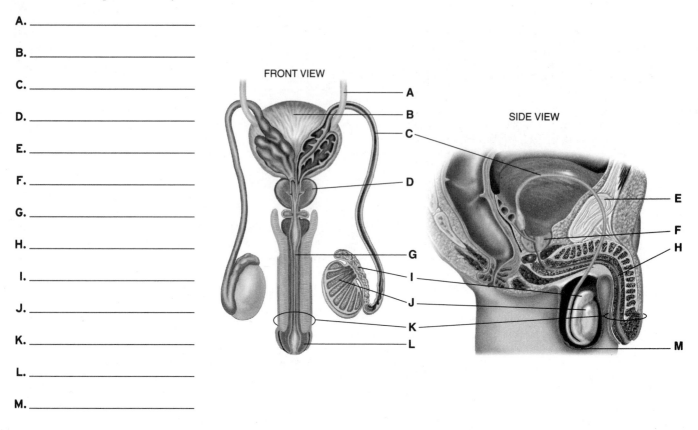

17. The Female Reproductive System

A. _____

B. _____

C. _____

D. _____

E. _____

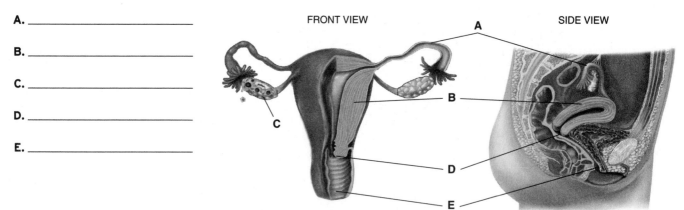

Crossword Puzzle

The following crossword puzzle is an activity provided to reinforce correct spelling and understanding of medical terminology associated with emergency care and the EMT. Use the clues in the column to complete the puzzle.

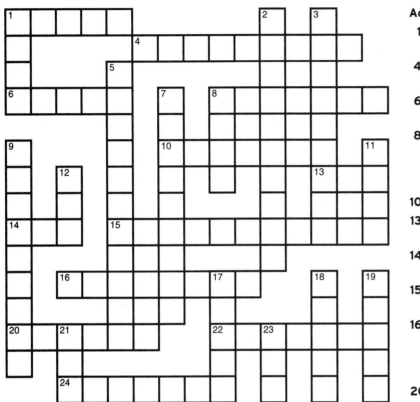

Across

1. One of three bones that fuse to form the pelvic ring
4. A collapsible tube that extends from the pharynx to the stomach
6. Seminal fluid ejaculated from the penis and containing sperm
8. The _____ magnum is a large opening at the base of the skull through which the brain connects to the spinal cord.
10. The bending of a joint
13. The nucleotide involved in energy metabolism
14. A portion of the medulla oblongata where the primary respiratory pacemaker is found
15. The part of the pharynx that lies above the level of the roof of the mouth
16. The _____ position is the position of reference in which the patient stands facing you, arms at the side, with the palms of the hands forward.
20. The last three or four vertebrae of the spine
22. One of three bones that fuse to form the pelvic ring
24. The breastbone

Down

1. An organ that lies below the midbrain and above the medulla and contains numerous important nerve fibers
2. The connection point between the pelvis and the vertebral column is known as the _____ joint.
3. The _____ artery leads from the right ventricle of the heart to the lungs; it carries oxygen-poor blood.
5. A(n) _____ muscle is a muscle over which a person has no conscious control.
7. Movement of a gas from an area of higher concentration to an area of lower concentration
8. To bend
9. Any portion of the airway that contains air and cannot participate in gas exchange
11. The pointed extremity of a conical structure
12. A portion of the medulla oblongata that is responsible for modulating breathing during speech
17. One of three bones that fuse to form the pelvic ring
18. The part of the skeleton comprising the skull, spinal column, and rib cage is known as the _____ skeleton.
19. The longest and one of the strongest bones in the body
21. The brain and spinal cord
23. Fluid produced in the ventricles of the brain that flows in the subarachnoid space and bathes the meninges

Critical Thinking

Multiple Choice

Read each critical-thinking item carefully and then select the best response.

Questions 1–5 are derived from the following scenario: Kory, a 16-year-old boy, attempted to jump down a flight of stairs on his skateboard but landed face down on his chest and stomach, where he stayed until found. He was not wearing a helmet, and he hit the pavement with his head. Two bones were protruding from his right ankle.

_____ 1. His open wound would be known as a(n):
  A. ulna/radial fracture.
  B. acromion/humerus fracture.
  C. tibia/fibula fracture.
  D. patella/fibula fracture.

_____ 2. What part of his spinal column do you want to keep immobilized, so as not to move any of its seven vertebrae?
  A. Cervical
  B. Thoracic
  C. Sacrum
  D. Coccyx

_____ 3. If the patient were to develop pain in his right upper quadrant, what organ may be causing the pain?
  A. Liver
  B. Stomach
  C. Spleen
  D. Appendix

_____ 4. Kory was found in what position?
  A. Prone
  B. Supine
  C. Shock
  D. Lateral recumbent

_____ 5. To keep his spinal column straight, in what position would you place him on the cot?
  A. Prone
  B. Supine
  C. Fowler's position
  D. Trendelenburg's position

Short Answer

Complete this section with short written answers using the space provided.

1. List the four components of blood and each of their functions.

_____

_____

2. List the five sections of the spinal column and indicate the number of vertebrae in each.

_____

_____

3. What organs are in each of the quadrants of the abdomen?

RUQ: _____

LUQ: _____

RLQ: _____

LLQ: _____

4. List in the proper order the parts of the heart that blood flows through.

1. _____

2. _____

3. _____

4. _____

5. _____

6. _____

7. _____

8. _____

9. _____

Ambulance Calls

The following case scenarios provide an opportunity to explore the concerns associated with patient management and to enhance critical-thinking skills. Read each scenario and answer each question to the best of your ability.

1. You are dispatched to the scene of a bar fight. A 34-year-old man has been stabbed in the right upper quadrant of the abdomen with a knife. Using medical terminology, indicate which organ(s) might be affected.

   How would you describe this patient's injuries?

   _____

   _____

   _____

2. You are dispatched to a one-vehicle motor vehicle collision, car versus telephone pole. You arrive to find an unrestrained driver who is complaining of chest pain. You notice the steering wheel is deformed.

   Based on the mechanism of injury and his chief complaint, what are the patient's potential injuries?

   _____

   _____

   _____

3. You are dispatched to a local BMX bike track just down the road from the fire station. You arrive to find a 14-year-old boy walking toward you, holding his left arm in place. He tells you that as he was turning a corner on the track he fell off his bike and landed on his shoulder.

   What possible injuries does this patient have?

   _____

   _____

   _____

Fill-in-the-Patient Care Report

Read the incident scenario and then complete the following patient care report (PCR).

You note that it has been far too quiet this evening as you and your partner sit overlooking the west end of the city. An approaching car's headlights briefly illuminate the cab of the ambulance before swinging around a curve, dropping you back into darkness again. The radio buzzes and you both snap to attention.

"Six-nineteen from central, I've got a priority-one call. Please proceed to the intersection of Alpha Street and 15th Avenue for an assault. Police reporting the scene as secure. I'm showing you assigned at 2312."

Your partner acknowledges the call as you pull out of the parking lot and begin the 17-minute cross-town trip to the scene location. Upon arrival, you are directed to a 38-year-old, 115-pound (52-kg) woman who is lying on the sidewalk, arms wrapped tightly around her torso.

"There was a fight over at Hank's bar," the police officer squatting next to the patient tells you. "Linda here was attacked by several other ladies and assaulted pretty severely in the street."

You kneel next to the moaning woman and explain that you are there to help her. After confirming a patent airway, you ask the police officer to hold the patient's head in a neutral, in-line position while you initiate high-flow oxygen therapy via a nonrebreathing mask set at 15 L/min. You and your partner then apply a cervical collar, secure the patient to a long backboard, and load her into the ambulance. You look at your watch and see that it has been 29 minutes since the initial dispatch.

Your partner jumps into the back of the ambulance with the patient while you slide into the cab, notify dispatch of your departure from the scene, and pull away, heading toward the university trauma center 13 minutes south on 15th Avenue. Your partner finds darkening bruises on the patient's upper arms, the left side of her chest, and down the fronts of both legs. Her stomach is distended and rigid, causing her to wince and cover her torso with her hands when touched.

By the time you pull to a stop in the hospital's ambulance bay, your partner has obtained two sets of vital signs—the first, 2 minutes following departure from the scene and the other 6 minutes later. The results were, in order: blood pressure, 108/56 mm Hg and 104/54 mm Hg; pulse, 96 beats/min and 104 beats/min; respirations, 16 breaths/min (good tidal volume but labored) and 18 breaths/min (adequate tidal volume and labored); and pulse oximetry 96% and 95%. The patient also seemed to be growing more anxious during the transport and was treated for shock with blankets and proper positioning.

You and your partner quickly transfer the patient to the open and waiting trauma room bed, provide the physician with a full report, and are back in service 15 minutes after initially arriving at the hospital.

Fill-in-the-Patient Care Report

EMS Patient Care Report (PCR)					
Date:	Incident No.:		Nature of Call:		Location:
Dispatched:	En Route:	At Scene:	Transport:	At Hospital:	In Service:
Patient Information					
Age: Sex: Weight (in kg [lb]):			Allergies: Medications: Past Medical History: Chief Complaint:		
Vital Signs					
Time:	BP:	Pulse:		Respirations:	Sao$_2$:
Time:	BP:	Pulse:		Respirations:	Sao$_2$:
Time:	BP:	Pulse:		Respirations:	Sao$_2$:
EMS Treatment (circle all that apply)					
Oxygen @ ___ L/min via (circle one): NC NRM Bag-Mask Device		Assisted Ventilation		Airway Adjunct	CPR
Defibrillation	Bleeding Control		Bandaging	Splinting	Other Shock Treatment
Narrative					

Life Span Development

General Knowledge

Matching

Match each of the items in the left column to the appropriate definition in the right column.

_____ **1.** Preschoolers

_____ **2.** Anxious-avoidant attachment

_____ **3.** Nephrons

_____ **4.** Toddlers

_____ **5.** Atherosclerosis

_____ **6.** School age

_____ **7.** Conventional reasoning

_____ **8.** Early adults

_____ **9.** Moro reflex

_____ **10.** Postconventional reasoning

_____ **11.** Rooting reflex

_____ **12.** Fontanelles

_____ **13.** Secure attachment

_____ **14.** Middle adults

A. The basic filtering units in the kidneys

B. Cholesterol and calcium buildup inside the walls of the blood vessels that forms plaque

C. Persons who are 19 to 40 years of age

D. Areas where the infant's skull has not fused together

E. Persons who are 1 to 3 years of age

F. A bond between an infant and his or her parents in which the infant understands that the parents will be responsive to his or her needs

G. Persons who are 41 to 60 years of age

H. An infant reflex in which the infant opens his or her arms wide, spreads the fingers, and seems to grab at things

I. A type of reasoning in which a child bases decisions on his or her conscience

J. A bond between an infant and his or her caregiver in which the infant is repeatedly rejected and develops an isolated lifestyle

K. A type of reasoning in which a child looks for approval from peers and society

L. Persons who are 3 to 6 years of age

M. An infant reflex that occurs when something touches an infant's cheek, and the infant instinctively turns his or her head toward the touch

N. A person who is 6 to 12 years of age

Multiple Choice

Read each item carefully and then select the one best response.

_____ **1.** Kidney function declines by _____ between the ages of 20 and 90 years.

   A. 10%

   B. 50%

   C. 45%

   D. 20%

_____ **2.** An adolescent is a person between the ages of:

   A. 6 and 12 years.

   B. 3 and 6 years.

   C. 12 and 18 years.

   D. 10 and 19 years.

_____ **3.** Stealing money from a parent's wallet and denying it when caught is an example of _____ reasoning.

   A. postconventional

   B. psychosocial

   C. conventional

   D. preconventional

_____ **4.** One consequence of the loss of neurons among elderly persons is a(n):

   A. change in sleep patterns.

   B. steady decline in intelligence.

   C. inability to reproduce.

   D. loss of physical skills.

_____ **5.** Maturation of the reproductive system usually takes place during:

   A. early adulthood.

   B. preschool.

   C. middle adulthood.

   D. adolescence.

_____ **6.** From birth to 1 month old, a person is called a(n):

   A. infant.

   B. toddler.

   C. neonate.

   D. newborn.

_____ **7.** The maximum life expectancy for humans is estimated to be _____ years.

   A. 120

   B. 78

   C. 67

   D. 56

_____ **8.** What do middle adults tend to focus their time and energy on?

   A. Raising a family

   B. Excelling in a career

   C. Achieving life goals

   D. Creating a self-image

_____ **9.** When encountering a patient with depressed fontanelles, you should suspect:

   A. respiratory distress.

   B. dehydration.

   C. atherosclerosis.

   D. nephrosis.

_____ **10.** What is "vital capacity"?

   A. The volume of blood moved by each contraction of the heart

   B. The maximum thickness of the meninges

   C. The volume of air moved during the deepest points of respiration

   D. The amount of air left in the lungs following exhalation

_____ **11.** Clingy behavior and the fear of unfamiliar people or places are normal among 10- to 18-month-old children and are commonly caused by _____ anxiety.

   A. bonding

   B. separation

   C. avoidant

   D. mistrust

_____ **12.** Diastolic blood pressure tends to _____ with age.
- **A.** decrease
- **B.** compensate
- **C.** increase
- **D.** decompensate

_____ **13.** In what age range do toddlers and preschoolers fit into?
- **A.** 1 to 6 years
- **B.** 2 to 8 years
- **C.** 2 to 7 years
- **D.** 0 to 5 years

_____ **14.** Work, family, and stress best describe the life stage known as:
- **A.** middle adulthood.
- **B.** adolescence.
- **C.** late adulthood.
- **D.** early adulthood.

_____ **15.** At what age can an infant normally start tracking objects with his or her eyes and recognizing familiar faces?
- **A.** 7 months
- **B.** 2 months
- **C.** 4 months
- **D.** 10 months

True/False

If you believe the statement to be more true than false, write the letter "T" in the space provided. If you believe the statement to be more false than true, write the letter "F."

_____ **1.** The majority of elderly people live in assisted-living facilities.

_____ **2.** The rooting reflex takes place when an infant's lips are stroked.

_____ **3.** Toddlers should have pulse rates between 90 and 150 beats/min.

_____ **4.** Men can produce sperm well into their 80s.

_____ **5.** The older the patient is the larger his pupils will be.

_____ **6.** Typically, antisocial behavior will peak around age 13.

_____ **7.** Language is usually mastered by the 24th month.

_____ **8.** Breastfeeding helps to boost an infant's immune system.

_____ **9.** Infant respirations should be counted by watching for abdominal rise.

_____ **10.** When questioning an adolescent about a medical issue, never ask questions without a parent present.

Fill-in-the-Blank

Read each item carefully and then complete the statement by filling in the missing words.

1. _____ adults are those who are age 19 to _____ years.

2. In toddlers, the pulse rate is _____ to _____ beats/min and the respiratory rate is

   _____ to _____ breaths/min.

3. Middle adults tend to focus on achieving their _____ _____.

4. Most elderly individuals can hear _____ and are able to see _____.

5. Rebellious behavior can be part of an adolescent trying to find his or her own _____.

6. A(n) _____ usually weighs 6 to _____ pounds at birth, and the head accounts for

   _____% of its body weight.

7. An infant's lungs are _____, and providing bag-mask ventilations that are too forceful can result in

   trauma from pressure, or _____.

8. By _____ to 24 months, toddlers begin to understand cause and _____.

9. Changes in gastric and intestinal function may inhibit _____ intake and utilization in

   _____ adults.

10. Among elderly persons, _____ function in the 5 years preceding death is presumed to decline, a theory

    referred to as the _____ _____ hypothesis.

Crossword Puzzle

The following crossword puzzle is an activity provided to reinforce correct spelling and understanding of medical terminology associated with emergency care and the EMT. Use the clues in the column to complete the puzzle.

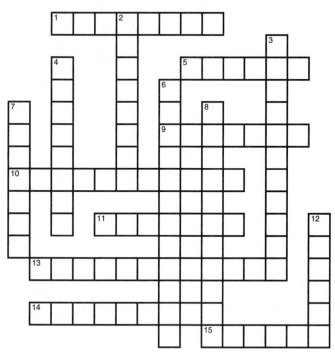

Across

1. The stage of development during which infants gain trust of their parents or caregivers if their world is planned, organized, and routine is known as "trust and _____."

5. _____ grasp is an infant reflex that occurs when something is placed in the infant's palm.

9. Person who is birth to 1 month of age

10. Persons who are 12 to 18 years of age

11. _____ reflex is an infant reflex that occurs when something touches an infant's cheek, and the infant instinctively turns his or her head toward the touch.

13. Persons who are 3 to 6 years of age

14. A person who is 6 to 12 years of age

15. _____ attachment is a bond in which an infant understands that his or her parents or caregivers will be responsive to his or her needs.

Down

2. Persons who are 1 to 3 years of age

3. Injury resulting from pressure disequilibrium across body surfaces

4. The basic filtering units in the kidneys

6. In _____ reasoning, a child looks for approval from peers and society.

7. Persons who are from 1 month to 1 year of age

8. Areas where the infant's skull has not fused together

12. Persons who are 41 to 60 years of age are known as _____ adults.

Critical Thinking

Multiple Choice

Read each critical-thinking item carefully and then select the one best response.

You are dispatched to a public park in the middle of a sprawling subdivision for an arm injury. You arrive to find a crying 8-year-old boy cradling his swollen and deformed left forearm. His friends tell you that he was holding onto the bars of the play structure and that his arm "snapped" when he jumped into the sand below.

_____ 1. You would expect this boy's pulse to be:

    A. between 60 and 80 beats/min.

    B. higher than 150 beats/min.

    C. most likely above 90 beats/min.

    D. around 70 beats/min.

_____ 2. An adult bystander tells you that the boy kept trying to impress his friends with more and more dangerous stunts on the play structure prior to the injury. This is an indication of _____ reasoning.

    A. conventional

    B. preconventional

    C. unconventional

    D. postconventional

_____ 3. You would expect to find a respiratory rate of between _____ and _____ breaths/min with this patient.

    A. 12; 20

    B. 15; 20

    C. 10; 15

    D. 20; 30

Short Answer

Complete this section with short written answers using the space provided.

1. Explain why breathing can become more labor intensive among the elderly.

_____

_____

2. Describe conventional reasoning.

_____

_____

3. Explain the stage of development known as "trust and mistrust."

_____

_____

4. What is the terminal drop hypothesis?

_____

_____

5. List the nine basic stages of life.

_____

_____

Ambulance Calls

The following case scenarios provide an opportunity to explore the concerns associated with patient management and to enhance critical-thinking skills. Read each scenario and answer each question to the best of your ability.

1. You are dispatched to a residential care facility for a "fall from bed" and arrive to find a 96-year-old man refusing assistance even though he has a large, darkening hematoma above his left ear. He keeps telling the care facility staff and you that he doesn't want any of you "yahoos" touching him.

What would you be most concerned about with this patient?

_____

_____

_____

2. You respond to a local residence for a toddler who burned her arm by knocking a lit candle off a shelf. You have responded to numerous abuse situations as an EMT and now find yourself suspicious of any child's injury. You would like to speak to this 16-month-old patient alone, but both parents stay nearby and seem very concerned about the child's well-being.

Would you try to speak to the child alone? Explain your reason.

_____

_____

_____

3. You and your partner are requested to a high school for a teenaged boy who fell from the stage while rehearsing a play. You arrive to find him surrounded by concerned classmates. He is guarding the left side of his chest and breathing shallowly, but he refuses assistance and insists that he is doing fine.

How would you best manage this patient?

_____

_____

_____

Fill-in-the-Patient Care Report

Read the incident scenario and then complete the following patient care report (PCR).

The dispatch tones awaken you from a light sleep and you instinctively pull a notepad from your pocket and write down the key components of the following dispatch.

0345

Geary Residential Home

16654 Geary St

Respiratory distress

Within 3 minutes you and your partner, Leticia, are pulling the ambulance from the fire station and moving off through the silent, early morning streets. At 0359 you arrive at the front entrance of the building and are escorted down several long, carpeted hallways to a small, dimly lit room.

"This is Mrs. Gershon," your escort tells you. "She started complaining about her breathing 20 minutes ago and it's just getting worse."

Mrs. Gershon is a 93-year-old woman who has been living at Geary for nearly 17 years. She used to share the room with her husband, Ronald, until his death 3 years ago. She has had three myocardial infarctions in the past and takes medication to regulate blood pressure. Based on her wristband, you see that she is allergic to penicillin. She is sitting on the edge of her bed in the tripod position, breathing through pursed lips, and you can clearly see accessory muscle use in her neck.

"Hello, Mrs. Gershon. We are from the fire department and we are here to help," you say to her. You speak loudly and clearly because her nurse told you that she has difficulty hearing. She looks up at you, inhales shallowly once, and then stops breathing.

"Mrs. Gershon, don't stop now," you say as Leticia quickly hands you the bag-mask device, hissing with 15 L/min of oxygen. You begin ventilating the elderly woman, who is obviously exhausted after struggling to breathe for such a long period. You find no resistance to your assisted ventilations, and Mrs. Gershon just stares up at you as you continue squeezing the bag. Leticia and several nurses from the facility move the 44-kg (97-lb) patient onto the gurney and out to the ambulance as you continue ventilations. Before climbing into the driver's seat, Leticia places the pulse oximetry finger clip onto the patient. She then calls in your departure for the hospital at 0410 and provides a brief report to the receiving facility through dispatch. Within 7 minutes you hear the truck's backup alarm and the patient care compartment is flooded with the bright yellow light of the hospital's ambulance bay. The SaO_2 readout is showing 95%.

Several nurses and the ED physician come out to the ambulance and assist with getting Mrs. Gershon inside, where she is quickly sedated and intubated while you provide a verbal report to the charge nurse.

Eighteen minutes after arriving at the hospital, your ambulance is cleaned, stocked, and ready for the next call.

Fill-in-the-Patient Care Report

EMS Patient Care Report (PCR)					
Date:	**Incident No.:**		**Nature of Call:**		**Location:**
Dispatched:	**En Route:**	**At Scene:**	**Transport:**	**At Hospital:**	**In Service:**
Patient Information					
Age:			**Allergies:**		
Sex:			**Medications:**		
Weight (in kg [lb]):			**Past Medical History:**		
			Chief Complaint:		
Vital Signs					
Time:	**BP:**	**Pulse:**	**Respirations:**	**Sao$_2$:**	
Time:	**BP:**	**Pulse:**	**Respirations:**	**Sao$_2$:**	
Time:	**BP:**	**Pulse:**	**Respirations:**	**Sao$_2$:**	
EMS Treatment **(circle all that apply)**					
Oxygen @ ___ L/min via (circle one): NC NRM Bag-Mask Device		**Assisted Ventilation**	**Airway Adjunct**		**CPR**
Defibrillation	**Bleeding Control**	**Bandaging**	**Splinting**		**Other Shock Treatment**
Narrative					

Principles of Pharmacology

General Knowledge

Matching

Match each of the items in the left column to the appropriate definition in the right column.

_____	**1.** Absorption	**A.** Lotions, creams, ointments
_____	**2.** Contraindication	**B.** Effect that a drug is expected to have
_____	**3.** Side effect	**C.** The study of the properties and effects of drugs and medications
_____	**4.** Adsorption	**D.** Amount of medication given
_____	**5.** Dose	**E.** Gelatin shells filled with powdered or liquid medication
_____	**6.** Indication	**F.** Any action of a drug other than the desired one
_____	**7.** Action	**G.** To bind or stick to a surface
_____	**8.** Pharmacology	**H.** Therapeutic use for a particular medication
_____	**9.** Capsules	**I.** Process by which medications travel through body tissues
_____	**10.** Topical medications	**J.** Situation in which a drug should not be given

Multiple Choice

Read each item carefully and then select the one best response.

_____ **1.** The proper dose of a medication depends on all of the following EXCEPT:

    A. the patient's age.

    B. the patient's size.

    C. generic substitutions.

    D. the desired action.

_____ **2.** Nitroglycerin relieves the squeezing or crushing pain associated with angina by:

    A. dilating the arteries to increase the oxygen supply to the heart muscle.

    B. causing the heart to contract harder and increase cardiac output.

    C. causing the heart to beat faster to supply more oxygen to the heart.

    D. all of the above.

_____ **3.** The brand name that a manufacturer gives to a medication is called the _____ name.

    A. trade

    B. generic

    C. chemical

    D. prescription

_____ **4.** The fastest way to deliver a chemical substance is by the _____ route.

    A. intravenous

    B. oral

    C. sublingual

    D. intramuscular

_____ **5.** The form the manufacturer chooses for a medication ensures:

    A. the proper route of the medication.

    B. the timing of the medication's release into the bloodstream.

    C. the medication's effects on target organs or body systems.

    D. all of the above.

_____ **6.** Solutions may be given:

    A. orally.

    B. intramuscularly.

    C. rectally.

    D. all of the above.

_____ **7.** In the prehospital setting, a(n) _____ is the preferred method of giving oxygen to patients who have sufficient tidal volume and can provide up to 90% inspired oxygen.

    A. nasal cannula

    B. nonrebreathing mask

    C. bag-mask device

    D. endotracheal tube

_____ **8.** Characteristics of epinephrine include:

    A. dilating passages in the lungs.

    B. constricting blood vessels.

    C. increasing the heart rate and blood pressure.

    D. all of the above.

_____ **9.** Epinephrine acts as a specific antidote to:

    A. adrenaline.

    B. histamine.

    C. asthma.

    D. bronchitis.

_____ **10.** Nitroglycerin relieves pain because its purpose is to increase blood flow by relieving the spasms or causing the arteries to:

    A. dilate.

    B. constrict.

    C. thicken.

    D. contract.

_____ **11.** Nitroglycerin affects the body in the following ways (select all that apply):

    A. It decreases blood pressure.

    B. It relaxes veins throughout the body.

    C. It often causes a mild headache after administration.

    D. It increases blood return to the heart.

Questions 12–16 are derived from the following scenario: You are called to a home of a known 34-year-old man with diabetes. When you arrive, you find the patient supine and unconscious on the living room floor with snoring respirations.

_____ **12.** Medications most EMTs carry in the ambulance that would pertain to this call include:

    A. insulin, oxygen, and oral glucose.

    B. nitroglycerin, oxygen, and oral glucose.

    C. activated charcoal, oxygen, and oral glucose.

    D. none of the above.

_____ **13.** Oral glucose:

    A. is a suspension.

    B. should be given to this patient.

    C. is placed between a patient's cheek and gum.

    D. is not carried by EMTs.

_____ **14.** The government publication listing all drugs in the United States is called the:

    A. *United States Pharmacopoeia.*

    B. *Department of Transportation Reference Guide.*

    C. *US Pharmacology.*

    D. *Nursing Drug Reference.*

_____ **15.** Oral glucose is _____ for this patient.

    A. indicated

    B. contraindicated

    C. not normally given

    D. prescribed

_____ **16.** Oxygen:

    A. is a controlled substance.

    B. should be applied to this patient.

    C. is not flammable.

    D. is considered a suspension.

True/False

If you believe the statement to be more true than false, write the letter "T" in the space provided. If you believe the statement to be more false than true, write the letter "F."

_____ **1.** Oxygen is a flammable substance.

_____ **2.** Glucose may be administered to an unconscious patient in order to save his or her life.

_____ **3.** Epinephrine is a hormone produced by the body to aid in digestion.

_____ **4.** Nitroglycerin decreases blood pressure.

_____ **5.** Sublingual medications are rapidly absorbed into the digestive tract.

_____ **6.** Vital signs should be taken before and after a medication is given.

_____ **7.** Even though medications can react with each other, this is not a potentially harmful condition for the patient.

_____ **8.** Nitroglycerin should be administered only when the patient's systolic blood pressure is below 100 mm Hg.

Fill-in-the-Blank

Read each item carefully and then complete the statement by filling in the missing words.

1. _____ is a simple sugar that is readily absorbed by the bloodstream.

2. _____ is the main hormone that controls the body's fight-or-flight response.

3. Nitroglycerin is usually taken _____.

4. In all but the _____ _____ route, the medication is absorbed into the bloodstream

through various body tissues.

5. When given by mouth, _____ may be absorbed from the stomach fairly quickly because the medication

is already dissolved.

6. A(n) _____ is a chemical substance that is used to treat or prevent disease or relieve pain.

Crossword Puzzle

The following crossword puzzle is an activity provided to reinforce correct spelling and understanding of medical terminology associated with emergency care and the EMT. Use the clues in the column to complete the puzzle.

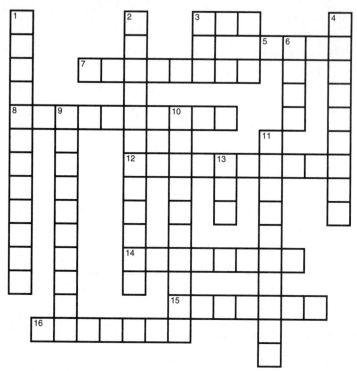

Across

3. A device that changes a liquid medication into a spray and pushes it into a nostril
5. The amount of medication given on the basis of the patient's size and age
7. A liquid mixture that cannot be separated by filtering or allowing the mixture to stand
8. The process by which medications travel through body tissues until they reach the bloodstream
12. A medication that binds to a receptor and blocks other medications
14. Activated _____ is an oral medication that binds and adsorbs ingested toxins in the gastrointestinal tract for treatment of some poisonings and medication overdoses.
15. A medication that causes stimulation of receptors
16. Medications that enter the body through the digestive system

Down

1. Into the bone
2. The use of multiple medications on a regular basis
3. A miniature spray canister through which droplets or particles of medication may be inhaled
4. Through the rectum
6. By mouth
9. A mixture of ground particles that are distributed evenly throughout a liquid but that do not dissolve
10. A delivery route in which a medication is pushed through a specialized atomizer device called a mucosal atomizer device (MAD) into the nare
11. Breathing into the lungs
13. A semiliquid substance that is administered orally in capsule form or through plastic tubes

Critical Thinking

Multiple Choice
Read each critical-thinking item carefully and then select the one best response.

_____ 1. You and your rookie partner are dispatched to a home on the east side of town for a possible poisoning. Upon arrival, you are met by a frantic mother who carries her crying 4-year-old boy up to your truck. "Please help him!" she pleads. "I was cleaning the garage and before I could stop him he drank a jar of gasoline that my husband uses to clean car parts." Your partner puts the truck in park and sets the parking brake. "I'll grab the activated charcoal," he says, climbing out of the cab. You should:

    A. administer the activated charcoal and transport the child immediately.

    B. ask to see the jar to determine how much gasoline was swallowed.

    C. contact online medical direction while administering the activated charcoal.

    D. not administer activated charcoal.

_____ 2. Your patient is a 73-year-old man who was struck with severe chest pressure with radiating pain while having dinner at a local diner. He has a small vial of nitroglycerin in his pocket but says through clenched teeth that he has not taken any in several days and needs you to help him to get the vial open. After administering oxygen, what is the first thing that you should do?

    A. Obtain the patient's blood pressure and ensure that his systolic pressure is not below 110 mm Hg.

    B. Begin assisting the patient's ventilations.

    C. Place him in a position of comfort for transport.

    D. Ask if he has taken any erectile dysfunction medications in the last 24 hours.

_____ 3. You are called to the beach for a 15-year-old boy who is having trouble breathing. He tells you between gasps that he was stung by something and that his body feels "swollen." Just then, a woman runs up to you and puts an EpiPen into your hand. "Here," she says breathlessly. "He needs this!" Would you administer epinephrine to this patient?

    A. Yes, by pushing the EpiPen firmly against the patient's thigh for several seconds.

    B. Not until you determine if it was prescribed for the patient.

    C. Yes, using the sublingual route.

    D. No, his signs and symptoms contraindicate an epinephrine injection.

_____ 4. "I think she's drunk!" a bystander yells, as you and your partner arrive on the scene of an unknown medical aid. You observe an approximately 45-year-old woman stumbling between several cars in the parking lot of a grocery store. As you catch up to the woman, you ask her clearly if she is diabetic. She nods clumsily and leans against one of the cars. You test her blood glucose and obtain a reading of 49 mg/dL. What should you do?

    A. Administer glucose gel orally.

    B. Ask the bystanders if anyone knows her medical history.

    C. Restrain her onto the gurney to keep her from hurting herself or others.

    D. Request an ALS response so glucose can be administered intravenously.

_____ 5. You are dispatched to the county fair for a 54-year-old woman complaining of chest pain. You arrive to find her pressing on the center of her chest and presenting with pale, clammy skin. You ask if she has any cardiac history and she tells you, "No, I just have asthma and my doctor says that I am prediabetic." Would you give this patient aspirin?

    A. No, nitroglycerin would be more appropriate.

    B. Yes, her signs and symptoms indicate cardiac compromise and aspirin could help.

    C. No, aspirin is contraindicated for asthmatics.

    D. Yes, its analgesic properties may help with the discomfort.

Short Answer

Complete this section with short written answers using the space provided.

1. List seven routes of medication administration.

_____

_____

2. Describe the general steps of administering medication.

_____

_____

3. Describe the action of activated charcoal and the steps of administration that are specific to this medication.

_____

_____

4. List three characteristics of epinephrine.

_____

_____

5. How is an epinephrine auto-injector activated?

_____

_____

6. List four side effects of nitroglycerin.

_____

_____

7. Explain why metered-dose inhalers are often used with a spacer.

_____

_____

Ambulance Calls

The following case scenarios provide an opportunity to explore the concerns associated with patient management and to enhance critical-thinking skills. Read each scenario and answer each question to the best of your ability.

1. You are dispatched to "difficulty breathing" at one of your town's many parks. As you near the park entrance, you see a crowd of people who frantically wave for you. You arrive to find a city employee who was apparently mowing the park grounds when he accidentally mowed over a yellow jacket nest. He was wearing coveralls, but he was repeatedly stung around his neck and face. He appears to be somewhat confused; you can hear stridor with each inspiration and his blood pressure is 80/40 mm Hg. Your local protocols allow EMTs to carry EpiPens.

    How do you best manage this patient?

    _____

    _____

    _____

2. You are dispatched to an "unknown medical problem" at the Crosstown Mall. You were called after police were summoned to subdue a combative male shopper. Police officers were able to calm him down, but felt that something was "not right" about him. You arrive to find a calm but confused man who is sweaty and pale. He has no complaints, but keeps repeating, "I have to get home now." You notice a medical ID bracelet indicating that this patient is an insulin-dependent diabetic.

    How do you best manage this patient?

    _____

    _____

    _____

3. You are dispatched to the residence of a 68-year-old man who is complaining of "crushing" chest pain radiating down his left arm for the past hour. He is pale, cool, diaphoretic, and is very nauseated. He tells you he had a heart attack several years ago and takes nitroglycerin, as needed. He took two tablets prior to your arrival and reports no relief.

    How would you best manage this patient?

    _____

    _____

    _____

Fill-in-the-Patient Care Report

Read the incident scenario and then complete the following patient care report (PCR).

"Hey you! Medic!" It's 1300, and you are just finishing lunch at one of the picnic tables in Northern Park when you hear someone yelling from across the small duck pond. "This lady needs help!"

You whistle at your partner who is sitting in the ambulance reading a biology textbook and then begin the short walk to where a small crowd is gathering near an ivy-covered gazebo.

"I think she's having trouble breathing," a man says, moving aside so you can see a 38-year-old woman sitting in the tripod position on a wooden park bench. Her eyes are bulging, her lips and fingernails are beginning to turn blue, and you can immediately see accessory muscles moving in her neck as she struggles to breathe. You kneel in front of the bench, making eye contact with the panicked woman and say, "I'm an EMT and I'm going to help you, okay?" She nods her head frantically.

"Does anyone know her?" you shout, looking around at the confused faces around you. A teenaged girl appears and says, "I don't know her but she dropped this when she first started to freak out." The girl then hands you a blue plastic metered-dose inhaler labeled for asthma.

Approximately 4 minutes since first being alerted to the problem you quickly shake the metered-dose inhaler and hand it to the woman, who claws for it and pumps it once into her mouth and inhales weakly. Right then your partner arrives with the gurney and the equipment bags from the ambulance, and you instruct him to initiate oxygen therapy immediately with a nonrebreathing mask.

As you are helping the 45-kg woman onto the gurney, you notice that her lips and fingernails are returning to normal and that although she is still struggling to breath she is moving more air with each respiratory cycle. The high-concentration oxygen, set at 15 L/min, seems to be helping. Four minutes after the patient first used her inhaler, you and your partner load her into the ambulance for the 10-minute drive to the closest emergency department.

You obtain the patient's vital signs as soon as the ambulance rolls away from the scene, noting a blood pressure of 142/98 mm Hg, a heart rate of 110 beats/min, 28 labored respirations per minute, and a pulse oximetry reading of 88%. You are able to complete two more sets of vitals at 5-minute intervals prior to pulling into the hospital ambulance bay (138/90 mm Hg, 102 beats/min, 24 breaths/min labored, 92%; and 132/88 mm Hg, 96 beats/min, 20 breaths/min with good tidal volume, 96%) and between one more puff from the inhaler and the high-flow oxygen, the patient has improved tremendously.

You and your partner transfer the patient to an emergency department bed, provide the charge nurse with a full report, and are ready to go back into service 48 minutes from first being alerted to the emergency.

Fill-in-the-Patient Care Report

EMS Patient Care Report (PCR)					
Date:	**Incident No.:**	**Nature of Call:**		**Location:**	
Dispatched:	**En Route:**	**At Scene:**	**Transport:**	**At Hospital:**	**In Service:**

Patient Information	
Age:	**Allergies:**
Sex:	**Medications:**
Weight (in kg [lb]):	**Past Medical History:**
	Chief Complaint:

Vital Signs				
Time:	**BP:**	**Pulse:**	**Respirations:**	**Sao$_2$:**
Time:	**BP:**	**Pulse:**	**Respirations:**	**Sao$_2$:**
Time:	**BP:**	**Pulse:**	**Respirations:**	**Sao$_2$:**

EMS Treatment

(circle all that apply)

Oxygen @ ___ L/min via (circle one): NC NRM Bag-Mask Device		**Assisted Ventilation**	**Airway Adjunct**	**CPR**
Defibrillation	**Bleeding Control**	**Bandaging**	**Splinting**	**Other Shock Treatment**

Narrative

Skills

Skill Drill

Test your knowledge of this skill by filling in the correct words in the photo caption.

Skill Drill 7-1: Oral Medication Administration

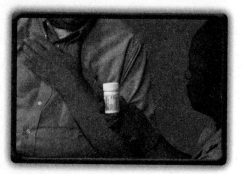

Take _____
precautions. Prepare the appropriate
amount of medication. Instruct the
patient to _____
(if appropriate) or swallow the
medication with water, if administering
a(n) _____ or
_____.

Patient Assessment

General Knowledge

Matching

Match each of the items in the left column to the appropriate definition in the right column.

_____ **1.** Triage
_____ **2.** Cyanosis
_____ **3.** Subcutaneous emphysema
_____ **4.** Tachycardia
_____ **5.** Conjunctiva
_____ **6.** Symptom
_____ **7.** Accessory muscles
_____ **8.** Breath sounds
_____ **9.** Chief complaint
_____ **10.** Diaphoretic
_____ **11.** Jaundice
_____ **12.** Orientation
_____ **13.** OPQRST
_____ **14.** Palpate

_____ **15.** Responsiveness
_____ **16.** Retractions
_____ **17.** Sclera
_____ **18.** Frostbite
_____ **19.** Crepitus
_____ **20.** Paradoxical motion

A. Indication of air movement in the lungs
B. Lining of the eyelid
C. Movements in which the skin pulls in around the ribs during inspiration
D. White of the eyes
E. The mental status of a patient
F. The six pain questions
G. Yellow skin color due to liver disease or dysfunction
H. A crackling sound
I. Examine by touch
J. Damage to tissues as the result of exposure to cold
K. The way in which a patient responds to external stimuli
L. Secondary muscles of respiration
M. Air under the skin
N. Motion of a segment of chest wall that is opposite the normal movement during breathing
O. The reason a patient called for help
P. The process of establishing treatment and transport priorities
Q. A bluish gray skin color associated with reduced oxygen levels
R. Profuse sweating
S. Subjective finding that the patient feels
T. A heart rate greater than 100 beats/min

Match the question with the corresponding assessment tool.

_____ **21.** What does the pain feel like?
_____ **22.** How long have you had the pain?
_____ **23.** Are you taking any medications?
_____ **24.** Did you eat this morning?
_____ **25.** Does anything make the pain feel better or worse?
_____ **26.** On a scale of 1 to 10, how do you rate your pain?
_____ **27.** What were you doing before this happened?
_____ **28.** What type of reaction do you have when you take medication?
_____ **29.** Does the pain move anywhere?
_____ **30.** When did the problem begin?
_____ **31.** Does your chest hurt?
_____ **32.** Have you been recently ill?

A. Signs and symptoms
B. Allergies
C. Medications
D. Past medical history
E. Last oral intake
F. Events leading up to illness
G. Onset
H. Provocation/palliation

I. Quality
J. Region/radiation
K. Severity
L. Timing

Multiple Choice

Read each item carefully and then select the one best response.

_____ 1. The scene size-up consists of all of the following EXCEPT:
   A. determining the mechanism of injury.
   B. requesting additional assistance.
   C. determining level of responsiveness.
   D. personal protective equipment (PPE)/standard precautions.

_____ 2. Your primary safety concern is for:
   A. yourself.
   B. your partner.
   C. your patient.
   D. the bystanders.

_____ 3. With _____, the force of the injury occurs over a broad area, and the skin is usually not broken.
   A. motor vehicle collisions
   B. blunt trauma
   C. penetrating trauma
   D. gunshot wounds

_____ 4. With _____, the force of the injury occurs at a small point of contact between the skin and the object piercing the skin.
   A. motor vehicle collisions
   B. blunt trauma
   C. penetrating trauma
   D. falls

_____ 5. _____ is the measure of the amount of air that is moved into and out of the lungs in one breath.
   A. Residual volume
   B. Tidal volume
   C. Vital capacity
   D. Minute volume

_____ 6. The physical examination consists of all of the following EXCEPT:
   A. puncture.
   B. inspection.
   C. palpation.
   D. auscultation.

_____ 7. When determining the initial general impression, you should note all of the following EXCEPT:
   A. the patient's age.
   B. the level of distress.
   C. the events leading up to the incident.
   D. the patient's sex.

_____ 8. When considering the need for additional resources, which of the following is NOT a question you should ask?
   A. How many patients are there?
   B. Is it raining?
   C. Who contacted EMS?
   D. Does the scene pose a threat to you or your patient's safety?

_____ **9.** The primary assessment includes evaluation of all of the following EXCEPT:

  A. mental status.

  B. pupils.

  C. airway.

  D. circulation.

_____ **10.** The best indicator of brain function is the patient's:

  A. pulse rate.

  B. papillary response.

  C. mental status.

  D. respiratory rate and depth.

_____ **11.** What does the "P" on the AVPU scale represent?

  A. Responsive to palpation

  B. Responsive to pain

  C. Responsive to provocation

  D. Responsive to palliation

_____ **12.** A normal respiratory rate for an adult is typically:

  A. 5 to 10 breaths per minute.

  B. 12 to 20 breaths per minute.

  C. 15 to 30 breaths per minute.

  D. 20 to 30 breaths per minute.

_____ **13.** For children younger than 1 year old, you should palpate the _____ artery when assessing the pulse.

  A. carotid

  B. radial

  C. femoral

  D. brachial

_____ **14.** The automated external defibrillator (AED) should be used on pediatric medical patients who are at least _____ year(s) old and who have been assessed to be unresponsive, apneic, and pulseless.

  A. 1

  B. 8

  C. 9

  D. 10

_____ **15.** When there are low levels of oxygen in the blood, the lips and mucous membranes appear blue or gray. This condition is called:

  A. cyanosis.

  B. pallor.

  C. jaundice.

  D. ashen.

_____ **16.** Your first consideration when assessing a pulse is to determine:

  A. how fast the rate is.

  B. the quality.

  C. if one is present.

  D. if the rhythm is regular.

_____ **17.** To obtain the pulse rate in most patients, you should count the number of pulses felt in a _____ period and then multiple by two.

  A. 15-second

  B. 20-second

  C. 25-second

  D. 30-second

_____ **18.** In deeply pigmented skin, you should look for changes in color in areas of the skin that have less pigment, including:

  A. the sclera.

  B. the conjunctiva.

  C. the mucous membranes of the mouth.

  D. all of the above.

_____ **19.** All of the following are conditions not related to the body's circulation that may slow capillary refill EXCEPT:

  A. local circulatory compromise.

  B. hypothermia.

  C. age.

  D. abdominal pain.

_____ **20.** Which of the following is NOT considered a method for controlling external bleeding?

  A. Direct pressure

  B. Tourniquet

  C. Cold water

  D. Elevation

_____ **21.** The _____ is/are the most serious thing that the patient is concerned about; the reason why they called 9-1-1.

  A. chief complaint

  B. pertinent negatives

  C. severity

  D. past medical history

_____ **22.** The four items used to assess the orientation of a patient's mental status include all the following EXCEPT:

  A. person.

  B. place.

  C. history.

  D. events.

_____ **23.** An integral part of the rapid scan is evaluation using the mnemonic:

  A. AVPU.

  B. DCAP-BTLS.

  C. OPQRST.

  D. SAMPLE.

_____ **24.** In the absence of light, the pupils will:

  A. constrict.

  B. stay fixed.

  C. dilate.

  D. become unequal.

_____ **25.** _____ cause the pupils to constrict to a pinpoint.

  A. Opiates

  B. Antidepressants

  C. Antihypertensive medications

  D. Diabetic medications

_____ **26.** When assessing breathing, you should obtain all of the following EXCEPT:

  A. respiratory rate.

  B. depth of breathing.

  C. quality/character of breathing.

  D. breath odor.

_____ **27.** Which of the following statements regarding assessment of the airway is TRUE?

    A. The body will not be supplied the necessary oxygen if the airway is not managed.

    B. You should use the head tilt–chin lift maneuver to open the airway in trauma patients.

    C. The tongue is generally not a cause of airway obstruction.

    D. A conscious patient who cannot speak or cry is most likely hyperventilating.

_____ **28.** Which of the following is NOT considered a type of breath sound?

    A. Rhonchi

    B. Vibration

    C. Wheeze

    D. Stridor

_____ **29.** The MOST important thing to consider in patients with multiple injuries in various stages of healing is that:

    A. this patient is rather clumsy.

    B. the patient could have an underlying cancer.

    C. the patient might be a victim of abuse.

    D. the patient probably has a high tolerance for pain.

_____ **30.** Which of the following questions should you ask yourself when dealing with a patient who is not answering your questions?

    A. Is the patient hungry?

    B. Is there a language problem?

    C. Is the patient tired?

    D. Is the patient angry with me?

_____ **31.** _____ is an assessment tool used to evaluate the effectiveness of oxygenation.

    A. Capnography

    B. Capnometry

    C. Pulse oximetry

    D. Blood glucose

_____ **32.** The pressure felt along the wall of the artery when the ventricles of the heart contract is referred to as the:

    A. asystolic pressure.

    B. diastolic pressure.

    C. idiopathic pressure.

    D. systolic pressure.

_____ **33.** A blood pressure cuff that's too large for the patient:

    A. may result in a falsely low reading.

    B. may result in a falsely high reading.

    C. will not affect the reading.

    D. should be used in patients with arm pain.

_____ **34.** When examining the abdomen, you should palpate for all of the following EXCEPT:

    A. guarding.

    B. crepitation.

    C. tenderness.

    D. rigidity.

_____ **35.** Crackling sounds produced by air bubbles under the skin are known as:

    A. subcutaneous ecchymosis.

    B. subcutaneous emphysema.

    C. subcutaneous erythema.

    D. subcutaneous emboli.

_____ **36.** Unstable patients should be reassessed every _____ minutes.
   A. 5
   B. 10
   C. 15
   D. 20

_____ **37.** In the _____ position, the patient sits leaning forward on outstretched arms with the head and chin thrust slightly forward.
   A. Fowler's
   B. tripod
   C. sniffing
   D. lithotomy

_____ **38.** In an unresponsive adult patient, the primary location to assess the pulse is the _____ artery.
   A. carotid
   B. femoral
   C. radial
   D. brachial

_____ **39.** Liver disease or dysfunction may cause _____, resulting in the patient's skin and sclera turning yellow.
   A. cyanosis
   B. jaundice
   C. diaphoresis
   D. lack of perfusion

_____ **40.** When obtaining a blood pressure by palpation in the arm, you should place your fingertips on the _____ artery.
   A. carotid
   B. brachial
   C. radial
   D. posterior tibial

_____ **41.** The first set of vital signs that you obtain is called the:
   A. original vital signs.
   B. baseline vital signs.
   C. actual vital signs.
   D. real vital signs.

_____ **42.** Which of the following is NOT considered a sign?
   A. Dizziness
   B. Marked deformities
   C. External bleeding
   D. Wounds

_____ **43.** When blood pressure drops, the body compensates to maintain perfusion to the vital organs by:
   A. decreasing the pulse rate.
   B. dilating the arteries.
   C. decreasing the respiratory rate.
   D. decreasing the blood flow to the skin and extremities.

_____ **44.** When assessing and treating a patient who is visually impaired, it is important that you do all of the following EXCEPT:
   A. speak loudly into the patient's ear, because he or she can't see you.
   B. announce yourself when entering the residence.
   C. put items that were moved back into their previous position.
   D. explain to the patient what is happening.

_____ **45.** Which of the following statements is FALSE regarding the assessment of patients with a language barrier?

    A. You should find an interpreter.

    B. Determine whether the patient understands you.

    C. Questioning should be lengthy and complex.

    D. Be aware of the language diversity in your community.

True/False

If you believe the statement to be more true than false, write the letter "T" in the space provided. If you believe the statement to be more false than true, write the letter "F."

_____ **1.** Responsiveness is evaluated with the mnemonic DCAP-BTLS.

_____ **2.** Reassessment is not necessary for stable patients.

_____ **3.** An assessment of the patient's musculoskeletal system typically is done because of a chief complaint associated with some type of trauma.

_____ **4.** The apparent absence of a palpable pulse in an unresponsive patient is not a cause for concern.

_____ **5.** A patient with a poor general impression is considered a priority patient.

_____ **6.** When assessing the head, you should assess the patient's ears and nose for fluid.

_____ **7.** Paradoxical motion of the chest wall is commonly associated with upper respiratory infections.

_____ **8.** The abdomen is broken into six areas for assessment.

_____ **9.** In the reassessment process, you should reevaluate everything that has been done to this point in the patient assessment process.

_____ **10.** Law enforcement personnel may be needed at scenes to control traffic or intervene in domestic violence situations.

_____ **11.** Determining the mental status and the level of consciousness of a patient take a great deal of time while on scene.

_____ **12.** Depressed brain function can result from trauma or stroke.

_____ **13.** PEARRL is used to describe skin color.

_____ **14.** You should consider providing positive-pressure ventilation in a conscious patient who has a respiratory rate of 14 breaths per minute.

_____ **15.** When documenting vital signs, you should note whether the patient's respirations are regular or irregular.

_____ **16.** Patients with difficulty breathing, severe chest pain, and signs of poor perfusion should be transported immediately.

_____ **17.** You should aim to assess, stabilize, and begin transport of trauma patients within 20 minutes.

_____ **18.** Correct identification of high-priority patients is an essential aspect of the primary assessment and helps to improve patient outcome.

_____ **19.** You should not interrupt patients when speaking, and you should be empathetic to their situation.

_____ **20.** Being openly judgmental of patients who may have a chemical dependency is acceptable as long as you remain professional.

_____ **21.** Scenes involving domestic violence can be extremely dangerous for EMS personnel.

_____ **22.** You should consider all females of childbearing age who are reporting lower abdominal pain to be pregnant unless ruled out by history or other information.

_____ **23.** Once you have allowed a talkative patient a chance to express himself or herself, you should allow the patient to continue talking about whatever he or she wants.

_____ **24.** Emergency medical technicians (EMTs) can expect anxious patients to exhibit signs of psychological shock.

_____ **25.** It is rather unusual for a patient, family member, or friend to vent hostility toward EMS.

_____ **26.** Information gathered from an intoxicated patient may be unreliable.

_____ **27.** Your presence may make a crying patient feel more secure.

_____ **28.** Depression is not a common reason for patients to call for EMS.

_____ **29.** When assessing a patient, you should inspect the pelvis for symmetry and any obvious signs of injury, bleeding, and deformity.

_____ **30.** Pulse and motor and sensory functions are typically assessed when examining a patient's extremities.

Fill-in-the-Blank

Read each item carefully and then complete the statement by filling in the missing words.

1. A(n) _____ is an objective condition that you can observe about the patient.

2. _____ _____ are protective measures for dealing with blood and bodily fluids.

3. When there are multiple patients, you should use the _____ _____ _____ to help organize the triage, logistics, and treatment of patients.

4. _____ _____ _____ should be requested for patients with severe injuries or complex medical problems.

5. Identifying and initiating treatment of immediate potentially life-threatening conditions is the goal of the _____ _____.

6. You should think of the _____ _____ as a visual assessment, gathering information as you approach the patient.

7. _____ is the circulation of blood within an organ or tissue.

8. _____ tests the mental status of the patient by checking memory and thinking ability.

9. When light is shined into the eyes, the pupils should _____.

10. A brassy, crowing sound that is prominent on inspiration, suggesting a mildly occluded airway, is referred to as _____.

11. If there is a potential for trauma, use the modified _____ to open the airway.

12. During _____ the chest muscles relax and air is released out of the lungs.

13. If a patient seems to develop difficulty breathing after your primary assessment, you should immediate reevaluate the _____.

14. If you hear fluid in the airway during your assessment, you should immediately _____ the airway to prevent aspiration.

15. A patient who coughs up thick, yellowish or greenish sputum most likely has a(n) _____

_____.

16. _____ _____ and see-saw breathing in a pediatric patient indicate inadequate

breathing.

17. If you cannot palpate a pulse in an unresponsive patient, you should begin _____.

18. _____ is a heart rate greater than 100 beats per minute.

19. The _____ is the delicate membrane lining the eyelids, and it covers the exposed surface of the eye.

20. Skin that is cool, clammy, and pale in your primary assessment typically indicates _____.

21. When the skin is bathed in sweat, it is described as _____.

22. A capillary refill time should be less than _____ second(s).

23. _____ patency is always your number one priority.

24. A rapid scan to identify immediate threats should take _____ to _____ second(s).

25. The _____ _____ refers to the time from injury to definitive care.

26. The goal of the primary assessment is to identify and treat _____ _____.

27. _____ _____ provides details about the patient's chief complaint and an account of the

patient's signs and symptoms.

28. You should use _____ questions when taking a history on a patient.

29. _____ is a mnemonic used to gather past medical or trauma history.

30. _____ _____ are negative findings that warrant no care or intervention.

31. One of the most common causes of patient confusion is _____.

32. _____ describes the process of touching or feeling the patient for abnormalities.

33. _____ is a noninvasive method that can quickly and efficiently provide information on a patient's

ventilatory status, circulation, and metabolism.

34. _____ _____ is the residual pressure that remains in the arteries during the relaxation

phase of the heart.

35. A(n) _____ assessment should be performed any time you are confronted with a patient who has a

change in mental status, a possible head injury, or syncope.

Crossword Puzzle

The following crossword puzzle is an activity provided to reinforce correct spelling and understanding of medical terminology associated with emergency care and the EMT. Use the clues in the column to complete the puzzle.

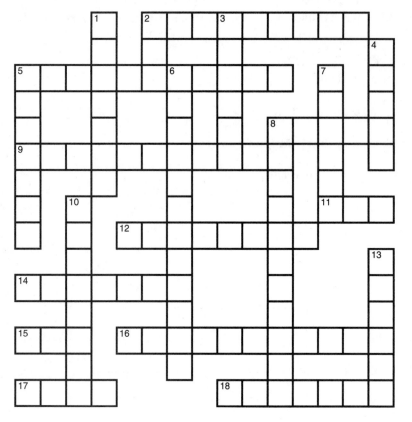

Across

2. Negative findings that warrant no care or intervention are known as _____ negatives.

5. Blood pressure that is lower than the normal range

8. The pressure wave that occurs as each heartbeat causes a surge in the blood circulating through the arteries

9. A rapid heart rate, more than 100 beats/min

11. The general type of illness a patient is experiencing

12. A(n) _____ scan is performed during the secondary assessment.

14. A harsh, high-pitched, crowing inspiratory sound

15. The way in which traumatic injuries occur

16. The delicate membrane that lines the eyelids and covers the exposed surface of the eye

17. Objective findings that can be seen, heard, felt, smelled, or measured

18. To examine by touch

Down

1. Coarse, low-pitched breath sounds heard in patients with chronic mucus in the upper airways

2. Clothing or specialized equipment that provides protection to the wearer

3. _____ position is an upright position in which the patient leans forward onto two arms stretched forward and thrusts the head and chin forward.

4. A crackling, rattling breath sound that signals fluid in the air spaces of the lungs

5. A step within the patient assessment process that provides details about the chief complaint is called _____ taking.

6. Flaring out of the nostrils, indicating that there is an airway obstruction

7. The _____ Period is the time from injury to definitive care.

8. _____ motion is the motion of the chest wall section that is detached in a flail chest.

10. Involuntary muscle contractions of the abdominal wall in an effort to protect an inflamed abdomen

13. The process of establishing treatment and transportation priorities according to severity of injury and medical need

Critical Thinking

Short Answer

Complete this section with short written answers using the space provided.

1. What is the single goal of primary assessment?

_____

_____

2. What is the general impression based on?

_____

_____

3. What do the letters ABC stand for in the assessment process?

_____

_____

4. What four kinds of questions are asked when assessing orientation, and what purpose do these questions serve?

_____

_____

5. What six questions should you ask yourself when assessing a patient's breathing?

_____

_____

6. List the elements of DCAP-BTLS.

_____

_____

7. List at least three mechanisms of injury and at least three natures of illness.

_____

_____

8. Define the acronym PEARRL.

_____

_____

9. Explain the difference between a sign and a symptom.

_____

_____

10. What four questions should you ask yourself when determining if additional resources are needed at the scene?

_____

_____

Ambulance Calls

The following case scenarios provide an opportunity to explore the concerns associated with patient management and to enhance critical-thinking skills. Read each scenario and answer each question to the best of your ability.

1. You are dispatched to a motor vehicle collision where you find a 32-year-old man with extensive trauma to the face and gurgling in his airway. He is responsive only to pain. You also note that the windshield is spider-webbed and that there is deformity to the steering wheel. He is not wearing a seatbelt.

   How would you best manage this patient? What clues tell you the transport status?

   _____

   _____

   _____

2. You are dispatched to a local residence for "difficulty breathing." You find a man standing in his kitchen, leaning against a counter, and holding a metered-dose inhaler. As you question him, you see that he is working very hard to breathe, hear wheezing, and note that he can answer you with only one- or two-word responses.

   How would you best manage this patient?

   _____

   _____

   _____

3. You are dispatched to "man fallen" at a private home. You arrive to find an older man who is semiconscious (responsive to painful stimuli) and has fallen down a flight of wooden stairs onto a cement basement floor. He has bruising and a small laceration above his left eye.

   How would you best manage this patient?

   _____

   _____

   _____

Skills

Skill Drills

Skill Drill 8-1: Rapid Scan
Test your knowledge of this skill by placing the photos below in the correct order. Number the first step with a "1," the second step with a "2," etc.

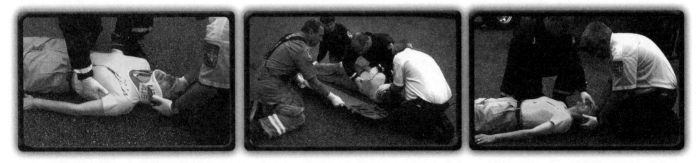

_____ Assess the chest. Listen to breath sounds on both sides of the chest.

_____ Assess the back. In trauma patients, roll the patient in one motion.

_____ Assess the head. Have your partner maintain in-line stabilization if trauma is suspected.

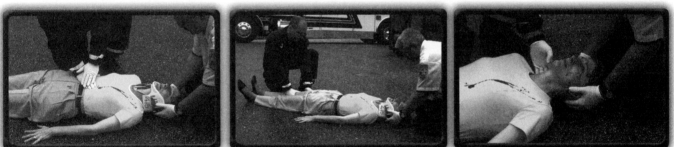

_____ Assess the abdomen.

_____ Assess all four extremities. Assess pulse and the motor and sensory function.

_____ Assess the neck.

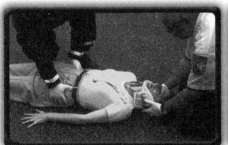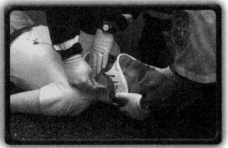

_____ Assess the pelvis. If there is no pain, gently compress the pelvis downward and inward to look for tenderness and instability.

_____ Apply a cervical spinal immobilization device on trauma patients.

Skill Drill 8-3: Obtaining Blood Pressure by Auscultation
Test your knowledge of this skill by placing the photos below in the correct order. Number the first step with a "1," the second step with a "2," etc.

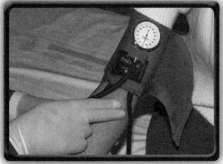

_____ Support the exposed arm at the level of the heart. Palpate the brachial artery.

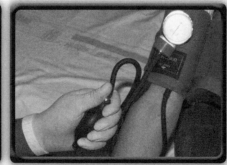

_____ Open the valve, and quickly release remaining air.

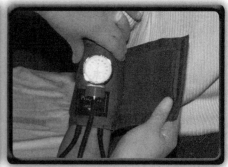

_____ Follow standard precautions. Check for ports, central lines, mastectomy, and injury to the arm. If any are present, use the other arm. Apply the cuff snugly. The lower border of the cuff should be about 1″ above the antecubital space.

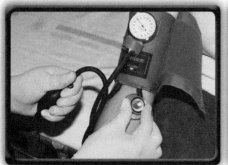

_____ Close the valve, and pump to 30 mm Hg above the point at which you stop hearing pulse sounds. Note the systolic and diastolic pressures as you let air escape slowly.

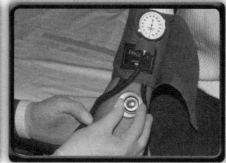

_____ Place the stethoscope over the brachial artery, and grasp the ball-pump and turn-valve.

Airway Management

General Knowledge

Matching

Match each of the items in the left column to the appropriate definition in the right column.

_____ **1.** Inhalation   **A.** Moves down slightly when it contracts

_____ **2.** Exhalation   **B.** Irregular breathing pattern with increased rate and depth followed by apnea

_____ **3.** Alveoli   **C.** Active part of breathing

_____ **4.** Mediastinum   **D.** Voice box

_____ **5.** Hypoxic drive   **E.** Amount of air moved during one breath

_____ **6.** Tidal volume   **F.** Raises ribs when it contracts

_____ **7.** Diaphragm   **G.** Space between the lungs

_____ **8.** Intercostal muscle   **H.** Site of oxygen diffusion

_____ **9.** Ventilation   **I.** Thorax size decreases

_____ **10.** Larynx   **J.** Insufficient oxygen for cells and tissues

_____ **11.** Hypoxia   **K.** Backup system to control respiration

_____ **12.** Cheyne-Stokes   **L.** Exchange of air between lungs and the environment

Multiple Choice

Read each item carefully and then select the one best response.

_____ **1.** What percentage of the air we breathe is made up of oxygen?

    A. 78%

    B. 12%

    C. 16%

    D. 21%

_____ **2.** Regarding the maintenance of the airway in an unconscious adult, which of the following is FALSE?

    A. Insertion of an oropharyngeal airway helps keep the airway open.

    B. The head tilt–chin lift maneuver should always be used to open the airway.

    C. Secretions should be suctioned from the mouth, as necessary.

    D. Inserting a rigid suction catheter beyond the tongue may cause gagging.

_____ **3.** The normal respiratory rate for an adult is:

    A. about equal to the person's heart rate.

    B. 12 to 20 breaths/min.

    C. faster when the person is sleeping.

    D. the same as in infants and children.

_____ **4.** All of the following are signs of hypoxia EXCEPT:

    A. tachycardia.

    B. dehydration.

    C. cyanosis.

    D. weak pulse.

_____ **5.** The brain stem normally triggers breathing by increasing respirations when:

    A. carbon dioxide levels increase.

    B. oxygen levels increase.

    C. carbon dioxide levels decrease.

    D. nitrogen levels decrease.

_____ **6.** Which of the following is NOT a sign of abnormal breathing?

    A. Warm, dry skin

    B. Speaking in two- or three-word sentences

    C. Unequal breath sounds

    D. Skin pulling in around the ribs during inspiration

_____ **7.** The proper technique for sizing an oropharyngeal airway before insertion is to measure the device from:

    A. the tip of the nose to the earlobe.

    B. the bridge of the nose to the tip of the chin.

    C. the corner of the mouth to the earlobe.

    D. the center of the jaw to the earlobe.

_____ **8.** What is the most common problem you may encounter when using a bag-mask device?

    A. Volume of the bag-mask device

    B. Positioning of the patient's head

    C. Environmental conditions

    D. Maintaining an airtight seal

_____ **9.** When ventilating a patient with a bag-mask device, you should:

    A. look for inflation of the cheeks.

    B. look for signs of the patient breathing on his or her own.

    C. look for rise and fall of the chest.

    D. listen for gurgling.

_____ **10.** Suctioning the oral cavity of an adult should be accomplished within:

    A. 5 seconds.

    B. 10 seconds.

    C. 15 seconds.

    D. 20 seconds.

_____ **11.** Which of the following is the preferred method of assisting ventilations?

    A. Mouth-to-mask with one-way valve

    B. Two-person bag-mask device with reservoir and supplemental oxygen

    C. Flow-restricted, oxygen-powered ventilation device

    D. One-person bag-mask device with oxygen reservoir and supplemental oxygen

_____ **12.** When a person goes _____ minutes without oxygen, brain damage is very likely.

    A. 0 to 4

    B. 4 to 6

    C. 6 to 10

    D. more than 10

_____ **13.** If your partner, while examining a patient, states that the patient's lungs are equal and bilateral, you would understand your partner to mean that:

    A. both lungs have labored breathing.

    B. both lungs are equally bad.

    C. the patient is not breathing.

    D. there are clear and equal lung sounds on both sides.

_____ **14.** What are agonal gasps?

    A. Occasional gasping breaths, but adequate to maintain life

    B. Occasional gasping breaths, unable to maintain life

    C. Painful respirations due to broken ribs

    D. Another name for ataxic respirations

_____ **15.** You come upon an unresponsive patient who is not injured and is breathing on her own with a normal rate and an adequate tidal volume. What would be the advantage of placing her in the recovery position?

    A. It's the preferred position of comfort for patients.

    B. It helps to protect their cervical spine when injuries are hidden.

    C. It helps to maintain a clear airway.

    D. It's easier to load them onto the cot from this position.

True/False

If you believe the statement to be more true than false, write the letter "T" in the space provided. If you believe the statement to be more false than true, write the letter "F."

_____ **1.** Nasal airways keep the tongue from blocking the upper airway and facilitate suctioning of the oropharynx.

_____ **2.** Nasal cannulas can deliver a maximum of 44% oxygen at 6 L/min.

_____ **3.** Oral airways should be measured from the tip of the nose to the earlobe.

_____ **4.** Compressed gas cylinders pose no unusual risk.

_____ **5.** The pin-indexing system is used to ensure compatibility between pressure regulators and oxygen flowmeters.

Fill-in-the-Blank

Read each item carefully and then complete the statement by filling in the missing words.

1. Air enters the body through the _____ _____ _____.

2. In exhalation, air pressure in the lungs is _____ than the pressure outside.

3. The air we breathe contains _____ percent oxygen and _____ percent nitrogen.

4. The primary mechanism for triggering breathing is the level of _____ _____ in the blood.

5. During inhalation, the _____ and _____ _____ contract, causing the thorax to enlarge.

6. Continuous _____ Airway _____ has proven to be immensely beneficial to patients experiencing respiratory distress from acute pulmonary edema or obstructive pulmonary disease.

7. Insufficient oxygen in the cells and tissues is called _____.

Labeling

Label the following diagrams with the correct terms.

1. Upper and Lower Airways

A. _____

B. _____

C. _____

D. _____

E. _____

F. _____

G. _____

H. _____

I. _____

J. _____

K. _____

L. _____

M. _____

N. _____

O. _____

P. _____

Q. _____

R. _____

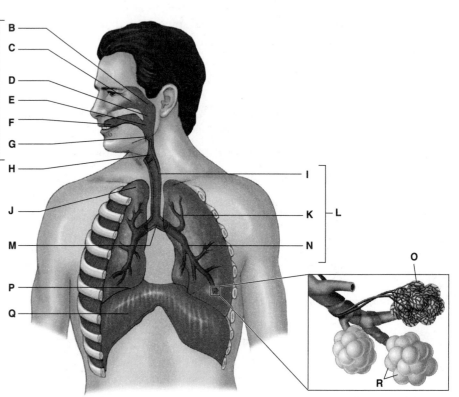

2. Oral Cavity

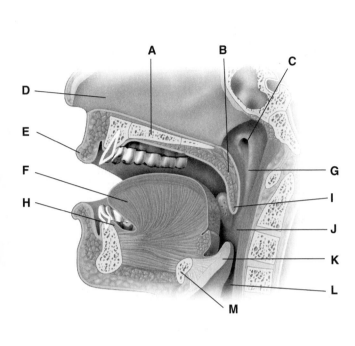

A. _____

B. _____

C. _____

D. _____

E. _____

F. _____

G. _____

H. _____

I. _____

J. _____

K. _____

L. _____

M. _____

3. Thoracic Cavity

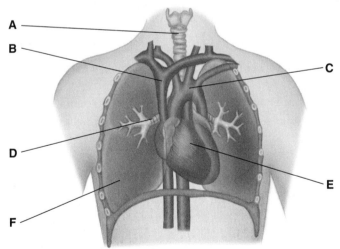

A. _____

B. _____

C. _____

D. _____

E. _____

F. _____

Crossword Puzzle

The following crossword puzzle is an activity provided to reinforce correct spelling and understanding of medical terminology associated with emergency care and the EMT. Use the clues in the column to complete the puzzle.

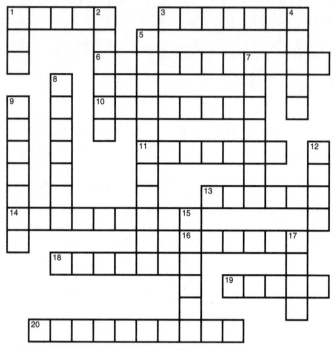

Across

1. Absence of spontaneous breathing
3. The space in between the vocal cords that is the narrowest portion of the adult's airway
6. The process of delivering oxygen to the blood by diffusion from the alveoli following inhalation into the lungs
10. A safety system for large oxygen cylinders, designed to prevent the accidental attachment of a regulator to a cylinder containing the wrong type of gas, is known as the _____ Standard System.
11. _____ pressure can be applied to occlude the esophagus to inhibit gastric distention and regurgitation of vomitus in the unconscious patient.
13. _____ ventilation is the volume of air moved through the lungs in 1 minute, minus the dead space, and is calculated by multiplying tidal volume (minus dead space) and respiratory rate.
14. The metabolism that takes place in the absence of oxygen is called _____ metabolism; the principle product is lactic acid.
16. _____ respirations are irregular, ineffective respirations that may or may not have an identifiable pattern.
18. _____ exchange is a term used to distinguish the degree of distress in a patient with a mild airway obstruction. The patient is still conscious and able to cough forcefully, although wheezing may be heard.
19. The amount of air that can be forcibly expelled from the lungs after breathing in as deeply as possible is known as the _____ capacity.
20. A liquid protein substance that coats the alveoli in the lungs, decreases alveolar surface tension, and keeps the alveoli expanded; a low level in a premature infant contributes to respiratory distress syndrome

Down

1. A ventilation device attached to a control box that allows the variables of ventilation to be set. It frees the EMT to perform other tasks while the patient is being ventilated.
2. Occasional, gasping breaths that occur after the heart has stopped are known as _____ respirations.
4. An opening through the skin and into an organ or other structure; one in the neck connects the trachea directly to the skin.
5. Increased carbon dioxide level in the bloodstream
7. A life-threatening collection of air within the pleural space is called a(n) _____ pneumothorax.
8. A dangerous condition in which the body tissues and cells do not have enough oxygen
9. The term used to describe the amount of gas in air or dissolved in fluid, such as blood, is _____ pressure.
12. Mechanical maintenance of pressure in the airway at the end of expiration to increase the volume of gas remaining in the lungs
15. Point at which the trachea divides into the left and right mainstem bronchi
17. A method of ventilation used primarily in the treatment of critically ill patients with respiratory distress; can prevent the need for endotracheal intubation

Critical Thinking

Multiple Choice

Read each critical-thinking item carefully and then select the one best response.

Questions 1–5 are derived from the following scenario: You respond to a construction site and find a worker lying supine in the dirt. He has been hit by a heavy construction vehicle and flew more than 15′ (4.6 m) before landing in his current position. There is discoloration and distention of his abdomen about the RUQ. He is unconscious and his respirations are 10 breaths/min and shallow, with noisy gurgling sounds.

_____   1. What airway technique will you use to open his airway?
   A. Head tilt–neck lift maneuver
   B. Jaw thrust
   C. Head tilt–chin lift maneuver
   D. None of the above

_____   2. After opening the airway, your next priority is to:
   A. provide oxygen at 6 L/min via nonrebreathing mask.
   B. provide oxygen at 15 L/min via nasal cannula.
   C. assist respirations.
   D. suction the airway.

_____   3. What method will you use to keep his airway open?
   A. Nasal cannula
   B. Jaw thrust
   C. Oropharyngeal airway
   D. Any of the above

_____   4. While assisting with respirations, you note gastric distention. In order to prevent or alleviate the distention, you should:
   A. ensure that the patient's airway is appropriately positioned.
   B. ventilate the patient at the appropriate rate.
   C. ventilate the patient at the appropriate volume.
   D. all of the above.

_____   5. The correct ventilation rate for assisting this adult patient is:
   A. one breath every 5 to 6 seconds.
   B. one breath every 3 to 5 seconds.
   C. one breath every 10 to 12 seconds.
   D. There is no need to assist with ventilations for this patient.

Short Answer

Complete this section with short written answers using the space provided.

1. List the five early signs of hypoxia.

_____

_____

2. What are the normal respiratory rates for adults, children, and infants?

_____

_____

3. How can you avoid gastric distention while performing artificial ventilation?

_____

_____

4. Identify the five ideal components of a manually triggered ventilation device.

_____

_____

5. List six signs of inadequate breathing.

_____

_____

6. What are accessory muscles? Name three.

_____

_____

7. When should medical control be consulted before inserting a nasal airway?

_____

_____

8. List the four steps in nasal airway insertion.

_____

_____

9. What is the best suction tip for suctioning the oropharynx, and why?

_____

_____

10. What is the time limit for each episode of suctioning an adult?

_____

_____

Ambulance Calls

The following case scenarios provide an opportunity to explore the concerns associated with patient management and to enhance critical-thinking skills. Read each scenario and answer each question to the best of your ability.

1. You are dispatched to a crash with multiple patients early one morning near the end of your shift. Your patient was the unrestrained driver of one of the vehicles. She is 38 years old and struck her face against the steering wheel and windshield. There is a large laceration on her nose and several teeth are missing. Although unconscious, she has vomited a large amount of food and blood, which is pooling in her mouth. You note gurgling noises as she attempts to breathe.

   How would you best manage this patient?

   _____

   _____

   _____

2. You are dispatched to a local restaurant for an unconscious woman. As you arrive, you are greeted by a frantic restaurant manager. She tells you that one of her staff members went into the restroom to complete the hourly cleaning routine and found a woman lying on the floor, motionless and apparently not breathing. You and your partner enter the cramped ladies' bathroom to find an older woman who is apneic, cyanotic, and has a carotid pulse. You attempt to ventilate the patient using a bag-mask device, but are unsuccessful.

   How should you manage this patient?

   _____

   _____

   _____

3. You are outside doing some yard work when you hear one of your neighbors call for help. As you cross the street, you see a husband standing over his wife, who is lying on the ground. He tells you that she complained of feeling lightheaded and then she suddenly passed out. He further tells you that he was able to help her to the ground without injury. When you assess her, you hear snoring sounds as she breathes.

   How do you manage this patient?

   _____

   _____

   _____

Fill-in-the-Patient Care Report

Read the incident scenario and then complete the following patient care report (PCR).

It is 1530, and you have just been dispatched to Market Street High School for a possible drug overdose. As your partner steers the ambulance into the nearly empty school parking lot at 1543, you see a woman waving her arms from near one of the low, gray buildings. You and your partner pull the equipment-laden gurney from the back of the truck and hurry across the grass.

"The janitor found her in the stall," the woman's voice trembles as you arrive at the restroom entrance where she is standing. "She's kind of breathing but I can't wake her up… she's had some troubles in the past with drugs."

You find the 14-year-old girl lying on her left side on the tile floor in the middle of three stalls, unresponsive to pain and with slow, snoring respirations.

"You see that?" your partner says, unzipping the airway bag and pointing toward the girl's bluish lips and fingernails.

"I'm going to drag her out here so we have room while you get the bag-mask device set up," you say, carefully pulling the 110-pound (50-kg) girl from the stall and resting her on her back. You immediately open her airway with the head tilt–chin lift maneuver, which stops the snoring sound, but you still note that her breathing is very shallow. Just then your partner finishes assembling the oxygen tank and bag-mask device and inserts an oropharyngeal airway. Within 2 minutes of the time that you got out of the ambulance, your partner is assisting the patient's respirations, getting adequate chest rise, and you are getting a quick set of vitals signs.

You note that her blood pressure is 124/86 mm Hg, pulse is 112 beats/min and regular, respirations (with assistance) are 12 breaths/min, and her oxygen saturation is 93%.

Just as you are finishing vitals, the local fire crew arrives and helps place the patient onto the gurney and into the back of the ambulance. One of the fire fighters even jumps into the back to continue assisting the girl's ventilations so your partner can complete the assessment and obtain a second set of vitals en route to the receiving hospital.

You notify dispatch at 1556 that you are pulling away from the scene and headed to the hospital 12 minutes south of the school. The patient's second set of vitals, obtained 4 minutes after going en route, were: blood pressure 122/86 mm Hg, pulse 110 beats/min, respirations 12 breaths/min (still being assisted), and a pulse oximetry reading of 96%.

Upon arrival at the hospital, you transfer the patient to the emergency department staff and clean and restock your equipment. Sixty-five minutes after receiving the initial dispatch, you go back in service.

Fill-in-the-Patient Care Report

EMS Patient Care Report (PCR)				
Date:	Incident No.:	Nature of Call:		Location:
Dispatched:	En Route:	At Scene:	Transport:	At Hospital:	In Service:

Patient Information	
Age: Sex: Weight (in kg [lb]):	Allergies: Medications: Past Medical History: Chief Complaint:

Vital Signs				
Time:	BP:	Pulse:	Respirations:	Sao$_2$:
Time:	BP:	Pulse:	Respirations:	Sao$_2$:
Time:	BP:	Pulse:	Respirations:	Sao$_2$:

EMS Treatment (circle all that apply)			
Oxygen @ ___ L/min via (circle one): NC NRM Bag-Mask Device	Assisted Ventilation	Airway Adjunct	CPR
Defibrillation	Bleeding Control	Bandaging	Splinting	Other Shock Treatment

Narrative

Skills

Skill Drills

Test your knowledge of these skills by filling in the correct words in the photo captions.

Skill Drill 9-2: Positioning the Unconscious Patient

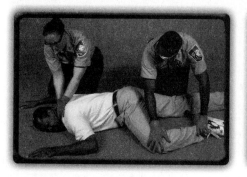

1. Support the _____ while your partner straightens the patient's legs.

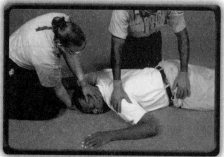

2. Have your partner place his or her _____ on the patient's far _____ and hip.

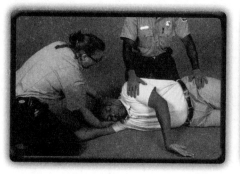

3. _____ the patient as a unit with the responder at the patient's _____ calling the count to begin the move.

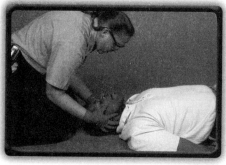
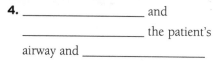

4. _____ and _____ the patient's airway and _____ status.

Skill Drill 9-3: Inserting an Oral Airway

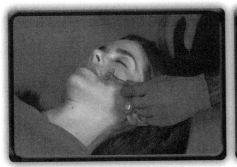 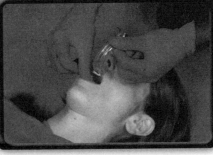 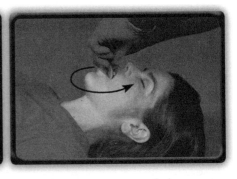

1. Size the _____ by measuring from the patient's _____ to the corner of the _____.

2. Open the patient's _____ with the _____-finger technique. Hold the _____ upside down with your other hand. Insert the airway with the tip facing the _____ of the mouth.

3. _____ the airway _____. Insert the airway until the _____ rests on the patient's lips and teeth. In this position, the airway will hold the _____ forward.

Skill Drill 9-7: Placing an Oxygen Cylinder Into Service

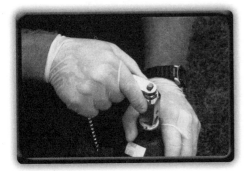 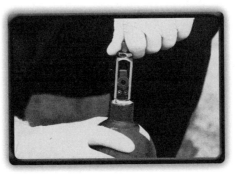

1. Using an oxygen _____, turn the valve _____ to slowly "crack" the cylinder.

2. Attach the regulator/flowmeter to the _____ stem using the two pin-_____ holes and make sure that the _____ is in place over the larger hole.

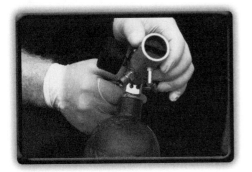 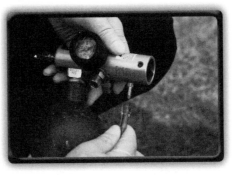

3. Align the _____ so that the pins fit snugly into the correct holes on the _____ stem, and hand tighten the _____.

4. Attach the _____ connective tubing to the _____.

Skill Drill 9-8: Performing Mouth-to-Mask Ventilation

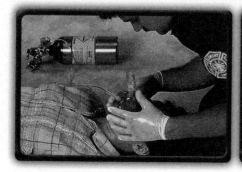

1. Once the patient's head is properly _____ and an airway _____ is inserted, place the mask on the patient's face. _____ the mask to the face using both hands (EC _____).

2. _____ into the one-way valve until you note visible _____ rise.

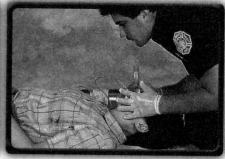

3. Remove your _____ and watch the patient's chest fall during _____.

General Knowledge

Matching

Match each of the items in the left column to the appropriate definition in the right column.

_____ **1.** Shock

_____ **2.** Perfusion

_____ **3.** Sphincters

_____ **4.** Autonomic nervous system

_____ **5.** Blood pressure

_____ **6.** Anaphylaxis

_____ **7.** Septic shock

_____ **8.** Syncope

_____ **9.** Compensated shock

A. Severe allergic reaction

B. Hypoperfusion

C. Regulates involuntary body functions

D. Early stage of shock

E. Provides a rough measure of perfusion

F. Severe bacterial infection

G. Sufficient circulation to meet cell needs

H. Regulate blood flow in capillaries

I. Fainting

Multiple Choice

Read each item carefully and then select the one best response.

_____ **1.** Shock:

    A. refers to a state of collapse and failure of the cardiovascular system.

    B. results in adequate flow of blood to the body's cells.

    C. creates an excess of cellular nutrients.

    D. all of the above.

_____ **2.** Blood flow through the capillary beds is regulated by:

    A. systolic pressure.

    B. the capillary sphincters.

    C. perfusion.

    D. diastolic pressure.

_____ **3.** The autonomic nervous system regulates involuntary functions such as:

    A. sweating.

    B. digestion.

    C. constriction and dilation of capillary sphincters.

    D. all of the above.

_____ **4.** Regulation of blood flow is determined by:

    A. oxygen intake.

    B. systolic pressure.

    C. cellular need.

    D. diastolic pressure.

_____ **5.** Perfusion requires having a working cardiovascular system as well as:
- **A.** adequate oxygen exchange in the lungs.
- **B.** adequate nutrients in the form of glucose in the blood.
- **C.** adequate waste removal.
- **D.** all of the above.

_____ **6.** The action of hormones such as epinephrine and norepinephrine stimulates _____ to maintain pressure in the system and, as a result, perfusion of all vital organs.
- **A.** an increase in heart rate
- **B.** an increase in the strength of cardiac contractions
- **C.** vasoconstriction in nonessential areas
- **D.** all of the above

_____ **7.** Basic causes of shock include:
- **A.** poor pump function.
- **B.** blood or fluid loss.
- **C.** blood vessel dilation.
- **D.** all of the above.

_____ **8.** Noncardiovascular causes of shock include respiratory insufficiency and:
- **A.** sepsis.
- **B.** metabolism.
- **C.** anaphylaxis.
- **D.** hypovolemia.

_____ **9.** _____ develops when the heart muscle can no longer generate enough pressure to circulate the blood to all organs.
- **A.** Pump failure
- **B.** Cardiogenic shock
- **C.** A myocardial infarction
- **D.** Congestive heart failure

_____ **10.** Neurogenic shock usually results from damage to the spinal cord at the:
- **A.** cervical level.
- **B.** thoracic level.
- **C.** lumbar level.
- **D.** sacral level.

_____ **11.** In septic shock:
- **A.** there is an insufficient volume of fluid in the container.
- **B.** the fluid that has leaked out often collects in the respiratory system.
- **C.** there is a larger-than-normal vascular bed to contain the smaller-than-normal volume of intravascular fluid.
- **D.** all of the above.

_____ **12.** Neurogenic shock is caused by:
- **A.** a radical change in the size of the vascular system.
- **B.** massive vasoconstriction.
- **C.** low volume.
- **D.** fluid collecting around the spinal cord causing compression of the cord.

_____ **13.** Hypovolemic shock is a result of:
- **A.** widespread vasodilation.
- **B.** low volume.
- **C.** massive vasoconstriction.
- **D.** pump failure.

_____ **14.** An insufficient concentration of _____ in the blood can produce shock as rapidly as vascular causes.

    A. oxygen

    B. hormones

    C. epinephrine

    D. histamine

_____ **15.** In anaphylactic shock, the combination of poor oxygenation and poor perfusion is a result of:

    A. widespread vasodilation.

    B. low volume.

    C. massive vasoconstriction.

    D. pump failure.

_____ **16.** You should suspect shock in all of the following except:

    A. a mild allergic reaction.

    B. multiple severe fractures.

    C. a severe infection.

    D. abdominal or chest injury.

_____ **17.** When treating a suspected shock patient, vital signs should be recorded approximately every _____ minutes.

    A. 2

    B. 5

    C. 10

    D. 15

_____ **18.** The Golden Period refers to the first 60 minutes after:

    A. medical help arrives on scene.

    B. transport begins.

    C. the injury occurs.

    D. 9-1-1 is called.

_____ **19.** Signs of cardiogenic shock include all of the following EXCEPT:

    A. cyanosis.

    B. strong, bounding pulse.

    C. nausea.

    D. anxiety.

_____ **20.** _____ is a sudden reaction of the nervous system that produces temporary vascular dilation and fainting.

    A. Neurogenic shock

    B. Psychogenic shock

    C. Vascular shock

    D. Cardiogenic shock

True/False

If you believe the statement to be more true than false, write the letter "T" in the space provided. If you believe the statement to be more false than true, write the letter "F."

_____   **1.** Life-threatening allergic reactions can occur in response to almost any substance that a patient may encounter.

_____   **2.** Bleeding is the most common cause of cardiogenic shock following an injury.

_____   **3.** Shock occurs when oxygen and nutrients cannot get to the body's cells.

_____   **4.** A person in shock, left untreated, will most likely survive.

_____   **5.** Compensated shock is related to the last stages of shock.

_____   **6.** An injection of epinephrine is the only really effective treatment for anaphylactic shock.

_____   **7.** Septic shock is a combination of vessel and content failure.

_____   **8.** Metabolism is the cardiovascular system's circulation of blood and oxygen to all cells in different tissues and organs of the body.

_____   **9.** Shock occurs only with massive blood loss from the body.

_____   **10.** Decompensated shock occurs when the systolic blood pressure falls below 120 mm Hg.

Fill-in-the-Blank

Read each item carefully and then complete the statement by filling in the missing words.

1. _____ refers to the failure of the cardiovascular system.

2. Pressure in the arteries during cardiac _____ is known as systolic pressure.

3. The body responds to shock by directing blood flow away from organs that are more _____ of low flow.

4. Blood pressure is a rough measurement of _____.

5. The cardiovascular system consists of the _____, _____, and _____.

6. Inadequate circulation that does not meet the body's needs is known as _____.

7. _____ are circular muscle walls in capillaries, causing the walls to _____ and

_____.

8. _____ pressure occurs during cardiac relaxation, while _____ pressure occurs during cardiac contractions.

9. _____ pressure is the pressure in the blood vessels at all times.

10. The autonomic nervous system controls the _____ actions of the body.

Crossword Puzzle

The following crossword puzzle is an activity provided to reinforce correct spelling and understanding of medical terminology associated with emergency care and the EMT. Use the clues in the column to complete the puzzle.

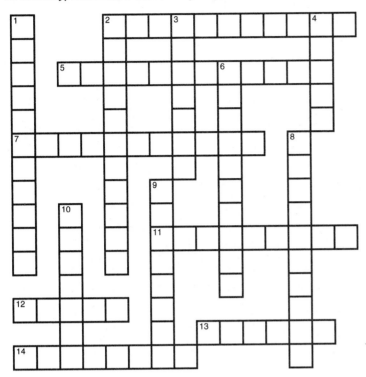

Across

2. The early stage of shock, in which the body can still compensate for blood loss, is called _____ shock.
5. The final stage of shock, resulting in death, is called _____ shock.
7. A balance of all systems of the body
11. The force or resistance against which the heart pumps
12. Hypoperfusion
13. Shock caused by severe infection is called _____ shock.
14. A swelling of a part of an artery, resulting from weakening of the arterial wall

Down

1. A condition in which the internal body temperature falls below 95°F (35°C)
2. Shock caused by inadequate function of the heart is called _____ shock.
3. The precontraction pressure in the heart as the volume of blood builds up
4. The presence of abnormally large amounts of fluid between cells in body tissues, causing swelling of the affected area
6. Circular muscles that encircle and, by contracting, constrict a duct, tube, or opening
8. Circulatory failure caused by paralysis of the nerves that control the size of the blood vessels is called _____ shock.
9. Bluish color of the skin resulting from poor oxygenation of the circulating blood
10. Fainting

Critical Thinking

Multiple Choice

Read each critical-thinking item carefully and then select the best response.

_____ 1. You are called to the residence of a 67-year-old man who is complaining of chest pain. He is alert and oriented. During your assessment, the patient tells you he has had two previous heart attacks. He is taking medication for fluid retention. As you listen to his lungs, you notice that he has fluid in his lungs. This is known as pulmonary:

    A. edema.

    B. overload.

    C. cessation.

    D. failure.

_____ **2.** You are called to a construction site where a 27-year-old worker has fallen from the second floor. He landed on his back and is drifting in and out of consciousness. A quick assessment reveals no bleeding or blood loss. His blood pressure is 90/60 mm Hg with a pulse rate of 110 beats/min. His airway is open and breathing is within normal limits. You realize the patient is in shock. The patient's shock is due to an injury to the:

A. cervical vertebrae.

B. skull.

C. spinal cord.

D. peripheral nerves.

_____ **3.** You respond to the local nursing home for an 85-year-old woman who has altered mental status. During your assessment, you notice that the patient has an elevated body temperature. She is hypotensive and her pulse is tachycardic. The nursing staff tells you that she has been sick for several days and that they called because her mental status continued to decline. You suspect the patient is in septic shock. The shock is due to:

A. pump failure.

B. massive vasoconstriction.

C. widespread dilation.

D. increased volume.

_____ **4.** You are called to a motor vehicle collision. Your patient is a 19-year-old woman who was not wearing her seatbelt. She is conscious but confused. Her airway is open and respirations are within normal limits. Her pulse is slightly tachycardic but regular. Her blood pressure is within normal limits. She is complaining of being thirsty and appears very anxious. You know that the last measurable factor to change to indicate shock is:

A. mental status.

B. blood pressure.

C. pulse rate.

D. respirations.

_____ **5.** You respond to a 17-year-old football player who was hit by numerous opponents and while walking off the field became unconscious. He is currently unconscious. You take c-spine control and start your assessment. You know that in the treatment of shock you must:

A. secure and maintain an airway.

B. provide respiratory support.

C. assist ventilations.

D. all of the above.

Short Answer

Complete this section with short written answers using the space provided.

1. List the causes, signs and symptoms, and treatment of anaphylactic shock.

_____

_____

2. List the causes, signs and symptoms, and treatment of cardiogenic shock.

_____

_____

3. List the causes, signs and symptoms, and treatment of hypovolemic shock.

_____

_____

4. List the causes, signs and symptoms, and treatment of neurogenic shock.

_____

_____

5. List the causes, signs and symptoms, and treatment of psychogenic shock.

_____

_____

6. List the causes, signs and symptoms, and treatment of septic shock.

_____

_____

7. List the three basic physiologic causes of shock.

_____

_____

8. List the signs and symptoms of decompensated shock.

_____

_____

Ambulance Calls

The following case scenarios provide an opportunity to explore the concerns associated with patient management and to enhance critical-thinking skills. Read each scenario and answer each question to the best of your ability.

1. You are dispatched to the victim of a fall at the local community college theater. One of the students involved in rigging the theater backgrounds fell from the platform above the stage. He landed directly on his back and is now complaining of numbness and tingling in his lower body.

How would you best manage this patient?

_____

_____

_____

2. You are dispatched to a local long-term care facility for an older man with a history of fever. You arrive to find an 80-year-old man who is responsive to painful stimuli and has the following vital signs: blood pressure of 80/40 mm Hg, weak radial pulse of 140 beats/min and irregular, respirations of 60 breaths/min and shallow, and pulse oximetry of 80% on 4 L/min nasal cannula.

How would you best manage this patient?

_____

_____

_____

3. You are dispatched to a residence where a 16-year-old girl was stung by a bee. Her mother tells you she is severely allergic to bees. She is voice responsive, covered in hives, and is wheezing audibly. She has a very weak radial pulse and is blue around the lips.

How would you best manage this patient?

_____

_____

_____

Fill-in-the-Patient Care Report

Read the incident scenario and then complete the following patient care report (PCR).

You look at the glowing face of your watch in the darkness of the ambulance cab and realize that you have 4 hours until the end of your shift at 0200. At that moment, the dispatcher's voice bursts from the radio with a call for a motorcyclist down in the eastbound lanes of Highway 62 at exit 19, a 5-minute drive from your current location. Your partner copies the dispatch as you activate the lights and sirens and pull out of the parking lot, en route to the scene.

As you pull past the highway patrol's vehicle barricade, you see pieces of metal and plastic scattered down the freeway and a man lying motionless across both closed lanes. You and your partner approach to find the man responsive and coherent but complaining of "feeling odd" and not being able to move his legs. Along with the help of a responding fire crew, you and your partner are able to quickly remove the patient's helmet, apply a cervical collar, and immobilize the approximately 143-pound (65-kg) 18-year-old man to a long backboard after initiating oxygen therapy.

"Eight minute scene time!" your partner whistles, shutting you into the back of the ambulance with the immobilized patient. As your partner pulls away from the accident scene en route to the local trauma center minutes away, you obtain a set of vital signs (blood pressure 98/62 mm Hg; pulse 110 beats/min and weak; respirations 18 breaths/min, shallow but adequate; a pulse oximetry reading of 94% on high-flow oxygen via nonrebreathing mask; and pale, cool, moist skin). You cut away the patient's clothing to look for concealed injuries and find that both of his legs are pale, cooler than his torso, and not diaphoretic.

"I'm really feeling weird," the man says, panic evident in his eyes. "Am I dying?"

"We're doing everything we can to make sure that doesn't happen," you say before asking your partner to upgrade to lights and sirens while you cover the patient with blankets. Exactly 5 minutes after leaving the scene you unload the patient and push him through the automatic doors of the university hospital where he is quickly enveloped by the trauma team.

Approximately 15 minutes later, you and your partner pull out of the ambulance bay and advise dispatch that you are back and available for another call.

Fill-in-the-Patient Care Report

EMS Patient Care Report (PCR)					
Date:	Incident No.:		Nature of Call:		Location:
Dispatched:	En Route:	At Scene:	Transport:	At Hospital:	In Service:
Patient Information					
Age: Sex: Weight (in kg [lb]):			Allergies: Medications: Past Medical History: Chief Complaint:		
Vital Signs					
Time:	BP:	Pulse:		Respirations:	Sao$_2$:
Time:	BP:	Pulse:		Respirations:	Sao$_2$:
Time:	BP:	Pulse:		Respirations:	Sao$_2$:
EMS Treatment (circle all that apply)					
Oxygen @ ___ L/min via (circle one): NC NRM Bag-Mask Device		Assisted Ventilation		Airway Adjunct	CPR
Defibrillation	Bleeding Control		Bandaging	Splinting	Other Shock Treatment
Narrative					

Skills

Skill Drills

Test your knowledge of this skill by placing the photos below in the correct order. Number the first step with a "1," the second step with a "2," etc.

Skill Drill 10-1: Treating Shock

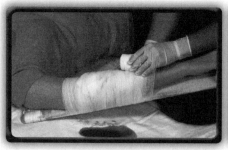

_____ Splint the patient on a backboard. Splint any broken bones or joint injuries during transport.

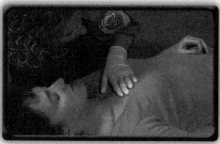

_____ Keep the patient supine, open the airway, and check breathing and pulse.

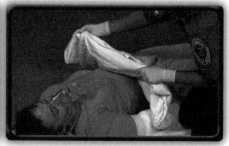

_____ Give high-flow oxygen if you have not already done so, and place blankets under and over the patient.

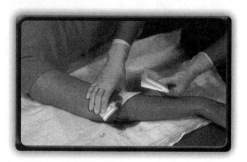

_____ Control obvious external bleeding. Apply a tourniquet, if necessary, to achieve rapid control of blood loss from extremities.

Assessment Review

Answer the following questions pertaining to the assessment of the types of emergencies discussed in this chapter.

_____ **1.** In the scene size-up for a patient(s) who you think may be susceptible to shock, you should:

    A. ensure scene safety.

    B. determine the number of patients.

    C. consider cervical spine stabilization.

    D. all of the above.

_____ **2.** During the primary assessment of a patient in shock, you should:

    A. treat any immediate life threats.

    B. obtain a SAMPLE history.

    C. get a complete set of vital signs.

    D. inform medical control of the situation.

_____ **3.** You have completed your primary assessment of an embarrassed patient who fainted after seeing a coworker injure himself. Your next step should be:

    A. a rapid secondary assessment.

    B. to obtain a medical history.

    C. a detailed physical examination.

    D. a reassessment.

_____ **4.** Interventions for the treatment of shock should include:

    A. giving the patient something to drink.

    B. maintaining normal body temperature.

    C. giving high-flow oxygen.

    D. delayed transport to splint fractures.

_____ **5.** You are transporting an unstable patient who you feel is going into shock. How often do you recheck his vital signs?

    A. Every 3 minutes

    B. Every 10 minutes

    C. Every 5 minutes

    D. Every 15 minutes

Emergency Care Summary

Fill in the following chart pertaining to the management of the types of emergencies discussed in this chapter.

NOTE: While the steps below are widely accepted, be sure to consult and follow your local protocol.

Treating Cardiogenic Shock

This type of shock is a failure of the pump (heart) and is often the result of a myocardial infarction. Since the heart is no longer an effective pump, fluid backs up in the body and the lungs.

1. Assess _____. Patient will often have _____ (fluid in the lungs).
2. Patient is often complaining of _____ pain.
3. Administer high-flow oxygen via a _____ _____.
4. Place the patient in a _____ or semi-_____ position to assist breathing.
5. Do not administer _____ if blood pressure is low; contact medical control.
6. Keep the patient calm, request _____ if available, and transport promptly.
7. Keep alert for the need to assist _____, perform cardiopulmonary resuscitation, or _____.

Treating Septic Shock

A systemic infection causes the blood vessels to become leaky and dilate, causing the container to enlarge. Patient requires complex management in the hospital.

1. Assess and manage _____ _____ to the ABCs.
2. Administer high-flow oxygen.
3. Prevent _____ loss.
4. _____ as promptly as possible.

Treating Anaphylactic Shock

Severe allergic reactions can rapidly progress to anaphylactic shock. The body's response to the allergen causes widespread vasodilation.

1. Request _____.
2. Be prepared to assist the patient with their prescribed _____ _____.
3. Oxygenate and ventilate the patient as necessary.
4. Prompt _____ to the closest emergency department is essential.

Treating Hypovolemic Shock

This type of shock is caused by a loss of blood or body fluids. It should be suspected first whenever a patient presents with signs and symptoms of shock. Blood loss may be external or internal secondary to a traumatic injury. Body fluids can be lost due to burns, excessive vomiting, or diarrhea.

1. Management of a patient with hypovolemic shock focuses on preventing further _____ or _____ loss.
2. Manage threats to the _____.
3. Control _____ _____ with direct pressure, pressure dressings, and _____.
4. _____ bleeding is difficult to manage. Splinting injured extremities may _____ blood loss.
5. Place the patient on a(n) _____ _____. The _____ or the shock position may be used to assist with perfusion.
6. High-flow oxygen should be administered to _____ hypovolemic patients.
7. Prompt transport to a(n) _____ center is required. Do not delay transport.

Treating Respiratory Insufficiency

Patients in shock as a result of respiratory insufficiency require immediate airway maintenance and oxygen.

1. Clear _____ and _____ airway as required.
2. Give supplemental _____ and assist ventilations if necessary.
3. _____ promptly.

BLS Resuscitation

General Knowledge

Matching

Match each of the items in the left column to the appropriate definition in the right column.

_____ **1.** Artificial ventilation

_____ **2.** Abdominal thrust

_____ **3.** Basic life support (BLS)

_____ **4.** Advanced life support (ALS)

_____ **5.** Cardiopulmonary resuscitation (CPR)

_____ **6.** Automated external defibrillation

_____ **7.** Impedance threshold device

_____ **8.** Head tilt–chin lift maneuver

_____ **9.** Jaw-thrust maneuver

_____ **10.** Recovery position

A. Steps used to establish artificial ventilation and circulation in a patient who is not breathing and has no pulse

B. Opening the airway without causing manipulation to the cervical spine

C. Noninvasive emergency lifesaving care used to treat airway obstructions, respiratory arrest, and cardiac arrest

D. Procedures such as cardiac monitoring, intravenous medications, and advanced airway adjuncts

E. Method of dislodging food or other material from the throat of a conscious choking victim

F. Emergency lifesaving device that is programmed to recognize and treat certain cardiac arrhythmias in cardiac arrest

G. Opening the airway and establishing breathing resuscitation by mouth-to-mask ventilation and by the use of mechanical devices

H. Used to maintain an open airway in an adequately breathing patient with a decreased level of consciousness

I. Opening the airway in a patient who has not sustained trauma to the cervical spine

J. Valve device that helps to draw more blood back to the heart during chest compressions

Multiple Choice

Read each item carefully and then select the one best response.

_____ **1.** Basic life support is noninvasive emergency lifesaving care that is used to treat:
   A. airway obstruction.
   B. respiratory arrest.
   C. cardiac arrest.
   D. all of the above.

_____ **2.** After _____ without oxygen, brain damage is likely.
   A. 1 minute
   B. 3 minutes
   C. 4 minutes
   D. 6 minutes

_____ **3.** All of the following are considered advanced lifesaving procedures EXCEPT:

    A. cardiac monitoring.

    B. mouth-to-mouth.

    C. administration of intravenous (IV) fluids and medications.

    D. use of advanced airway adjuncts.

_____ **4.** In a conscious infant who is choking, you would first give five back slaps, followed by:

    A. attempting to breathe.

    B. five chest thrusts.

    C. checking a pulse.

    D. five abdominal thrusts.

_____ **5.** In addition to checking level of consciousness, it is also important to protect the _____ from further injury while assessing the patient and performing CPR.

    A. spinal cord

    B. ribs

    C. internal organs

    D. facial structures

_____ **6.** In most cases, cardiac arrest in children younger than 9 years results from:

    A. choking.

    B. aspiration.

    C. congenital heart disease.

    D. respiratory arrest.

_____ **7.** Causes of respiratory arrest in infants and children include:

    A. aspiration of foreign bodies.

    B. airway infections.

    C. sudden infant death syndrome (SIDS).

    D. all of the above.

_____ **8.** Signs of irreversible or biologic death include clinical death along with:

    A. rigor mortis.

    B. dependent lividity.

    C. decapitation.

    D. all of the above.

_____ **9.** Once you begin CPR in the field, you must continue until:

    A. the fire department arrives.

    B. the funeral home arrives.

    C. a person of equal or higher training relieves you.

    D. law enforcement arrives and assumes responsibility.

_____ **10.** Once the patient is properly positioned, you can easily assess:

    A. the airway.

    B. consciousness.

    C. disability.

    D. all of the above.

_____   **11.** To perform a _____, place your fingers behind the angles of the patient's lower jaw and then move the jaw forward.

    A. head tilt–chin lift maneuver

    B. jaw-thrust maneuver

    C. tongue–jaw lift maneuver

    D. all of the above

_____   **12.** Providing fast, aggressive ventilations could result in:

    A. excessive bleeding.

    B. rupture of the bronchial tree.

    C. gastric distention.

    D. damage to the oral pharynx.

_____   **13.** A _____ is an opening that connects the trachea directly to the skin.

    A. tracheostomy

    B. stoma

    C. laryngectomy

    D. none of the above

_____   **14.** _____ position helps to maintain a clear airway in a patient with a decreased level of consciousness who has not had traumatic injuries and is breathing on his or her own.

    A. The recovery

    B. The lithotomy

    C. Trendelenburg's

    D. Fowler's

_____   **15.** Cardiac arrest is determined by the absence of the pulse at the _____ artery.

    A. femoral

    B. radial

    C. ulnar

    D. carotid

_____   **16.** The proper hand placement for chest compressions is accomplished by placing the heel of one hand on the sternum:

    A. between the nipples.

    B. near the clavicles.

    C. over the xiphoid process.

    D. none of the above.

_____   **17.** Complications from chest compressions can include:

    A. fractured ribs.

    B. a lacerated liver.

    C. a fractured sternum.

    D. all of the above.

_____   **18.** When checking for a pulse in an infant, you should palpate the _____ artery.

    A. radial

    B. brachial

    C. carotid

    D. femoral

_____   **19.** The rate of compressions for an infant is at least _____ compressions per minute.
    A. 70
    B. 80
    C. 90
    D. 100

_____   **20.** The ratio of compression to ventilation for infants and children is _____ for two-rescuer CPR.
    A. 1:5
    B. 5:1
    C. 15:2
    D. 2:15

_____   **21.** Sudden airway obstruction is usually easy to recognize in someone who is eating or has just finished eating because they suddenly:
    A. are unable to speak or cough.
    B. turn cyanotic.
    C. make exaggerated efforts to breathe.
    D. all of the above.

_____   **22.** You should suspect an airway obstruction in the unresponsive patient if:
    A. the patient is breathing.
    B. you feel resistance when blowing into the patient's lungs.
    C. there is no pulse.
    D. you have adequate chest rise with each ventilation.

_____   **23.** You should use _____ for women in advanced stages of pregnancy, patients who are very obese, and children younger than 1 year.
    A. the blind finger sweep
    B. back slaps
    C. the abdominal-thrust maneuver
    D. chest thrusts

_____   **24.** For a patient with a mild airway obstruction, you should:
    A. begin chest compressions.
    B. attempt a finger sweep to remove the foreign body.
    C. not interfere with the patient's attempt to expel the foreign body.
    D. immediately perform abdominal thrusts.

True/False

If you believe the statement to be more true than false, write the letter "T" in the space provided. If you believe the statement to be more false than true, write the letter "F."

_____   **1.** During the primary assessment, you need to quickly evaluate the patient's airway, breathing, circulation, and level of consciousness.

_____   **2.** All unconscious patients need all elements of BLS.

_____   **3.** A person who is unresponsive may or may not need CPR.

_____   **4.** The recovery position should be used to maintain an open airway in a patient with a head or spinal injury.

_____   **5.** A barrier device should be used in performing ventilation because it will prevent aspiration of foreign objects.

_____   **6.** You should not start CPR if the patient has obvious signs of irreversible death.

_____   **7.** After you apply pressure to depress the sternum, you must follow with an equal period of relaxation so that the chest returns to normal position.

_____   **8.** The ratio of compressions to ventilations for one-person CPR on an adult is 2:1.

_____   **9.** Short, jabbing compressions are more effective than rhythmic compressions.

_____   **10.** For infants, the preferred technique of artificial ventilation is mouth-to-nose-and-mouth ventilation with a mask or other barrier device.

_____   **11.** You need to use less ventilatory pressure to inflate a child's lungs because the airway is smaller than that of an adult.

_____   **12.** AEDs are approved for use in children younger than 1 month of age.

_____   **13.** In the adult, the sternum should be depressed 1″ to 1.5″ (2.5 to 3.8 cm) during chest compressions.

_____   **14.** In adults, the compression-to-breath ratio is always 30:2 in two-rescuer CPR.

Fill-in-the-Blank

Read each item carefully and then complete the statement by filling in the missing words.

1. Permanent brain damage may occur if the brain is without oxygen for _____ to _____ minutes.

2. CPR does not require any equipment; however, you should use a(n) _____ device to perform rescue breathing.

3. Because of the urgent need to start CPR in a pulseless, nonbreathing patient, you must complete a primary assessment as soon as possible and begin CPR with _____.

4. If you encounter a patient who has a hard lump beneath the skin in the chest near the heart, you should assume the patient has a _____.

5. _____ _____, such as living wills, may express the patient's wishes, but these documents are not binding for all health care providers.

6. For CPR to be effective, the patient must be lying supine on a(n) _____ surface.

7. Without an open _____, rescue breathing will not be effective.

8. The _____ _____ _____ should be applied to an adult cardiac arrest patient as soon as it is available.

9. Assess for a pulse in an adult patient by palpating the _____ artery.

10. A(n) _____ _____ _____ is a device that depresses the sternum via a compressed gas-powered plunger mounted on a backboard.

Crossword Puzzle

The following crossword puzzle is an activity provided to reinforce correct spelling and understanding of medical terminology associated with emergency care and the EMT. Use the clues in the column to complete the puzzle.

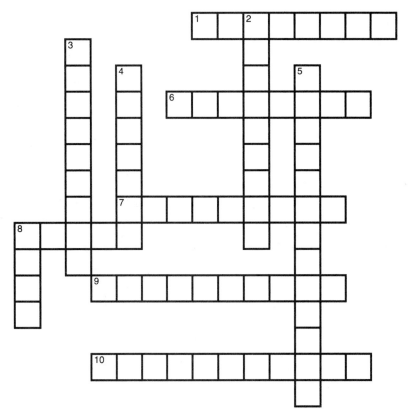

Across

1. The _____–chin lift maneuver is a combination of two movements to open the airway by tilting the forehead back and lifting the chin.

6. The _____ position is used to maintain a clear airway in unconscious patients without injuries who are breathing adequately.

7. _____ threshold device limits the amount of air entering the lungs during the recoil phase between chest compressions.

8. _____ life support is noninvasive emergency lifesaving care that is used to treat medical conditions.

9. A(n) _____ piston device depresses the sternum via a compressed gas-powered plunger mounted on a backboard.

10. Advanced lifesaving procedures are known as advanced _____.

Down

2. The _____-thrust maneuver is the preferred method to dislodge a severe airway obstruction in adults and children.

3. The _____ maneuver is a technique to open the airway by placing the fingers behind the angle of the jaw and bringing the jaw forward.

4. _____ distention is a condition in which air fills the stomach.

5. Cardiopulmonary _____ is the combination of rescue breathing and chest compressions to establish adequate ventilation and circulation in a patient.

8. A load-distributing _____ is a circumferential chest compression device that puts inward pressure on the thorax.

Critical Thinking

Short Answer

Complete this section with short written answers using the space provided.

1. List the four obvious signs of death, in addition to absence of pulse and breathing, that are used as a general rule against starting CPR.

_____

_____

2. List the five components to the American Heart Association's chain of survival.

_____

_____

3. List five respiratory problems leading to cardiac arrest in children.

_____

_____

4. Describe how to perform the head tilt–chin lift maneuver.

_____

_____

5. Describe how to perform the jaw-thrust maneuver.

_____

_____

6. Describe the process of chest compressions during one-rescuer adult CPR.

_____

_____

7. List and describe the method for "switching positions" during two-rescuer adult CPR.

_____

_____

8. Describe the process of abdominal thrusts for a standing patient and a supine patient.

_____

_____

9. Describe the process for chest thrusts on a standing and a supine patient.

_____

_____

10. Describe the process for removing a foreign body airway obstruction in an infant.

_____

_____

Ambulance Calls

The following case scenarios provide an opportunity to explore the concerns associated with patient management and to enhance critical-thinking skills. Read each scenario and answer each question to the best of your ability.

1. You are dispatched to a "person down." The dispatcher informs you that the caller said the patient is not breathing. Upon arrival, you find a 78-year-old woman in bed, apneic and pulseless. In the process of moving the patient to place a CPR board underneath her, you note the discoloration of her back and hips known as dependent lividity.

How would you best manage this patient?

_____

_____

_____

2. You are off duty when you hear a dispatch for "chest pain" at a private residence near you. You arrive to find the patient's family members attempting to apply an AED they bought over the Internet. The patient currently has a pulse and is breathing.

How would you best manage this situation?

_____

_____

_____

3. You are dispatched to an "unconscious man" at a private residence. You arrive to find the man lying in the grass in the backyard. Due to the ladder and equipment on the rooftop, it appears he was working on the roof of his two-story home. No one witnessed the event.

How would you best manage this patient?

_____

_____

_____

Skills

Skill Drills

Skill Drill 11-1: Positioning the Patient
Test your knowledge of this skill by placing the photos below in the correct order. Number the first step with a "1," the second step with a "2," etc.

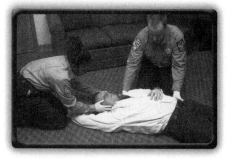

_____ Move the patient to a supine position with legs straight and arms at the sides.

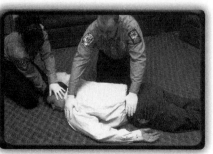

_____ Grasp the patient, stabilizing the cervical spine if needed.

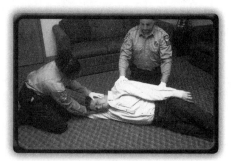

_____ Move the head and neck as a unit with the torso as your partner pulls on the distant shoulder and hip.

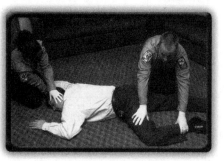

_____ Kneel beside the patient, leaving room to roll the patient toward you.

Skill Drill 11-2: Performing Chest Compressions
Test your knowledge of this skill by filling in the correct words in the photo captions.

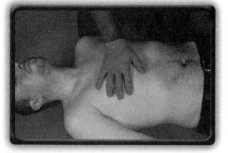

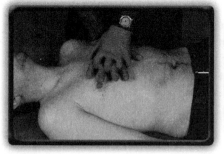

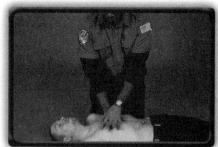

1. Place the _____ of one hand on the _____ between the nipples.

2. Place the _____ of your other _____ over the first hand.

3. With you arms straight, lock your _____, and position your shoulders directly over your _____. Depress the sternum _____ to _____ using a direct downward movement. Allow the chest to return to its normal position. _____ and relaxation should be of equal duration.

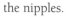

Skill Drill 11-3: Performing One-Rescuer Adult CPR
Test your knowledge of this skill by placing the photos below in the correct order. Number the first step with a "1," the second step with a "2," etc.

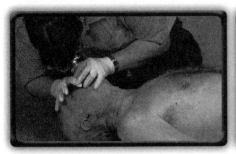

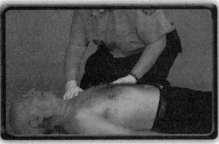

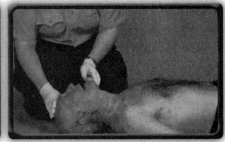

_____ Give two ventilations of 1 second each and observe for visible chest rise. Continue cycles of 30 chest compressions and two ventilations until additional personnel arrive or the patient starts to move.

_____ Determine unresponsiveness and breathlessness and call for help.

_____ Open the airway according to your suspicion of spinal injury.

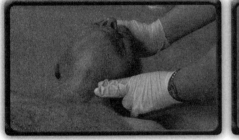

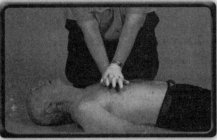

_____ Check for a carotid pulse for no more than 10 seconds.

_____ If there is no pulse, begin CPR until an AED is available. Give 30 chest compressions at a rate of at least 100 per minute.

Skill Drill 11-4: Performing Two-Rescuer Adult CPR
Test your knowledge of this skill by filling in the correct words in the photo captions.

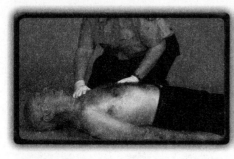

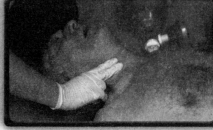

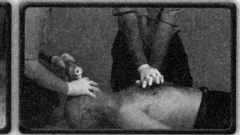

1. Determine _____ and breathlessness and take positions.

2. Check for a(n) _____ pulse. If there is no pulse but a(n) _____ is available, apply it now.

3. Begin CPR, starting with _____. Give 30 chest compressions at a rate of _____ per minute.

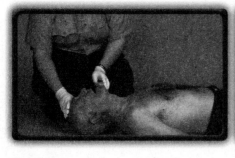

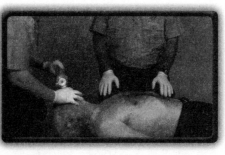

4. _____ the airway according to your suspicion of spinal injury.

5. Give _____ of 1 second each and observe for _____. Continue cycles of 30 chest compressions and two ventilations (switch roles every 2 minutes) until ALS personnel take over or the patient starts to move.

Medical Overview

General Knowledge

Matching
Match each of the items in the left column to the related term in the right column.

_____ 1. Asthma
_____ 2. Hemophilia
_____ 3. Congestive heart failure
_____ 4. Substance abuse
_____ 5. Chronic bronchitis
_____ 6. Diabetes mellitus
_____ 7. Pelvic inflammatory disease
_____ 8. Syncope
_____ 9. Depression
_____ 10. Kidney stones
_____ 11. Emphysema
_____ 12. Appendicitis
_____ 13. Anaphylactic reaction
_____ 14. Heart attack
_____ 15. Sickle cell disease
_____ 16. Pancreatitis
_____ 17. Vaginal bleeding
_____ 18. Diverticulitis
_____ 19. Plant poisoning
_____ 20. Seizure

A. Respiratory
B. Cardiovascular
C. Neurologic
D. Gastrointestinal
E. Urologic
F. Endocrine
G. Hematologic
H. Immunologic
I. Toxicologic
J. Psychiatric
K. Gynecologic

Multiple Choice
Read each item carefully and then select the one best response.

_____ 1. The most important aspect of the scene size-up is:
  A. determining the number of patients.
  B. calling for additional resources.
  C. ensuring scene safety.
  D. determining the nature of the illness.

_____ 2. The _____ is your awareness and concern for potentially serious underlying and unseen injuries or illnesses.
  A. nature of illness
  B. index of suspicion
  C. general impression
  D. clinical impression

_____   **3.** If your patient is alone and unresponsive, in order to obtain some form of medical history you should:

        A. ask people in the neighborhood.

        B. go through the patient's wallet.

        C. search the scene for medication containers or medical devices.

        D. search through the patient's bedroom drawers for hidden illegal drugs.

_____   **4.** "Why did you call for EMS today?" helps to determine the:

        A. chief complaint.

        B. past medical history.

        C. medications.

        D. provocation of pain.

_____   **5.** You should assess pulse, motor, and sensation in all of the extremities and check for pupillary reactions if you suspect a(n) _____ problem.

        A. cardiovascular

        B. endocrine

        C. neurologic

        D. psychological

_____   **6.** When palpating the chest and abdomen, you are attempting to identify areas of:

        A. bruising.

        B. tenderness.

        C. crepitus.

        D. nausea.

_____   **7.** Patients with altered mental status should be considered _____ when determining transport options.

        A. nonemergency

        B. low priority

        C. moderate priority

        D. high priority

_____   **8.** A patient suffering from a heart attack should be transported to:

        A. a local clinic, 5 minutes away.

        B. a community hospital with no catheterization lab, 10 minutes away.

        C. a university hospital with a catheterization lab, 15 minutes away.

        D. a trauma center, 20 minutes away.

_____   **9.** Which statement regarding HIV is FALSE?

        A. It is not easily transmitted in your work environment.

        B. It is not considered a hazard when deposited on mucous membranes.

        C. You should always wear gloves when treating a patient with HIV.

        D. Many patients with HIV do not show symptoms.

_____   **10.** If you have been exposed to an HIV-positive patient's blood, you should:

        A. not worry about it, because transmission rates are low.

        B. seek medical advice as soon as possible.

        C. wait until your next doctor visit to seek evaluation.

        D. wash the area thoroughly and get an updated tetanus shot.

_____   **11.** Patients who are being treated with penicillin for a syphilis infection are considered:

        A. communicable for the rest of their life.

        B. noncommunicable in about 4 weeks.

        C. noncommunicable within 28 to 48 hours.

        D. noncommunicable right from the initial infection.

_____ **12.** The incubation period for hepatitis B is typically
    A. 1 to 2 weeks.
    B. 5 to 10 weeks.
    C. 4 to 12 weeks.
    D. 1 to 10 weeks.

_____ **13.** Vaccinations are NOT available for which form of hepatitis?
    A. Hepatitis A
    B. Hepatitis B
    C. Hepatitis C
    D. None of the above

_____ **14.** Which of the following statements about tuberculosis is FALSE?
    A. It is found in open, uncrowded living spaces.
    B. It can be found in crowded environments with poor ventilation.
    C. It is spread through the air via droplets.
    D. The primary infection is typically not serious.

_____ **15.** _____ is a bacterium that causes infections and is resistant to most antibiotics.
    A. Meningitis
    B. Tuberculosis
    C. Hepatitis C
    D. MRSA

True/False

If you believe the statement to be more true than false, write the letter "T" in the space provided. If you believe the statement to be more false than true, write the letter "F."

_____ **1.** You are obligated as a medical professional to refrain from labeling patients and displaying personal biases.

_____ **2.** In an unconscious adult patient, you should assess for a pulse in the carotid artery.

_____ **3.** If it is unclear if the patient needs oxygen, you should avoid giving it until clearer indications arise.

_____ **4.** History-taking may be the only way to determine what the problem is or what may be causing the problem.

_____ **5.** Conscious medical patients will always need a full-body, or head-to-toe, examination.

_____ **6.** A patient should be transported with lights and sirens activated when there is a life-threatening condition.

_____ **7.** Exposure to the virus that causes AIDS is the most feared infection risk for EMTs.

_____ **8.** EMTs can receive a vaccination against HIV to protect them from exposure.

_____ **9.** Chancres from a syphilis infection are commonly located on the face.

_____ **10.** Hepatitis A can only be transmitted from a patient who has an acute infection.

_____ **11.** HIV is far more contagious than hepatitis B.

_____ **12.** If you are exposed to a patient with pulmonary tuberculosis, you should be tested with a tuberculin skin test to see if you have been infected.

_____ **13.** MRSA is believed to be transmitted from patient to patient via the unwashed hands of health care providers.

_____ **14.** Whooping cough is an airborne disease caused by a virus.

_____ **15.** SARS is a serious, potentially life-threatening viral infection caused by a recently discovered family of viruses.

_____ **16.** The transmission risk for humans with Avian flu is very high.

_____ **17.** When examining the neck, you should assess for jugular vein distention and tracheal deviation.

_____ **18.** You should avoid asking family members for information regarding patient allergies and medication.

_____ **19.** Cardiac arrest patients should be transported to the closest appropriate facility.

_____ **20.** Differentiating a high-priority transport from a low-priority transport is often a skill developed with experience.

Fill-in-the-Blank
Read each item carefully and then complete the statement by filling in the missing words.

1. _____ _____ may be the result of sickle cell disease or various blood-clotting

   disorders, such as hemophilia.

2. _____ _____ occurs when you become focused on one aspect of the patient's condition

   and exclude all others.

3. As you approach a patient, you should determine the level of consciousness by using the _____ scale.

4. You should assess vital signs every _____ minutes in an unstable patient and every

   _____ minutes in a stable patient.

5. Permission to administer certain medication is usually obtained from _____ _____.

6. A(n) _____ should be used on a patient who is apneic and pulseless.

7. _____ patients include those with altered mental status, airway and breathing difficulties, or any sign of

   circulatory compromise.

8. Modes of transportation ultimately come in two categories: _____ or _____.

9. A(n) _____ _____ is a medical condition caused by the growth and spread of small

   harmful organisms within the body.

10. _____ refers to inflammation of the liver.

11. _____ _____ is transmitted orally through oral or fecal contamination.

12. You should note any _____ _____ along the veins that indicate potential IV drug use

    when examining the extremities.

13. _____ is the strength or ability of a pathogen to produce disease.

14. _____ is a chronic mycobacterial disease that usually strikes the lungs.

15. Patients with a fever, headache, stiff neck, and altered mental status may be suffering from _____.

Fill-in-the-Table

Fill in the missing parts of the table.

Read each section of the chart and complete the missing areas.

Causes of Infectious Disease		
Type of Organism	**Description**	**Example**
Bacteria		*Salmonella*
	Smaller than bacteria; multiply only inside a host and die when exposed to the environment	
Fungi		
Protozoa (parasites)		Amoebas
	Invertebrates with long, flexible, rounded, or flattened bodies	

Crossword Puzzle

The following crossword puzzle is an activity provided to reinforce correct spelling and understanding of medical terminology associated with emergency care and the EMT. Use the clues in the column to complete the puzzle.

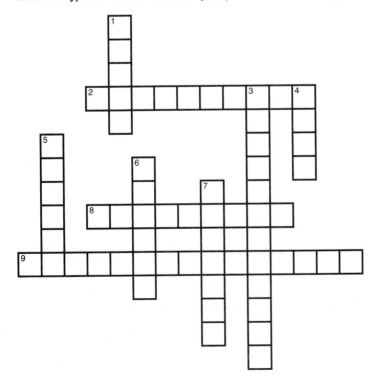

Across

2. An inflammation of the meningeal coverings of the brain and spinal cord
8. The strength or ability of a pathogen to produce disease
9. The general type of illness a patient is experiencing

Down

1. Awareness that unseen life-threatening injuries or illness may exist is known as _____ of suspicion.
3. A chronic bacterial disease that usually affects the lungs but can also affect other organs, such as the brain and kidneys
4. Potentially life-threatening viral infection that usually starts with flulike symptoms
5. _____ emergencies are injuries that are the result of physical forces applied to the body.
6. _____ simplex is a virus characterized by small blisters whose location depends on the type of virus.
7. _____ emergencies are life threats that require EMS attention because of illnesses or conditions not caused by an outside force.

Critical Thinking

Short Answer

Complete this section with short written answers using the space provided.

1. List four examples of how you can contract HIV while taking care of patients in EMS.

_____

_____

2. What are the five major components of patient assessment for medical emergencies?

_____

_____

3. Define each component of the acronym TACOS, which is used when determining factors that could complicate the chief complaint.

_____

_____

4. List three conditions that are deemed serious and require rapid transport.

_____

_____

Ambulance Calls

The following case scenarios provide an opportunity to explore the concerns associated with patient management and to enhance critical-thinking skills. Read each scenario and answer each question to the best of your ability.

1. You respond to a local apartment building in the downtown area for a 42-year-old man with respiratory distress. Upon arrival, you notice the patient sitting in a chair with pale, diaphoretic skin. The patient tells you that he has been sick for several days and is too sick to drive himself to the hospital. When taking a history, the patient tells you that he has had night sweats and has been coughing up blood. His only complaint is fever and slight shortness of breath. He has no other significant history.

   How would you best manage this patient?

_____

_____

_____

2. While driving back from a call, your unit is dispatched to a local recreation area for a 58-year-old woman with chest pain. Upon arrival, you notice a woman lying on the ground with several bystanders assisting her. The patient is alert and oriented and complains of chest pain.

   What history-taking questions can you ask to help with your assessment of this patient?

_____

_____

_____

Respiratory Emergencies

General Knowledge

Matching

Match each of the items in the left column to the appropriate definition in the right column.

_____ **1.** Respiration

_____ **2.** Pulmonary edema

_____ **3.** Epiglottitis

_____ **4.** Emphysema

_____ **5.** Pleural effusion

_____ **6.** Tuberculosis

_____ **7.** Dyspnea

_____ **8.** Pneumonia

_____ **9.** Hypoxia

_____ **10.** Bronchitis

_____ **11.** Hyperventilation

_____ **12.** Allergen

_____ **13.** Embolus

_____ **14.** Asthma

_____ **15.** Pneumothorax

A. An acute or chronic inflammation of the major lung passageways

B. Acute spasm of the bronchioles, associated with excessive mucus production and swelling of the mucous lining

C. Accumulation of air in the pleural space

D. Fluid build-up within the alveoli and lung tissue

E. An infection of the lung that damages lung tissue

F. A substance that causes an allergic reaction

G. Difficulty breathing

H. Bacterial infection that can produce severe swelling

I. A blood clot or other substance in the circulatory system that travels to a blood vessel where it causes blockage

J. Disease of the lungs in which the alveoli lose elasticity due to chronic stretching

K. Overbreathing to the point that the level of carbon dioxide in the blood falls below normal

L. Fluid outside of the lung

M. Condition in which the body's cells and tissues do not have enough oxygen

N. The exchange of oxygen and carbon dioxide

O. A disease that can lay dormant in the lungs for decades, then reactivate

Multiple Choice

Read each item carefully and then select the one best response.

_____ **1.** A blood clot lodged in the pulmonary artery is referred to as:

    A. a myocardial infarction.

    B. a stroke.

    C. a pulmonary embolism.

    D. a pulmonary effusion.

_____ **2.** The oxygen–carbon dioxide exchange takes place in the:

    A. trachea.

    B. bronchial tree.

    C. alveoli.

    D. blood.

_____ **3.** The letter "S" in the pneumonic PASTE refers to:

    A. symptoms.

    B. sputum.

    C. severity.

    D. sickness.

_____ **4.** If carbon dioxide levels drop too low, the person automatically breathes:

    A. normally.

    B. rapidly and deeply.

    C. slower and less deeply.

    D. fast and shallow.

_____ **5.** If the level of carbon dioxide in the arterial blood rises above normal, the patient breathes:

    A. normally.

    B. rapidly and deeply.

    C. slower, less deeply.

    D. fast and shallow.

_____ **6.** Inflammation and swelling of the pharynx, larynx, and trachea resulting in a "seal bark" is typically caused by:

    A. emphysema.

    B. chronic bronchitis.

    C. croup.

    D. epiglottitis.

_____ **7.** The rate of breathing is typically increased when:

    A. oxygen levels increase.

    B. oxygen levels decrease.

    C. carbon dioxide levels increase.

    D. carbon dioxide levels decrease.

_____ **8.** _____ is a sign of hypoxia to the brain.

    A. Altered mental status

    B. Decreased pulse rate

    C. Decreased respiratory rate

    D. Delayed capillary refill time

_____ **9.** An obstruction to the exchange of gases between the alveoli and the capillaries may result from:

    A. epiglottitis.

    B. pneumonia.

    C. a cold.

    D. all of the above.

_____ **10.** Pulmonary edema can develop quickly after a major:

    A. heart attack.

    B. episode of syncope.

    C. brain injury.

    D. all of the above.

_____ **11.** Pulmonary edema may also be produced by:

    A. cigarette smoking.

    B. seasonal allergies.

    C. inhaling toxic chemical fumes.

    D. carbon monoxide poisoning.

_____ **12.** _____ is a loss of the elastic material around the air spaces as a result of chronic stretching of the alveoli.

    A. Emphysema

    B. Bronchitis

    C. Pneumonia

    D. Diphtheria

_____ **13.** _____ is a genetic disorder that affects the lungs and digestive system.

    A. Chronic obstructive pulmonary disease

    B. Cystic fibrosis

    C. Pertussis

    D. Bronchiolitis

_____ **14.** The patient with COPD usually presents with:

    A. bloody sputum.

    B. a green or yellow productive cough.

    C. a decreased pulse rate.

    D. pulmonary edema.

_____ **15.** A pneumothorax is a partial or complete accumulation of air in the:

    A. pleural space.

    B. alveoli.

    C. abdomen.

    D. subcutaneous tissue.

_____ **16.** Asthma produces a characteristic _____ as patients attempt to exhale through partially obstructed air passages.

    A. rhonchi

    B. stridor

    C. wheezing

    D. rattle

_____ **17.** An allergic response to certain foods or some other allergen may produce an acute:

    A. bronchodilation.

    B. asthma attack.

    C. vasoconstriction.

    D. insulin release.

_____ **18.** Treatment for anaphylaxis and acute asthma attacks includes:

    A. epinephrine.

    B. high-flow oxygen.

    C. antihistamines.

    D. all of the above.

_____ **19.** A collection of fluid outside the lungs on one or both sides of the chest is called a:

    A. pulmonary edema.

    B. subcutaneous emphysema.

    C. pleural effusion.

    D. tension pneumothorax.

_____ **20.** Always consider _____ in patients who were eating just before becoming short of breath.

    A. upper airway obstruction

    B. anaphylaxis

    C. lower airway obstruction

    D. bronchoconstriction

_____ **21.** _____ is defined as overbreathing to the point that the level of arterial carbon dioxide falls below normal.

    A. Reactive airway syndrome

    B. Hyperventilation

    C. Tachypnea

    D. Pleural effusion

_____ **22.** Which of the following is NOT an indication of inadequate breathing?

    A. Accessory muscle use

    B. Cyanosis

    C. A regular pattern of inspiration and expiration

    D. Unequal chest expansion

Questions 23-27 are derived from the following scenario: You respond to a home of a 78-year-old man having difficulty breathing. He is sitting at the kitchen table in a classic tripod position, wearing a nasal cannula. He is cyanotic, smoking, and has his shirt unbuttoned. His respirations are 30 breaths/min and shallow, his pulse rate is 110 beats/min, and his blood pressure is 136/88 mm Hg.

_____ **23.** Your first thought as an EMT should be to:

    A. apply a nonrebreathing mask at 15 L/min.

    B. call for back-up.

    C. assess the airway status.

    D. determine scene safety.

_____ **24.** His brain stem senses the level of _____ in the arterial blood, causing the rapid respirations.

    A. carbon dioxide

    B. oxygen

    C. insulin

    D. none of the above

_____ **25.** Proper management of this patient should include:

    A. supplemental oxygen.

    B. chest compressions.

    C. suctioning.

    D. all the above.

_____ **26.** Which of the following is NOT a sign or symptom of his inadequate breathing?

    A. He was cyanotic.

    B. His shirt was unbuttoned.

    C. He was in a tripod position.

    D. His pulse rate was over 100 beats/min (tachycardia).

_____ **27.** What should you do during the reassessment?

    A. Assess vital signs every 5 minutes.

    B. Repeat the initial and focused assessments.

    C. Reassess interventions performed.

    D. All of the above.

_____ **28.** Which of the following is a question you would NOT ask during the history taking and the secondary assessment of a patient with dyspnea?

    A. What has the patient already done for the breathing problem?

    B. Does the patient use a prescribed inhaler?

    C. Does the patient have any allergies?

    D. What time did the patient wake up this morning?

_____ **29.** Generic names for popular inhaled medications include:

    A. ventolin.

    B. flovent.

    C. albuterol.

    D. atrovent.

_____ **30.** Contraindications to helping a patient self-administer a metered-dose inhaler include all of the following EXCEPT:

    A. failure to obtain permission from medical control.

    B. noticing that the patient is in the tripod position.

    C. noticing that the patient has already taken the maximum dose of the medication.

    D. noticing that the medication has expired.

_____ **31.** Contraindications for continuous positive airway pressure (CPAP) include:

    A. being alert and able to follow commands.

    B. a pulse oximetry reading of less than 90%.

    C. a respiratory rate greater than 26 breaths/min.

    D. hypotension.

_____ **32.** A prolonged asthma attack that is unrelieved by epinephrine may progress into a condition known as:

    A. pleural effusion.

    B. status epilepticus.

    C. status asthmaticus.

    D. reactive airway disease.

_____ **33.** Which of following statements is FALSE regarding influenza?

    A. It may worsen chronic medical conditions.

    B. It is primarily a human respiratory disease that has mutated to infect animals.

    C. It is transmitted by direct contact with nasal secretions and aerosolized droplets.

    D. It has the potential to become a pandemic.

_____ **34.** Pulse oximeters measure the percentage of hemoglobin saturated with:

    A. carbon dioxide.

    B. carbon monoxide.

    C. oxygen.

    D. iron.

_____ **35.** An acute spasm of the smaller airways associated with excessive mucus production and swelling is characteristic of:

    A. asthma.

    B. chronic bronchitis.

    C. emphysema.

    D. severe acute respiratory syndrome (SARS).

True/False

If you believe the statement to be more true than false, write the letter "T" in the space provided. If you believe the statement to be more false than true, write the letter "F."

_____ **1.** Chronic bronchitis is characterized by spasm and narrowing of the bronchioles due to exposure to allergens.

_____ **2.** With pneumothorax, the lung collapses because the negative vacuum pressure in the pleural space is lost.

_____ **3.** Anaphylactic reactions occur only in patients with a previous history of asthma or allergies.

_____ **4.** Decreased breath sounds in asthma occur because fluid in the pleural space has moved the lung away from the chest wall.

_____ **5.** Patients with carbon monoxide poisoning initially complain of headache, fatigue, and nausea.

_____ **6.** Pulmonary edema is commonly associated with congestive heart failure.

_____ **7.** The distinction between hyperventilation and hyperventilation syndrome is straightforward and should guide the EMT's treatment choices.

_____ **8.** COPD most often results from cigarette smoking.

_____ **9.** Asthma and COPD are characterized by long inspiratory times.

_____ **10.** MRSA is a bacterium that most commonly infects people with weak immune systems.

_____ **11.** When assessing a patient, the general impression will help you decide whether the patient's condition is stable or unstable.

_____ **12.** Skin color, capillary refill, level of consciousness, and respiratory pattern are key in evaluating the respiratory patient.

_____ **13.** Oxygen is typically withheld from COPD patients regardless of their breathing status.

_____ **14.** Side effects of inhalers used for acute shortness of breath include increased pulse rate, nervousness, and muscle tremors.

_____ **15.** Patients who are hyperventilating should be treated by having them breathe into a paper bag.

_____ **16.** Epiglottitis is more predominant in the adult population.

_____ **17.** An RSV infection can cause respiratory illnesses such as bronchiolitis and pneumonia.

_____ **18.** When assisting a patient with a small-volume nebulizer, the oxygen flowmeter should be set to 10 L/min.

_____ **19.** Snoring sounds are indicative of a partial upper airway obstruction.

_____ **20.** Signs and symptoms of pulmonary emboli include dyspnea, hemoptysis, and tachycardia.

Fill-in-the-Blank

Read each item carefully and then complete the statement by filling in the missing words.

1. The level of _____ _____ sensed by the brain stem stimulates respiration.

2. The level of _____ in the blood is a secondary stimulus for respiration.

3. _____ passes from the blood through capillaries to tissue cells.

4. Carbon dioxide and oxygen are exchanged in the _____.

5. If you suspect a patient has tuberculosis, you should wear gloves, eye protection, and a(n) _____

_____.

6. Abnormal breathing is indicated by a rate slower than _____ breaths/min or faster than _____ breaths/min.

7. _____ _____ is an odorless, highly poisonous gas that results from incomplete oxidation of carbon in combustion.

8. High-pitched sounds heard on inspiration as air tries to pass through an obstruction in the upper airway is commonly referred to as _____.

9. _____ are the sounds of air trying to pass through fluid in the alveoli.

10. When asking questions about the present illness during the history and secondary assessment, use the mnemonics _____ and _____ to guide you in your general questioning.

11. One sign of foreign body aspiration in a child may be an abnormality in the _____.

12. A patient with a seizure lasting longer than 30 minutes is said to be experiencing _____ _____.

13. _____ is an airborne bacterial infection that is highly contagious and results in coughing attacks lasting longer than a minute.

14. _____ are lower pitched sounds caused by secretions or mucus in the larger airways.

15. A patient with a barrel chest and a "puffing" style of breathing most likely has _____.

Labeling
Label the following diagrams with the correct terms.

1. Obstruction, Scarring, and Dilation of the Alveolar Sac

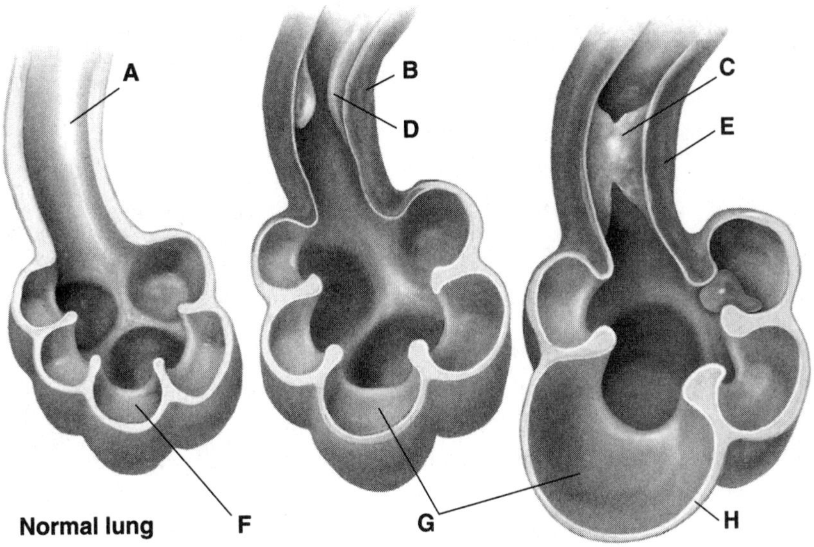

A. _____

B. _____

C. _____

D. _____

E. _____

F. _____

G. _____

H. _____

Normal lung

Crossword Puzzle

The following crossword puzzle is an activity provided to reinforce correct spelling and understanding of medical terminology associated with emergency care and the EMT. Use the clues in the column to complete the puzzle.

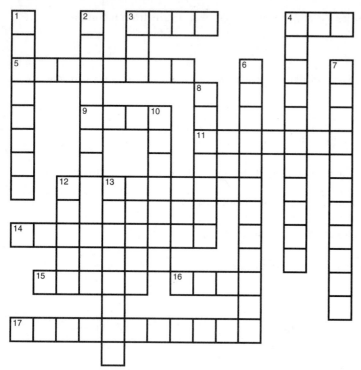

Across

3. A bacterium that can cause infections in different parts of the body and is particularly dangerous because of its resistance to methicillin

4. A virus that causes an infection of the lungs and breathing passages. This virus is highly contagious and spreads through droplets.

5. Pulmonary _____ is a blood clot that breaks off from a large vein and travels to the blood vessels of the lung, causing obstruction of blood flow.

9. A slow process of dilation and disruption of the airways and alveoli caused by chronic bronchial obstruction

11. _____ effusion is a collection of fluid between the lung and chest wall that may compress the lung.

13. A backup system to control respirations when oxygen levels fall is known as the _____ drive.

14. A disease of the lungs in which there is extreme dilation and eventual destruction of the pulmonary alveoli with poor exchange of oxygen and carbon dioxide; it is one form of chronic obstructive pulmonary disease.

15. Crackling, rattling breath sounds signaling fluid in the air spaces of the lungs

16. Potentially life-threatening viral infection that usually starts with flulike symptoms

17. Collapse of the alveolar air spaces of the lungs

Down

1. A high-pitched, whistling breath sound, characteristically heard on expiration in patients with asthma or chronic obstructive pulmonary disease

2. Coarse breath sounds heard in patients with chronic mucus in the airways

3. A miniature spray canister used to direct medications through the mouth and into the lungs

4. The exchange of oxygen and carbon dioxide

6. A disease that can lay dormant in a person's lungs for decades, then reactivate; many strains are resistant to many antibiotics

7. A(n) _____ nebulizer is a respiratory device that holds liquid medicine that is turned into a fine mist.

8. A condition in which the body's cells and tissues do not have enough oxygen

10. Shortness of breath or difficulty breathing

12. Influenza _____ is a virus that has crossed the animal/human barrier and has infected humans, recently reaching a pandemic level with the H1N1 strain.

13. An allergic response usually to outdoor airborne allergens such as pollen or sometimes indoor allergens such as dust mites or pet dander

Critical Thinking

Short Answer

Complete this section with short written answers using the space provided.

1. List five characteristics of normal breathing.

_____

_____

2. List six conditions where wheezing can be found.

_____

_____

3. Under what conditions should you not assist a patient with a metered-dose inhaler?

_____

_____

4. Describe chronic bronchitis.

_____

_____

5. List complications associated with a tracheostomy tube.

_____

_____

6. Explain carbon dioxide retention.

_____

_____

7. When ventilating a patient, how would you determine whether your ventilations are adequate?

_____

_____

Ambulance Calls

The following case scenarios provide an opportunity to explore the concerns associated with patient management and to enhance critical-thinking skills. Read each scenario and answer each question to the best of your ability.

1. You are called to the home of a young boy who is reportedly experiencing difficulty swallowing. You arrive to find concerned parents who tell you that their son seems to "be sick." He can't swallow, has a high fever, and refuses to lie down. As you enter the child's bedroom, you find him standing with arms outstretched onto the footboard of the bed, drooling and with a very frightened look on his face.

How do you best manage this patient?

_____

_____

_____

2. You are dispatched to a 36-year-old woman complaining of shortness of breath. You arrive to find a slightly overweight woman who tells you she "can't catch her breath." She is a smoker whose only medication is birth control pills.

How would you best manage this patient?

_____

_____

_____

3. You are called to the home of a 73-year-old man complaining of severe dyspnea. The patient has a history of COPD and is on home oxygen at 2 L/min via nasal cannula. His family tells you he has a long history of breathing problems and emphysema. He is cyanotic around his lips, and his respirations are 36 breaths/min and shallow.

How would you best manage this patient?

_____

_____

_____

4. You respond to a skilled nursing facility to find an 82-year-old man complaining of shortness of breath. The nursing staff tells you the patient has a cardiac history. The patient is using accessory muscles and can speak in two- to three-word sentences. You notice pink froth produced when the patient coughs and hear crackles when listening to the lungs.

How would you best manage this patient?

_____

_____

_____

Skills

Skill Drills

Skill Drill 13-1: Assisting a Patient With a Metered-Dose Inhaler
Test your knowledge of this skill by filling in the correct words in the photo captions.

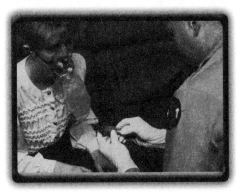

1. Check to make sure you have the correct medication for the correct patient. Check the expiration date. Ensure inhaler is at room temperature or _____.

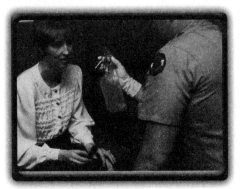

2. Remove oxygen mask. Hand inhaler to patient. Instruct about breathing and _____ _____.

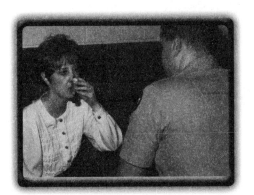

3. Instruct patient to press inhaler and inhale one puff. Instruct about _____ _____.

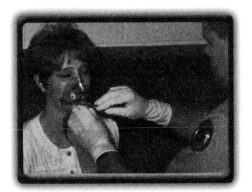

4. Reapply _____. After a few _____, have patient repeat _____ if order or protocol allows.

Skill Drill 13-2: Assisting a Patient With a Small-Volume Nebulizer
Test your knowledge of this skill by placing the photos below in the correct order. Number the first step with a "1," the second step with a "2," etc.

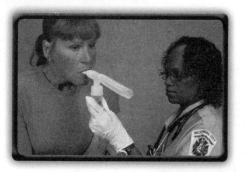

_____ Instruct the patient on how to breathe.

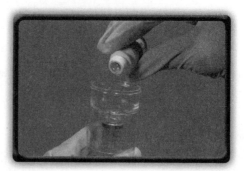

_____ Insert the medication into the container on the nebulizer. In some cases, sterile saline may be added (about 3 mL) to achieve the optimum volume of fluid for the nebulized application.

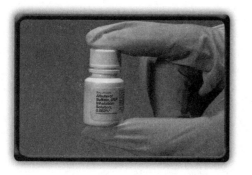

_____ Check to make sure you have the correct medication for the correct patient. Check the expiration date. Confirm you have the correct patient.

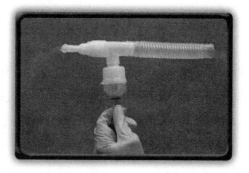

_____ Attach the medication container to the nebulizer, mouthpiece, and tubing. Attach oxygen tubing to the oxygen tank. Set the flowmeter at 6 L/min.

Assessment Review

Answer the following questions pertaining to the assessment of the types of emergencies discussed in this chapter.

_____ 1. You have been assessing a 17-year-old girl in respiratory distress and you have just obtained her baseline vital signs. Your next step is to:

    A. make a transport decision.

    B. consider a secondary assessment.

    C. contact medical control.

    D. make interventions.

_____ 2. You have determined that the patient in question 1 is hyperventilating. Your emergency care would include:

    A. having her breathe into a small paper sack.

    B. providing oxygen.

    C. have her run in place until the hyperventilation subsides.

    D. none of the above.

_____ 3. You have been called to a patient who resides in a long-term care facility and who is having difficulty breathing. After assessing and treating life threats to the patient's airway, breathing, and circulation, your next step is to:

    A. make a transport decision.

    B. obtain a SAMPLE history.

    C. obtain an OPQRST history.

    D. obtain baseline vital signs.

_____ 4. During the reassessment, vital signs should be taken every _____ minutes for the unstable patient.

    A. 3

    B. 5

    C. 10

    D. 15

_____ 5. During the reassessment, vital signs should be taken every _____ minutes for the stable patient.

    A. 3

    B. 5

    C. 10

    D. 15

Emergency Care Summary

Complete the statements pertaining to emergency care for the types of emergencies discussed in this chapter by filling in the missing word(s).

NOTE: While the steps below are widely accepted, be sure to consult and follow your local protocol.

General Management of Respiratory Emergencies

Managing life threats to the patient's _____ and ensuring the delivery of high-flow oxygen are the primary concerns with any respiratory emergency. Patients breathing at a rate of less than _____ breaths/min or greater than _____ breaths/min should have ventilations assisted with a(n) _____ _____ . Continually assess the patient's mental status, and provide emotional support as needed. Transport in the position of comfort. For all respiratory emergencies, make sure you have taken the appropriate standard precautions, including the use of a(n) _____ _____ .

Upper or Lower Airway Infection

Dyspnea from an upper airway infection may be from _____ or _____. Patients should receive _____ oxygen if available. Patients who are sitting forward, seem lethargic, or are drooling may have _____. Do not force the patient to lie down or attempt to suction or insert a(n) _____ airway because this may cause a spasm and a complete airway obstruction. Transport should be rapid.

Lower airway infections may be from the common cold, bronchitis, or _____. Patients need supplemental oxygen, monitoring of vital signs, and transport to the hospital.

Asthma, Hay Fever, and Anaphylaxis

Not all wheezing is the result of asthma! Obtain a thorough _____ from the patient or family. If the patient is wheezing and has asthma, assist with the patient's prescribed _____ or administer a small-volume nebulizer containing _____. Provide supplemental oxygen and provide ventilatory support as needed. Patients whose asthma progresses to _____ _____ require immediate transportation. Be prepared to assist their ventilations because they may become too exhausted to breathe.

Hay fever usually requires only support and transport, but if the condition has worsened from generalized cold symptoms, the patient may require supplemental oxygen and _____ support.

Anaphylaxis is a true emergency that requires rapid intervention and _____. Airway, oxygen, and ventilatory support are paramount. Determine if the patient has a prescribed _____ _____ and assist with administration by placing it in the patient's hand. Guide the _____ _____ to the patient's thigh (lateral aspect) at a _____ angle and administer the medication. Hold the _____ in place for _____ seconds. Transport promptly. Reassess the patient's condition en route to the hospital.

Pneumothorax

A pneumothorax may occur spontaneously or may be the result of a(n) _____ _____. Place the patient in a position of comfort, and support the _____. Provide prompt transport, monitor the patient carefully, and be prepared to assist ventilations and provide _____ _____ if necessary.

Obstruction of the Airway

Managing an airway obstruction is a priority. Use age-appropriate _____ life support foreign body airway obstruction _____ to clear the airway. Administer supplemental oxygen, and transport the patient to the closest hospital. Some patients do not want to go to a hospital after the obstruction is cleared. Encourage them to be transported for evaluation of possible _____ to the airway.

Hyperventilation

Gather a thorough _____, and attempt to determine the _____ _____ because the hyperventilation may be the result of a serious problem. Do not have the patient breathe into a(n) _____ _____; this maneuver could make things worse. Instead, _____ the patient, administer supplemental oxygen, and provide prompt transport to the hospital.

Cardiovascular Emergencies

General Knowledge

Matching

Match each of the items in the left column to the appropriate definition in the right column.

_____ **1.** Atria

_____ **2.** Coronary arteries

_____ **3.** Atrioventricular node

_____ **4.** Myocardium

_____ **5.** Sinus node

_____ **6.** Venae cavae

_____ **7.** Ventricles

_____ **8.** Aorta

_____ **9.** Atherosclerosis

_____ **10.** Arrhythmia

_____ **11.** Ischemia

_____ **12.** Infarction

_____ **13.** Tachycardia

_____ **14.** Asystole

_____ **15.** Bradycardia

_____ **16.** Thromboembolism

A. Absence of heart electrical activity

B. Calcium and cholesterol buildup inside blood vessels

C. Blood vessels that supply blood to the myocardium

D. Abnormal heart rhythm

E. Unusually slow heart rhythm, less than 60 beats/min

F. Lack of oxygen

G. Heart muscle

H. Lower chambers of the heart

I. Tissue death

J. Rapid heart rhythm, greater than 100 beats/min

K. Carry oxygen-poor blood back to the heart

L. Upper chambers of the heart

M. Body's main artery

N. Electrical impulses begin here

O. Electrical impulses slow here to allow blood to move from the atria to the ventricles

P. Blood clot floating through blood vessels until it reaches a narrow area and blocks blood flow

Match each of the medical conditions in the left column to the appropriate description in the right column.

_____ **17.** Acute myocardial infarction

_____ **18.** Cardiac arrest

_____ **19.** Angina pectoris

_____ **20.** Cardiogenic shock

_____ **21.** Congestive heart failure

_____ **22.** Hypertensive emergency

_____ **23.** Dissecting aneurysm

A. Swollen ankles, rales

B. Sudden tearing, separation of lining, potential for great blood loss

C. Heart lacks pumping power, low blood pressure

D. Severe headache, bounding pulses, ringing in ears

E. Pulseless, apneic

F. Exertional chest pain, relieved by nitroglycerin

G. Complete blockage of coronary artery

Multiple Choice

Read each item carefully and then select the one best response.

_____ **1.** _____ allows a cardiac muscle cell to contract spontaneously without a stimulus from a nerve source.

A. Repetition

B. Reactivity

C. Automaticity

D. Autonomy

_____ **2.** The aorta receives its blood supply from the:

    A. right atrium.

    B. left atrium.

    C. right ventricle.

    D. left ventricle.

_____ **3.** Blood enters the right atrium from the body through the:

    A. vena cava.

    B. aorta.

    C. pulmonary artery.

    D. pulmonary vein.

_____ **4.** The only vein(s) in the body that carry oxygenated blood is/are the:

    A. external jugular veins.

    B. pulmonary veins.

    C. subclavian veins.

    D. inferior vena cava.

_____ **5.** Normal electrical impulses originate in the sinus node, just above the:

    A. atria.

    B. ventricles.

    C. AV junction.

    D. bundle of His.

_____ **6.** Dilation of the coronary arteries _____ blood flow.

    A. shuts off

    B. increases

    C. decreases

    D. regulates

_____ **7.** The _____ are tiny blood vessels that are approximately one cell thick.

    A. arterioles

    B. venules

    C. capillaries

    D. ventricles

_____ **8.** _____ carry oxygen to the body's tissues and then remove carbon dioxide.

    A. Red blood cells

    B. White blood cells

    C. Platelets

    D. Veins

_____ **9.** _____ is the maximum pressure exerted by the left ventricle as it contracts.

    A. Cardiac output

    B. Diastolic blood pressure

    C. Systolic blood pressure

    D. Stroke volume

_____ **10.** Atherosclerosis can lead to a complete _____ of a coronary artery.

    A. occlusion

    B. disintegration

    C. dilation

    D. contraction

_____ **11.** The lumen of an artery may be partially or completely blocked by the blood-clotting system due to a _____ that exposes the inside of the atherosclerotic wall.

   A. tear

   B. crack

   C. clot

   D. rupture

_____ **12.** Tissues downstream from a blood clot will suffer from lack of oxygen. If blood flow is resumed in a short time, the _____ tissues will recover.

   A. dead

   B. ischemic

   C. necrosed

   D. dry

_____ **13.** Risk factors for myocardial infarction include all of the following EXCEPT:

   A. male gender.

   B. high blood pressure.

   C. stress.

   D. increased activity level.

_____ **14.** When, for a brief period of time, heart tissues do not get enough oxygen, the pain is called:

   A. AMI.

   B. angina.

   C. ischemia.

   D. CAD.

_____ **15.** Angina pain may be felt in the:

   A. epigastrium.

   B. legs.

   C. lower back.

   D. lower abdomen.

_____ **16.** The underlying cause of a dissecting aortic aneurysm is:

   A. controlled hypertension.

   B. uncontrolled hypertension.

   C. malignant hypertension.

   D. benign hypertension.

_____ **17.** Because the oxygen supply to the heart is diminished with angina, the _____ can become compromised, putting the person at risk for significant cardiac rhythm problems.

   A. circulation

   B. cardiac output

   C. electrical system

   D. vasculature

_____ **18.** About _____ minutes after blood flow is cut off, some heart muscle cells begin to die.

   A. 10

   B. 20

   C. 30

   D. 40

_____ **19.** An acute myocardial infarction is more likely to occur in the larger, thick-walled left ventricle, which needs more _____ than the right ventricle.

   A. oxygen and glucose

   B. force to pump

   C. blood and oxygen

   D. electrical activity

_____ **20.** Which of the following statements regarding CHF is FALSE?

    A. Stridor is a common lung sound heard on exam.

    B. It can be caused by diseased heart valves.

    C. It can be treated with nitroglycerin.

    D. Ankle edema is a common finding.

_____ **21.** Cardiogenic shock can occur within 24 hours of a(n):

    A. hypertensive emergency.

    B. acute myocardial infarction.

    C. aortic aneurysm.

    D. unstable angina attack.

_____ **22.** Sudden death is usually the result of _____, in which the heart fails to generate an effective blood flow.

    A. AMI

    B. atherosclerosis

    C. PVCs

    D. cardiac arrest

_____ **23.** Disorganized, ineffective quivering of the ventricles is known as:

    A. ventricular fibrillation.

    B. asystole.

    C. ventricular stand still.

    D. ventricular tachycardia.

_____ **24.** Which of the following is NOT a cause of congestive heart failure?

    A. Chronic hypotension

    B. Heart valve damage

    C. A myocardial infarction

    D. Longstanding high blood pressure

_____ **25.** Signs and symptoms of shock include all of the following EXCEPT:

    A. elevated heart rate.

    B. pale, clammy skin.

    C. air hunger.

    D. elevated blood pressure.

_____ **26.** Which of the following changes in heart function occur in patients with CHF?

    A. A decrease in heart rate

    B. Enlargement of the left ventricle

    C. Enlargement of the right ventricle

    D. A decrease in blood pressure

_____ **27.** Physical findings of AMI include skin that is _____ because of poor cardiac output and the loss of perfusion.

    A. pink

    B. white

    C. gray

    D. red

_____ **28.** All patient assessments begin by determining whether the patient:

    A. is breathing.

    B. can talk.

    C. is responsive.

    D. has a pulse.

_____ **29.** To assess chest pain, use the mnemonic:

   A. AVPU.

   B. OPQRST.

   C. SAMPLE.

   D. CHART.

_____ **30.** When using the mnemonic OPQRST, the "P" stands for:

   A. parasthesia.

   B. pain.

   C. provocation.

   D. predisposing factors.

_____ **31.** In addition to angina and myocardial infarction, nitroglycerin can be used to treat:

   A. congestive heart failure.

   B. cardiogenic shock.

   C. aortic aneurysm.

   D. hypertensive emergency.

_____ **32.** When administering nitroglycerin to a patient, you should make sure the patient has not taken any medications for _____ in the last 24 hours.

   A. angina

   B. erectile dysfunction

   C. migraine headaches

   D. gallbladder dysfunction

_____ **33.** In general, a maximum of _____ dose(s) of nitroglycerin is/are given for any one episode of chest pain.

   A. one

   B. two

   C. three

   D. four

_____ **34.** _____ are inserted when the electrical-control system of the heart is so damaged that it cannot function properly.

   A. Stents

   B. Pacemakers

   C. Balloon angioplasties

   D. Defibrillations

_____ **35.** When the battery wears out in a pacemaker, the patient may experience:

   A. syncope.

   B. chest pain.

   C. nausea.

   D. tachycardia.

_____ **36.** The computer inside the AED is specifically programmed to recognize rhythms that require defibrillation to correct, most commonly:

   A. asystole.

   B. ventricular tachycardia.

   C. ventricular fibrillation.

   D. supraventricular tachycardia.

_____ **37.** The AED should be applied only to unresponsive patients with no:

   A. significant medical problems.

   B. cardiac history.

   C. pulse.

   D. brain activity.

_____ **38.** _____ usually refers to a state of cardiac arrest despite an organized electrical complex.

    A. Asystole

    B. Pulseless electrical activity

    C. Ventricular fibrillation

    D. Ventricular tachycardia

_____ **39.** The links in the chain of survival include all of the following EXCEPT:

    A. early access and CPR.

    B. early ACLS.

    C. early administration of nitroglycerin.

    D. early defibrillation.

_____ **40.** Defibrillation works best if it takes place within _____ minutes of the onset of cardiac arrest.

    A. 2

    B. 4

    C. 6

    D. 10

Questions 41–45 are derived from the following scenario: At 0500, you respond to the home of a 76-year-old man complaining of chest pain. Upon arrival, the patient states that he had been sleeping in the recliner all night due to indigestion, when the pain woke him up. He also tells you he has taken two nitroglycerin tablets.

_____ **41.** Your first priority is to:

    A. apply an AED.

    B. provide high-flow oxygen.

    C. evaluate the need to administer a third nitroglycerin tablet.

    D. size up the scene.

_____ **42.** His vital signs are as follows: respirations, 16 breaths/min; pulse, 98 beats/min; blood pressure, 92/76 mm Hg. He is still complaining of chest pain. What actions should you take to intervene?

    A. Provide high-flow oxygen.

    B. Administer a third nitroglycerin tablet.

    C. Apply an AED.

    D. Begin chest compressions.

_____ **43.** When operating an AED, what is the first step in the defibrillation sequence?

    A. Plug the pads connector to the AED.

    B. Apply the AED pads to the patient's chest.

    C. Remove clothing from the patient's chest.

    D. Turn on the AED.

_____ **44.** After applying an AED to this patient, the AED states, "No shock advised." What is your next step of action?

    A. Load and transport the patient.

    B. Push to reanalyze.

    C. Perform CPR for 2 minutes starting with chest compressions, then have the AED reanalyze.

    D. Consider termination.

_____ **45.** Your patient is now conscious, and you are en route to the hospital. You are six blocks away when the patient stops breathing and no longer has a pulse. You should:

    A. continue to the hospital.

    B. continue to the hospital and analyze the rhythm.

    C. stop the vehicle and analyze the rhythm.

    D. none of the above.

True/False

If you believe the statement to be more true than false, write the letter "T" in the space provided. If you believe the statement to be more false than true, write the letter "F."

_____ **1.** The right side of the heart pumps oxygen-rich blood to the body.

_____ **2.** In the normal heart, the need for increased blood flow to the myocardium is easily met by an increase in heart rate.

_____ **3.** Atherosclerosis results in narrowing of the lumen of coronary arteries.

_____ **4.** Infarction is a temporary interruption of the blood supply to the tissues.

_____ **5.** Angina can result from a spasm of the artery.

_____ **6.** The pain of angina and the pain of AMI are easily distinguishable.

_____ **7.** Nitroglycerin works in most patients within 5 minutes to relieve the pain of AMI.

_____ **8.** If an AED malfunctions during use, you must report that problem to the manufacturer and the Department of Human Resources.

_____ **9.** Angina occurs when the heart's need for oxygen exceeds its supply.

_____ **10.** White blood cells are the most numerous cells in the blood and help the blood to clot.

_____ **11.** Cardiac arrest in younger children is less common than in older children and is usually caused by a breathing problem.

_____ **12.** An AED with special pediatric pads may be used on pediatric medical patients between the ages of 1 month and 8 years who have been assessed to be unresponsive, not breathing, and pulseless.

_____ **13.** Dissecting aortic aneurysms are rarely considered life threatening.

_____ **14.** Heart disease is the number one killer of women in the United States.

_____ **15.** If a patient complaining of chest pain has a history of a previous AMI, you should ask if this pain feels similar to the previous AMI.

Fill-in-the-Blank

Read each item carefully and then complete the statement by filling in the missing words.

1. The heart is divided down the middle by a wall called the _____.

2. The _____ is the body's main artery.

3. The _____ ventricle pumps blood in through the pulmonary circulation.

4. Electrical impulses spread from the _____ node to the ventricles.

5. Blood supply to the heart is increased by _____ of the coronary arteries.

6. _____ _____ cells remove carbon dioxide from the body's tissues.

7. _____ blood pressure reflects the pressure on the walls of the arteries when the ventricle is at rest.

8. The heart has _____ chambers.

9. The _____ side of the heart is more muscular because it must pump blood into the aorta and all the other arteries of the body.

10. _____ is the most effective way to assist a person with CHF to breathe effectively and to prevent an invasive airway management technique.

11. The collection of fluid in the part of the body that is closest to the ground is called _____ _____.

12. A hypertensive emergency usually occurs only with a systolic pressure greater than _____.

13. In CHF, blood tends to back up in the _____ _____, increasing the pressure in the capillaries of the lungs.

14. A late finding in cardiogenic shock would be a systolic blood pressure of less than _____.

15. Damage to the _____ area of the heart often presents with bradycardia.

Labeling

Label the following diagrams with the correct terms.

1. Right and Left Sides of the Heart

Where arrows appear, also indicate the origin and destination of the blood.

A. _____

B. _____

C. _____

D. _____

E. _____

F. _____

G. _____

H. _____

I. _____

J. _____

K. _____

L. _____

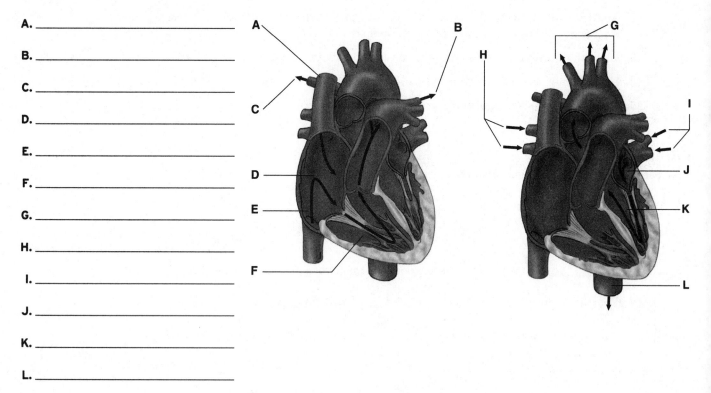

2. Electrical Conduction System

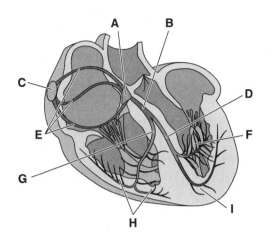

A. _____

B. _____

C. _____

D. _____

E. _____

F. _____

G. _____

H. _____

I. _____

3. Pulse Points

State the name of the artery that is being assessed at each pulse point below:

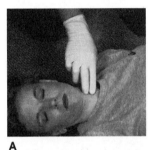

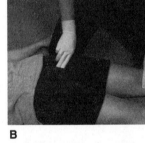

A

B

A. _____

B. _____

C. _____

D. _____

E. _____

F. _____

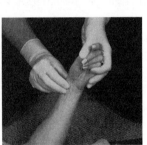

C

D

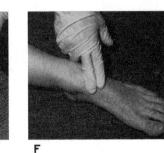

E

F

Crossword Puzzle

The following crossword puzzle is an activity provided to reinforce correct spelling and understanding of medical terminology associated with emergency care and the EMT. Use the clues in the column to complete the puzzle.

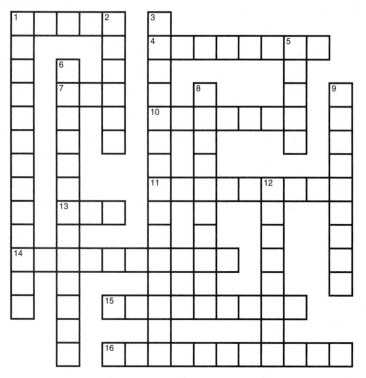

Across

1. The main artery, which receives blood from the left ventricle and delivers it to all the other arteries
4. The complete absence of heart electrical activity
7. Death of heart muscle following obstruction of blood flow to it
10. A fainting spell or transient loss of consciousness
11. The flow of blood through body tissues and vessels
13. A disorder in which the heart loses part of its ability to effectively pump blood
14. An irregular or abnormal heart rhythm
15. The _____ nervous system controls the involuntary activities of the body, such as the heart rate, blood pressure, and digestion of food.
16. A rapid heart rate, greater than 100 beats/min

Down

1. _____ syndrome is a term used to describe a group of symptoms caused by myocardial ischemia.
2. One of two (right and left) upper chambers of the heart
3. The _____ nervous system controls vegetative functions, such as digestion of food and relaxation.
5. The inside diameter of an artery or other hollow structure
6. A state in which the heart fails to generate effective and detectable blood flow
8. Death of a body tissue, usually caused by interruption of its blood supply
9. _____ edema is swelling in the part of the body closest to the ground, caused by collection of fluid in the tissues.
12. Any body part nearer to the head

Critical Thinking

Short Answer

Complete this section with short written answers using the space provided.

1. Explain the differentiating features between an AMI and a dissecting aortic aneurysm.

_____

_____

2. What are the three most common errors of AED use?

_____

_____

3. If ALS is not responding to the scene, what are the three points at which transport should be initiated for a cardiac arrest patient?

_____

_____

4. List four safety considerations for operating an AED.

_____

_____

5. Explain the difference between stable angina and unstable angina.

_____

_____

6. List three ways in which AMI pain differs from angina pain.

_____

_____

7. List three serious consequences of AMI.

_____

_____

8. Name at least five signs and symptoms associated with AMI.

_____

_____

9. List six steps in the treatment of a patient with CHF.

_____

_____

Ambulance Calls

The following case scenarios provide an opportunity to explore the concerns associated with patient management and to enhance critical-thinking skills. Read each scenario and answer each question to the best of your ability.

1. You are dispatched to the residence of a 58-year-old man complaining of chest pain. He states that it feels like "somebody is standing on my chest." He sat down when it started and took a nitroglycerin tablet. He is still a little nauseated and sweaty, but feels better. He is very anxious.

   How would you best manage this patient?

   _____

   _____

   _____

2. You are dispatched to the home of a 45-year-old man experiencing chest pain. He told his wife that he was fine, but she decided to call 9-1-1. When you arrive, you find your patient sitting in the living room looking anxious. He is sweaty and pale and admits the pain is worse than just a few moments ago. He tells you that he is a very athletic person, so the pain must just be stress related and it will go away after he relaxes for a while. He tells you he does not want to be taken to the hospital.

   How would you best manage this patient?

   _____

   _____

   _____

3. You are dispatched to the home of a 60-year-old woman complaining of sudden weakness. She tells you that she usually has enough energy to perform daily tasks around the house, but today she's suddenly very tired, has some pain in her jaw, and has some nausea. She denies any history of recent illness including cough, cold, or fever. She is otherwise healthy and does not take any medications.

   How would you best manage this patient?

   _____

   _____

   _____

Fill-in-the-Patient Care Report

Read the incident scenario and then complete the following patient care report (PCR).

Your shift ends at 1900 and you have 10 minutes to go. As you sit there daydreaming about your plans for the evening, the tones go off. "Unit 6291, respond to 1574 S. Main St for a 58-year-old man with chest pain; time 1901."

You immediately acknowledge the call and note the incident number of 011543. You arrive on the scene 8 minutes later and notice a woman standing on the front porch. Your partner grabs the gear as you approach the woman on the porch. She tells you that her husband has had chest pain for about 30 minutes and has taken two nitroglycerin tablets, but is not feeling any better.

As you enter the residence, you see a man sitting up on the living room couch. The man looks like he is having difficulty breathing. You introduce yourself to the patient and ask what is wrong. "I have horrible pressure in my chest," the patient replies. "Please help me." Because you are less than 5 minutes from the hospital, you elect not to request ALS.

"I was just sitting here on the couch when I began to feel incredible constant pressure in my chest. Then I began to get short of breath. I initially thought it was my angina, but this feels different and my nitro doesn't seem to be helping."

Your partner applies 15 L/min of oxygen via nonrebreathing mask, and you note that you have been on scene for 2 minutes. You note that the patient has an intact airway, and although he is a little short of breath he seems to be breathing adequately.

As you continue with your assessment, you note clear lung sounds and good pulses in all of his extremities.

"Does your pressure go anywhere?" you ask. "No," replies the patient.

"On a scale from 1 to 10, can you rate that pressure for me?" The patient responds with a 5 out of 10.

Your partner hands you a piece of paper indicating the vital signs: pulse, 88 beats/min; respirations, 22 breaths/min; blood pressure, 136/88 mm Hg; Sao_2, 99%; time, 1914.

The patient tells you he has a history of hypertension, angina, and diabetes. He takes lisinopril, nitroglycerin, metformin, and metoprolol. When you ask him about allergies, he says, "I can't have aspirin—my throat closes up."

Your local protocol allows you to assist with administration of nitroglycerin. You check the patient's nitro and verify that it is indeed prescribed to him and that it is not expired. Because his systolic blood pressure is above 100 mm Hg, you elect to give the patient a nitro tablet. You explain to the patient that he is to place the tablet under his tongue and that he is not to chew or swallow it. You note the time as 1916.

You finish your secondary assessment and package the patient onto your litter.

The patient is loaded into your ambulance and transported to the local hospital. Just as you start en route to the hospital, you notice that it has been 5 minutes since you administered the nitro. You reassess his vital signs: pulse, 84 beats/min; respirations, 18 breaths/min; blood pressure, 122/74 mm Hg; Sao_2, 98%. The patient now rates his pain as a 4 out of 10.

In 5 minutes you arrive at the local hospital with a stable patient and transfer care to the ED staff.

After giving your report to the ED staff and restocking/cleaning the unit, your partner looks at you and says, "Hey, you're only 35 minutes late." After his comment, you mark your unit available and return to the station.

Fill-in-the-Patient Care Report

EMS Patient Care Report (PCR)					
Date:	**Incident No.:**	**Nature of Call:**		**Location:**	
Dispatched:	**En Route:**	**At Scene:**	**Transport:**	**At Hospital:**	**In Service:**
Patient Information					
Age:			**Allergies:**		
Sex:			**Medications:**		
Weight (in kg [lb]):			**Past Medical History:**		
			Chief Complaint:		
Vital Signs					
Time:	**BP:**	**Pulse:**	**Respirations:**	**Sao$_2$:**	
Time:	**BP:**	**Pulse:**	**Respirations:**	**Sao$_2$:**	
Time:	**BP:**	**Pulse:**	**Respirations:**	**Sao$_2$:**	
EMS Treatment **(circle all that apply)**					
Oxygen @ ___ L/min via (circle one): NC NRM Bag-Mask Device		**Assisted Ventilation**	**Airway Adjunct**	**CPR**	
Defibrillation	**Bleeding Control**	**Bandaging**	**Splinting**	**Other Shock Treatment**	
Narrative					

Skills

Skill Drill

Skill Drill 14-1: Administration of Nitroglycerin
Test your knowledge of this skill by filling in the correct words in the photo captions.

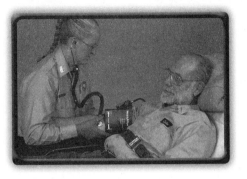

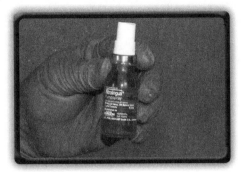

1. Obtain an order from _____
_____. Take the
patient's blood pressure. Administer
_____ only if the
_____ blood pressure is
greater than 100 mm Hg.

2. Check the medication and expiration
date. Ask the patient about the last dose
and its _____. Make
sure that the patient understands the
route of _____. Prepare
to have the patient lie down to prevent
_____.

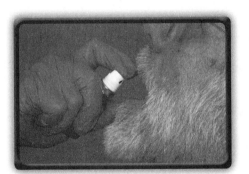

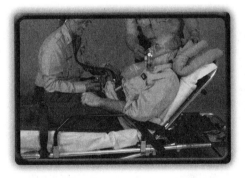

3. Ask the patient to lift his or her
_____. Place the
tablet or spray the dose under the
_____ (while wearing gloves),
or have the patient do so. Have the patient
keep his or her mouth _____
with the tablet or spray under the tongue
until it is dissolved and absorbed. Caution
the patient against _____ or
swallowing the tablet.

4. Recheck the blood pressure within
_____ minutes.
Record each medication and the
time of administration. Reevaluate
the _____
_____ and blood pressure,
and repeat treatment, if necessary.

Skill Drill 14-2: AED and CPR

Test your knowledge of this skill by placing the photos below in the correct order. Number the first step with a "1," the second step with a "2," etc.

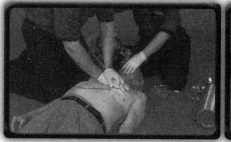 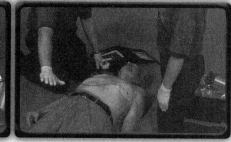 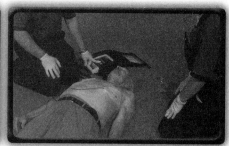

_____If a shock is advised, clear the patient, push the Shock button, and immediately resume CPR compressions. If no shock is advised, immediately resume CPR compressions. After five cycles (2 minutes) of CPR, reanalyze the cardiac rhythm. Repeat the cycle of five cycles (2 minutes) of CPR, one shock (if indicated), and 2 minutes of CPR. Transport, and contact medical control as needed.

_____ Verbally and visually clear the patient. Push the Analyze button, if there is one. Wait for the AED to analyze the cardiac rhythm. If no shock is advised, perform five cycles (about 2 minutes) of CPR and then reanalyze the cardiac rhythm. If a shock is advised, recheck that all are clear, and push the Shock button. After the shock is delivered, immediately resume CPR, beginning with chest compressions.

_____ Turn on the AED. Apply the AED pads to the chest and attach the pads to the AED. Stop CPR.

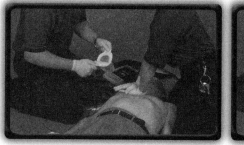 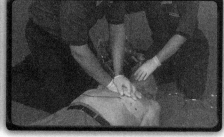

_____ Assess compression effectiveness if CPR is already in progress. If the patient is unresponsive and CPR has not been started yet, begin providing chest compressions and rescue breaths at a rate of 30 compressions to two breaths, continuing until an AED arrives and is ready for use.

_____ After five cycles (about 2 minutes) of CPR, reanalyze the cardiac rhythm. Do not interrupt chest compressions for more than 10 seconds.

Assessment Review

Answer the following questions pertaining to the assessment of the types of emergencies discussed in this chapter.

_____ 1. What type of additional resource is typically required for someone with chest pain?

    A. Lift assistance

    B. Advanced life support

    C. Police

    D. Rescue team

_____ 2. When taking a SAMPLE history of a conscious person with chest pain, what specific question should the EMT ask of the patient?

    A. Has he or she had a heart attack before?

    B. How long does he or she want to stay in the hospital?

    C. Did his or her physician inform him or her of risk factors associated with heart disease?

    D. Does he or she exercise on a regular basis?

_____ 3. Which step should NOT be taken to complete a history and physical exam on an unconscious patient with a suspected cardiac problem?

    A. Perform a full-body scan.

    B. Obtain vital signs.

    C. Obtain history from family or bystanders.

    D. Look through the patient's wallet for medical information.

_____ 4. A patient taking medications such as Lasix or digoxin is likely to have which of the following underlying medical conditions?

    A. Hypertension

    B. Hyperglycemia

    C. Congestive heart failure

    D. Cerebral vascular accident

_____ 5. When assessing a cardiac arrest patient, you notice what appears to be a pacemaker implanted in the upper left chest. Care for this patient should include:

    A. attempting to deactivate the device by placing a magnet over it.

    B. making sure the AED patches are not directly over the pacemaker device.

    C. waiting for ALS to arrive before applying the AED.

    D. not using the AED in this situation.

Emergency Care Summary

Fill in the following chart pertaining to the management of the types of emergencies discussed in this chapter.

Note: While the steps below are widely accepted, be sure to consult and follow your local protocol.

General Management of Cardiovascular Emergencies

Managing life threats to the patient's ABCs and ensuring the delivery of high-flow oxygen are primary concerns with any cardiovascular emergency. If the patient is unconscious, determine whether CPR is needed. In conscious patients, obtain a thorough history. "Time is _____," so rapid transport will be needed to a _____ _____ facility for patients presenting with signs and symptoms of a(n) _____ infarction. If local protocols allow, administer aspirin and assist the patient in taking his or her prescribed nitroglycerin. Be prepared to _____ if the patient becomes pulseless.

Cardiogenic Shock

Shock is a state of hypoperfusion. The hypoperfusion from cardiogenic shock is due to failure of the pump (heart). The container (blood vessels) is intact, and the fluid (blood) is still present within the container. EMTs need to be able to recognize cardiogenic shock over other types of shock because the management is different. The first clue is that there is no _____ _____ _____. _____ _____ is usually the chief complaint. The pulse may be irregular. The patient may have respiratory distress due to fluid buildup in the lungs (_____ _____) due to poor cardiac output. As with other shocks, the blood pressure is low. Do not place this patient in the shock or _____ position because it will increase the workload of the heart and cause increased fluid collection in the lungs. Place the patient in a position of comfort. Administer high-concentration oxygen. Request ALS support if transport is delayed. *Do not* give _____; the blood pressure is already low. If a specialty center is close by, transport there; if not, transport to the nearest hospital.

Congestive Heart Failure

Fluid in the lungs is called pulmonary edema. Pulmonary edema can be caused by cardiac failure after an AMI (CHF) or a noncardiogenic cause such as a toxic inhalation. In either case, the outcome is the same: fluid in the lungs prevents the efficient exchange of oxygen and carbon dioxide. The patient will present with respiratory distress, usually severe, and appear very anxious. The skin will be cool, pale, and _____. The patient's blood pressure is often high unless the AMI is so severe as to cause _____ _____. Patients with a history of CHF will often sleep with multiple pillows or upright in a recliner. Jugular vein distention is common. The patient needs high-flow oxygen. Assisted ventilation or CPAP is often helpful. Assist the patient in taking his or her prescribed nitroglycerin if medical control or protocol allows, ensuring the systolic blood pressure is more than _____ mm Hg before giving the nitroglycerin. Patients experiencing pulmonary edema may require positive-pressure ventilation with a bag-mask device or CPAP. _____ is the most effective way to assist a person with CHF to breathe effectively and prevent an invasive airway management technique. Transport promptly to the closest emergency department.

Neurologic Emergencies

General Knowledge

Matching

Match each of the items in the left column to the appropriate definition in the right column.

_____ 1. Aneurysm

_____ 2. Aphasia

_____ 3. Aura

_____ 4. Brain stem

_____ 5. Cerebellum

_____ 6. Cerebrum

_____ 7. Hemiparesis

_____ 8. Hypoglycemia

_____ 9. Incontinence

_____ 10. Ischemia

_____ 11. Postictal state

_____ 12. Seizure

_____ 13. Status epilepticus

_____ 14. Stroke

_____ 15. Transient ischemic attack

A. A period following a seizure that typically includes labored respirations and altered mental status

B. Low blood glucose levels

C. A temporary alteration in consciousness, classified as generalized, partial, or status epilepticus

D. Experiencing a warning sense prior to an event

E. Part of the brain located above the cerebellum; divided into right and left hemispheres

F. Loss of bowel or bladder control

G. Stroke symptoms that go away in less than 24 hours

H. Weakness of one side of the body

I. A seizure lasting longer than 30 minutes

J. An interruption of blood flow to the brain that results in a loss of brain function

K. Controls muscle and body coordination

L. A lack of oxygen that causes cells to not function properly

M. A swelling or enlargement of part of an artery resulting from weakness of the arterial wall

N. An inability to produce or understand speech

O. Controls basic functions of the body, such as breathing and blood pressure

Multiple Choice

Read each item carefully and then select the one best response.

_____ 1. A _____ is typically characterized by unconsciousness and a generalized severe twitching of all of the body's muscles that lasts several minutes or longer.

    A. stroke

    B. postictal state

    C. simple partial seizure

    D. generalized seizure

_____ 2. The _____ controls the most basic functions of the body, such as breathing, blood pressure, swallowing, and pupil constriction.

    A. brain stem

    B. cerebellum

    C. cerebrum

    D. spinal cord

_____ **3.** At each vertebra in the neck and back, _____ nerves, called spinal nerves, branch out from the spinal cord and carry signals to and from the body.

    A. two

    B. three

    C. four

    D. five

_____ **4.** All of the following are associated with altered mental status EXCEPT:

    A. coma.

    B. seizure.

    C. incontinence.

    D. intoxication.

_____ **5.** When blood flow to a particular part of the brain is cut off by a blockage inside a blood vessel, the result is:

    A. a hemorrhagic stroke.

    B. atherosclerosis.

    C. an ischemic stroke.

    D. a cerebral embolism.

_____ **6.** Patients who are at the highest risk of hemorrhagic stroke are those who have:

    A. untreated hypertension.

    B. an aneurysm.

    C. a berry aneurysm.

    D. atherosclerosis.

_____ **7.** Patients with a subarachnoid hemorrhage typically complain of a sudden severe:

    A. bout of dizziness.

    B. headache.

    C. altered mental status.

    D. thirst.

_____ **8.** The plaque that builds up in atherosclerosis obstructs blood flow and interferes with the vessel's ability to:

    A. constrict.

    B. dilate.

    C. diffuse.

    D. exchange gases.

_____ **9.** A TIA, or mini-stroke, is the name given to a stroke when symptoms go away on their own in less than:

    A. half an hour.

    B. 1 hour.

    C. 12 hours.

    D. 24 hours.

_____ **10.** Patients with a decreased level of consciousness:

    A. should not be given anything by mouth.

    B. should be given glucose regardless of the underlying condition.

    C. do not require medical care.

    D. require immediate assessment of their pupils.

_____ **11.** Hypoglycemia can mimic conditions such as:

    A. cystic fibrosis.

    B. myocardial infarction.

    C. high fevers.

    D. stroke.

_____ 12. When assessing a patient with a history of seizure activity, it is important to:

     A. determine whether this episode differs from any previous ones.

     B. ask if the patient has had any recent surgeries.

     C. assess whether the patient has swallowed his or her tongue.

     D. ask whether anyone else in the household has had a seizure.

_____ 13. Signs and symptoms of possible seizure activity include all the following EXCEPT:

     A. altered mental status.

     B. incontinence.

     C. muscle rigidity and twitching.

     D. petechiae.

_____ 14. Common causes of altered mental status include all of the following EXCEPT:

     A. body temperature abnormalities.

     B. hypoxia.

     C. unequal pupils.

     D. hypoglycemia.

_____ 15. The principal difference between a patient who has had a stroke and a patient with hypoglycemia almost always has to do with the:

     A. papillary response.

     B. mental status.

     C. blood pressure.

     D. capillary refill time.

_____ 16. Consider the possibility of _____ in a patient who has had a seizure.

     A. hyperkalemia

     B. hyperglycemia

     C. hypoglycemia

     D. hypertension

_____ 17. _____ are the second most common type of headache and are thought to be caused by changes in blood vessel size in the base of the brain.

     A. Sinus headaches

     B. Tension headaches

     C. Migraine headaches

     D. Compression headaches

_____ 18. Headache, vomiting, altered mental status, and seizures are all considered early signs of:

     A. increased intracranial pressure.

     B. decreased intracranial pressure.

     C. increased extracranial pressure.

     D. decreased extracranial pressure.

_____ 19. People with _____ have a higher risk of hemorrhagic stroke.

     A. uncontrolled hyperglycemia

     B. uncontrolled hypertension

     C. high fevers

     D. meningitis

_____ 20. Headaches caused by muscle contractions in the head and neck are typically associated with:

     A. sinus headaches.

     B. migraine headaches.

     C. compression headaches.

     D. tension headaches.

_____ **21.** The following conditions may simulate a stroke EXCEPT:

    A. hyperglycemia.

    B. a postictal state.

    C. hypoglycemia.

    D. subdural bleeding.

_____ **22.** When assessing a patient with a possible CVA, you should check the _____ first.

    A. pulse

    B. airway

    C. pupils

    D. blood pressure

_____ **23.** A _____ is usually a warning sign that a larger, significant stroke may occur in the future.

    A. heart attack

    B. seizure

    C. transient ischemic attack

    D. migraine headache

_____ **24.** Which mnemonic is used to check a patient's mental status?

    A. OPQRST

    B. SAMPLE

    C. AVPU

    D. PEARRL

Questions 25–29 are derived from the following scenario: You are called to a home and find a 56-year-old woman supine in her bed. She appears alert, but has slurred speech. Her family tells you she has a history of TIAs and hypertension.

_____ **25.** How would you BEST determine the probability of this patient having a stroke?

    A. By using AVPU

    B. By using the Cincinnati Prehospital Stroke Scale

    C. By using the Glasgow Coma Scale

    D. By assessing her blood glucose

_____ **26.** Which of the following would NOT be pertinent information regarding her condition?

    A. Knowing the time of onset of symptoms

    B. Gathering a list of patient medications

    C. Determining if the patient has a facial droop

    D. Asking the patient about childhood illnesses

_____ **27.** You ask the patient, "What day is it today?" Her reply is "butterfly." Which area of the brain is likely affected?

    A. Occipital lobe

    B. Left hemisphere

    C. Cerebellum

    D. Right hemisphere

_____ **28.** If the receiving facility told you the cause of her stroke was due to a build-up of calcium and cholesterol, forming a plaque inside the walls of her blood vessels, you would know that this patient has:

    A. atherosclerosis.

    B. multiple sclerosis.

    C. polyarteritis.

    D. liver dysfunction.

_____ **29.** Treatment for this patient should include all the following EXCEPT:

    A. providing high-flow oxygen.

    B. providing rapid transport.

    C. continuously talking to the patient.

    D. providing oral glucose.

True/False

If you believe the statement to be more true than false, write the letter "T" in the space provided. If you believe the statement to be more false than true, write the letter "F."

_____ 1. The postictal state following a seizure commonly lasts only about 3 to 5 minutes.

_____ 2. A low oxygen level can affect the entire brain, often causing anxiety, restlessness, and confusion.

_____ 3. Febrile seizures result from sudden high fevers and are generally well tolerated by children.

_____ 4. Hemiparesis is the inability to speak or understand speech.

_____ 5. Patients with migraine headaches are sometimes sensitive to light and sound.

_____ 6. Right-sided facial droop is most likely an indication of a problem in the right cerebral hemisphere.

_____ 7. Serious conditions that include headache as a symptom are hemorrhagic stroke, brain tumors, and meningitis.

_____ 8. A cerebral embolism is an obstruction of a cerebral artery caused by a clot that was formed somewhere else and traveled to the brain.

_____ 9. Hemorrhagic stroke is the most common type of stroke.

_____ 10. Patients with a stroke affecting the right hemisphere of the brain can usually understand language, but their speech may be slurred.

_____ 11. Patients who have bleeding in their brain may have very low blood pressures.

_____ 12. All seizures involve muscle twitching and general convulsions.

_____ 13. A patient having a seizure may become cyanotic from a lack of oxygen.

_____ 14. Patients with a decreased level of consciousness should not be given anything by mouth.

_____ 15. Hyperglycemia should be considered in a patient following an MVC with an altered mental status.

_____ 16. Psychological problems and complications of medications can cause altered mental status.

_____ 17. Patients who have had a stroke can lose their airway or stop breathing without warning.

_____ 18. You should wait until you get an accurate pulse oximeter reading on a seizure patient before administering oxygen.

_____ 19. Letting the hospital know the specifics regarding the patient's neurologic symptoms is generally not important.

_____ 20. A key piece of information to document is the time of onset of the patient's signs and symptoms.

Fill-in-the-Blank

Read each item carefully and then complete the statement by filling in the missing words.

1. There are _____ cranial nerves.

2. Playing the piano is coordinated by the _____.

3. The two main types of strokes are _____ and _____.

4. The brain is most sensitive to _____, _____, and _____ levels.

5. An incident in which you have more than one patient complaining of a headache may indicate _____ _____ _____.

6. A(n) _____ _____ seizure may cause twitching of the extremity muscles that may spread slowly to another body part.

7. Each hemisphere of the cerebrum controls activities on the _____ side of the body.

8. Complex partial seizures result from abnormal discharges from the _____ lobe of the brain.

9. _____ is a loss of bowel and bladder control and can be due to a generalized seizure.

10. Dilantin and Tegretol are medicines used to control _____ _____.

11. A period following a seizure in which the muscles relax and the breathing becomes labored is called a(n)

    _____ _____.

12. Weakness on one side of the body is known as _____.

13. A person who was eating prior to having a seizure may have a(n) _____ _____

    _____.

14. All patients with an altered mental status should have a(n) _____ _____

    _____ score calculated.

15. _____ _____ may reverse stroke symptoms and even stop the stroke if given within

    2 to 3 hours of onset of symptoms.

Labeling

Label the following diagrams with the correct terms.

1. Brain

A. _____

B. _____

C. _____

D. _____

E. _____

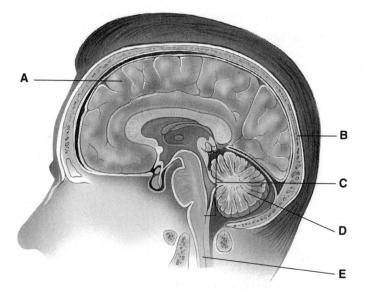

2. Spinal Cord

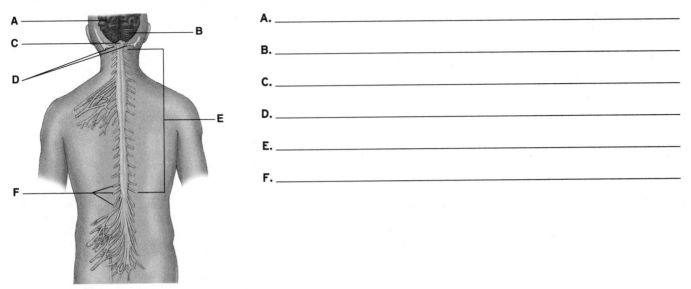

A. _____

B. _____

C. _____

D. _____

E. _____

F. _____

Crossword Puzzle

The following crossword puzzle is an activity provided to reinforce correct spelling and understanding of medical terminology associated with emergency care and the EMT. Use the clues in the column to complete the puzzle.

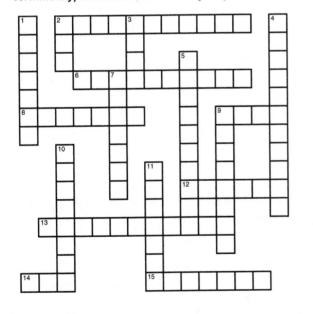

Across

2. A(n) _____ seizure features rhythmic back-and-forth motion of an extremity and body stiffness.

6. Slurred speech

8. The inability to understand and/or produce speech

9. A sensation that serves as a warning sign that a seizure is about to occur

12. An interruption of blood flow to the brain that results in the loss of brain function

13. Weakness on one side of the body

14. A stroke

15. Clotting that forms in a remote area and travels to the site of blockage

Down

1. A(n) _____ seizure affects a limited portion of the brain.

2. A disorder of the brain in which brain cells temporarily stop working because of insufficient oxygen, causing strokelike symptoms that resolve completely within 24 hours of onset

3. A state of profound unconsciousness from which one cannot be roused

4. A(n) _____ seizure is characterized by severe twitching of all of the body's muscles that may last several minutes or more.

5. Clotting of the cerebral arteries that may result in the interruption of cerebral blood flow and subsequent stroke

7. Generalized, uncoordinated muscular activity associated with loss of consciousness

9. A swelling or enlargement of part of a blood vessel, resulting from weakening of the vessel wall

10. A lack of oxygen in the cells of the brain that causes them not to function properly

11. _____ seizures result from sudden high fevers, particularly in children.

Critical Thinking

Short Answer

Complete this section with short written answers using the space provided.

1. Discuss the Cincinnati Prehospital Stroke Scale, including normal and abnormal findings.

_____

_____

2. Why is prompt transport of stroke patients critical?

_____

_____

3. Describe the characteristics of a postictal state.

_____

_____

4. What is the difference between a simple partial and a complex partial seizure?

_____

_____

5. List three conditions that may simulate stroke.

_____

_____

6. Determine the Glasgow Coma Scale score for the following patients.

_____ **A.** You respond to the scene of a 45-year-old woman with hypoglycemia. As you walk into the room, the patient looks at you and smiles. The patient is oriented to place, but does not know the day of the week or the year. When you ask the patient to raise her arms, she smiles at you. When you pinch her hand, she pushes your hand away and says, "Ouch."

_____ **B.** You are at a nursing home where an 84-year-old man was found on the floor next to his bed having a seizure. The patient is now postictal and opens his eyes when you pinch his hand. When you ask the patient whether he remembers what happened, he responds with garbled speech. The patient is unable to follow your commands, but pulls away when you pinch his hand.

_____ **C.** You respond to the scene of an MVC. Upon arrival you find a 25-year-old man who was ejected from his vehicle as it rolled down an embankment. The patient fails to open his eyes to any external stimuli. The bystanders state that he has been unresponsive since the crash and has not moved. You place an oral airway into the patient and continue to manage his airway and provide cervical spine immobilization. You attempt multiple times to elicit a painful response; however, the patient does not move his extremities or open his eyes.

_____ **D.** You and your partner are eating at a local restaurant when your server tells you the manager is not feeling well. As you approach the manager, he apologizes to you for interrupting your meal. The patient tells you that he has not felt right since he opened the restaurant this morning. The manager is able to tell you the daily specials on the menu and is able to roll up his sleeves so you can take a blood pressure.

Ambulance Calls

The following case scenarios provide an opportunity to explore the concerns associated with patient management and to enhance critical-thinking skills. Read each scenario and answer each question to the best of your ability.

1. You are dispatched to a private residence for a "confused man." You arrive to find an older man sitting in a recliner. As you begin your assessment, you notice that he has right-sided weakness and does not seem to understand your questions. He is alone in the home, and it appears that no one lives with him in the residence.

   How would you best manage this patient?

   _____

   _____

   _____

2. You are dispatched to a 36-year-old man who had seizure activity at least an hour ago. The patient is incontinent, cold, clammy, and unresponsive. His friends tell you that the "shaking" stopped and he has not woken up. They thought he might just be tired until they discovered they could not wake him. He has no history of seizure activity. He has diabetes for which he takes medication.

   How would you best manage this patient?

   _____

   _____

   _____

3. You are dispatched to a local business for "woman with severe headache." The 55-year-old patient states that she has had headaches in the past, but this headache is the worst she has ever had in her life. She feels like the room is spinning around, she is seeing "double," and she feels sick to her stomach. She has a history of hypertension. She tells you that she stopped taking her blood pressure medicine about 6 to 8 months ago because she could no longer afford it.

   How would you best manage this patient?

   _____

   _____

   _____

4. You are dispatched to a local shopping center for a 42-year-old woman who is having a seizure. Upon arrival, you find your patient alert and sitting in a chair. The patient has a GCS score of 15 and states that it has been a few months since she has had a seizure. The patient states that she feels fine and does not want to go to the hospital.

   How would you manage this situation?

   _____

   _____

   _____

Skills

Assessment Review

Answer the following questions pertaining to the types of emergencies discussed in this chapter.

Questions 1–4 are derived from the following scenario: You are dispatched to a local residence for a change in mental status. Upon arrival, you find a 67-year-old man sitting at his kitchen table. The patient seems to be having trouble speaking and is leaning to his left. The patient's wife called 9-1-1 because she thought her husband was having a stroke.

_____ 1. Which of the following is NOT part of the Cincinnati Prehospital Stroke Scale criteria?

    A. Facial droop

    B. Speech

    C. Gait

    D. Arm drift

_____ 2. The patient's wife tells you the patient has a history of hypertension, myocardial infarction, renal failure, diabetes, and GERD. Based on the patient's history, what are possible conditions that could explain his symptoms?

    A. Heart attack

    B. Hypoglycemia

    C. Hyperglycemia

    D. Hyperkalemia

_____ 3. As you are packaging the patient, the wife says she called 9-1-1 right away because she read about how time was an important factor with stroke patients. With regard to thrombolytic therapy at the hospital, what is the timeline that will allow this therapy to be most effective?

    A. Given within 2 to 3 hours of symptom onset

    B. Given within 6 to 12 hours of symptom onset

    C. Given within the first 24 hours of symptom onset

    D. There is no optimal time requirement for this treatment.

_____ 4. While transporting the patient to the hospital, his left-sided weakness and speech improve. By the time you reach the hospital, the patient appears almost normal. Which of the following is MOST likely to be the underlying cause of the patient's condition?

    A. Hemorrhagic stroke

    B. Ischemic stroke

    C. Transient ischemic attack

    D. Partial simple seizure

Gastrointestinal and Urologic Emergencies

General Knowledge

Matching

Match each of the items in the left column to the appropriate definition in the right column.

_____ **1.** Aneurysm	**A.** Paralysis of the bowel
_____ **2.** Cholecystitis	**B.** Pain felt in an area of the body other than the actual source
_____ **3.** Retroperitoneal	**C.** Protective, involuntary abdominal muscle contractions
_____ **4.** Ulcer	**D.** Inflammation of the gallbladder
_____ **5.** Hernia	**E.** Behind the peritoneum
_____ **6.** Ileus	**F.** Vomiting
_____ **7.** Guarding	**G.** A condition of sudden onset of pain within the abdomen
_____ **8.** Uremia	**H.** A membrane lining the abdomen
_____ **9.** Emesis	**I.** Swelling or enlargement of a weakened arterial wall
_____ **10.** Referred pain	**J.** Build up of waste products in the blood as a result of kidney failure
_____ **11.** Acute abdomen	**K.** Protrusion of a loop of an organ or tissue through an abnormal body opening
_____ **12.** Cystitis	**L.** Obstruction of blood circulation resulting from compression or entrapment of organ tissue
_____ **13.** Strangulation	**M.** Erosion of the stomach or small intestinal lining
_____ **14.** Peritonitis	**N.** Inflammation of the bladder
_____ **15.** Peritoneum	**O.** Inflammation of the peritoneum

Match the condition in the left column with the appropriate localization of pain in the right column.

_____ **16.** Appendicitis	**A.** Lower midabdomen (retropubic)
_____ **17.** Cholecystitis	**B.** Right upper quadrant (direct); right shoulder (referred)
_____ **18.** Ulcer	**C.** Upper abdomen (both quadrants); back
_____ **19.** Diverticulitis	**D.** Costovertebral angle
_____ **20.** Abdominal aortic aneurysm	**E.** Low part of back and lower quadrants
_____ **21.** Cystitis	**F.** Right lower quadrant (direct); around navel (referred); rebounding pain
_____ **22.** Kidney infection	**G.** Anywhere in the abdominal area
_____ **23.** Kidney stone	**H.** Right or left flank, radiating to genitalia
_____ **24.** Pancreatitis	**I.** Left lower quadrant
_____ **25.** Peritonitis	**J.** Upper midabdomen or upper part of back

Multiple Choice

Read each item carefully and then select the one best response.

_____ **1.** Peritonitis, with associated fluid loss, is the result of:

    A. abnormal shift of fluid from body tissue into the bloodstream.

    B. abnormal shift of fluid from bloodstream into body tissue.

    C. normal shift of fluid from body tissue into the bloodstream.

    D. normal shift of fluid from bloodstream into body tissue.

_____ **2.** Distention of the abdomen is gauged by:

  A. visualization.

  B. auscultation.

  C. palpation.

  D. the patient's complaint of pain around the umbilicus.

_____ **3.** A hernia that returns to its proper body cavity is said to be:

  A. reducible.

  B. extractable.

  C. incarcerated.

  D. replaceable.

_____ **4.** A patient who presents with vomiting, signs of shock, and history of eating disorder and alcohol abuse is likely to be suffering from:

  A. diverticulitis.

  B. Mallory-Weiss Syndrome.

  C. appendicitis.

  D. cholecystitis.

_____ **5.** When an organ of the abdomen is enlarged, rough palpation may cause _____ of the organ.

  A. distention

  B. nausea

  C. swelling

  D. rupture

_____ **6.** Severe back pain may be associated with which of the following conditions?

  A. Abdominal aortic aneurysm

  B. PID

  C. Appendicitis

  D. Mittelschmerz

_____ **7.** The _____ are found in the retroperitoneal space.

  A. stomach and gallbladder

  B. kidneys, ovaries, and pancreas

  C. liver and pancreas

  D. adrenal glands and uterus

_____ **8.** _____ can be caused by an obstructing gallstone, alcohol abuse, and other diseases.

  A. Appendicitis

  B. A peptic ulcer

  C. Pancreatitis

  D. Diverticulitis

_____ **9.** _____ commonly produces symptoms about 30 minutes after a particularly fatty meal and usually at night.

  A. A peptic ulcer

  B. Cholecystitis

  C. Appendicitis

  D. Pancreatitis

_____ **10.** Which of the following is NOT a common disease that produces signs of an acute abdomen?

  A. Diverticulitis

  B. Cholecystitis

  C. Acute appendicitis

  D. Glomerulonephritis

_____ **11.** _____ occur(s) when there is excess pressure within the portal system and surrounding vessel; may lead to life-threatening bleeding.

    A. Esophageal rupture

    B. Esophageal varices

    C. Esophageal ulcers

    D. Esophageal reflux

Questions 12–16 are derived from the following scenario: You have been dispatched to the home of a 52-year-old woman with severe flank pain.

_____ **12.** Which of the following would be an appropriate question to ask regarding the pain?

    A. Have you experienced any belching?

    B. Do you feel nauseous?

    C. Is the pain constant or intermittent?

    D. Have you been urinating more or less?

_____ **13.** The patient tells you that she has right flank pain that radiates into her groin. What is the MOST likely cause of her condition?

    A. Cholecystitis

    B. Ileus

    C. Appendicitis

    D. Kidney stone

_____ **14.** In addition to the patient's presentation, which of the following would NOT be an additional expected sign or symptom?

    A. Diarrhea

    B. Hematuria

    C. Nausea

    D. Vomiting

_____ **15.** You should transport her:

    A. in a position of comfort.

    B. supine.

    C. left lateral recumbent.

    D. in the recovery position.

_____ **16.** Which of the following is NOT a function of the liver?

    A. It filters toxic substances.

    B. It creates glucose stores.

    C. It acts as a reservoir for bile.

    D. It produces substances for blood clotting.

_____ **17.** A patient presents with lower quadrant abdominal pain, tenderness above the pubic bone, and frequent urination with urgency. What is the MOST likely underlying condition?

    A. Cholecystitis

    B. Cystitis

    C. Gastroenteritis

    D. Diverticulitis

_____ **18.** Infected pouches in the lining of the colon are associated with:

    A. cholecystitis.

    B. cystitis.

    C. gastroenteritis.

    D. diverticulitis.

_____ **19.** Pregnancy, straining at stool, and chronic constipation cause increased pressure that could result in:

A. Mallory-Weiss Syndrome.

B. diverticulitis.

C. hemorrhoids.

D. gallstones.

_____ **20.** Diarrhea is the principal symptom in:

A. gastroenteritis.

B. esophagitis.

C. pancreatitis.

D. peptic ulcers.

_____ **21.** Bowel inflammation, diverticulitis, and hemorrhoids are common causes of bleeding in the:

A. upper GI tract.

B. middle GI tract.

C. lower GI tract.

D. all of the above.

_____ **22.** A patient complains of heartburn, pain with swallowing, and feeling like an object is stuck in the throat. Which of the following is the MOST likely cause?

A. Esophageal varices

B. Esophagitis

C. Peptic ulcer

D. Gastroenteritis

_____ **23.** Pain that initially starts in the umbilical area and then later moves to the lower right quadrant is typically associated with:

A. gastroenteritis.

B. pancreatitis.

C. appendicitis.

D. diverticulitis.

_____ **24.** When the abdominal muscles become rigid in an effort to protect the abdomen from further irritation, this is referred to as:

A. guarding.

B. tenderness.

C. rebound tenderness.

D. referred pain.

_____ **25.** If a patient misses a dialysis treatment, weakness and _____ can be the first in a series of conditions that can become progressively more serious.

A. diarrhea

B. chest pain

C. vomiting

D. pulmonary edema

_____ **26.** _____ regulates the amount of glucose in the bloodstream.

A. Bicarbonate

B. Amylase

C. Insulin

D. Bile

_____ **27.** Regulation of acidity and blood pressure is largely attributed to the:

    A. liver.

    B. kidneys.

    C. gallbladder.

    D. pancreas.

_____ **28.** Which of the following organs is part of the lymphatic system and plays a role in regulation of red blood cells and the immune system?

    A. Bladder

    B. Liver

    C. Spleen

    D. Pancreas

_____ **29.** Which of the following is NOT part of the male reproductive system?

    A. Epididymis

    B. Prostate gland

    C. Seminal vesicles

    D. Fallopian tubes

_____ **30.** _____ is responsible for the breakdown of starches into sugar.

    A. Insulin

    B. Bile

    C. Amylase

    D. Bicarbonate

True/False

If you believe the statement to be more true than false, write the letter "T" in the space provided. If you believe the statement to be more false than true, write the letter "F."

_____ **1.** Referred pain is a result of connection between ligaments in the abdominal and chest cavities.

_____ **2.** The adverse effects of dialysis include hypotension, muscle cramps, nausea and vomiting, and hemorrhage and infection at the access site.

_____ **3.** Questioning about bowel habits and flatulence is not necessary and considered unprofessional.

_____ **4.** If a female is of childbearing age, you should question her about her last menstrual period.

_____ **5.** The parietal peritoneum lines the walls of the abdominal cavity.

_____ **6.** Peritonitis is associated with a loss of blood from the abdominal cavity.

_____ **7.** When palpating the abdomen, always start with the quadrant where the patient complains of the most severe pain.

_____ **8.** Massive hemorrhaging is associated with rupture of an abdominal aortic aneurysm.

_____ **9.** Peptic ulcer disease affects both men and women equally.

_____ **10.** Patients with abdominal pain should be placed in a position of comfort, but should not be given oxygen unless they show signs of shock.

Labeling

Label the following diagrams with the correct terms.

1. Solid Organs

A. _____

B. _____

C. _____

D. _____

E. _____

F. _____

2. Hollow Organs

A. _____

B. _____

C. _____

D. _____

E. _____

F. _____

G. _____

H. _____

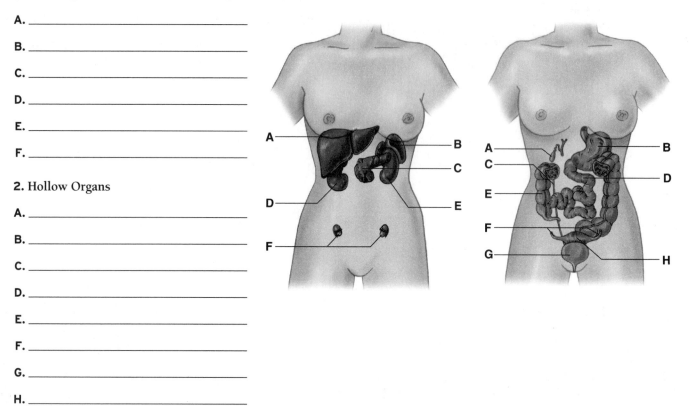

3. Urinary System

A. _____

B. _____

C. _____

D. _____

E. _____

F. _____

G. _____

H. _____

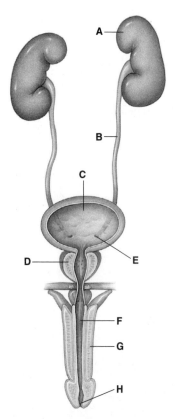

Crossword Puzzle

The following crossword puzzle is an activity provided to reinforce correct spelling and understanding of medical terminology associated with emergency care and the EMT. Use the clues in the column to complete the puzzle.

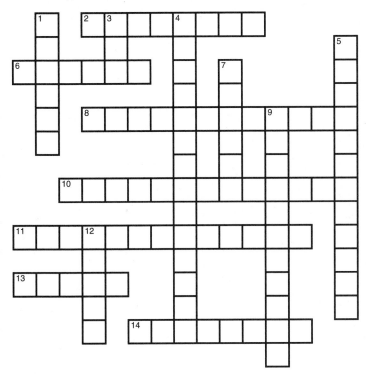

Across

2. Involuntary muscle contractions (spasm) of the abdominal wall

6. The protrusion of a loop of an organ or tissue through an abnormal body opening

8. Pain felt in an area of the body other than the area where the cause of pain is located

10. Inflammation of the gallbladder

11. Complete obstruction of blood circulation in a given organ as a result of compression or entrapment

13. Paralysis of the bowel; stops contractions that move material through the intestine

14. Inflammation of the bladder

Down

1. Severe kidney failure resulting in the buildup of waste products within the blood

3. An infection, usually of the lower urinary tract (urethra and bladder), that occurs when normal bacterial flora enter the urethra and grow

4. Inflammation in small pockets at weak areas in the muscle walls

5. Solid crystalline masses formed in the kidney, resulting from an excess of insoluble salts or uric acid crystallizing in the urine

7. Vomiting

9. Inflammation of the peritoneum

12. _____ abdomen is a condition of sudden onset of pain within the abdomen, usually indicating peritonitis.

Critical Thinking

Short Answer

Complete this section with short written answers using the space provided.

1. Explain the phenomenon of referred pain.

_____

_____

2. List questions to ask yourself when reassessing a patient with abdominal pain.

_____

_____

3. Why does abdominal distention accompany ileus?

_____

_____

4. Explain the steps used to physically assess the abdomen.

_____

_____

Ambulance Calls

The following case scenarios provide an opportunity to explore the concerns associated with patient management and to enhance critical-thinking skills. Read each scenario and answer each question to the best of your ability.

1. You are called to the local high school nurse's office for a 16-year-old girl complaining of fever and abdominal pain that started around the umbilicus, but now is localized to the right lower quadrant. The patient also complains of nausea and vomiting.

How would you best manage this patient?

_____

_____

_____

2. You are dispatched to a long-term care facility for a geriatric man with abdominal pain. Upon your arrival, one of the staff members tells you that this patient has been bedridden and taking pain medications for the last several weeks and has recently had problems passing a normal bowel movement. He now has a distended, tender abdomen with nausea, vomiting, and tachycardia.

How would you best manage this patient?

_____

_____

_____

3. You are dispatched to the home of another responder for "severe back pain." You arrive to find your coworker writhing in pain on the floor. He tells you that when he tried to urinate (unsuccessfully), he immediately experienced a sharp, cramping sensation in his right side. As you are talking to him he throws up. After vomiting, he tells you the pain is worse and is now spreading to his groin.

How would you best manage this patient?

_____

_____

_____

Skills

Assessment Review

Answer the following questions pertaining to the assessment of the types of emergencies discussed in this chapter.

Questions 1–5 are derived from the following scenario: You respond to the home of a 6-year-old boy complaining of severe back pain. You find the boy in the fetal position crying and in obvious pain. As you ask questions of the child, he remains silent and his dad answers your questions.

_____ **1.** What will you determine during the primary assessment?

   A. The priority of care

   B. The child's level of consciousness

   C. Finding and treating any life threats

   D. All of the above

_____ **2.** Your partner takes the father to a separate room to obtain a SAMPLE history. Which question(s) should she ask?

   A. "Do you know what medications he is currently taking?"

   B. "Where is his mother?"

   C. "Sir, we need to know, did you or your wife hurt him?"

   D. All of the above

_____ **3.** As you take a SAMPLE history of the boy, he admits to you that his father kicked him in the stomach a few days ago and it has been hurting since. How should you proceed?

   A. Confront the father to see if this is true.

   B. Call for police backup.

   C. Take the child without the father's knowledge.

   D. All of the above

_____ **4.** Upon examination, you note that his abdomen is distended. The likely cause of the distention is:

   A. strangulation.

   B. cholecystitis.

   C. ileus.

   D. none of the above.

_____ **5.** During your reassessment, you should:

   A. repeat the primary assessment.

   B. repeat the secondary assessment.

   C. reassure the patient.

   D. all of the above.

Emergency Care Summary

Complete the statements pertaining to emergency care for the types of emergencies discussed in this chapter by filling in the missing words.

Note: While the steps below are widely accepted, be sure to consult and follow your local protocol.

General Management of Gastrointestinal and Urologic Emergencies

1. Explain to the patient what you are going to do in terms of assessing the abdomen.

2. Establish and maintain a patent airway. Provide oxygen (_____-flow reduces nausea). Monitor for vomiting and protect the airway against _____.

3. Allow the patient to assume a position of comfort. You will find that most patients want to be _____ with their _____ drawn up to relax the abdominal muscles, unless there is any trauma, in which case the patient will remain supine and stabilized.

4. Obtain SAMPLE history and vital signs.

5. Palpate the _____ quadrants of the abdomen gently to determine whether each quadrant is tense (_____) or soft when palpated.

6. Determine whether the patient can relax the _____ _____ on command.

7. Request ALS support when intravenous fluids or pain management is necessary.

Endocrine and Hematologic Emergencies

General Knowledge

Matching

Match each of the items in the left column to the appropriate definition in the right column.

_____ **1.** Hormone

_____ **2.** Sickle cell disease

_____ **3.** Type 1 diabetes

_____ **4.** Acidosis

_____ **5.** Insulin

_____ **6.** Diabetic coma

_____ **7.** Polyuria

_____ **8.** Thrombophilia

_____ **9.** Polyphagia

_____ **10.** Insulin shock

_____ **11.** Glucose

_____ **12.** Kussmaul respirations

_____ **13.** Hyperglycemia

_____ **14.** Diabetes

_____ **15.** Polydipsia

_____ **16.** Hemophilia

_____ **17.** Type 2 diabetes

A. Inherited disease that affects red blood cells

B. Altered level of consciousness caused by insufficient glucose

C. Diabetes that usually starts in childhood; requires insulin

D. Excessive eating

E. Deep, rapid breathing

F. Excessive urination

G. A tendency to develop blood clots

H. Excessive thirst persisting for a long period of time

I. Diabetes with onset later in life; may be controlled by diet and oral medication

J. Chemical produced by a gland that regulates body organs

K. Literal meaning: "A passer through; a siphon"

L. Extremely high blood glucose level

M. Pathologic condition resulting from the accumulation of acids in the body

N. Disorder that causes an inability to develop blood clots

O. Hormone that enables glucose to enter the cells

P. Primary fuel, along with oxygen, for cellular metabolism

Q. State of unconsciousness resulting from several problems, including ketoacidosis, dehydration, and hyperglycemia

Multiple Choice

Read each item carefully and then select the one best response.

_____ **1.** Patients with which type of diabetes are more likely to have metabolic problems and organ damage?

A. Type 1

B. Type 2

C. Sugar diabetes

D. HHNC

_____ **2.** Normal blood glucose levels range from _____ mg/dL.

A. 80 to 120

B. 90 to 140

C. 70 to 110

D. 60 to 100

_____ **3.** A sickle cell crisis caused by an acute drop in hemoglobin levels is know as a(n):

A. hemolytic crisis.

B. aplastic crisis.

C. splenic sequestration crisis.

D. vaso-occlusive crisis.

_____ **4.** Diabetes is a metabolic disorder in which the hormone _____ is missing or ineffective.
   A. estrogen
   B. adrenaline
   C. insulin
   D. epinephrine

_____ **5.** Emergency care of a patient with hemophilia includes all of the following EXCEPT:
   A. rapid transport.
   B. bleeding control.
   C. oxygen at 4 L/min.
   D. ventilations, if needed.

_____ **6.** The accumulation of ketones and fatty acids in blood tissue can lead to a dangerous condition in diabetic patients known as:
   A. diabetic ketoacidosis.
   B. insulin shock.
   C. HHNC.
   D. hypoglycemia.

_____ **7.** The term for excessive eating as a result of cellular "hunger" is:
   A. polyuria.
   B. polydipsia.
   C. polyphagia.
   D. polyphony.

_____ **8.** Insulin is produced by the:
   A. adrenal glands.
   B. hypothalamus.
   C. spleen.
   D. pancreas.

_____ **9.** Factors that may contribute to diabetic coma include:
   A. infection.
   B. alcohol consumption.
   C. insufficient insulin.
   D. all of the above.

_____ **10.** The only organ that does not require insulin to allow glucose to enter its cells is the:
   A. liver.
   B. brain.
   C. pancreas.
   D. heart.

_____ **11.** The sweet or fruity odor on the breath of a diabetic patient is caused by _____ in the blood.
   A. acetone
   B. ketones
   C. alcohol
   D. insulin

_____ **12.** It is uncommon to encounter _____ patients with thrombophilia.
   A. bed-ridden
   B. surgical
   C. obese
   D. pediatric

_____ **13.** Oral diabetic medications include:

    A. Micronase.

    B. Glucotrol.

    C. Diabinese.

    D. all of the above.

_____ **14.** _____ is one of the basic sugars in the body.

    A. Dextrose

    B. Sucrose

    C. Fructose

    D. Syrup

_____ **15.** _____ is the hormone that is normally produced by the pancreas that enables glucose to enter the cells.

    A. Insulin

    B. Adrenaline

    C. Estrogen

    D. Epinephrine

_____ **16.** The term for excessive urination is:

    A. polyuria.

    B. polydipsia.

    C. polyphagia.

    D. polyphony.

_____ **17.** When fat is used as an immediate energy source, _____ and fatty acids are formed as waste products.

    A. dextrose

    B. sucrose

    C. ketones

    D. bicarbonate

_____ **18.** An African American patient complaining of severe, generalized pain may have undiagnosed:

    A. sickle cell disease.

    B. type 1 diabetes.

    C. thrombopenia.

    D. hemophilia.

_____ **19.** The onset of hypoglycemia can occur within:

    A. seconds.

    B. minutes.

    C. hours.

    D. days.

_____ **20.** Without _____, or with very low levels, brain cells rapidly suffer permanent damage.

    A. epinephrine

    B. ketones

    C. bicarbonate

    D. glucose

_____ **21.** _____ is/are a potentially life-threatening complication of insulin shock.

    A. Kussmaul respirations

    B. Hypotension

    C. Seizures

    D. Polydipsia

_____ **22.** Blood glucose levels are measured in:

    A. micrograms per deciliter.

    B. milligrams per deciliter.

    C. milliliters per decigram.

    D. microliters per decigram.

_____ **23.** Diabetic coma may develop as a result of:

    A. too little insulin.

    B. too much insulin.

    C. overhydration.

    D. metabolic alkalosis.

_____ **24.** Always suspect hypoglycemia in any patient with:

    A. Kussmaul respirations.

    B. an altered mental status.

    C. nausea and vomiting.

    D. all of the above.

_____ **25.** The most important step in caring for the unresponsive diabetic patient is to:

    A. give oral glucose immediately.

    B. perform a focused assessment.

    C. open the airway.

    D. obtain a SAMPLE history.

_____ **26.** Determination of diabetic coma or insulin shock should:

    A. be made before transport of the patient.

    B. be made before administration of oral glucose.

    C. be determined by a urine glucose test.

    D. be based upon your knowledge of the signs and symptoms of each condition.

_____ **27.** When obtaining the medical history of a patient experiencing a sickle cell crisis, you should:

    A. determine the patient's level of consciousness.

    B. ask the patient if he has been compliant with his medications.

    C. take the patient's vital signs.

    D. avoid asking about previous sickle cell crises.

_____ **28.** Contraindications for the use of oral glucose include:

    A. unconsciousness.

    B. known alcoholism.

    C. insulin shock.

    D. all of the above.

_____ **29.** When reassessing the diabetic patient after administration of oral glucose, watch for:

    A. airway problems.

    B. seizures.

    C. sudden loss of consciousness.

    D. all of the above.

_____ **30.** Signs and symptoms associated with hypoglycemia include:

    A. warm, dry skin.

    B. rapid, weak pulse.

    C. Kussmaul respirations.

    D. anxious or combative behavior.

_____ **31.** The patient in insulin shock is experiencing:

    A. hyperglycemia.

    B. hypoglycemia.

    C. diabetic ketoacidosis.

    D. low insulin production.

_____ **32.** Signs of dehydration include:

    A. good skin turgor.

    B. elevated blood pressure.

    C. sunken eyes.

    D. all of the above.

_____ **33.** Hospital interventions for hemophilia may include:

    A. blood transfusions.

    B. analgesics for pain.

    C. intraveneous (IV) therapy.

    D. all of the above.

_____ **34.** Causes of insulin shock include:

    A. taking too much insulin.

    B. vigorous exercise without sufficient glucose intake.

    C. nausea, vomiting, and anorexia.

    D. all of the above.

_____ **35.** Insulin shock can develop more often and more severely in children than in adults due to their:

    A. high activity level and failure to maintain a strict schedule of eating.

    B. genetic makeup.

    C. smaller body size.

    D. all of the above.

_____ **36.** Because diabetic coma is a complex metabolic condition that usually develops over time and involves all the tissues of the body, correcting this condition may:

    A. be accomplished quickly through the use of oral glucose.

    B. require rapid infusion of IV fluid to prevent permanent brain damage.

    C. take many hours in a hospital setting.

    D. include a reduction in the amount of insulin normally taken by the patient.

_____ **37.** A patient in insulin shock or a diabetic coma may appear to be:

    A. having a heart attack.

    B. perfectly normal.

    C. intoxicated.

    D. having a stroke.

True/False

If you believe the statement to be more true than false, write the letter "T" in the space provided. If you believe the statement to be more false than true, write the letter "F."

_____ 1. When patients use fat for energy, the fat waste products increase the amount of acid in the blood and tissue.

_____ 2. The level of consciousness can be affected if a patient has not exercised enough.

_____ 3. People with sickle cell disease have red blood cells that survive for only 120 days.

_____ 4. If blood glucose levels remain low, a patient may lose consciousness or have permanent brain damage.

_____ 5. Signs and symptoms can develop quickly in children because their level of activity can exhaust their glucose levels.

_____ 6. Hemophilia types A and B have the exact same signs and symptoms.

_____ 7. Diabetic emergencies can occur when a patient's blood glucose level gets too high or drops too low.

_____ 8. Diabetic patients may require insulin to control their blood glucose.

_____ 9. Insulin is one of the basic sugars essential for cell metabolism in humans.

_____ 10. A clot that forms deep in a vein is called an aplastic crisis.

_____ 11. Diabetes can cause kidney failure, blindness, and damage to blood vessels.

_____ 12. Most children with diabetes are insulin dependent.

_____ 13. Within the red blood cells, leukocytes are responsible for carrying oxygen.

_____ 14. Many adults with diabetes can control their blood glucose levels with diet alone.

Fill-in-the-Blank

Read each item carefully and then complete the statement by filling in the missing words.

1. The full name of diabetes is _____ _____.

2. A(n) _____ crisis is an acute accelerated _____ in the patient's hemoglobin level.

3. Type 1 diabetes is considered to be a(n) _____ problem, in which the body becomes allergic to its own tissues and literally destroys them.

4. An African American patient or any patient of _____ descent who complains of severe pain may have undiagnosed _____ _____ disease.

5. Diabetes is defined as a lack of or _____ action of insulin.

6. Too much blood glucose by itself does not always cause _____ _____, but on some occasions it can lead to it.

7. _____ is the study and prevention of blood-_____ diseases.

8. A patient in insulin shock needs _____ immediately, and a patient in a diabetic coma needs _____ and IV fluid therapy.

Fill-in-the-Table

Fill in the missing parts of the table.

	Hyperglycemia	Hypoglycemia
History		
Food intake		
Insulin dosage		
Onset		
Skin		
Infection		
Gastrointestinal Tract		
Thirst		
Hunger		
Vomiting		
Respiratory System		
Breathing		
Odor of breath		
Cardiovascular System		
Blood pressure		
Pulse		
Nervous System		
Consciousness		
Urine		
Sugar		
Acetone		
Treatment		
Response		

Crossword Puzzle

The following crossword puzzle is an activity provided to reinforce correct spelling and understanding of medical terminology associated with emergency care and the EMT. Use the clues in the column to complete the puzzle.

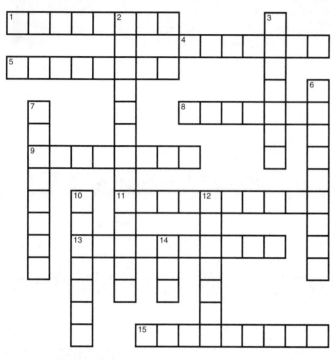

Across

1. A condition in which the body stops producing red blood cells is known as _____ crisis.
4. A hormone produced by the islets of Langerhans that enables glucose in the blood to enter cells
5. The passage of an unusually large volume of urine in a given period
8. A chemical substance produced by a gland that regulates the activity of organs and tissues
9. A pathologic condition that results from the accumulation of acids in the body
11. The study and prevention of blood-related disorders
13. Excessive thirst that persists for long periods, despite reasonable fluid intake
15. Glands that secrete or release chemicals that are used inside the body are known as _____ glands.

Down

2. A tendency to develop blood clots as a result of an abnormality of the coagulation system
3. The primary fuel, in conjunction with oxygen, for cellular metabolism
6. _____ crisis is a rapid destruction of red blood cells that occurs faster than the body's ability to create new cells.
7. _____ mellitus is a metabolic disorder in which the ability to metabolize carbohydrates is impaired.
10. _____ diabetes typically develops in childhood and requires synthetic insulin for proper treatment and control.
12. _____ diabetes typically develops in later life and often can be controlled through diet and oral medications.
14. A form of hyperglycemia in uncontrolled diabetes in which certain acids accumulate when insulin is not available

Critical Thinking

Multiple Choice

Read each critical-thinking item carefully and then select the best response.

Questions 1–5 are derived from the following scenario: A 54-year-old golfer collapsed on the 17th green at the golf course. His friend said he wasn't feeling well after the eighth hole, but insisted on walking and finishing out the game. His skin is pale, cool, and diaphoretic, and he provides incoherent answers to your questions.

_____ 1. During your rapid full-body scan, you discover a medical alert necklace around his neck that reads "Type 2 Diabetic." This tells you that he most likely:

    A. developed diabetes later in life.

    B. produces inadequate amounts of insulin.

    C. takes noninsulin-type oral medications.

    D. all of the above.

_____ **2.** His blood glucose level is 65 mg/dL. You:

    A. do not suspect hypoglycemia and begin to think that his condition is cardiac in nature.

    B. suspect hyperglycemia and proceed to give oral glucose.

    C. suspect hypoglycemia and proceed to give oral glucose.

    D. suspect hypoglycemia but oral glucose is contraindicated for him.

_____ **3.** The patient loses consciousness and a second blood glucose level reads 48 mg/dL. You should:

    A. call for, or rendezvous with, an ALS unit.

    B. ensure a patent airway.

    C. provide high-flow oxygen.

    D. all of the above.

_____ **4.** Because of his blood glucose level and rapid respirations, you suspect:

    A. insulin shock.

    B. diabetic coma.

    C. renal failure.

    D. mittelschmerz.

_____ **5.** Because the patient is unconscious and his blood glucose level is 48 mg/dL, how should the glucose be delivered?

    A. Between the cheek and gum

    B. Placed on the back of the tongue

    C. Placed on the tip of the tongue

    D. None of the above

Short Answer

Complete this section with short written answers using the space provided.

1. What is insulin, and what is its role in metabolism?

_____

_____

2. What are two trade names for oral glucose?

_____

_____

3. What two basic complications are caused by the shape of the red blood cells in people with sickle cell disease?

_____

_____

4. When should you NOT give oral glucose to a patient experiencing a suspected diabetic emergency?

_____

_____

5. How can thrombophilia lead to a pulmonary embolism?

_____

_____

6. What are the three problems that result in the development of diabetic coma?

_____

_____

7. List the physical signs of diabetic coma.

_____

_____

8. If a diabetic patient was "fine" 2 hours ago and now is unconscious and unresponsive, which diabetes-related condition would you suspect and why?

_____

_____

9. What is a major cause of death among hemophiliacs?

_____

_____

Ambulance Calls

The following case scenarios provide an opportunity to explore the concerns associated with patient management and to enhance critical-thinking skills. Read each scenario and answer each question to the best of your ability.

1. You are called to a local residence where you find a 22-year-old woman supine in bed, unresponsive to your attempts to rouse her. She is cold and clammy with gurgling respirations. Her mother tells you that her only history is diabetes, which she has had since she was a small child.

How would you best manage this patient?

_____

_____

_____

2. You are requested to respond to a local convenience store for an unknown medical problem. Upon arrival, you find a young African American man sitting on the curb, clutching his torso and crying. He tells you that he is in severe pain and has a history of sickle cell disease.

How would you best manage this patient?

_____

_____

_____

3. You are dispatched to assist with a diabetic patient well known in your department for being noncompliant with his medications and diet. You have responded numerous times to his residence, all for instances of low blood sugar. Family members greet you at the door and say, "It's Jon again. Just give him some sugar like you usually do." You walk into the patient's bedroom to discover him unconscious with snoring respirations.

How would you best manage this patient?

_____

_____

_____

Fill-in-the-Patient Care Report

Read the incident scenario and then complete the following patient care report (PCR).

"Truck nine, trauma emergency," the dispatcher's voice bursts from the radio on your hip, drawing glances from several people around you in the grocery store.

"Go ahead to nine," your partner, Jerry, responds over the radio from somewhere else in the store.

"Truck nine, trauma emergency at 12556 Old Lake House Drive, for a laceration with uncontrolled bleeding. Showing you dispatched at 1752."

Within 3 minutes, both of you converge on the ambulance parked outside under a line of spruce trees and are en route through rush hour traffic to the subdivision on the east end of the town lake.

"Central, truck nine, we are on scene," you say quickly into the mic before opening your door and climbing from the truck.

"Showing you on scene at 1803," comes the muffled reply from the cab radio.

You are quickly ushered into the home and led by a frantic woman to an upstairs bedroom. As you press through the door, you see a 14-year-old boy holding a blood-soaked T-shirt against his forearm. In front of him on a desk is a half-completed wooden model of an old pirate ship, now sprinkled with darkening blood.

"The blade slipped and he cut his arm," the boy's mother says rapidly. "Oh please help him, he's got hemophilia!"

You gently move the soaked T-shirt and see a 1″ (3-cm) laceration that is bleeding profusely, running steadily down his arm and onto the carpet. You immediately apply pressure to the wound and direct Jerry to start high-flow oxygen therapy. You position the patient onto the stair chair and move him down to the wheeled stretcher in the living room, happy that he weighs only 132 pounds (60 kg).

Once on the gurney, you and Jerry cover the boy with a blanket and load him into the ambulance. You look at your watch (1813) and ask Jerry to get a quick blood pressure on the patient while you continue holding pressure on the wound.

"108 over 60," he says before closing you in with the patient and climbing into the cab of the truck while you check his pulse and count 98 beats/min, get a respiratory rate of 16 breaths/min with good tidal volume, and a pulse oximetry reading of 96%. While en route to the hospital, you realize that the bleeding is just not going to stop with pressure, so you apply a tourniquet on the patient's arm and clearly document the time.

At 1819, Jerry backs into the trauma center's ambulance parking and you both roll the patient into the waiting trauma bay, where you turn him over to the waiting team and provide a verbal report.

Approximately 20 minutes later, after thoroughly cleaning and decontaminating the ambulance, you call yourselves back on duty and available for the next call.

Fill-in-the-Patient Care Report

EMS Patient Care Report (PCR)					
Date:	**Incident No.:**		**Nature of Call:**		**Location:**
Dispatched:	**En Route:**	**At Scene:**	**Transport:**	**At Hospital:**	**In Service:**

Patient Information	
Age:	**Allergies:**
Sex:	**Medications:**
Weight (in kg [lb]):	**Past Medical History:**
	Chief Complaint:

Vital Signs				
Time:	**BP:**	**Pulse:**	**Respirations:**	**Sao$_2$:**
Time:	**BP:**	**Pulse:**	**Respirations:**	**Sao$_2$:**
Time:	**BP:**	**Pulse:**	**Respirations:**	**Sao$_2$:**

EMS Treatment (circle all that apply)				
Oxygen @ ___ L/min via (circle one): **NC NRM Bag-Mask Device**	**Assisted Ventilation**	**Airway Adjunct**		**CPR**
Defibrillation	**Bleeding Control**	**Bandaging**	**Splinting**	**Other Shock Treatment**

Narrative

Skills

Skill Drills

Test your knowledge of this skill by filling in the correct words in the photo captions.

Skill Drill 17-1: Administering Glucose

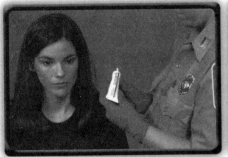

1. Make sure that the tube of glucose is intact and has not _____.

2. Squeeze a generous amount of oral glucose onto the _____ _____ of a _____ _____ or tongue depressor.

3. Open the patient's _____. Place the tongue depressor on the _____ _____ between the cheek and the gum with the _____ _____ next to the cheek. Repeat until the entire tube has been used.

Assessment Review

Answer the following questions pertaining to the assessment of the types of emergencies discussed in this chapter.

Questions 1–5 are derived from the following scenario: While driving back to the station, you and your partner find an unconscious person lying on the grass in front of a home.

_____ **1.** After completing scene size-up, your first step is to:
- **A.** take appropriate BSI precautions.
- **B.** form a general impression of the patient.
- **C.** apply oxygen.
- **D.** none of the above.

_____ **2.** The patient appears to be a woman in her mid-30s, and she is unresponsive to verbal or painful stimulus. Because there is no one around, you are unable to complete a patient history. Which physical examination should you perform first?
- **A.** Focused physical examination
- **B.** Rapid full-body scan
- **C.** Detailed physical examination
- **D.** Blood glucose level

_____ **3.** Her respirations are 28 breaths/min, her pulse is 110 beats/min, and her blood pressure is 94/52 mm Hg. How should you intervene for her?

A. Give her oral glucose.

B. Give her insulin.

C. Provide high-flow oxygen.

D. All of the above.

_____ **4.** Your protocols do not allow you to measure blood glucose levels, and you are unsure as to the nature of her illness. You should:

A. provide oral glucose anyway.

B. provide insulin found in her purse.

C. provide nitroglycerin found in her purse.

D. none of the above.

_____ **5.** When relaying information to medical control, you should inform them of:

A. the patient's condition.

B. any changes of consciousness.

C. any difficulty the patient may experience in breathing.

D. all of the above.

Immunologic Emergencies

General Knowledge

Matching

Match each of the items in the left column to the appropriate definition in the right column.

_____ **1.** Allergic reaction

_____ **2.** Leukotrienes

_____ **3.** Wheezing

_____ **4.** Urticaria

_____ **5.** Stridor

_____ **6.** Allergen

_____ **7.** Wheal

_____ **8.** Toxin

A. Substance made by body; released in anaphylaxis

B. Harsh, high-pitched inspiratory sound, usually resulting from upper airway obstruction

C. Raised, swollen area on skin resulting from an insect bite or allergic reaction

D. An exaggerated immune response to any substance

E. Multiple raised areas on the skin that itch or burn

F. A poison or harmful substance

G. Substance that causes an allergic reaction

H. High-pitched, whistling breath sound usually resulting from blockage of the airway and typically heard on expiration

Multiple Choice

Read each item carefully and then select the one best response.

_____ **1.** Steps for assisting a patient with administration of an EpiPen include:
  A. taking body substance isolation precautions.
  B. placing the tip of the auto-injector against the medial part of the patient's thigh.
  C. recapping the injector before placing it in the trash.
  D. all of the above.

_____ **2.** Allergens may include:
  A. food.
  B. animal bites.
  C. semen.
  D. all of the above.

_____ **3.** Anaphylaxis is not always life threatening, but it typically involves:
  A. multiple organ systems.
  B. wheezing.
  C. urticaria.
  D. wheals.

_____ **4.** Signs and symptoms of insect stings or bites include:
  A. swelling.
  B. wheals.
  C. localized heat.
  D. all of the above.

_____ **5.** Prolonged respiratory difficulty can cause _____, shock, and even death.
  A. tachypnea
  B. pulmonary edema
  C. tachycardia
  D. airway obstruction

_____ **6.** Speed is essential because in severe cases of anaphylaxis, _____ can occur rapidly.
  A. urticaria
  B. compensation
  C. death
  D. recovery

_____ **7.** Questions to ask when obtaining a history from a patient appearing to have an allergic reaction include:
  A. whether the patient has a history of allergies.
  B. what the patient was exposed to.
  C. how the patient was exposed.
  D. all of the above.

_____ **8.** The dosage of epinephrine in an adult EpiPen is:
  A. 0.10 mg.
  B. 0.15 mg.
  C. 0.30 mg.
  D. 0.50 mg.

_____ **9.** Epinephrine, whether made by the body or by a drug manufacturer, works rapidly to:
  A. raise the pulse rate and blood pressure.
  B. inhibit an allergic reaction.
  C. relieve bronchospasm.
  D. all of the above.

_____ **10.** Because the stinger of the honeybee is barbed and remains in the wound, it can continue to inject venom for up to:
  A. 1 minute.
  B. 15 minutes.
  C. 20 minutes.
  D. several hours.

_____ **11.** You should not use tweezers or forceps to remove an embedded stinger because:
  A. squeezing may cause the stinger to inject more venom into the wound.
  B. the stinger may break off in the wound.
  C. the tweezers are not sterile and may cause infection.
  D. removing the stinger may cause bleeding.

_____ **12.** Your assessment of the patient experiencing an allergic reaction should include evaluations of the:
  A. respiratory system.
  B. circulatory system.
  C. skin.
  D. all of the above.

_____ **13.** Eating certain foods, such as shellfish or nuts, may result in a relatively _____ reaction that still can be quite severe.
  A. mild
  B. fast
  C. slow
  D. rapid

_____ **14.** In dealing with allergy-related emergencies, you must be aware of the possibility of acute
_____ and cardiovascular collapse.

    A. hypotension

    B. tachypnea

    C. airway obstruction

    D. shock

_____ **15.** Wheezing occurs because excessive _____ and mucus are secreted into the bronchial passages.

    A. fluid

    B. carbon dioxide

    C. blood

    D. all of the above

True/False

If you believe the statement to be more true than false, write the letter "T" in the space provided. If you believe the statement to be more false than true, write the letter "F."

_____ **1.** Allergic reactions can occur in response to almost any substance.

_____ **2.** An allergic reaction occurs when the body has an immune response to a substance.

_____ **3.** Wheezing is a high-pitched breath sound, usually resulting from blockage of the airway, and is heard on expiration.

_____ **4.** For a patient appearing to have an allergic reaction, give 100% oxygen via nasal cannula.

Fill-in-the-Blank

Read each item carefully and then complete the statement by filling in the missing words.

1. Wheezing occurs because excessive fluid and mucus are secreted into the _____ _____.

2. Small areas of generalized itching or burning that appear as multiple, small, raised areas on the skin are called

_____.

3. The stinger of the honeybee is _____, so the bee cannot withdraw it.

4. A reaction involving the entire body is called _____.

5. The presence of _____ or respiratory distress indicates that the patient is having a severe enough

allergic reaction to lead to death.

6. Epinephrine inhibits the allergic reaction by constricting the _____ _____.

7. Your ability to recognize and manage the many signs and symptoms of allergic reactions may be the only thing standing

between a patient and _____ _____.

Crossword Puzzle

The following crossword puzzle is an activity provided to reinforce correct spelling and understanding of medical terminology associated with emergency care and the EMT. Use the clues in the column to complete the puzzle.

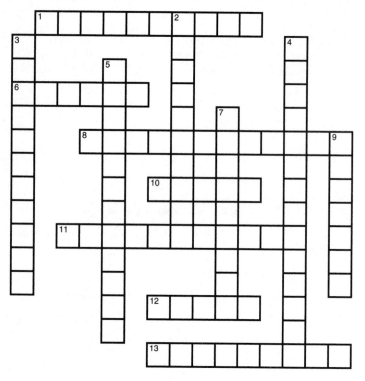

Across

1. Substances released by the immune system that are responsible for many of the symptoms of anaphylaxis, such as vasodilation
6. The _____ system includes all of the structures and processes designed to mount a defense against foreign substances and disease-causing agents.
8. Chemical substances that contribute to anaphylaxis
10. A poison or harmful substance
11. An extreme, life-threatening systemic allergic reaction that may include shock and respiratory failure
12. A raised, swollen, well-defined area on the skin resulting from an insect bite or allergic reaction
13. Substances that cause an allergic reaction

Down

2. The study of the body's immune system
3. A substance produced by the body (commonly called adrenaline) and a drug produced by pharmaceutical companies that increases pulse rate and blood pressure
4. The body's response to substances perceived by the body as foreign
5. The act of injecting venom
7. Small spots of generalized itching and/or burning that appear as multiple raised areas on the skin
9. A harsh, high-pitched respiratory sound, generally heard during inspiration, that is caused by partial blockage or narrowing of the upper airway

Critical Thinking

Multiple Choice

Read each critical-thinking item carefully and then select the one best response.

You have been called to a park where a local church is holding a potluck dinner. As you exit your ambulance, a woman approaches you holding her 7-year-old son who is wheezing and having difficulty breathing. She informs you that he had inadvertently eaten a brownie with nuts, and he is allergic to nuts.

_____ 1. You lift the child's shirt and find small, raised areas that he is trying to scratch. They are likely to be:

    A. leukotrienes.

    B. histamines.

    C. urticaria.

    D. none of the above.

_____ 2. Why is this patient wheezing?

    A. He has had an envenomation.

    B. His bronchioles are constricting.

    C. His bronchioles are dilating.

    D. His uvula has swollen.

_____ 3. The child's mother has an EpiPen that contains the appropriate dose of epinephrine for a child. What dose would that be?

    A. 0.8 mg

    B. 0.5 mg

    C. 0.4 mg

    D. 0.15 mg

_____ 4. When assisting with an auto-injector, how long should you hold the pen against the thigh?

    A. 3 seconds

    B. 5 seconds

    C. 10 seconds

    D. None of the above

_____ 5. After removing the auto-injector from the child's thigh, you should:

    A. record the time.

    B. record the dose.

    C. reassess his vital signs.

    D. all of the above.

Short Answer

Complete this section with short written answers using the space provided.

1. List the common side effects of epinephrine.

_____

_____

2. What are the five stimuli that most often cause allergic reactions?

_____

_____

3. What are the steps for administering or assisting with administration of an epinephrine auto-injector?

_____

_____

4. What are the common respiratory and circulatory signs and symptoms of an allergic reaction?

_____

_____

Ambulance Calls

The following case scenarios provide an opportunity to explore the concerns associated with patient management and to enhance critical-thinking skills. Read each scenario and answer each question to the best of your ability.

1. You are dispatched to assist a 12-year-old child who was climbing a tree and apparently disturbed a wasp nest. When you arrive, the child is lying under the tree, and the nest is on the ground next to her.

How would you best manage this patient?

_____

_____

_____

2. You are dispatched to a local seafood restaurant for a person who is having difficulty breathing. Upon arrival, you find a 22-year-old woman with facial edema, cyanosis around the lips, audible wheezing, and urticaria on her face and upper body. Her boyfriend tells you she ate shrimp and she is allergic to them. He also tells you she has some medicine in her purse and hands you an EpiPen prescribed to her.

How would you best manage this patient?

_____

_____

_____

_____

Fill-in-the-Patient Care Report

Read the incident scenario and then complete the following patient care report (PCR).

"Unit six-twelve, emergency assignment, you're headed to Crab Town Restaurant at 231 Seaside Parkway for an allergic reaction. Showing you dispatched at 1734."

Your partner, Ed, confirms the dispatch over the radio as you activate the lights and sirens and steer toward Seaside Parkway.

"Six-twelve is on scene," Ed says, snapping the microphone back into its holder as you shift the ambulance into park and pull on a pair of exam gloves.

"Unit six-twelve, copying you on scene at 1742."

As you roll the gurney into the restaurant, you are met by a frantic waitress who leads you to a small table at the rear of the bustling restaurant. A 37-year-old man is holding the edge of the table so tightly that his knuckles are white as he struggles to breathe. His face, neck, and hands are obviously swollen; bright hives are visible just above the collar of his shirt; and there is a bluish tinge to his lips and fingernails.

"Get some oxygen on him, Ed, and get the bag-valve ready," you say, pulling the portable radio from your belt. "I'm going to call for an ALS crew."

As Ed places a nonrebreathing mask onto the patient with 15 L/min of oxygen, you request an ALS rendezvous and then turn to the small group of terrified diners who were sitting with the patient. "Does he have an EpiPen or anything for this allergy?"

"No," a woman says, tears smearing the mascara down her cheeks. "He's my husband and I've never seen him react like this to anything."

"Let's load him, Ed!" You pull the gurney over, and the two of you help the 63-kg (138-lb) patient onto it as he sucks noisily on the oxygen. About 6 minutes after arriving, Ed is pulling the ambulance out of the parking lot while you get a baseline set of vitals on the patient.

His blood pressure is 100/64 mm Hg, pulse is 116 beats/min, and you note that it is strong and rapid. His respirations are 26 breaths/min and becoming more labored by the minute, coupled with an obvious anxiety; the patient is becoming very restless. The digital pulse oximeter screen shows 92%.

"Okay sir, I'm going to help you to breathe," you grab the bag-mask device and show it to him. "I'm going to help your breathing with this. Try and relax, although I know that's tough right now."

You remove the nonrebreathing mask and attach the bag-mask device to the truck oxygen supply and begin gently forcing air into the patient with every inhalation. He is beginning to panic, so you have to reassure him loudly and constantly every time that you squeeze the bag.

The back door suddenly pops open and a paramedic that you know climbs aboard with his jump kit. You feel the ambulance start rolling again.

"Great job, my friend," he says to you. "Keep it up while I get my stuff together." The paramedic quickly assembles a syringe and jabs it into the patient's upper arm and then begins to monitor his pulse and breathing. Within a minute, you can see that the swelling is reversing and the patient starts to take deeper breaths, exhaling in relieved yells. You look at your watch (1755) and get another set of vitals while the paramedic talks calmly to the patient. His blood pressure is now 140/94 mm Hg, pulse rate is 128 beats/min, and breathing is 18 breaths/min and much less labored. The SaO₂ is showing 96%, and you reconnect the nonrebreathing mask and place it onto the patient.

You call in a quick, but thorough, verbal report to the receiving facility and provide the ETA given by Ed.

At 1801, you arrive at the hospital followed closely by the ALS ambulance that the paramedic had come from and wheel the deeply breathing patient through the emergency department doors. You and the paramedic provide verbal reports to the physician, and he assumes care of the quickly recovering patient.

At 1814, your unit goes back into service.

Fill-in-the-Patient Care Report

EMS Patient Care Report (PCR)					
Date:	Incident No.:		Nature of Call:		Location:
Dispatched:	En Route:	At Scene:	Transport:	At Hospital:	In Service:
Patient Information					
Age:			Allergies:		
Sex:			Medications:		
Weight (in kg [lb]):			Past Medical History:		
			Chief Complaint:		
Vital Signs					
Time:	BP:	Pulse:	Respirations:		Sao_2:
Time:	BP:	Pulse:	Respirations:		Sao_2:
Time:	BP:	Pulse:	Respirations:		Sao_2:
EMS Treatment **(circle all that apply)**					
Oxygen @ ___ L/min via (circle one): NC NRM Bag-Mask Device		Assisted Ventilation	Airway Adjunct		CPR
Defibrillation	Bleeding Control	Bandaging	Splinting		Other Shock Treatment
Narrative					

Skills

Skill Drill

Test your knowledge of this skill by filling in the correct words in the photo captions.

Skill Drill 18-2: Using a Twinject Auto-injector

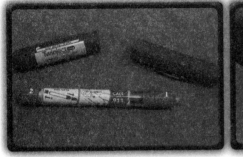 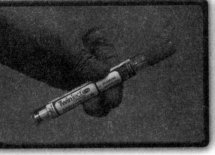 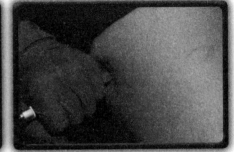

1. Remove the _____ from the container.

2. Clean the administration site with a(n) _____ preparation. Pull off _____ cap "1" to expose a round _____ tip. Do not cover the rounded tip with your _____. Pull off green cap "2."

3. Place the _____ red tip against the _____ part of the thigh. The injection can be administered outside of _____, if necessary. Once the needle has entered the skin, press hard for _____ second(s). Remove the Twinject. Check to make sure the _____ is visible. If the _____ is not visible, repeat the steps.

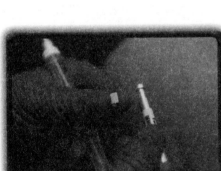 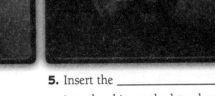

4. If symptoms recur or have not improved within _____ minute(s), repeat the dose. Carefully unscrew and remove the _____ tip. Hold the _____ plastic, pulling the syringe out of the barrel without touching the _____. Slide the yellow collar off the plunger without pulling on the _____.

5. Insert the _____ into the skin on the lateral part of the _____ and push the plunger down.

Assessment Review

Answer the following questions pertaining to the assessment of the types of emergencies discussed in this chapter.

_____ **1.** As you begin to assess a patient suspected of anaphylactic shock, which of these steps would be done first?

    A. Assist with an EpiPen.

    B. Record epinephrine administration time.

    C. Provide high-flow oxygen.

    D. Obtain a pulse oximetry reading.

_____ **2.** After assisting with an EpiPen:

    A. apply high-flow oxygen, if it has not been done already.

    B. take a set of vital signs.

    C. place the used EpiPen in a biohazard container.

    D. all of the above.

_____ **3.** When using the Twinject auto-injector:

    A. remove the safety cap.

    B. wipe the thigh with antiseptic.

    C. push the autoinjector firmly against the thigh for about 10 seconds.

    D. all of the above.

_____ **4.** What does the "M" stand for in SAMPLE?

    A. Mechanism—what substance caused the reaction?

    B. Maintenance—has the patient been compliant with his or her medications?

    C. Medications—what medications is the patient currently taking?

    D. None of the above

_____ **5.** What does the "P" stand for in SAMPLE?

    A. Pain—rate your pain from 1–10

    B. Probable cause—what caused this to happen?

    C. Priority—is this a high or low priority patient?

    D. Past pertinent history

Emergency Care Summary

Fill in the following chart pertaining to the management of the types of emergencies discussed in this chapter.

Note: While the steps below are widely accepted, be sure to consult and follow your local protocol.

Using an Auto-injector

1. Remove the auto-injector's _____ _____, and quickly wipe the _____ with antiseptic.
2. Place the tip of the auto-injector against the _____ part of the _____.
3. Push the auto-injector firmly against the _____, and hold it in place until all the medication is injected (about _____ second[s]).

Using Twinject

1. Remove the injector from the container.
2. Clean the administration site with a(n) _____ preparation. Pull off _____ _____ "1" to expose a(n) _____ _____ tip. Do not cover the rounded tip with your hand.
3. Pull off green cap "2."
4. Place the round red tip against the lateral part of the thigh. The injection can be administered outside of clothing if necessary. Once the needle has entered the skin, press hard for 10 seconds.
5. Remove the Twinject. Check to see whether the needle is visible. If the needle is **not** visible, the dose was not administered and all the steps should be repeated.
6. If symptoms recur or have not improved within 10 minutes, repeat the dose. Carefully unscrew and remove the _____ _____. Hold the blue plastic, pulling the syringe out of the barrel without touching the _____. Slide the yellow collar off the plunger without pulling on the _____.
7. Insert the needle into the skin on the lateral part of the thigh and push the plunger down.

CHAPTER

Toxicology

19

General Knowledge

Matching

Match each of the items in the left column to the appropriate definition in the right column.

_____ 1. Poison

_____ 2. Substance abuse

_____ 3. Antidote

_____ 4. Tolerance

_____ 5. Cholinergic

_____ 6. Ingestion

_____ 7. Hematemesis

_____ 8. Stimulant

_____ 9. Opioid

_____ 10. Sedative

_____ 11. Anticholinergic

A. Xanax, Librium, Valium

B. Drug or agent with actions similar to morphine

C. Atropine, Benadryl, some cyclic antidepressants

D. Need for increasing amounts of a drug to obtain the same effect

E. Agent that produces an excited state

F. Substance whose chemical action can damage body structures or impair body functions

G. Substance that will counteract the effects of a particular poison

H. Misuse of any substance to produce a desired effect

I. Taking a substance by mouth

J. Overstimulates body functions controlled by parasympathetic nerves

K. Vomiting blood

Multiple Choice

Read each item carefully and then select the one best response.

_____ 1. Activated charcoal is in the form of a(n):

    A. elixir.

    B. suspension.

    C. syrup.

    D. emulsion.

_____ 2. The presence of burning or blistering of the mucous membranes suggests:

    A. ingestion of depressants.

    B. ingestion of poison.

    C. overdose of heroin.

    D. that the patient may be a heavy smoker.

_____ 3. Treatment for ingestion of poisonous plants includes all of the following EXCEPT:

    A. assessing the patient's airway and vital signs.

    B. taking the plant to the emergency department.

    C. administering activated charcoal.

    D. prompt transport.

_____ 4. The MOST important consideration in caring for a patient who has been exposed to an organophosphate insecticide or some other cholinergic agent is to:

    A. maintain the airway.

    B. apply high-flow oxygen.

    C. avoid exposure yourself.

    D. initiate CPR.

_____ **5.** Which of the following would NOT provide clues to the nature of the poison?
   A. Open windows
   B. Scattered pills
   C. Chemicals
   D. A needle or syringe

_____ **6.** The MOST worrisome avenue of poisoning is:
   A. ingestion.
   B. inhalation.
   C. injection.
   D. absorption.

_____ **7.** The major side effect of ingesting activated charcoal is:
   A. depressed respirations.
   B. overproduction of stomach acid.
   C. black stools.
   D. increased blood pressure.

_____ **8.** Alcohol is a powerful CNS depressant. It:
   A. sharpens the sense of awareness.
   B. slows reflexes.
   C. increases reaction time.
   D. increases reflexes.

_____ **9.** Which of the following is a frequently abused synthetic opioid?
   A. Heroin
   B. Morphine
   C. Meperidine (Demerol)
   D. Codeine

_____ **10.** Which of the following is NOT part of treatment of patients who have overdosed with sedative-hypnotics and have respiratory depression?
   A. Provide airway clearance.
   B. Provide ventilatory assistance.
   C. Provide prompt transport.
   D. Administer syrup of ipecac.

_____ **11.** Anticholinergic medications have properties that block the _____ nerves.
   A. parasympathetic
   B. sympathetic
   C. adrenergic
   D. parasympatholytic

_____ **12.** _____ crack produces the most rapid means of absorption and therefore the most potent effect.
   A. Injected
   B. Absorbed
   C. Smoked
   D. Ingested

_____ **13.** "Nerve gases" overstimulate normal body functions that are controlled by parasympathetic nerves, causing:
   A. increased salivation.
   B. pupil dilation.
   C. decreased urination.
   D. decreased lacrimation.

_____ **14.** Signs and symptoms of staphylococcal food poisoning include:

    A. difficulty speaking.

    B. nausea, vomiting, and diarrhea.

    C. blurred vision.

    D. respiratory distress.

_____ **15.** Inhalant effects range from mild drowsiness to coma, but unlike most other sedative-hypnotics these agents may often cause:

    A. seizures.

    B. vomiting.

    C. swelling of the tongue.

    D. rashes.

_____ **16.** Cocaine may be taken which of the following ways?

    A. Inhalation

    B. Injection

    C. Absorption

    D. All of the above

_____ **17.** Which of the following is NOT considered an abusable substance?

    A. Alcohol

    B. Nasal decongestants

    C. Detergents

    D. Food

_____ **18.** A person who has been using marijuana rarely needs transport to the hospital. Exceptions may include all of the following EXCEPT a patient who is:

    A. intoxicated.

    B. very anxious.

    C. paranoid.

    D. hallucinating.

_____ **19.** Sympathomimetics are CNS stimulants that frequently cause:

    A. hypotension.

    B. tachycardia.

    C. pinpoint pupils.

    D. muscle weakness.

_____ **20.** Carbon monoxide:

    A. is odorless.

    B. produces severe hypoxia.

    C. does not damage or irritate the lungs.

    D. all of the above.

_____ **21.** Chlorine:

    A. is odorless.

    B. does not damage or irritate the lungs.

    C. causes pulmonary edema.

    D. all of the above.

_____ **22.** Localized signs and symptoms of absorbed poisoning include:

    A. a history of exposure.

    B. burns, irritation of the skin.

    C. dyspnea.

    D. muscle weakness.

_____ **23.** Which of the following statements regarding injected poisons is FALSE?

    A. They may result in dizziness, fever, and chills.

    B. They are frequently caused by a drug overdose.

    C. They are easily diluted once in the bloodstream.

    D. You should remove rings, watches, and bracelets in areas of swelling.

_____ **24.** When dealing with substances such as phosphorous and elemental sodium, you should do all of the following EXCEPT:

    A. brush the chemical off the patient.

    B. remove contaminated clothing.

    C. apply a dry dressing to the burn area.

    D. irrigate with water.

_____ **25.** Injected poisons are impossible to dilute or remove, because they are usually _____ or cause intense local tissue destruction.

    A. absorbed quickly into the body

    B. bound to hemoglobin

    C. large compounds

    D. combined with the cerebrospinal fluid

_____ **26.** Medical problems that may cause the patient to present as intoxicated include all of the following EXCEPT:

    A. head trauma.

    B. syncope.

    C. uncontrolled diabetes.

    D. toxic reactions.

_____ **27.** Which of the following is NOT considered a sign or symptom of alcohol withdrawal?

    A. Agitation and restlessness

    B. Fever and sweating

    C. Seizures

    D. Chest pain

_____ **28.** Treatments for inhaled poisons include:

    A. moving the patient into fresh air.

    B. applying an SCBA to the patient.

    C. covering the patient to prevent spread of the poison.

    D. considering CPAP application.

_____ **29.** Signs and symptoms of chlorine exposure include all of the following EXCEPT:

    A. cough.

    B. chest pain.

    C. rales.

    D. wheezing.

_____ **30.** Which of the following is NOT a typical ingested poison?

    A. Aerosol propellants

    B. Household cleaners

    C. Plants

    D. Contaminated food

_____ **31.** Ingestion of an opiate, sedative, or barbiturate can cause depression of the CNS and:

    A. paralysis of the extremities.

    B. dilation of the pupils.

    C. carpopedal spasms.

    D. slow breathing.

_____ **32.** Inhaled poisons include:

   A. chlorine.

   B. venom.

   C. dieffenbachia.

   D. salmonella.

_____ **33.** Which of the following is NOT considered part of the standard treatment of poisonings?

   A. Administering a specific antidote

   B. Providing high-flow oxygen

   C. Diluting the agent

   D. Administering syrup of ipecac

Questions 34-38 are derived from the following scenario: You have responded to the home of a 26-year-old woman who has reportedly taken a large number of pills in an attempt to commit suicide. As you enter the living room, you see her sleeping in her chair, with several empty alcohol containers. She is breathing heavily.

_____ **34.** You are able to arouse her consciousness for a short period of time. Which course of action takes priority?

   A. Administer syrup of ipecac.

   B. Cover her with a blanket to maintain body temperature.

   C. Have her take activated charcoal while she is conscious.

   D. Ask her why she attempted suicide.

_____ **35.** You have determined to give her activated charcoal. How much should you give her?

   A. Half a glass

   B. 12.5 to 25 g

   C. 25 to 50 g

   D. 25 to 50 mL

_____ **36.** What would be the desired goal of giving her activated charcoal?

   A. To vomit the drugs and alcohol

   B. To bind the toxin and prevent absorption

   C. To teach her a lesson

   D. To prevent excretion

_____ **37.** If she does not want to take the activated charcoal, you should:

   A. restrain her, pinch her nose, and make her drink it.

   B. have her sign a patient refusal form.

   C. attempt to persuade her.

   D. all of the above.

_____ **38.** Side effects of ingesting activated charcoal include all of the following EXCEPT:

   A. vomiting.

   B. hematemesis.

   C. nausea.

   D. black stools.

_____ **39.** Which of the following is not commonly associated with an overdose from a cardiac medication?

   A. Cardiac arrhythmia

   B. Bleeding

   C. Unconsciousness

   D. Urinary incontinence

_____ **40.** Ringing in the ears is associated with an overdose of:

   A. acetaminophen.

   B. aspirin.

   C. ethylene alcohol.

   D. methyl alcohol.

True/False

If you believe the statement to be more true than false, write the letter "T" in the space provided. If you believe the statement to be more false than true, write the letter "F."

_____ 1. The usual adult dose of activated charcoal is 25 to 50 g.

_____ 2. The general treatment of a poisoned patient is to induce vomiting.

_____ 3. Activated charcoal is a standard of care in all ingestions.

_____ 4. Inhaled chlorine produces profound hypoxia without lung irritation.

_____ 5. Shaking activated charcoal decreases its effectiveness.

_____ 6. Opioid overdose typically presents with pinpoint pupils.

_____ 7. Cholinergics include nerve gases, organophosphate insecticides, and certain wild mushrooms.

_____ 8. Alcohol is a stimulant.

_____ 9. Demerol, Dilaudid, and Vicodin are all examples of opioids.

_____ 10. Cocaine is one of the most addicting substances known.

_____ 11. Ethyl alcohol (typical drinking alcohol) can cause respiratory arrest if taken in too high a dose.

_____ 12. Ingestion of the plant dieffenbachia can cause irritation of the lower airway.

Fill-in-the-Blank

Read each item carefully and then complete the statement by filling in the missing words.

1. When dealing with exposure to chemicals, treatment focuses on support, including assessing and maintaining the

   patient's _____.

2. The most commonly abused drug in the United States is _____.

3. Activated charcoal works by _____, or sticking to, many commonly ingested poisons, preventing the

   toxin from being absorbed into the body.

4. If the patient has a chemical agent in the eyes, you should irrigate the eyes quickly and thoroughly for at least

   _____ _____ _____ minutes for acid substances and _____ _____ _____ minutes

   for alkali substances.

5. Opioid analgesics are CNS depressants and can cause severe _____ _____.

6. Severe acute alcohol ingestion may cause _____.

7. Your primary responsibility to the patient who has been poisoned is to _____ that a poisoning

   occurred.

8. The usual dosage for activated charcoal for an adult or child is _____ _____ of activated charcoal

   per _____ of body weight.

9. As you irrigate the eyes, make sure that the fluid runs from the bridge of the nose _____.

10. Approximately 80% of all poisoning is by _____, including plants, contaminated food, and most drugs.

11. Patients experiencing alcohol withdrawal may develop _____ _____ if they no longer

 have their daily source of alcohol.

12. Phosphorus and elemental sodium _____ when they come in contact with water.

13. Increasing tolerance of a substance can lead to _____.

14. _____ may develop from sweating, fluid loss, insufficient fluid intake, or vomiting associated with

 delirium tremens.

Fill-in-the-Table

Fill in the missing parts of the table.

Toxidromes: Typical Signs and Symptoms of Specific Overdoses	
Agent	Signs and Symptoms
Opioid (Examples: heroin, oxycodone)	• Hypoventilation or respiratory arrest • _____ • Sedation or coma • _____
_____ (Examples: epinephrine, albuterol, cocaine, methamphetamine)	• Hypertension • _____ • Dilated pupils • Agitation or seizures • _____
Sedative-hypnotics (Examples: diazepam [Valium], secobarbital [Seconal], flunitrazepam, [Rohypnol])	• _____ • Sedation or coma • Hypoventilation • _____
_____ (Examples: atropine, Jimson weed)	• _____ • _____ • Hypertension • Dilated pupils • _____ • Sedation, agitation, seizures, coma, or delirium • _____
_____ (Examples: pilocarpine, nerve gas)	• _____ • _____ • Pinpoint pupils • Excess lacrimation (tearing) or salivation • _____ • _____

Crossword Puzzle

The following crossword puzzle is an activity provided to reinforce correct spelling and understanding of medical terminology associated with emergency care and the EMT. Use the clues in the column to complete the puzzle.

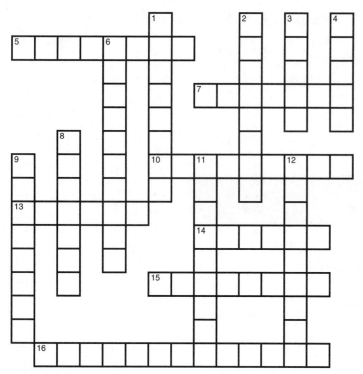

Across

5. A substance that decreases activity and excitement
7. Any drug or agent with actions similar to morphine
10. An agent that produces an excited state
13. A substance whose chemical action could damage structures or impair function when introduced into the body
14. Vomiting
15. A substance that is used to neutralize or counteract a poison
16. Agents that produce false perceptions in any one of the five senses

Down

1. An excessive quantity of a drug that can have toxic or lethal consequences
2. _____ tremens is a severe withdrawal syndrome seen in alcoholics who are deprived of ethyl alcohol.
3. A poison or harmful substance produced by bacteria, animals, or plants
4. Substance _____ is the misuse of any substance to produce some desired effect.
6. The study of toxic or poisonous substances
8. Vomited material
9. A sleep-inducing effect or agent
11. Swallowing; taking a substance by mouth
12. A state of overwhelming obsession or physical need to continue the use of a drug or agent

Critical Thinking

Short Answer

Complete this section with short written answers using the space provided.

1. How does activated charcoal work to counteract ingested poison?

_____

_____

2. What are four routes of contact for poisoning?

_____

_____

3. List the typical signs and symptoms of an overdose of sympathomimetics.

_____

_____

4. What are the two main types of food poisoning?

_____

_____

5. What differentiates the presentation of acetaminophen poisoning from that of other substances? What does this mean to the prehospital caregiver?

_____

_____

6. What condition do the mnemonics DUMBELS and SLUDGE pertain to, and what do they mean?

_____

_____

7. In addition to alcohol and marijuana, what are the eight categories of drugs seen in overdoses and/or poisoning?

_____

_____

8. What five questions should you ask a possible poisoning victim?

_____

_____

9. Why should phosphorous or elemental sodium poisoning victims not be irrigated?

_____

_____

Ambulance Calls

The following case scenarios provide an opportunity to explore the concerns associated with patient management and to enhance critical-thinking skills. Read each scenario and answer each question to the best of your ability.

1. You are dispatched to a private residence for "accidental ingestion." You arrive to find a 3-year-old whose parents tell you "got into some rat poison." The child is alert, crying, and responding appropriately to parents and environmental stimuli.

   How would you best manage this patient?

   _____

   _____

   _____

2. You are dispatched to the sidewalk in front of a small business for "an intoxicated man." You arrive to find a 60-year-old man sitting on the curb, holding a bottle inside a paper bag. He is not fully alert and can only tell you that his name is Andy. He allows you to take his blood pressure, and as you roll up his sleeve you notice needle marks along his veins.

   How would you best manage this patient?

   _____

   _____

   _____

3. You are called to a possible suicide attempt. You arrive on the scene to find police and a neighbor in the home of a 25-year-old woman who is unresponsive, supine on her bed. The neighbor tells you that the patient recently broke up with her boyfriend and has been very distraught. There is an empty pill bottle on the nightstand. When you look at the label, you see that the prescription was filled yesterday and that 30 tablets were dispensed. An empty liquor bottle is on the floor.

   How would you best manage this patient?

   _____

   _____

   _____

Skills

Assessment Review

Answer the following questions pertaining to the assessment of the types of emergencies discussed in this chapter.

_____ 1. Which of the following would NOT be an appropriate question to ask regarding an ingested poison?

    A. What is the substance?

    B. How much did the patient ingest?

    C. What color was the substance?

    D. Have any interventions been performed?

_____ 2. "Hot as a hare, blind as a bat, dry as a bone, red as a beet, and mad as a hatter" describes which of the following conditions?

    A. Cholinergic poisoning

    B. Anticholinergic poisoning

    C. Delirium tremens

    D. Sympathomimetic poisoning

_____ 3. _Shigella_, _Campylobacter_, and _Enterococcus_ are associated with what type of poisoning?

    A. Plant

    B. Food

    C. Hallucinogen

    D. Sympathomimetic

_____ 4. Ice, crank, speed, uppers, and meth are all street names for which type of poison?

    A. Hallucinogens

    B. Sympathomimetics

    C. Sedative-hypnotics

    D. Anticholinergics

_____ 5. When would you NOT give activated charcoal?

    A. If the patient drank gasoline

    B. If the patient overdosed on aspirin

    C. If the patient overdosed on antidepressants

    D. If the patient overdosed on opiates

Emergency Care Summary

Fill in the following chart pertaining to the management of the types of emergencies discussed in this chapter.

Note: While the steps below are widely accepted, be sure to consult and follow your local protocol.

General Management of Toxicologic Emergencies

1. Rescues from a toxic environment should only be performed by trained rescuers wearing appropriate

   _____ _____ _____.

2. Establish and maintain a patent airway. Provide high-flow oxygen. Monitor for vomiting and protect against

   _____.

3. Obtain _____ history and _____ _____. Ascertain what toxin may be

   involved.

4. Request _____ when necessary.

5. Take all containers, bottles, and labels of poisons to the receiving hospital.

6. For patients who have taken alcohol, opioids, sedative-hypnotics, or abused inhalants, monitor the level of consciousness

   and airway patency because these drugs produce _____ _____ _____

   depression and respiratory depression.

7. For abused inhalants, patients are prone to _____ and ventricular fibrillation.

8. For stimulants and anticholinergics, it is critical to monitor patients for hypertension and/or other _____

   effects.

9. For _____ agents, decontamination is a necessity. Monitor the patient for excessive _____

   secretions and seizures.

10. For patients who have plant poisoning, contact the regional poison center for assistance in identifying the plant.

11. For patients who have _____ poisoning, transport the food suspected to be responsible for the poisoning.

Administer _____ _____ for poisonous ingestions according to local protocol. Follow these

steps:

1. Do not give activated charcoal if the patient exhibits a(n) _____ _____

   _____, has ingested a substance for which charcoal is contraindicated, or is unable to

   _____.

2. Obtain an order from medical direction or follow protocol.

3. Shake the activated charcoal container well.

4. Place the activated charcoal suspension in a covered cup with a straw and ask the patient to drink. The dose for infants

   and children is _____ to 25 g and the dose for adults is 25 to _____ g.

Psychiatric Emergencies

General Knowledge

Matching

Match each of the items in the left column to the appropriate definition in the right column.

_____ 1. Psychosis

_____ 2. Psychogenic

_____ 3. Delirium

_____ 4. Depression

_____ 5. Psychiatric disorder

_____ 6. Behavior

_____ 7. Functional disorder

_____ 8. Psychiatric emergency

_____ 9. Behavioral crisis

_____ 10. Organic brain syndrome

A. What you can see of a person's response to the environment; his or her actions

B. Temporary or permanent dysfunction of the brain caused by a disturbance in brain tissue function

C. Any reaction to events that interferes with activities of daily living or is unacceptable to the patient or others

D. A persistent feeling of sadness or despair

E. Abnormal operation of an organ that cannot be traced to an obvious change in structure or physiology of the organ

F. A symptom or illness caused by mental factors as opposed to physical ones

G. An illness with psychological or behavioral symptoms that may result in impaired functioning

H. The patient may show agitation or violence or become a threat to self or others

I. A state of delusion in which the person is out of touch with reality

J. Condition of impairment in cognitive function that can present with disorientation, hallucinations, or delusions

Multiple Choice

Read each item carefully and then select the one best response.

_____ 1. Which of the following is NOT typically linked to a psychological or behavioral crisis?

   A. Mind-altering substances

   B. An underlying medical problem

   C. History of smoking

   D. Stress

_____ 2. Which of the following is a normal reaction to a crisis situation?

   A. Monday morning blues that last until Friday

   B. Feeling "blue" after the break up of a long-term relationship

   C. Feeling depressed week after week with no discernible cause

   D. Thoughts of suicide

_____ 3. Which of the following statements is FALSE?

   A. You may be able to predict whether a person will become violent.

   B. Scene safety is always your primary concern.

   C. Behavior problems may be the result of drug or alcohol abuse.

   D. Most people with a mental illness are dangerous.

_____ **4.** Learning to adapt to a variety of situations in daily life, including stresses and strains, is called:

    A. disruption.

    B. adjustment.

    C. behavior.

    D. functional.

_____ **5.** If the interruption of daily routine tends to recur on a regular basis, the behavior is also considered a _____ crisis.

    A. mental health

    B. functional

    C. behavioral

    D. psychogenic

_____ **6.** If an abnormal or disturbing pattern of behavior lasts for at least _____, it is regarded as a matter of concern from a mental health standpoint.

    A. 6 weeks

    B. 1 month

    C. 6 months

    D. 1 year

_____ **7.** Patients may show agitation, violence, or become a threat to themselves or others when they experience a(n) _____ emergency.

    A. psychiatric

    B. behavioral

    C. functional

    D. adjustment

_____ **8.** Which of the following is NOT considered a possible cause of a psychiatric disorder?

    A. Social disturbance

    B. Chemical disturbance

    C. Biologic disturbance

    D. Emotional disturbance

_____ **9.** An altered mental status may arise from:

    A. an oxygen saturation of 98%.

    B. moderate temperatures.

    C. an inadequate blood flow to the brain.

    D. adequate glucose levels in the blood.

_____ **10.** Organic brain syndrome may be caused by:

    A. daily stress.

    B. seizure disorders.

    C. myocardial infarction.

    D. thoracic spinal cord injury.

_____ **11.** All of the following are examples of a functional disorder EXCEPT:

    A. anxiety.

    B. depression.

    C. organic brain syndrome.

    D. schizophrenia.

_____ **12.** When documenting abnormal behavior, it is important to:

    A. document restraints only when leather restraints are used.

    B. document everything that happened on the call.

    C. avoid quoting the patient's own words.

    D. interject your interpretations of the patient's thoughts.

_____ **13.** Safety guidelines for behavioral emergencies include the following EXCEPT:

    A. assessing the scene.

    B. being prepared to spend extra time.

    C. encouraging purposeful movement.

    D. determining the underlying psychiatric disorder.

_____ **14.** In evaluating a situation that is considered a behavioral emergency, the first things to consider are:

    A. airway and breathing.

    B. scene safety and patient response.

    C. history of medications.

    D. respiratory and circulatory status.

_____ **15.** _____ is a behavior that is characterized by restlessness and irregular physical activity.

    A. Agitation

    B. Aggression

    C. Anxiety

    D. Apathy

_____ **16.** Which of the following is NOT considered a risk factor for suicide?

    A. Alcohol abuse

    B. Recent marriage

    C. Family history of suicide

    D. Depression

_____ **17.** Which of the following is NOT a risk factor to consider when assessing a suicidal patient?

    A. Does the patient appear to be well groomed?

    B. Is the environment unsafe?

    C. Is there an imminent threat to the patient or others?

    D. Is there evidence of self-destructive behavior?

_____ **18.** Signs and symptoms of agitated delirium include all of the following EXCEPT:

    A. hyperventilation.

    B. tachycardia.

    C. vivid hallucinations.

    D. dilated pupils.

_____ **19.** You should request the assistance of a _____ when a mentally impaired patient refuses to go to the hospital.

    A. physician

    B. court order

    C. law enforcement officer

    D. psychologist

_____ **20.** When restraining a patient without an appropriate order, legal actions may involve charges of:

    A. abandonment.

    B. negligence.

    C. battery.

    D. breach of duty.

_____ **21.** When restraining a patient on a stretcher, it is necessary to constantly reassess the patient's:

    A. level of consciousness.

    B. respiration and circulation status.

    C. emotional status.

    D. pain status.

Questions 22-26 are derived from the following scenario: Dean, a man in his 50s, is acting irrationally. His wife states that he thinks he is the dictator of a small country, and he is wearing nothing but a baseball cap and a belt with a small handgun attached to it.

_____ **22.** What is your best course of action?

    A. Call ALS.

    B. Assess Dean from a distance.

    C. Have his wife take the gun from him.

    D. Call for police back-up.

_____ **23.** The scene is safe. Dean now tells you he is "God" and can do anything he wants to. Which of the following should you NOT consider?

    A. He is probably not a threat to you.

    B. He may have a history of psychiatric problems.

    C. He could be suffering from an underlying medical problem.

    D. Alcohol or drugs could be a factor in his behavior.

_____ **24.** What are some tactics you can use to have Dean cooperate with your assessment?

    A. Reflective listening

    B. Threatening him with restraints

    C. Aggressive communication

    D. Passive listening

_____ **25.** Dean becomes agitated and states, "You'll never take me alive." Ordinarily, who can order restraint?

    A. Physician

    B. Court

    C. Law enforcement officer

    D. All of the above

_____ **26.** How many people should be present to restrain Dean?

    A. Two

    B. Four

    C. Six

    D. Eight

True/False

If you believe the statement to be more true than false, write the letter "T" in the space provided. If you believe the statement to be more false than true, write the letter "F."

_____ **1.** Depression lasting 8 months after being fired from a job is a normal mental health response.

_____ **2.** Low blood glucose or lack of oxygen to the brain may cause behavioral changes to the degree that a psychiatric emergency could exist.

_____ **3.** From a mental health standpoint, a pattern of abnormal behavior must last at least 3 months to be a matter of concern.

_____ **4.** A disturbed patient should always be transported with restraints.

_____ **5.** It is sometimes helpful to allow a patient with a behavioral emergency some time alone to calm down and collect his or her thoughts.

_____ **6.** It is important to maintain eye contact with the patient when dealing with a behavioral crisis.

_____ **7.** A patient should never be asked if he or she is considering suicide.

_____ **8.** Urinary tract infections can cause behavioral changes in elderly patients.

_____ **9.** All individuals with mental health disorders are dangerous, violent, or otherwise unmanageable.

_____ **10.** When completing the documentation, it is important to record the reasons why you restrained a patient.

_____ **11.** When restraining a patient, at least four people should be present to carry out the restraint.

_____ **12.** A patient should be placed face down when being restrained to a litter.

_____ **13.** Reassessment of restrained patients should take place every 5 minutes.

_____ **14.** Tears, sweating, and blushing may be significant indicators of state of mind such as sadness, nervousness, or embarrassment.

_____ **15.** Almost every situation, medical or trauma, will have some behavioral component.

Fill-in-the-Blank

Read each item carefully and then complete the statement by filling in the missing words.

1. _____ is what you can see of a person's response to the environment; his or her actions.

2. A(n) _____ _____ or emergency is any reaction to events that interferes with the activities of daily living or has become unacceptable to the patient, family, or community.

3. Chronic _____, or a persistent feeling of sadness or despair, may be a symptom of a mental or physical disorder.

4. _____ _____ _____ is a temporary or permanent dysfunction of the brain caused by a disturbance in the physical or physiologic functioning of the brain.

5. Any time you encounter an emotionally depressed patient, you must consider the possibility of _____.

6. People with _____ may experience symptoms including delusions, hallucinations, a lack of interest in pleasure, and erratic speech.

7. Violent or dangerous people should be managed by _____ _____ before emergency care is rendered.

8. When a patient is not mentally competent to grant consent, the law assumes that there is _____ _____.

9. The most common cause of dementia is primary progressive dementia, also known as _____ _____.

10. In subduing a disturbed patient, use the _____ force necessary.

Crossword Puzzle

The following crossword puzzle is an activity provided to reinforce correct spelling and understanding of medical terminology associated with emergency care and the EMT. Use the clues in the column to complete the puzzle.

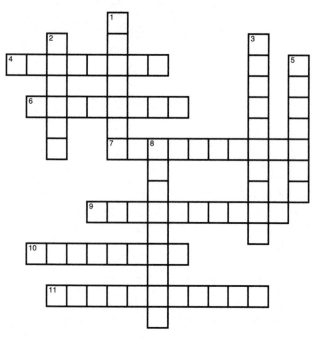

Across

4. _____ delirium is a condition of disorientation, confusion, and possible hallucinations coupled with purposeless, restless physical activity.

6. A psychiatric _____ is an illness with psychological or behavioral symptoms and/or impairment in functioning.

7. A persistent mood of sadness, despair, and discouragement

9. A(n) _____ disorder has no known physiologic reason for the abnormal functioning of an organ or organ system.

10. How a person functions or acts in response to his or her environment

11. An emergency in which abnormal behavior threatens a person's own health and safety or the health and safety of another person is known as a(n) _____ emergency.

Down

1. A change in the way a person thinks and behaves that may signal disease in the central nervous system or elsewhere in the body is known as _____ mental status.

2. Activities of daily _____ are the basic activities a person usually accomplishes during a day.

3. _____ crisis is the point at which a person's reactions to events interfere with activities of daily living.

5. _____ brain syndrome is temporary or permanent dysfunction of the brain, caused by a disturbance in the physical or physiologic functioning of brain tissue.

8. A mental disorder characterized by the loss of contact with reality

Critical Thinking

Short Answer

Complete this section with short written answers using the space provided.

1. What is the distinction between a behavioral crisis and a psychiatric emergency?

_____

_____

2. What three major areas should be considered in evaluating the possible source of a behavioral crisis?

_____

_____

3. What are three factors to consider in determining the level of force required to restrain a patient?

_____

_____

4. List 10 safety guidelines for dealing with behavioral emergencies.

_____

_____

_____

5. List 10 risk factors for suicide.

_____

_____

_____

6. Explain the process for "reflective listening."

_____

_____

_____

7. List five risk factors to consider when dealing with a potentially violent patient.

_____

_____

_____

Ambulance Calls

The following case scenarios provide an opportunity to explore the concerns associated with patient management and to enhance critical-thinking skills. Read each scenario and answer each question to the best of your ability.

1. You are dispatched to a nonemergency transport of a girl from a local hospital emergency department to a care facility that provides treatment for emotionally disturbed teenagers. She became violent in the emergency department and was placed in four-point restraints. As you begin transporting the patient, she begins to cry and asks you to remove the restraints.

How would you best manage this patient?

_____

_____

_____

2. You are dispatched to a "suicide attempt" at a private residence. When you arrive on scene, you are greeted by a calm, middle-aged man who appears to have been crying. He tells you that he was on the phone with his sister who lives out of state and that she must have called for the ambulance. The patient tells you that he was just upset, but he's fine now. Dispatch informed you via cellular phone that this man recently lost his wife of 15 years to breast cancer.

How would you best manage this patient?

_____

_____

_____

3. You are dispatched to the residence of a 40-year-old woman who is upset over the loss of her mother 5 weeks ago. She tells you that she has no family and has cared for her elderly mother for the past 7 years. She has not eaten for several days and is severely depressed.

How would you best manage this patient?

_____

_____

_____

Assessment Review

Answer the following questions pertaining to the assessment of the types of emergencies discussed in this chapter. Questions 1–5 are based on risk factors in assessing the level of danger in a behavior call.

_____ 1. When assessing the history, what past behavior(s) do you want to know the patient has exhibited?
   A. Hostile behavior
   B. Overly aggressive behavior
   C. Violent behavior
   D. All of the above

_____ 2. Physical tension is often a warning signal of impending hostility. What sign might warn you of physical tension?
   A. Posture
   B. Eye movement
   C. Facial expression
   D. Laughter

_____ 3. What warning signs can be detected from the scene?
   A. Hunting magazines on the table
   B. Known weapons in the outside shed
   C. Guns or knives near the patient
   D. Photos of hunting trips on the wall

_____ 4. What kind of speech may be an indicator of emotional distress?
   A. Quiet speech
   B. Obscene speech
   C. Rational speech
   D. Organized speech

_____ 5. What type of physical activity may be an indicator of risk to the EMT?
   A. Tense muscles
   B. Continuous stretching
   C. Lying down
   D. Vigorous exercise

Skills

Emergency Care Summary

Fill in the following chart pertaining to the management of the types of emergencies discussed in this chapter.
Note: While the steps below are widely accepted, be sure to consult and follow your local protocol.

General Management of Psychiatric Emergencies

Managing life threats to the patient's _____ and ensuring the delivery of high-flow oxygen are primary concerns with any psychiatric emergency. Without an underlying medical or trauma cause, there is usually little _____ care for the EMT to perform. Competent adults have the right to refuse treatment and transport, but in the case of psychiatric emergencies, you may have a reasonable belief that the patient may harm himself, herself, or others. If this is the case, contact _____ _____ to take the patient into custody. If _____ is required, consult with medical control, ensure law enforcement personnel are at the scene, and make sure that there are at least _____ people present. Use only approved restraint devices. Do not transport the patient in a(n) _____ position because the patient may experience severe respiratory distress or cardiac arrest, often called _____.

CHAPTER

Gynecologic Emergencies

21

General Knowledge

Matching

Match each of the items in the left column to the appropriate definition in the right column.

_____ **1.** Ovaries

_____ **2.** Fallopian tubes

_____ **3.** Uterus

_____ **4.** Cervix

_____ **5.** Vagina

_____ **6.** Labia

_____ **7.** Perineum

_____ **8.** Chlamydia

_____ **9.** Pelvic inflammatory disease

_____ **10.** Bacterial vaginosis

_____ **11.** Gonorrhea

A. Folds of tissue that surround the urethral and vaginal openings

B. Narrowest portion of the uterus; opens to the vagina

C. Disease causing lower abdominal and back pain, nausea, fever, pain during intercourse, and/or bleeding between menstrual cycles

D. Area of skin between the vagina and the anus

E. Connect(s) each ovary with the uterus

F. Infection of the uterus, ovaries, and fallopian tubes

G. Produce(s) an ovum, or an egg.

H. Outermost cavity of a woman's reproductive system; forms the lower part of the birth canal

I. Condition in which bacteria can grow and multiply rapidly in the reproductive tract, mouth, throat, eyes, and anus

J. Condition in which normal bacteria is replaced by an overgrowth of other bacterial forms

K. Muscular organ where the fetus grows

Multiple Choice

Read each item carefully and then select the one best response.

_____ **1.** Possible causes of vaginal bleeding include all of the following EXCEPT:

    A. ectopic pregnancy.

    B. cervical polyps.

    C. vaginal trauma.

    D. peptic ulcer.

_____ **2.** Painful urination associated with burning and a yellowish discharge is associated with:

    A. chlamydia.

    B. gonorrhea.

    C. endometriosis.

    D. syphilis.

_____ **3.** Which of the following statements is FALSE regarding assessment and treatment of a woman who was the victim of sexual assault?

    A. You may be called to testify in court regarding the incident.

    B. You should question the victim thoroughly about the assaulter in case the police missed any details.

    C. The patient should be given the option of being treated by a female responder.

    D. The patient should be discouraged from urinating or changing her clothes prior to examination at the hospital.

_____ **4.** The onset of menstruation usually occurs between the ages of:
    A. 8 and 10 years.
    B. 11 and 16 years.
    C. 16 and 18 years.
    D. 17 and 20 years.

_____ **5.** The most common presenting sign of PID is:
    A. vaginal discharge.
    B. fever.
    C. nausea and vomiting.
    D. lower abdominal pain.

_____ **6.** In rare cases, _____ causes arthritis that may be accompanied with skin lesions and inflammation of the eyes and urethra.
    A. chlamydia
    B. gonorrhea
    C. PID
    D. vaginal bleeding

_____ **7.** Left untreated, _____ can lead to premature birth or low birth weight in pregnant women.
    A. chlamydia
    B. gonorrhea
    C. bacterial vaginosis
    D. vaginal bleeding

_____ **8.** If a patient with vaginal bleeding presents with a rapid pulse and pale or cool skin, you should:
    A. attempt to locate the source of bleeding and correct it.
    B. place the patient in a supine position with her legs elevated.
    C. consider this to be a normal sign in a menstruating woman.
    D. inquire about recent problems with urination.

_____ **9.** When taking a history on a patient experiencing a gynecologic emergency, you should consider asking all of the following EXCEPT:
    A. Are you taking birth control?
    B. When was your last menstrual period?
    C. How many sexual partners have you had in the past?
    D. Do you have any history of sexually transmitted diseases?

_____ **10.** The "PID shuffle" refers to:
    A. a distinctive gait when the patient walks.
    B. rotation of the microorganisms that cause PID.
    C. symptoms that come and go.
    D. a structural abnormality in a patient's cervix.

_____ **11.** EMTs treating a patient of a sexual assault may not only be dealing with medical issues, but with _____ issues as well.
    A. psychological
    B. physiological
    C. educational
    D. sociological

_____ **12.** When performing a physical exam on a victim of sexual assault, you should:
    A. expose and evaluate the patient's vaginal area regardless of whether there is bleeding.
    B. allow multiple people to observe the examination in case you have to testify.
    C. limit your examination to a brief survey for life-threatening injuries.
    D. place the patient's clothes into a paper bag.

_____ **13.** Rape is considered to be a _____ diagnosis, not a medical diagnosis.

    A. psychological

    B. surgical

    C. sociological

    D. legal

_____ **14.** Often the most important intervention for a sexual assault patient is _____ and transport to a facility with a staff specially trained to deal with this scenario.

    A. comforting reassurance

    B. excellent assessment skills

    C. bandaging skills

    D. emotional sympathy

_____ **15.** Your _____ is the best tool to gain the patient's confidence to seek medical help.

    A. professionalism

    B. content knowledge

    C. compassion

    D. empathy

Questions 16-18 are derived from the following scenario: You are called to the scene of a possible assault. Upon arrival, you are directed by police to a dark room where you find a 22-year-old woman who says she was sexually assaulted by a coworker this afternoon.

_____ **16.** Your first course of action should be to:

    A. determine whether the patient is physically injured.

    B. establish the exact events of what took place.

    C. allow the patient to use the restroom.

    D. let the police question the patient before conducting a primary assessment.

_____ **17.** The second course of action involves the psychological care the patient. You should avoid:

    A. making attempts to get a female EMT to examine the patient.

    B. examination of the vaginal canal, even if active bleeding is taking place.

    C. attempting to gather information to assist the police.

    D. granting the patient's wishes for refusing care and transport.

_____ **18.** The patient tells you that she would really like to be transported to the hospital but refuses a physical examination. You should:

    A. explain to her that she cannot be transported without a physical exam.

    B. have the police take the patient into custody in order to legally force a physical exam.

    C. explain to her that this is a criminal case and that she must be examined.

    D. follow your system's refusal of treatment policy and respect the patient's wishes without judgment.

True/False

If you believe the statement to be more true than false, write the letter "T" in the space provided. If you believe the statement to be more false than true, write the letter "F."

_____ **1.** Chlamydial infection of the cervix can spread to the rectum, leading to rectal pain, discharge, or bleeding.

_____ **2.** If gonorrhea is not treated, the bacteria may enter the bloodstream and spread to other parts of the body, including the brain.

_____ **3.** Because menstrual bleeding is a monthly occurrence, it is not necessary to assess for other causes of vaginal bleeding.

_____ **4.** Obtaining an accurate and detailed patient assessment is critical when dealing with gynecologic issues.

_____ **5.** Most cases of gynecologic emergencies are not life threatening.

_____ **6.** Gynecologic emergencies are typically not embarrassing for women.

_____ **7.** When taking a history of a woman with a gynecologic complaint, you should inquire about the possibility of pregnancy and exposure to sexually transmitted diseases.

_____ **8.** Most presentations of tachycardia and hypotension are related to anxiety.

_____ **9.** Any report of syncope in a woman complaining of vaginal bleeding is considered significant.

_____ **10.** It is acceptable to place dressings into the vaginal canal to stop significant bleeding.

_____ **11.** When examining a female, you should limit the number of people involved.

_____ **12.** Gynecologic emergencies can occur at any age during a woman's lifetime.

_____ **13.** Injuries to the external genitals are typically not painful due to the very sparse nerve supply.

_____ **14.** When completing documentation of a sexual assault incident, adding your personal thoughts can help with the investigation.

_____ **15.** Determining the cause of vaginal bleeding should be of less importance than treating for shock and transporting the patient to an appropriate facility.

Fill-in-the-Blank

Read each item carefully and then complete the statement by filling in the missing words.

1. The _____ are located on each side of the lower abdomen and produce the ovum, or egg.

2. When a female reaches _____, she begins to ovulate and experience menstruation.

3. _____ _____ _____ is the most common gynecologic reason why women call for EMS.

4. _____ _____ can be very messy, sometimes involving large amounts of blood and bodily fluids.

5. _____ _____ and _____ _____ are two conditions that can cause vaginal bleeding in women who do not appear to be pregnant and who may not realize they are pregnant.

6. Make sure to use _____ _____ when attempting to control vaginal bleeding.

7. _____ _____ can cause significant blood loss and lead to hypovolemia.

8. You will need to work together with _____ _____ when dealing with a victim of sexual assault.

9. Symptoms of _____ appear approximately 2 to 10 days after exposure.

10. Women will continue to experience menstruation until they reach _____.

Labeling

Label the following diagrams with the correct terms.

1. Female Reproductive System

FRONT VIEW   SIDE VIEW

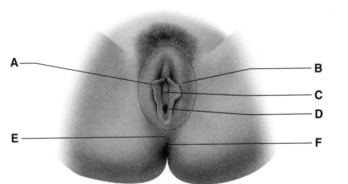

A. _____

B. _____

C. _____

D. _____

E. _____

2. External Genitalia

A. _____

B. _____

C. _____

D. _____

E. _____

F. _____

Crossword Puzzle

The following crossword puzzle is an activity provided to reinforce correct spelling and understanding of medical terminology associated with emergency care and the EMT. Use the clues in the column to complete the puzzle.

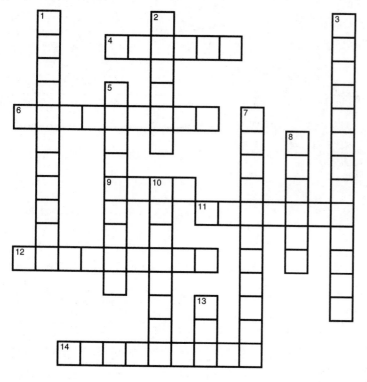

Across

4. The muscular organ where the fetus grows

6. _____ tubes connect each ovary with the uterus and are the primary location for fertilization of the ovum.

9. Sexual intercourse inflicted forcibly on another person, against that person's will

11. The primary female reproductive organs that produce an ovum, or egg

12. _____ vaginosis is an overgrowth of bacteria in the vagina.

14. A sexually transmitted disease caused by the bacterium Chlamydia trachomatis

Down

1. Outer fleshy "lips" covered with pubic hair that protect the vagina

2. The lower third, or neck, of the uterus

3. An attack against a person that is sexual in nature, the most common of which is rape

5. A sexually transmitted disease caused by Neisseria gonorrhoeae

7. Inner fleshy "lips" devoid of pubic hair that protect the vagina

8. The outermost cavity of a woman's reproductive system; the lower part of the birth canal

10. The area of skin between the vagina and the anus

13. An infection of the fallopian tubes and the surrounding tissues of the pelvis

Critical Thinking

Short Answer

Complete this section with short written answers using the space provided.

1. When performing your scene size-up, what questions should you ask yourself when dealing with a gynecologic emergency?

_____

_____

2. List at least five signs and symptoms commonly found with a gonorrhea infection.

_____

_____

3. Explain the general treatment strategies for vaginal bleeding.

_____

_____

Ambulance Calls

The following case scenarios provide an opportunity to explore the concerns associated with patient management and to enhance critical-thinking skills. Read each scenario and answer each question to the best of your ability.

1. You are dispatched to a local college campus for a 21-year-old woman with abdominal pain. The dispatcher tells you the patient has lower abdominal pain, fever, nausea, and vomiting. When you arrive on the campus, you are directed by campus police to the health center. There you find your patient lying supine on a bed. The patient tells you she has had lower abdominal pain and a fever for the past 24 hours. She describes the pain as "achy" and says it gets worse with walking. She believes she has a "stomach virus" due to the fever and vomiting. Your partner obtains vital signs as you continue with your assessment. After finishing your SAMPLE history, you casually ask if she has had any other recent illnesses or if she has any other complaints. The patient says, "Well, since you mentioned it, I've been having some rather foul vaginal discharge lately. But I just thought it would go away." The patient denies pregnancy because she just finished her menstrual period last week.

What is the likely cause of this patient's condition and how is it treated?

_____

_____

_____

2. You are dispatched to an apartment complex at 538 N. 10th Street, Apartment 4-C, for an assault. You look at your watch and note the time as 2101. On the way to the unit your partner remarks, "689th call for the year so far. No doubt we'll hit 700 before the end of the night." You make note of the incident number at 011689, and mark responding 2 minutes after dispatch. The additional information states this is for a 32-year-old woman who was sexually assaulted.

You arrive on scene 8 minutes after the initial dispatch, and notice the apartment is very well kept and is not cluttered. The police lead you to the back bedroom where you find your patient sitting up on the side of the bed speaking to the investigator. The patient appears alert, and you notice bleeding from the nose along with bruises to the patient's face. The patient tells you that she was raped by a maintenance worker at the apartment complex. She complains of pain to the nose, face, and groin. The patient says she is not sure whether she wants to go to the hospital, but definitely wants to take a shower and change her clothes.

Explain the key issues to consider when treating a victim of sexual assault.

_____

_____

_____

Fill-in-the-Patient Care Report

Using the previous case (Ambulance Call 2) and the additional information provided, complete the patient care report for this incident.

You explain to the patient that she should refrain from changing her clothes or washing because she could disrupt any potential evidence. The police agree with your statement.

As the police continue with some questions, you complete an initial assessment while your partner obtains the following vital signs at 2114: pulse, 102 beats/min; respirations, 22 breaths/min; blood pressure, 144/98 mm Hg; pulse oximetry, 98%.

You ask the patient if she would be more comfortable with a female EMT. Her response is a simple "No." The patient appears withdrawn and emotionally traumatized. You notice no obvious life-threatening injuries and ask the patient if she has bleeding anywhere. Her response, "No." The only visible external injuries you can find are multiple contusions to the face.

The patient does not make eye contact with you while questioning her medical history (diabetes), medications (lispro, Lantus, lisinopril), and allergies (none). When you ask her if she would like to tell you "what happened," she responds by saying, "Can't we just get going to the hospital? I would rather speak to the doctor."

You smile and say, "Absolutely."

Your partner applies oxygen at 2 L/min via nasal cannula. The patient is packaged on the litter and is loaded into the unit. Your partner verifies with the police the hospital destination, so they can continue with their investigation. You note that you were on scene a total of 11 minutes.

During transport, you notice that it has been 11 minutes since the vitals were assessed and ask the patient if she is having any pain. Her response, "No." You reassess the patient's vital signs: pulse, 108 beats/min; respirations, 20 breaths/min; blood pressure, 148/92 mm Hg; pulse oximetry, 97%.

Instead of calling in a report to the hospital, your partner calls in a basic update from the front of the cab so the patient does not relive the experience.

You arrive at the hospital about 6 minutes after you reassessed the vitals. Care is transferred over to the hospital staff, with no change in the patient's status. The nurse asks for a report, and you motion for her to leave the room with you. You give the report to the nurse away from the patient and any potential unnecessary personnel.

You and your partner don't have much to say to each other. The unit is cleaned and restocked, and you put yourself back in service at 2147.

Fill-in-the-Patient Care Report

EMS Patient Care Report (PCR)					
Date:	Incident No.:		Nature of Call:		Location:
Dispatched:	En Route:	At Scene:	Transport:	At Hospital:	In Service:
Patient Information					
Age: Sex: Weight (in kg [lb]):			Allergies: Medications: Past Medical History: Chief Complaint:		
Vital Signs					
Time:	BP:	Pulse:	Respirations:	Sao$_2$:	
Time:	BP:	Pulse:	Respirations:	Sao$_2$:	
Time:	BP:	Pulse:	Respirations:	Sao$_2$:	
EMS Treatment (circle all that apply)					
Oxygen @ ___ L/min via (circle one): NC NRM Bag-Mask Device		Assisted Ventilation	Airway Adjunct		CPR
Defibrillation	Bleeding Control	Bandaging	Splinting		Other Shock Treatment
Narrative					

Trauma Overview

General Knowledge

Matching

Match each of the items in the left column to the appropriate definition in the right column.

_____ **1.** Cavitation

_____ **2.** Multisystem trauma

_____ **3.** Kinetic energy

_____ **4.** Mechanism of injury (MOI)

_____ **5.** Potential energy

_____ **6.** Blunt trauma

_____ **7.** Penetrating trauma

_____ **8.** Work

A. Result of force to the body that causes injury but does not penetrate soft tissue or internal organs and cavities

B. Force acting over a distance

C. Product of mass, gravity, and height

D. Injury caused by objects that pierce the surface of the body

E. How trauma occurs

F. Energy of a moving object

G. Significant MOI that causes injuries to more than one body system

H. Emanation of pressure waves that can damage nearby structures

Multiple Choice

Read each item carefully and then select the one best response.

_____ **1.** Your awareness and concern for potentially serious obvious and underlying injuries is referred to as the:

   A. mechanism of injury.

   B. index of suspicion.

   C. scene size-up.

   D. general impression.

_____ **2.** The energy of a moving object is called:

   A. potential energy.

   B. thermal energy.

   C. kinetic energy.

   D. work.

_____ **3.** Energy can be:

   A. created.

   B. destroyed.

   C. converted.

   D. all of the above.

_____ **4.** The amount of kinetic energy that is converted to do work on the body dictates the _____ of the injury.

   A. location

   B. severity

   C. cause

   D. speed

_____ **5.** All of the following are considered types of motorcycle impacts EXCEPT:

    A. head-on collision.

    B. angular collision.

    C. controlled crash.

    D. rear collision.

_____ **6.** Which of the following is considered a type of impact from a motor vehicle collision?

    A. Ejection

    B. Rollover

    C. Crush

    D. Penetration

_____ **7.** The three collisions in a frontal impact include all of the following EXCEPT:

    A. car striking object.

    B. passenger striking vehicle.

    C. air bag striking passenger.

    D. internal organs striking solid structures of the body.

_____ **8.** Which of the following is NOT considered appropriate use of air medical services?

    A. The distance to a trauma center is greater than 25 miles.

    B. Traffic/road conditions make it unlikely to get the patient to the hospital in a timely manner.

    C. There is a mass-casualty incident.

    D. The closest trauma center is 10 minutes away by ground transport.

_____ **9.** Medium-velocity penetrating injuries may be caused by a:

    A. knife.

    B. military assault rifle.

    C. handgun.

    D. sling-shot.

_____ **10.** In a motor vehicle collision, as the passenger's head hits the windshield, the brain continues to move forward until it strikes the inside of the skull, resulting in a _____ injury.

    A. compression

    B. laceration

    C. lateral

    D. motion

_____ **11.** Your quick primary assessment of the patient and evaluation of the _____ can help to direct lifesaving care and provide critical information to the hospital staff.

    A. environment

    B. index of suspicion

    C. mechanism of injury

    D. abdominal area

_____ **12.** A contusion to a patient's forehead along with a spider-webbed windshield suggests possible injury to the:

    A. nose.

    B. brain.

    C. face.

    D. heart.

_____ 13. Which of the following is the MOST common cause of death from a blast injury?

    A. Amputation

    B. Burns

    C. Chest trauma

    D. Head trauma

_____ 14. Significant clues to the possibility of severe injuries in motor vehicle collisions include:

    A. death of a passenger.

    B. a blown out tire.

    C. broken glass.

    D. a deployed air bag.

_____ 15. Damage to the body that resulted from a pressure wave generated by an explosion is found in what type of blast injury?

    A. Primary

    B. Secondary

    C. Tertiary

    D. Miscellaneous

_____ 16. Air bags decrease injury to all of the following EXCEPT:

    A. chest.

    B. heart.

    C. face.

    D. head.

_____ 17. Optimally, on-scene time for critically injured patients should be less than _____ minutes.

    A. 5

    B. 10

    C. 15

    D. 20

_____ 18. _____ impacts are probably the number one cause of death associated with motor vehicle collisions.

    A. Frontal

    B. Lateral

    C. Rear-end

    D. Rollover

_____ 19. The most common life-threatening event in a rollover is _____ or partial ejection of the passenger from the vehicle.

    A. vehicle intrusion

    B. centrifugal force

    C. ejection

    D. spinal cord injury

_____ 20. A fall from more than _____ times the patient's height is considered to be significant.

    A. two

    B. three

    C. four

    D. five

Questions 21-24 are derived from the following scenario: A young boy was riding his bicycle down the street when he hit a parked car.

_____ **21.** How many collisions took place?
- **A.** 1
- **B.** 2
- **C.** 3
- **D.** 4

_____ **22.** What was the first collision?
- **A.** The bike hitting the car
- **B.** The bike rider hitting his bike or the car
- **C.** The bike rider's internal organs against the solid structures of the body
- **D.** The bike rider striking the pavement

_____ **23.** What was the second collision?
- **A.** The bike hitting the car
- **B.** The bide rider hitting his bike or the car
- **C.** The bike rider's internal organs against the solid structures of the body
- **D.** The bike rider striking the pavement

_____ **24.** What will raise your index of suspicion for this collision?
- **A.** The mechanism of injury
- **B.** The type of bike
- **C.** How loudly he's crying
- **D.** A quick visual assessment

_____ **25.** "For every action, there is an equal and opposite reaction" is:
- **A.** Newton's first law.
- **B.** Newton's second law.
- **C.** Newton's third law.
- **D.** a false statement.

_____ **26.** "A comprehensive regional resource capable of providing every aspect of trauma care from prevention through rehabilitation" is the definition of a _____ trauma center.
- **A.** Level I
- **B.** Level II
- **C.** Level III
- **D.** Level IV

_____ **27.** Which of the following is not considered a type of impact associated with a motorcycle crash?
- **A.** Head-on
- **B.** Rotational
- **C.** Controlled
- **D.** Ejection

_____ **28.** Burns from hot gases and respiratory injuries from inhaling toxic gas are associated with which type of blast injury?
- **A.** Primary
- **B.** Secondary
- **C.** Tertiary
- **D.** Miscellaneous

_____ **29.** A patient complaining of chest tightness, coughing up blood, and subcutaneous emphysema following an explosion may be suffering from a:

    A. myocardial blast injury.

    B. ruptured tympanic membrane.

    C. ruptured peritoneal cavity.

    D. pulmonary blast injury.

_____ **30.** Patients suffering from an open wound to the neck may suffer from all of the following EXCEPT:

    A. significant bleeding.

    B. air embolism.

    C. tension pneumothorax.

    D. subcutaneous crepitation.

True/False

If you believe the statement to be more true than false, write the letter "T" in the space provided. If you believe the statement to be more false than true, write the letter "F."

_____ **1.** Work is defined as force acting over distance.

_____ **2.** Energy can be both created and destroyed.

_____ **3.** The energy of a moving object is called potential energy.

_____ **4.** Rear-end collisions often cause whiplash injuries.

_____ **5.** Penetration or perforation to the chest wall is called an open chest wound.

_____ **6.** The injury potential of a fall is related to the height from which the patient fell.

_____ **7.** In the United States, traumatic injuries are the leading cause of death for people younger than 40 years of age.

_____ **8.** Rapid transport of an unstable trauma patient takes priority over assessing and managing the ABCs.

_____ **9.** Injuries to the aorta are relatively common in lateral impacts from a motor vehicle collision.

_____ **10.** Headrests are the major cause of whiplash-type injuries in rear-impact collisions.

_____ **11.** In car-versus-pedestrian collisions, the speed of the vehicle should be the first step in determining the mechanism of injury.

_____ **12.** Helmets are reliable at protecting against cervical spine injuries.

_____ **13.** Tertiary blast injuries result from flying debris, such as glass or shrapnel, striking the patient.

_____ **14.** You should perform frequent neurologic assessments in patients with a presumed head injury.

_____ **15.** All patients with chest trauma, regardless of the injury, should be reassessed every 5 minutes.

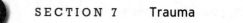

Fill-in-the-Blank

Read each item carefully and then complete the statement by filling in the missing words.

1. Energy that is available to cause injury _____ when an object's weight doubles, but

   _____ when its speed doubles.

2. _____ _____ causes injury by objects that pierce the surface of the body and cause

   damage to soft tissues, internal organs, and body cavities.

3. A compression injury to the anterior portion of the brain and stretching of the posterior portion is called a(n)

   _____ brain injury.

4. The formula for calculating kinetic energy is _____.

5. Whiplash-type injuries are typically caused by _____ impacts.

6. Air bags provide the final capture point of the passengers and decrease the severity of _____ injuries.

7. The top five causes of trauma death are motor vehicle collisions, falls, poisonings, _____, and

   drowning.

8. A "T-bone" collision typically refers to a(n) _____ impact.

9. The most common life-threatening event in a rollover collision is _____.

10. The liver, spleen, pancreas, and kidneys are all considered _____ organs in the abdomen.

11. The _____ _____ Scale uses eye opening, verbal response, and motor response to rate a

    patient's level of consciousness.

12. Air collecting between the lung tissue and the chest wall is commonly referred to as a(n) _____.

13. _____ _____ describes the limited on-scene time for patients with multisystem trauma.

14. _____ _____ _____ states that an object at rest tends to stay at rest,

    and an object in motion tends to stay in motion, unless acted on by some force.

15. A(n) _____ emergency occurs when the patient has an illness or condition that is not caused by an

    outside force.

Fill-in-the-Table

Fill in the missing parts of the table.

Recognizing Developing Problems in Trauma Patients		
Mechanism of Injury	**Signs and Symptoms**	**Index of Suspicion**
Blunt or penetrating trauma to the neck		• Significant bleeding or foreign bodies in the upper or lower airway, causing obstruction • Be alert for airway compromise.
Significant chest wall trauma from motor vehicle crashes, car-versus-pedestrian, and other crashes; penetrating trauma to the chest wall		• Cardiac or pulmonary contusion • Pneumothorax or hemothorax • Broken ribs, causing breathing compromise
Any significant blunt force trauma from motor vehicle crashes or penetrating injury		• Injuries in these regions may tear and cause damage to the large blood vessels located in these body areas, resulting in significant internal and external bleeding. • Be alert to the possibility of bruising to the brain and bleeding in and around the brain tissue, which may cause the development of excess pressure inside the skull around the brain.
Any significant blunt force trauma, falls from a significant height, or penetrating trauma		• Injuries to the bones of the spinal column or to the spinal cord

Crossword Puzzle

The following crossword puzzle is an activity provided to reinforce correct spelling and understanding of medical terminology associated with emergency care and the EMT. Use the clues in the column to complete the puzzle.

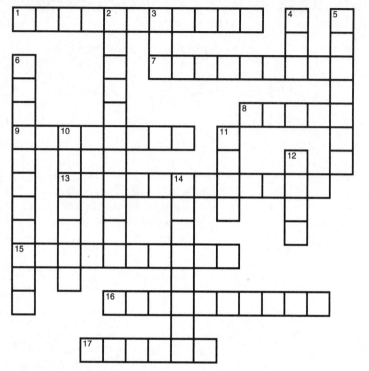

Across

1. An impact on the body without penetrating soft tissues or internal organs and cavities
7. Index of _____ is an awareness that unseen life-threatening injuries may exist.
8. Pulmonary trauma resulting from short-range exposure to the detonation of explosives is known a pulmonary _____ injury.
9. The _____ membrane is the eardrum.
13. The slowing of an object
15. The path a projectile takes once it is propelled
16. A phenomenon in which speed causes a bullet to generate pressure waves
17. Emergencies that are the result of physical forces applied to a patient's body are known as _____ emergencies.

Down

2. A score that takes into account the GCS score, respiratory rate, respiratory expansion, systolic blood pressure, and capillary refill
3. A scoring system used for patients with head trauma
4. The forces or energy transmission that cause injury
5. _____ energy is the energy of a moving object.
6. _____ trauma affects more than one body system.
10. _____ emergencies are illnesses or conditions not caused by an outside force.
11. Resistance that slows a projectile, such as air
12. The product of force times distance
14. Air bubbles in the arterial blood vessels are known as an arterial air _____.

Critical Thinking

Short Answer

Complete this section with short written answers using the space provided.

1. Describe potential energy.

_____

_____

2. List the series of collisions typical with motor vehicles.

_____

_____

3. List the three factors to consider when evaluating a fall.

_____

_____

4. Describe the phenomenon of cavitation as it relates to an injury from a bullet.

_____

_____

5. Why is it important to try to determine the type of gun and ammunition used when you are caring for a gunshot victim?

_____

_____

6. What type of injuries can you expect from a motor vehicle collision with a lateral impact and substantial intrusion?

_____

_____

7. List the information you should gather when determining the MOI of a motorcycle crash.

_____

_____

8. List the American College of Surgeons criteria for a Level I trauma patient.

_____

_____

Ambulance Calls

The following case scenarios provide an opportunity to explore the concerns associated with patient management and to enhance critical-thinking skills. Read each scenario and answer each question to the best of your ability.

1. You are dispatched to a one-car MVC. As you arrive, you notice that the car hit a large deer, which is lying in the road, dead. Highway speed limits on this road are 65 mph (105 kph). The driver was restrained with a lap belt only, and his vehicle was not equipped with air bags. He is complaining of head and neck pain and tells you that he doesn't remember what happened.

How would you best manage this patient?

_____

_____

_____

2. You are dispatched to assist a man who fell from a ladder as he was repairing shingles on the roof of his two-story home. You arrive to find an unconscious middle-aged man lying on the ground. He is breathing and has a pulse. The call to 9-1-1 was placed after the man was found by a neighbor.

How would you best manage this patient?

_____

_____

_____

3. You are called to the residence of a 19-year-old man who was stabbed in the abdomen with an ice pick. The scene is safe, and the patient is lying on the floor with the ice pick impaled in his left lower quadrant. Bystanders tell you he did not fall. He is alert and complaining of severe pain.

How would you best manage this patient?

_____

_____

_____

4. You are called to the scene of a pedestrian struck by a motor vehicle in a residential neighborhood. As you approach the scene, you notice a vehicle pulled off to the side with damage to its bumper and hood and what appears to be a person lying unresponsive in the roadway.

What factors do you need to consider when determining the mechanism of injury?

_____

_____

_____

CHAPTER

Bleeding

23

General Knowledge

Matching

Match each of the items in the left column to the appropriate definition in the right column.

_____ **1.** Pulmonary artery

_____ **2.** Heart

_____ **3.** Ventricle

_____ **4.** Aorta

_____ **5.** Atrium

_____ **6.** Pulmonary vein

_____ **7.** Coagulation

_____ **8.** Ecchymosis

_____ **9.** Epistaxis

_____ **10.** Hematoma

_____ **11.** Hemophilia

_____ **12.** Hemorrhage

_____ **13.** Hypovolemic shock

A. Mass of blood in the soft tissues beneath the skin

B. Formation of clot to plug opening in injured blood vessel, stopping blood flow

C. Upper chamber

D. A congenital condition in which a patient lacks one or more of the blood's normal clotting factors

E. Hollow muscular organ

F. Largest artery in body

G. A condition in which low blood volume results in inadequate perfusion

H. Oxygenated blood travels through this

I. Bruising

J. Deoxygenated blood travels through this

K. Lower chamber

L. Bleeding

M. Nosebleed

Multiple Choice

Read each item carefully and then select the one best response.

_____ **1.** The function of the blood is to _____ all of the body's cells and tissues.

    A. remove oxygen from

    B. deliver nutrients to

    C. carry waste products to

    D. all of the above

_____ **2.** The cardiovascular system consists of:

    A. a pump.

    B. a container.

    C. fluid.

    D. all of the above.

_____ **3.** Blood leaves each chamber of a normal heart through a(n):

    A. vein.

    B. artery.

    C. one-way valve.

    D. capillary.

_____ **4.** Blood enters the right atrium from the:
   A. coronary arteries.
   B. lungs.
   C. vena cava.
   D. coronary veins.

_____ **5.** Blood enters the left atrium from the:
   A. coronary arteries.
   B. lungs.
   C. vena cava.
   D. coronary veins.

_____ **6.** The only arteries in the body that carry deoxygenated blood are the:
   A. pulmonary arteries.
   B. coronary arteries.
   C. femoral arteries.
   D. subclavian arteries.

_____ **7.** The _____ is the thickest chamber of the heart.
   A. right atrium
   B. right ventricle
   C. left atrium
   D. left ventricle

_____ **8.** The _____ link(s) the arterioles and the venules.
   A. aorta
   B. capillaries
   C. vena cava
   D. valves

_____ **9.** At the arterial end of the capillaries, the muscles dilate and constrict in response to conditions such as:
   A. fright.
   B. a specific need for oxygen.
   C. a need to dispose of metabolic wastes.
   D. all of the above.

_____ **10.** Blood contains all of the following EXCEPT:
   A. white blood cells.
   B. plasma.
   C. cerebrospinal fluid.
   D. platelets.

_____ **11.** _____ is the circulation of blood within an organ or tissue in adequate amounts to meet the cells' current needs for oxygen, nutrients, and waste removal.
   A. Anatomy
   B. Perfusion
   C. Physiology
   D. Conduction

_____ **12.** The _____ only require(s) a minimal blood supply when at rest.
   A. lungs
   B. kidneys
   C. muscles
   D. heart

_____ 13. The term _____ means "constantly adapting to changing conditions."

    A. perfusion

    B. conduction

    C. dynamic

    D. autonomic

_____ 14. _____ is inadequate tissue perfusion.

    A. Shock

    B. Hyperperfusion

    C. Hypertension

    D. Contraction

_____ 15. The brain and spinal cord usually cannot go for more than _____ minutes without perfusion, or the nerve cells will be permanently damaged.

    A. 30 to 45

    B. 12 to 20

    C. 8 to 10

    D. 4 to 6

_____ 16. An organ or tissue that is considerably _____ is much better able to resist damage from hypoperfusion.

    A. warmer

    B. colder

    C. younger

    D. older

_____ 17. The body will not tolerate an acute blood loss of greater than _____ of blood volume.

    A. 10%

    B. 20%

    C. 30%

    D. 40%

_____ 18. If the typical adult loses more than 1 L of blood, significant changes in vital signs, such as _____, will occur.

    A. decreased heart rate

    B. increased respiratory rate

    C. increased blood pressure

    D. all of the above

_____ 19. _____ shock is a condition in which low blood volume results in inadequate perfusion or even death.

    A. Hypovolemic

    B. Metabolic

    C. Septic

    D. Psychogenic

_____ 20. You should consider bleeding to be serious if all of the following conditions are present EXCEPT:

    A. blood loss is rapid.

    B. there is no mechanism of injury.

    C. the patient has a poor general appearance.

    D. assessment reveals signs and symptoms of shock.

_____ **21.** Significant blood loss demands your immediate attention as soon as the _____ has been managed.
   A. fracture
   B. extrication
   C. airway
   D. none of the above

_____ **22.** The process of blood clotting and plugging the hole is called:
   A. conglomeration.
   B. configuration.
   C. coagulation.
   D. coalition.

_____ **23.** Even though the body is very efficient at controlling bleeding on its own, it may fail in situations such as:
   A. when medications interfere with normal clotting.
   B. when damage to the vessel may be so large that a clot cannot completely block the hole.
   C. when only part of the vessel wall is cut, preventing it from constricting.
   D. all of the above.

_____ **24.** A lack of one or more of the blood's clotting factors is called:
   A. a deficiency.
   B. hemophilia.
   C. platelet anomaly.
   D. anemia.

_____ **25.** You respond to a 25-year-old man who has cut his arm with a circular saw. The bleeding appears to be bright red and spurting. The patient is alert and oriented and converses with you freely. He appears to be stable at this point. What is your first step in controlling his bleeding?
   A. Direct pressure
   B. Maintain the airway
   C. Standard precautions
   D. Elevation

_____ **26.** When applying a bandage to hold a dressing in place, stretch the bandage tight enough to control the bleeding but not so tight as to decrease _____ to the extremity.
   A. blood flow
   B. pulses
   C. oxygen
   D. CRTs

_____ **27.** If bleeding continues after applying a pressure dressing, you should do all of the following EXCEPT:
   A. remove the dressing and apply another sterile dressing.
   B. apply manual pressure through the dressing.
   C. add more gauze pads over the first dressing.
   D. secure both dressings tighter with a roller bandage.

_____ **28.** When using an air splint to control bleeding in a fractured extremity, you should reassess the _____ frequently.
   A. airway
   B. breathing
   C. circulation in the injured extremity
   D. fracture site

_____ **29.** When treating a patient with signs and symptoms of hypovolemic shock and no outward signs of bleeding, always consider the possibility of bleeding into the:

   A. thoracic cavity.

   B. abdomen.

   C. skull.

   D. chest.

_____ **30.** Nontraumatic internal bleeding may be caused by a(n):

   A. ulcer.

   B. ruptured ectopic pregnancy.

   C. aneurysm.

   D. all of the above.

_____ **31.** The most common symptom of internal abdominal bleeding is:

   A. bruising around the abdomen.

   B. distention of the abdomen.

   C. rigidity of the abdomen.

   D. acute abdominal pain.

_____ **32.** Signs and symptoms of internal bleeding in both trauma and medical patients include:

   A. hematemesis.

   B. melena.

   C. hemoptysis.

   D. all of the above.

_____ **33.** The first sign of hypovolemic shock is a change in:

   A. respirations.

   B. heart rate.

   C. mental status.

   D. blood pressure.

True/False

If you believe the statement to be more true than false, write the letter "T" in the space provided. If you believe the statement to be more false than true, write the letter "F."

_____ **1.** Venous blood tends to spurt and is difficult to control.

_____ **2.** The human body is tolerant of blood losses greater than 20% of blood volume.

_____ **3.** The first step in controlling external bleeding is applying pressure to the proximal artery.

_____ **4.** The first step in preparing to treat a bleeding patient is standard precautions.

_____ **5.** A properly applied tourniquet should be loosened by the EMT every 10 minutes.

_____ **6.** A patient who has swallowed a lot of blood may become nauseated and vomit.

_____ **7.** You should contact medical control every time serious bleeding is encountered.

_____ **8.** If a wound continues to bleed after it is bandaged, you should remove the bandage and start over again.

_____ **9.** A tourniquet is always required for massive spurting blood loss.

_____ **10.** You should provide high-flow oxygen whenever you suspect internal bleeding.

Fill-in-the-Blank

Read each item carefully and then complete the statement by filling in the missing words.

1. The _____ side of the heart receives oxygen-poor blood from the veins.

2. _____ is the circulation of blood within an organ or tissue in adequate amounts to meet the cells' current needs for oxygen, nutrients, and waste removal.

3. A(n) _____ is also called a contusion.

4. _____ bleeding is any bleeding in a cavity or space inside the body.

5. A systolic blood pressure of less than _____ mm Hg with a weak, rapid pulse suggests the presence of hypoperfusion in a patient who may have significant bleeding.

6. _____ is vomited blood.

7. _____ blood is dark red and oozes from a wound steadily but slowly.

8. The _____ _____ system monitors the body's needs from moment to moment and adjusts blood flow by changing the vascular tone, as needed.

9. _____ are small tubes that are about the same diameter as a single red blood cell.

10. The heart is a(n) _____ muscle that is under the control of the autonomic nervous system.

Labeling

Label the following diagrams with the correct terms.

1. The Left and Right Sides of the Heart

A. _____

B. _____

C. _____

D. _____

E. _____

F. _____

G. _____

H. _____

I. _____

J. _____

K. _____

L. _____

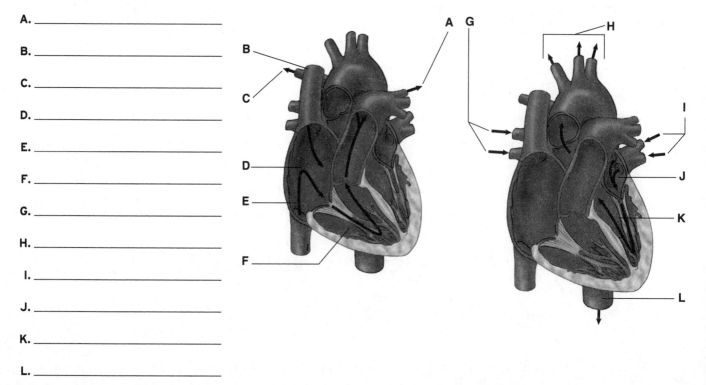

2. Perfusion

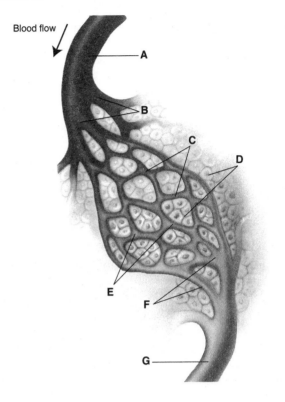

Blood flow

A. _____

B. _____

C. _____

D. _____

E. _____

F. _____

G. _____

3. Arterial Pressure Points

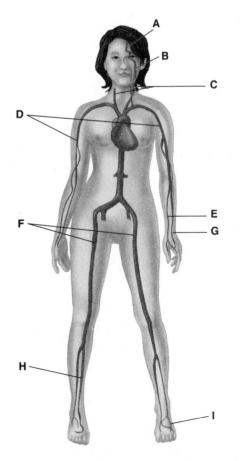

A. _____

B. _____

C. _____

D. _____

E. _____

F. _____

G. _____

H. _____

I. _____

Crossword Puzzle

The following crossword puzzle is an activity provided to reinforce correct spelling and understanding of medical terminology associated with emergency care and the EMT. Use the clues in the column to complete the puzzle.

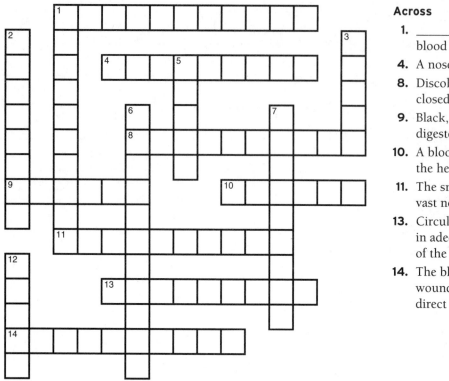

Across

1. _____ shock is a condition in which low blood volume results in inadequate perfusion.

4. A nosebleed

8. Discoloration of the skin associated with a closed wound

9. Black, foul-smelling, tarry stool containing digested blood

10. A blood vessel that carries blood away from the heart

11. The smallest branches of arteries leading to the vast network of capillaries

13. Circulation of blood within an organ or tissue in adequate amounts to meet the current needs of the cells

14. The bleeding control method used when a wound continues to bleed despite the use of direct pressure and elevation.

Down

1. A congenital condition in which the patient lacks one or more of the blood's normal clotting factors

2. A mass of blood in the soft tissues beneath the skin

3. The blood vessels that carry blood from the tissues to the heart

5. A condition in which the circulatory system fails to provide sufficient circulation so that every body part can perform its function

6. Vomited blood

7. A bruise, or ecchymosis

12. The main artery that receives blood from the left ventricle and delivers it to all the other arteries that carry blood to the tissues of the body

Critical Thinking

Multiple Choice
Read each critical-thinking item carefully and then select the one best response.

_____ 1. You and your partner respond to a patient who has had his hand nearly severed by a drill press. As you approach, you note that the patient is pale and there appears to be a lot of blood on the floor. The wound continues to bleed copiously. After applying a tourniquet, you write _____ and _____ on a piece of adhesive tape and apply it to the patient's forehead.

    A. the patient's name; tourniquet location

    B. your last name; unit number

    C. the letters "TK"; the exact time applied

    D. the date and time; estimated amount of blood loss

_____ 2. In the above call, when applying the tourniquet you know you must be sure to:

    A. use the narrowest bandage possible to minimize the area restricted.

    B. cover the tourniquet with a bandage.

    C. never pad underneath the tourniquet.

    D. not loosen the tourniquet after you have applied it.

_____ 3. You are called to a playground for an 8-year-old girl who has an uncontrolled nosebleed. The child is crying and will not talk to you. The babysitter and other children present did not witness any trauma, but there is a bump on the temporal portion of the girl's head. The babysitter does state that the girl has had a cold for several days but can give you no further information on her medical history. What could be the possible cause(s) of the bleeding?

    A. A skull fracture

    B. Sinusitis

    C. Coagulation disorder

    D. All of the above

_____ 4. You respond to a 33-year-old man who was hit in the ear by a line drive during a softball game. He is complaining of a severe headache, ringing in his ears, and dizziness. He has blood draining from his ear. Why would you not apply pressure to control bleeding?

    A. It should be collected to be reinfused at the hospital.

    B. It could collect within the head and increase the pressure on the brain.

    C. It is contaminated.

    D. You could fracture the skull with the pressure needed to staunch the flow of blood.

_____ 5. You are dispatched to a store in the downtown mall for an arm injury. When you arrive, you are directed to a small stock room where you find a teenaged girl holding a blood-soaked cloth tightly onto her left forearm. You notice blood droplets high up the wall and on the floor several feet from where she is sitting. "I was opening a shipment with a box-cutter," she says, her skin noticeably pale. "And it slipped and cut my arm." What type of bleeding should you anticipate?

    A. You should suspect heavy venous bleeding.

    B. She most likely has arterial bleeding.

    C. Internal bleeding is probably causing her skin to appear pale.

    D. Very sharp blades usually only cause capillary bleeding.

Short Answer

Complete this section with short written answers using the space provided.

1. Describe how the autonomic nervous system responds to severe bleeding.

   _____

   _____

2. Describe the characteristics of bleeding from each type of vessel (artery, vein, capillary).

   _____

   _____

3. List, in the proper sequence, the methods by which an EMT should attempt to control external bleeding.

   _____

   _____

4. List 10 signs and symptoms of hypovolemic shock.

   _____

   _____

5. List, in the proper sequence, the general EMT emergency care for patients with internal bleeding.

   _____

   _____

Ambulance Calls

The following case scenarios provide an opportunity to explore the concerns associated with patient management and to enhance critical-thinking skills. Read each scenario and answer each question to the best of your ability.

1. You arrive at a local school playground for a 9-year-old boy with a minor laceration on his left wrist. The teacher, who is holding a blood-soaked dressing on the boy's wound, tells you that she cannot stop the bleeding and that the boy has a history of hemophilia. The blood is steady, but not spurting, and dark in color.

   How would you best manage this patient?

   _____

   _____

   _____

2. You are dispatched to a local lumberyard for some sort of machinery accident. When you arrive, you observe a man sitting on the ground, surrounded by coworkers. The very pale foreman runs up to you as you get out of the truck and says, "His shirt got caught in a chop saw. His arm got cut off just below the elbow." As you approach, you see that the man is holding a blood-soaked towel to the shortened end of his right arm.

   How would you best manage this patient?

   _____

   _____

   _____

3. Your team is called to the local jail for an inmate who has injured his arm with a ballpoint pen. You find that he is bleeding continuously from a wound that is in the area of the antecubital vein of his left arm.

   How would you best manage this patient?

   _____

   _____

   _____

Fill-in-the-Patient Care Report

Read the incident scenario and then complete the following patient care report (PCR).

You and your partner are posted at the corner of Seventh Street and Brogan Avenue, completing the paperwork for a recent respiratory distress call, when emergency tones burst from the radio.

"Two-fifty-three, priority traffic," the dispatcher says immediately.

"Go ahead two-fifty-three," you respond.

"Two-fifty-three, code-three call to 1-4-6-7 Abner Lane for a leg laceration. Show your time of dispatch at sixteen-fifty-three."

You copy the assignment and slowly roll out into traffic after activating the lights and siren, proceeding to the address about six blocks away.

Five minutes later, you pull up outside of a well-kept home in a newly completed subdivision and are met by woman frantically waving her arms.

"Please hurry!" she shouts as you open your door. "My husband was chopping wood in the backyard and hit himself with the axe. He's bleeding real bad!"

You and your partner grab your bags and walk quickly to the home's backyard. The man, whom you estimate to be about 170 pounds (76.5 kg), is sitting on the redwood deck, pale and shaking, holding an old bloody T-shirt against his lower left leg; a huge circle of blood is soaking into the wood deck under him.

"Sir, we're from the city ambulance service and we're here to help you," you say, kneeling next to the man. "Can you tell me what happened?"

As the 42-year-old man describes how the axe glanced off a knot in the log that he was chopping, sending it deep into the flesh of his leg, you remove the T-shirt from the wound, observing a jagged laceration approximately 3.5″ (9-cm) long, and replace it with a wide trauma dressing. Your partner then places a nonrebreathing mask on the patient with the supplemental oxygen set to 15 L/min and begins assessing vitals.

At 1704, your partner reports the patient's vitals as: blood pressure 136/86 mm Hg; pulse 88 beats/min, strong and regular; respirations 16 breaths/min with good tidal volume; pale, cool, and diaphoretic skin; and pulse oximetry is 97%.

About 5 minutes after obtaining vitals, you have stopped the bleeding using a pressure bandage and are loading the patient into the ambulance, keeping him covered with a blanket and positioning him in Trendelenburg's position.

His wife tells you that he is allergic to amoxicillin and that he has been taking a cholesterol medication called Crestor ever since he suffered a transient ischemic attack in the spring of last year. You thank her for the information and climb into the patient compartment while your partner jumps into the driver's seat. Within a minute, you are en route to the Southside Medical Center emergency department and taking the patient's vitals again. This time they are: blood pressure, 122/76 mm Hg; pulse, 102 beats/min, weak and regular; respirations, 20 breaths/min and shallow, but with adequate tidal volume; skin is still pale, cool, and diaphoretic; and pulse oximetry is 94%.

At 1715 you arrive at the ambulance bay of the Southside Medical Center, quickly move the patient inside, and transfer his care to the emergency department staff. After giving a full report to the receiving nurse and properly cleaning and preparing the ambulance, you and your partner go back available at 1735.

EMS Patient Care Report (PCR)

Date:	Incident No.:	Nature of Call:		Location:	
Dispatched:	En Route:	At Scene:	Transport:	At Hospital:	In Service:

Patient Information

Age: Sex: Weight (in kg [lb]):	Allergies: Medications: Past Medical History: Chief Complaint:

Vital Signs

Time:	BP:	Pulse:	Respirations:	Sao$_2$:
Time:	BP:	Pulse:	Respirations:	Sao$_2$:
Time:	BP:	Pulse:	Respirations:	Sao$_2$:

EMS Treatment
(circle all that apply)

Oxygen @ ___ L/min via (circle one): NC NRM Bag-Mask Device	Assisted Ventilation	Airway Adjunct	CPR
Defibrillation	Bleeding Control	Bandaging	Splinting	Other Shock Treatment

Narrative

Skills

Skill Drills

Test your knowledge of these skills by filling in the correct words in the photo captions.

Skill Drill 23-1: Controlling External Bleeding

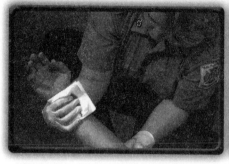 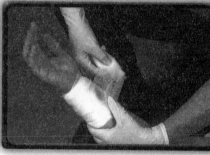 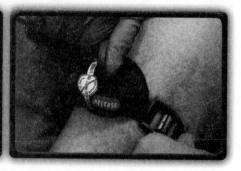

1. Apply _____
_____ over the
wound. Elevate the injury above
the _____ of
the _____ if no
_____ is suspected.

2. Apply a(n) _____
_____.

3. If direct pressure with a(n)
_____
_____ does not
control the bleeding, apply a(n)
_____ above the
level of the _____.

Skill Drill 23-2: Applying a Commercial Tourniquet

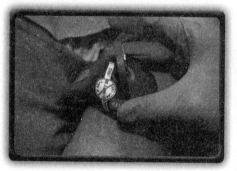 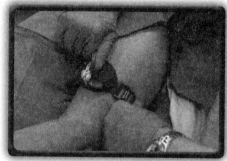

1. Hold _____
over the bleeding site and
place the tourniquet just
_____ the injury.

2. Click the buckle into place, pull the
strap tight, and turn the tightening
dial _____ until
pulses are no longer palpable
_____ to the
tourniquet or until bleeding has been
_____.

Assessment Review

Answer the following questions pertaining to the assessment of the types of emergencies discussed in this chapter.

_____ **1.** When you are performing a scene size-up on a patient with external bleeding, the minimum standard precautions that should be taken are:

    A. gloves and gown.

    B. gown and eye protection.

    C. gloves and eye protection.

    D. gown and face mask.

_____ **2.** For a patient with suspected internal bleeding, you should assess circulation by checking the pulse for:

    A. rate and quality.

    B. rate and rhythm.

    C. quality and rhythm.

    D. presence.

_____ **3.** If you have completed your primary assessment and transport decision on an unresponsive patient with a significant mechanism of injury, what components should be included in the secondary assessment?

    A. Quick check for life-threatening injuries

    B. Systemic body scan

    C. Determination of scene safety

    D. A comprehensive reassessment

_____ **4.** Your external bleeding patient needs a detailed physical exam. When should it be performed?

    A. Immediately after the primary assessment

    B. During the reassessment

    C. When you arrive at the patient's side

    D. En route to the hospital

_____ **5.** What should be included in the communications to the hospital when dealing with a patient with suspected internal bleeding?

    A. Amount of blood loss

    B. Location of the bleeding

    C. Interventions performed

    D. Patient's blood type

Emergency Care Summary

Fill in the following chart pertaining to the management of the types of emergencies discussed in this chapter.

NOTE: Although the following steps are widely accepted, be sure to consult with and follow your local protocol.

External Bleeding

Steps to Caring for Patient With External Bleeding
1. Follow standard precautions—at least gloves and eye protection.
2. Maintain cervical stabilization if MOI suggests possible _____ _____.
3. Administer high-flow oxygen as necessary, once significant bleeding is controlled.
4. Control external bleeding using as many of the following means as necessary:
- _____ _____, elevation, and pressure dressings
- Tourniquets
- _____
5. Apply direct local pressure to bleeding site, elevate the bleeding extremity, and apply a(n) _____ dressing.
6. If bleeding is not immediately controlled with the use of direct pressure, apply a(n) _____. Follow local protocol for approved methods of bleeding control.

Applying a Commercial Tourniquet
1. Follow standard precautions.
2. Hold direct pressure over the bleeding site.
3. Place the tourniquet around the extremity just _____ the bleeding site.
4. Click the _____ into place and pull the strap tight.
5. Turn the tightening dial _____ until pulses are no longer palpable distal to the tourniquet or until bleeding is controlled.

Treating Epistaxis
1. Follow standard precautions.
2. Help the patient to sit, leaning forward.
3. Apply direct pressure for at least _____ minutes by pinching nostrils together.
4. Keep the patient calm and quiet.
5. Apply ice over the nose.
6. Maintain the pressure until bleeding is completely controlled.
7. Provide prompt transport.
8. If bleeding cannot be controlled, transport patient immediately. Treat for _____ and administer oxygen via nonrebreathing mask if necessary.

Internal Bleeding

Steps to Caring for Patient with Internal Bleeding
1. Follow standard precautions.
2. Maintain the airway with cervical immobilization if MOI suggests possible spinal injury.
3. Administer high-flow oxygen and provide artificial ventilation as necessary.
4. Control all obvious external bleeding.
5. Apply a(n) _____ to an extremity where internal bleeding is suspected.
6. Monitor and record vital signs at least every 5 minutes.
7. Give the patient _____ by mouth.
8. Elevate the legs 6" to 12" (15 to 31 cm) in nontrauma patients.
9. Keep the patient warm.
10. Provide immediate transport for patients with signs and symptoms of shock. Report changes in the patient's condition to hospital personnel.

Soft-Tissue Injuries

General Knowledge

Matching

Match each of the items in the left column to the appropriate definition in the right column.

_____ 1. Dermis

_____ 2. Sweat glands

_____ 3. Epidermis

_____ 4. Mucous membranes

_____ 5. Sebaceous glands

_____ 6. Abrasion

_____ 7. Laceration

_____ 8. Penetrating wound

_____ 9. Avulsion

_____ 10. Evisceration

A. Gunshot wound

B. Cool the body by discharging a substance through the pores

C. Tissue hanging as a flap from a wound

D. Tough external layer forming a watertight covering for the body

E. Razor cut

F. Secrete a watery substance that lubricates the openings of the mouth and nose

G. Inner layer of skin that contains the structures that give skin its characteristic appearance

H. Produce oil, which waterproofs the skin and keeps it supple

I. Exposed intestines

J. Skinned knee

Multiple Choice

Read each item carefully and then select the one best response.

_____ 1. The _____ is (are) our first line of defense against external forces.

A. extremities

B. hair

C. skin

D. lips

_____ 2. The skin covering the _____ is quite thick.

A. lips

B. scalp

C. ears

D. eyelids

_____ 3. As the cells on the surface of the skin are worn away, new cells form in the _____ layer.

A. dermal

B. germinal

C. epidermal

D. subcutaneous

_____ 4. The hair follicles, sweat glands, and sebaceous glands are found in the:

A. dermis.

B. germinal layer.

C. epidermis.

D. subcutaneous layer.

_____ 5. The skin regulates temperature in a cold environment by:
   A. secreting sweat through sweat glands.
   B. constricting the blood vessels.
   C. dilating the blood vessels.
   D. increasing the amount of heat that is radiated from the body's surface.

_____ 6. Closed soft-tissue injuries are characterized by all of the following EXCEPT:
   A. pain at the site of injury.
   B. swelling beneath the skin.
   C. damage of the protective layer of skin.
   D. a history of blunt trauma.

_____ 7. A(n) _____ occurs whenever a large blood vessel is damaged and bleeds.
   A. contusion
   B. hematoma
   C. crushing injury
   D. avulsion

_____ 8. A(n) _____ is usually associated with extensive tissue damage.
   A. contusion
   B. hematoma
   C. crushing injury
   D. avulsion

_____ 9. A hematoma can result from:
   A. a soft-tissue injury.
   B. a fracture.
   C. any injury to a large blood vessel.
   D. all of the above.

_____ 10. A(n) _____ occurs when a great amount of force is applied to the body for a long period of time.
   A. contusion
   B. hematoma
   C. crushing injury
   D. avulsion

_____ 11. More extensive closed injuries may involve significant swelling and bleeding beneath the skin, which could lead to:
   A. compartment syndrome.
   B. contamination.
   C. hypovolemic shock.
   D. hemothorax.

_____ 12. Open soft-tissue wounds include all of the following EXCEPT:
   A. abrasions.
   B. contusions.
   C. lacerations.
   D. avulsions.

_____ 13. A laceration may be:
   A. linear.
   B. deep.
   C. jagged.
   D. all of the above.

_____ **14.** Because shootings usually end up in court, it is important to factually and completely document:

  A. the circumstances surrounding any gunshot injury.

  B. the patient's condition.

  C. the treatment given.

  D. all of the above.

_____ **15.** All open wounds are assumed to be _____ and present a risk of infection.

  A. contaminated

  B. life-threatening

  C. minimal

  D. extensive

_____ **16.** Before you begin caring for a patient with an open wound, you should:

  A. survey the scene.

  B. follow standard precautions.

  C. be sure the patient has an open airway.

  D. all of the above.

_____ **17.** Splinting an extremity even when there is no fracture can help to:

  A. reduce pain.

  B. minimize damage to an already-injured extremity.

  C. make it easier to move the patient.

  D. all of the above.

_____ **18.** Treatment for an abdominal evisceration includes:

  A. pushing the exposed organs back into the abdominal cavity.

  B. covering the organs with dry dressings.

  C. flexing the knees and legs to relieve pressure on the abdomen.

  D. applying moist, adherent dressings.

_____ **19.** An open neck injury may result in _____ if enough air is sucked into a blood vessel.

  A. hypovolemic shock

  B. tracheal deviation

  C. air embolism

  D. subcutaneous emphysema

_____ **20.** Burns may result from:

  A. heat.

  B. toxic chemicals.

  C. electricity.

  D. all of the above.

_____ **21.** Factors that can aid in determining the severity of a burn include:

  A. the depth of the burn.

  B. the extent of the burn.

  C. whether critical areas are involved.

  D. all of the above.

_____ **22.** _____ burns involve only the epidermis.

  A. Full-thickness

  B. Second-degree

  C. Superficial

  D. Third-degree

_____ 23. _____ burns cause intense pain.
   A. First-degree
   B. Second-degree
   C. Superficial
   D. Third-degree

_____ 24. _____ burns may involve the subcutaneous layers, muscle, bone, or internal organs.
   A. Superficial
   B. Partial-thickness
   C. Full-thickness
   D. Second-degree

_____ 25. Significant airway burns may be associated with:
   A. singeing of the hair within the nostrils.
   B. hoarseness.
   C. hypoxia.
   D. all of the above.

_____ 26. The most important consideration when dealing with electrical burns is:
   A. standard precautions.
   B. scene safety.
   C. level of responsiveness.
   D. airway.

_____ 27. Treatment of electrical burns includes:
   A. maintaining the airway.
   B. monitoring the patient closely for respiratory or cardiac arrest.
   C. splinting any suspected injuries.
   D. all of the above.

_____ 28. Which of the following should NOT be used as an occlusive dressing?
   A. Gauze pads
   B. Vaseline gauze
   C. Aluminum foil
   D. Plastic

_____ 29. Using elastic bandages to secure dressings may result in _____ if the injury swells or if the bandages are applied improperly.
   A. additional tissue damage
   B. loss of a limb
   C. impaired circulation
   D. all of the above

_____ 30. Burns are diffuse soft-tissue injuries created by destructive energy transfers from all of the following sources EXCEPT:
   A. thermal sources.
   B. kinetic sources.
   C. radiation sources.
   D. electrical sources.

_____ 31. _____ is an acute, potentially fatal viral infection of the central nervous system that affects all warm-blooded animals.
   A. Streptococcus
   B. Rabies
   C. Tuberculosis
   D. Emboli

True/False

If you believe the statement to be more true than false, write the letter "T" in the space provided. If you believe the statement to be more false than true, write the letter "F."

_____   **1.** Partial-thickness burns involve the epidermis and some portion of the dermis.

_____   **2.** Blisters are commonly seen with superficial burns.

_____   **3.** Severe burns are usually a combination of superficial, partial-thickness, and full-thickness burns.

_____   **4.** The rule of nines allows you to estimate the percentage of body surface area that has been burned.

_____   **5.** Two factors, depth and extent, are critical in assessing the severity of a burn.

_____   **6.** Your first responsibility with a burn patient is to stop the burning process.

_____   **7.** Burned areas should be immersed in cool water for up to 30 minutes.

_____   **8.** Electrical burns are always more severe than the external signs indicate.

_____   **9.** The hallmark sign of compartment syndrome is severe but painless swelling.

_____   **10.** Occlusive dressings are usually made of Vaseline gauze, aluminum foil, or plastic.

_____   **11.** Gauze pads prevent air and liquids from entering or exiting the wound.

_____   **12.** Elastic bandages can be used to secure dressings.

_____   **13.** Soft roller bandages are slightly elastic and the layers adhere somewhat to one another.

_____   **14.** Ecchymosis is associated with open wounds.

_____   **15.** A laceration is considered a closed wound.

Fill-in-the-Blank

Read each item carefully and then complete the statement by filling in the missing words.

1. There are three types of ionizing radiation: _____, _____, and _____.

2. A person will sweat in an effort to _____ the body.

3. Nerve endings are located in the _____.

4. When an area of the body is trapped for longer than 4 hours and arterial blood flow is compromised,

_____ _____ can develop.

5. In cold weather, blood vessels in the skin will _____.

6. The only exceptions to the rule of not removing an impaled object are an object in the _____ that

obstructs breathing and an object in the _____ that interferes with CPR.

7. _____ burns can occur when skin is exposed to temperatures higher than _____°F.

8. A(n) _____ is an injury in which part of the body is completely severed.

9. The external layer of skin is the _____ and the inner layer is the _____.

10. When the vessels of the skin dilate, heat is _____ from the body.

Labeling

1. Skin
Label the following diagram with the correct terms.

A. _____

B. _____

C. _____

D. _____

E. _____

F. _____

G. _____

H. _____

I. _____

J. _____

K. _____

L. _____

M. _____

N. _____

O. _____

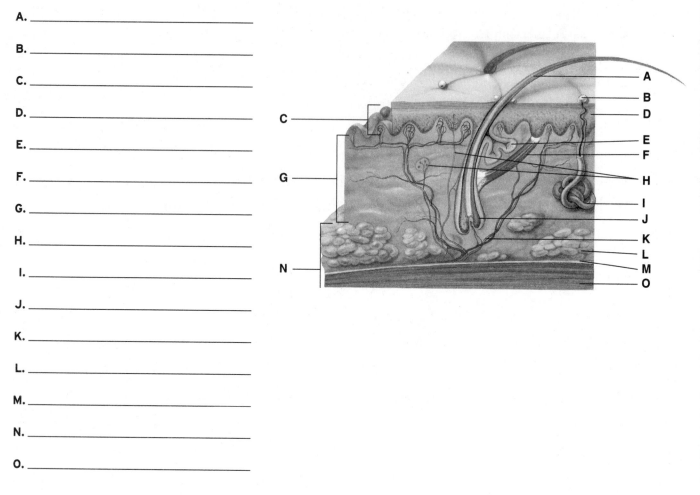

2. Rule of Nines

Label the following diagram with the correct percentage numbers.

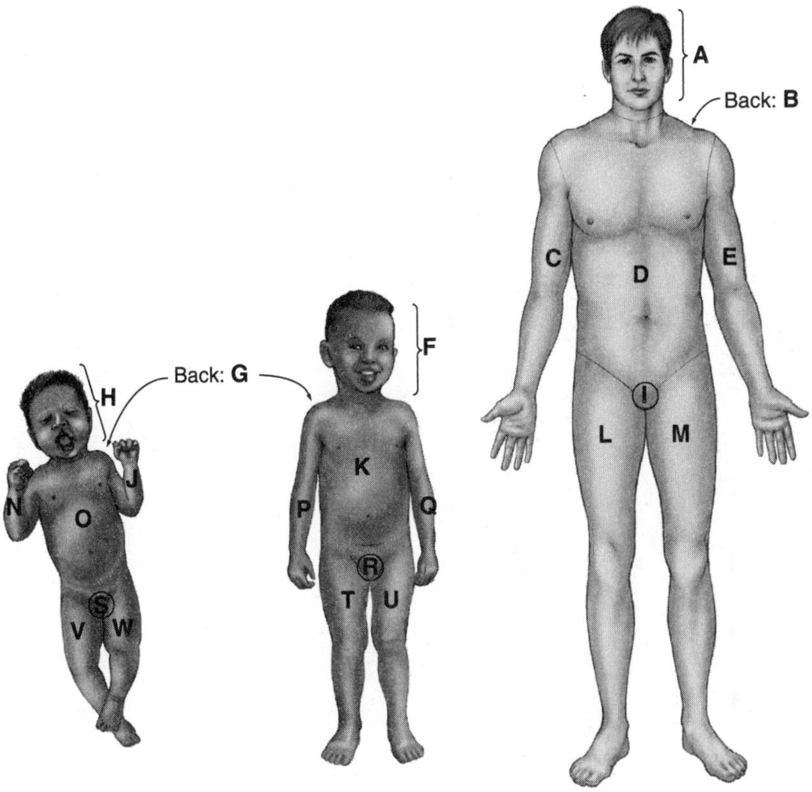

A. _____

B. _____

C. _____

D. _____

E. _____

F. _____

G. _____

H. _____

I. _____

J. _____

K. _____

L. _____

M. _____

N. _____

O. _____

P. _____

Q. _____

R. _____

S. _____

T. _____

U. _____

V. _____

W. _____

Crossword Puzzle

The following crossword puzzle is an activity provided to reinforce correct spelling and understanding of medical terminology associated with emergency care and the EMT. Use the clues in the column to complete the puzzle.

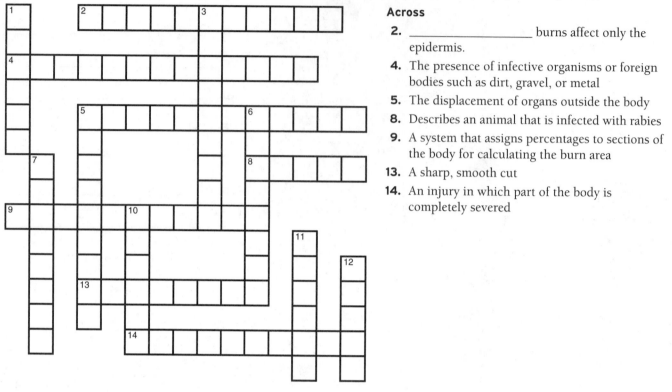

Across

2. _____ burns affect only the epidermis.

4. The presence of infective organisms or foreign bodies such as dirt, gravel, or metal

5. The displacement of organs outside the body

8. Describes an animal that is infected with rabies

9. A system that assigns percentages to sections of the body for calculating the burn area

13. A sharp, smooth cut

14. An injury in which part of the body is completely severed

Down

1. The linings of body cavities and passages that are in direct contact with the outside environment are known as _____ membranes.

3. A burn caused by an open flame

5. The outer layer of skin that acts as a watertight protective covering

6. Loss or damage of the superficial layer of skin as a result of a body part rubbing or scraping across a rough or hard surface

7. An injury in which soft tissue is torn completely loose or is hanging as a flap

10. The fiberlike connective tissue that covers arteries, veins, tendons, and ligaments

11. The inner layer of the skin; contains hair follicles, sweat glands, nerve endings, and blood vessels

12. Injuries in which damage occurs as a result from thermal heat, frictional heat, toxic chemicals, electricity, or nuclear radiation

Critical Thinking

Multiple Choice

Read each critical-thinking item carefully and then select the one best response.

_____ 1. You respond to a house fire with the local fire department. They bring a 48-year-old woman out of the house. She is unconscious but her airway is open. Her breathing is shallow at 30 breaths/min. Her pulse is 110 beats/min, strong and regular. Her blood pressure is 108/72 mm Hg. She has been burned over 40% of her body. The burned area appears to be dry and leathery. It looks charred and has pieces of fabric embedded in the flesh. You know that this type of burn is considered a:

   A. first-degree burn.

   B. second-degree burn.

   C. partial-thickness burn.

   D. third-degree burn.

_____ 2. You respond to a scene where a 24-year-old man has been shot. Law enforcement is on scene, and the scene is safe. As you approach the patient, you notice that he is bleeding from the lower-right abdominal area. He is alert and oriented but seems confused. His airway is open, and he is breathing at a normal rate. His pulse is 120 beats/min, weak, and regular. His blood pressure is 98/60 mm Hg. You ask the police officer about the weapon. You need this information because the amount of damage is related to the:

   A. size of the entrance wound.

   B. size of the bullet.

   C. size of the exit wound.

   D. speed of the bullet.

_____ 3. You respond to a scene where a 14-year-old girl was playing softball and slid into second base. She states she felt and heard a loud pop. There is no obvious bleeding, but swelling is present. Her pulse is 86 beats/min, and her blood pressure is 114/74 mm Hg. You decide you can manage this situation and decide to use the RICES method of treatment. The S stands for:

   A. swelling.

   B. soft tissue.

   C. splinting.

   D. shock.

_____ 4. In doing a more detailed examination on the patient in question 3, you notice that she has an abrasion on her left knee that she sustained when she slid. The abrasion is covered with dirt and is oozing blood. You know that this injury is classified as:

   A. superficial.

   B. deep.

   C. full thickness.

   D. none of the above.

_____ 5. You decide to manage the injury found in question 4. You flush the site with sterile water, and it continues to bleed. What would be the best way to control the bleeding from the site?

   A. Elevation

   B. Pressure dressings

   C. Tourniquets

   D. Pressure points

Short Answer

Complete this section with short written answers using the space provided.

1. List the three major classifications of depth of burns.

_____

_____

2. List the three general classifications of soft-tissue injuries.

_____

_____

3. Define the acronym RICES.

R: _____

I: _____

C: _____

E: _____

S: _____

4. Describe the classifications of a critical burn for an infant or child.

_____

_____

5. What treatment should be used with a patient who has been burned by a dry chemical?

_____

_____

6. Why are electrical burns particularly dangerous to a patient?

_____

_____

7. Identify the three general types of blast injuries.

_____

_____

8. List the three primary functions of dressings and bandages.

_____

_____

9. List the four types of open soft-tissue injuries.

_____

_____

10. List the five factors used to determine the severity of a burn.

_____

_____

Ambulance Calls

The following case scenarios provide an opportunity to explore the concerns associated with patient management and to enhance critical-thinking skills. Read each scenario and answer each question to the best of your ability.

1. You are dispatched to a residence where a 10-year-old girl fell onto a jagged piece of metal. She has a gaping laceration to the right upper arm that is spurting bright red blood. The mother tried to control bleeding with a towel, but it kept soaking through.

How would you best manage this patient?

_____

_____

_____

2. You are dispatched to the home of a 3-year-old boy for an unknown problem. You arrive to find a young mother screaming for your help. Apparently, she was cooking a meal for her other children when the phone rang. While she was talking, the 3-year-old child grabbed the pot handle, pulling boiling hot water onto his body.

How would you best manage this patient?

_____

_____

_____

3. You are watching television at the station when a fire fighter comes into the room holding his left hand. His wedding ring got caught in a piece of small machinery at the stationhouse, resulting in an avulsion of his ring finger.

How would you best manage this patient?

_____

_____

_____

Fill-in-the-Patient Care Report

Read the incident scenario and then complete the following patient care report (PCR).

You are just getting back into the ambulance after throwing your lunch bag away when the dispatcher's voice comes across the radio. "Medic nineteen, priority call, police officer shot at 14th and Berry. Showing you dispatched and responding at 1321."

Your partner, Alicia, fastens her seatbelt as you start the truck, and 8 minutes later you arrive at the scene of a traffic stop gone wrong. The intersection is in chaos, police cars block every lane, and you see an obviously dead man hanging from the driver-side door of an old, rusted sedan on the opposite side of the street. You are met by a shaken sergeant who leads you over to a 24-year-old officer who is on the pavement, leaning against the flattened tire of a bullet-riddled patrol car. A motorcycle officer in tall, shining boots is kneeling next to him, holding his hand to the side of the other man's neck; his normally light blue uniform shirt now looks dark purple due to the blood saturation.

"Hang in there, officer," Alicia says, pulling a nonrebreathing mask from the airway bag and assembling the oxygen cylinder.

You place your gloved hand over the neck wound, and the sergeant has to make the motorcycle officer move away. You use your free hand to fish an occlusive dressing from the jump kit and apply it to the large hole in the officer's neck.

"Am I dying?" the officer asks quietly. His eyes are nearly closed and his face is pale and sweaty.

"I don't think so," you say as you place a pressure dressing over the occlusive pad while Alicia places the nonrebreathing mask over the man's mouth and nose after setting the flow to 15 L/min. "We're going to do everything that we can for you, though."

Several fire fighters on scene help you secure the injured 73-kg (161-lb) officer to a long backboard and load him into the ambulance. You climb into the back, and Alicia slides behind the steering wheel, preparing to drive behind a string of police cars that will be blocking intersections for the entire 9-minute drive to the trauma center.

A quick assessment of the patient shows that he has no injuries other than the apparent gunshot wound to the neck, so you take a baseline set of vital signs as the ambulance begins rolling, a mere 5 minutes after arriving on scene. His blood pressure is 92/60 mm Hg, pulse is 120 beats/min, respirations are 20 breaths/min and shallow, and pulse oximetry is 92%.

"We need to move it, Al," you say to your partner, and you hear the engine grow louder as you cover the officer with blankets and check to make sure that no blood is seeping through the dressing. You then make contact with the trauma center and provide a verbal report and ETA. Four minutes before arriving, you obtain a second set of vital signs and find his blood pressure at 92/58 mm Hg, pulse at 124 beats/min, respirations still at 20 breaths/min and shallow, and the pulse oximetry at 94%.

Alicia pulls into the hospital ambulance zone 2 minutes sooner than normal for this transport and unloads the patient. You wheel him into the facility, flanked by grim-faced officers, and pass him to the capable trauma team, providing a brief verbal report to the trauma physician and the charge nurse.

Thirty minutes later, after cleaning and disinfecting the ambulance, you call yourselves back available and pull back into the traffic around the downtown medical center.

EMS Patient Care Report (PCR)

Date:	Incident No.:		Nature of Call:		Location:	
Dispatched:	En Route:	At Scene:	Transport:		At Hospital:	In Service:

Patient Information

Age:		Allergies:
Sex:		Medications:
Weight (in kg [lb]):		Past Medical History:
		Chief Complaint:

Vital Signs

Time:	BP:	Pulse:	Respirations:	Sao$_2$:
Time:	BP:	Pulse:	Respirations:	Sao$_2$:
Time:	BP:	Pulse:	Respirations:	Sao$_2$:

EMS Treatment
(circle all that apply)

Oxygen @ ___ L/min via (circle one): NC NRM Bag-Mask Device		Assisted Ventilation	Airway Adjunct	CPR
Defibrillation	Bleeding Control	Bandaging	Splinting	Other Shock Treatment

Narrative

Skills

Skill Drills

Test your knowledge of these skills by filling in the correct words in the photo captions.

Skill Drill 24-1: Controlling Bleeding From an Open Soft-Tissue Injury

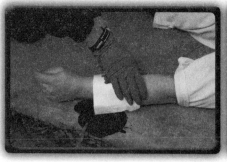
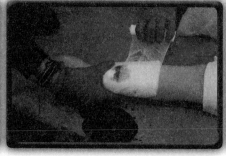
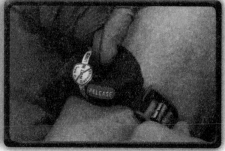

1. Apply _____ _____ with a sterile _____.

2. Apply a(n) _____ dressing.

3. If bleeding continues or recurs, apply a(n) _____ above the level of _____.

Skill Drill 24-3: Caring for Burns

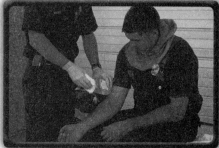
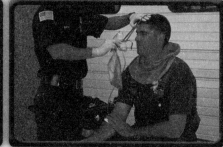
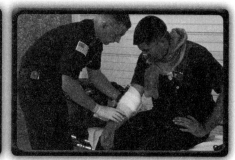

1. Follow _____ precautions to help prevent _____. If safe to do so, remove the _____ from the burning area; extinguish or _____ hot clothing and jewelry as necessary. If the wound(s) is (are) still burning or hot, _____ the hot area in _____, sterile _____, or cover with a wet, cool _____.

2. Provide high-flow _____, and continue to assess the _____.

3. Estimate the _____ of the burn, and then cover the area with a(n) _____, sterile dressing or clean _____. Assess and treat the patient for any other _____.

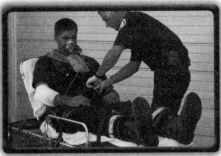

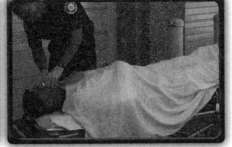

4. Prepare for transport. Treat for

_____.

5. Cover the patient with

_____ to prevent

loss of _____

_____. Transport

promptly.

Assessment Review

Answer the following questions pertaining to the assessment of the types of emergencies discussed in this chapter.

_____   **1.** During the primary assessment of burns, it is important to remember to:

    A. determine scene safety.

    B. obtain vital signs.

    C. prevent heat loss.

    D. estimate the amount of body surface injuries.

_____   **2.** You have been dispatched to a residence for a 24-year-old woman who splashed grease on her arm while cooking. As you approach her, she is crying and yelling that it hurts. Her pulse is 130 beats/min and regular. Her blood pressure is 126/86 mm Hg. You decide that she does not require immediate transport. The secondary assessment would include:

    A. proper interventions.

    B. an examination of the burned arm.

    C. deciding on the patient's priority for transport.

    D. an investigation of the chief complaint.

_____   **3.** During the reassessment of a burn patient with a significant MOI you should:

    A. splint all fractures.

    B. determine the transport decision.

    C. open all blisters.

    D. treat the patient for shock.

_____   **4.** During the intervention step of patient assessment for a burn patient, the first intervention should be to:

    A. stop the burning process.

    B. provide complete spinal stabilization.

    C. treat for shock.

    D. cover burns with moist sterile dressings.

_____   **5.** You respond to a patient who has been stabbed in the neck. You arrive to find the patient in police custody and bleeding moderately from the neck wound. The patient is alert, oriented, and swearing loudly. His pulse is 120 beats/min. His blood pressure is 124/76 mm Hg. You start to bandage the wound. What type of bandage should you use?

    A. Triangular bandage

    B. Adhesive bandage

    C. Roller bandage

    D. Occlusive bandage

Emergency Care Summary

Fill in the following chart pertaining to the management of the types of emergencies discussed in this chapter.

Note: While the steps below are widely accepted, be sure to consult and follow your local protocol.

General Management of Closed Injuries

1. Ensure an open airway and adequate _____. Treat as required.

2. Be alert for and treat for shock (hypoperfusion) by raising the legs or backboard 6″ to 12″, maintain _____ temperature, and administer high-concentration oxygen.

3. Treat a closed soft-tissue injury by applying the mnemonic RICES:

- Rest to keep patient quiet and comfortable

- Ice to _____ blood vessels and reduce _____

- Compression to compress blood vessels to slow _____

- Elevation to raise injured part above level of the heart to decrease _____

- _____ of extremity to decrease bleeding and pain

General Management of Open Injuries

1. Ensure you have followed standard precautions.

2. Ensure an open airway and adequate ventilations. Treat as required.

3. Apply a(n) _____ dressing to open chest injuries.

4. Apply direct pressure over the wound with a dry, _____ dressing.

5. Apply a(n) _____ dressing.

6. If bleeding continues or recurs, apply a tourniquet to an extremity _____ the level of bleeding.

7. Be alert for and treat for _____ (hypoperfusion) by raising legs or backboard 6″ to 12″, maintain body temperature, and administer high-concentration oxygen.

General Management of Burn Injuries

1. Stop the _____ process.

2. Take appropriate standard precautions.

3. Treat life threats involving the ABCs.

4. Cool the burned area with sterile water or _____. Immerse or continuously irrigate the affected area, following local treatment protocols.

5. Cover the burned area with a(n) _____ dressing. Dressing will be moist or dry, depending on local protocol.

6. Maintain body temperature and treat for shock.

Face and Neck Injuries

General Knowledge

Matching

Match each of the items in the left column to the appropriate definition in the right column.

_____ **1.** Anisocoria

_____ **2.** Cornea

_____ **3.** Eustachian tube

_____ **4.** Globe

_____ **5.** Iris

_____ **6.** Lens

_____ **7.** Mastoid process

_____ **8.** Pinna

_____ **9.** Pupil

_____ **10.** Retina

_____ **11.** Sclera

_____ **12.** Tragus

13. Turbinates

_____ **14.** Tympanic membrane

_____ **15.** Optic nerve

A. Layers of bone within the nasal cavity

B. Light-sensitive area of the eye where images are projected

C. Eyeball

D. Eardrum

E. External visible part of the ear

F. Tough, fibrous, white portion of the eye

G. Naturally occurring unequal pupils

H. Transparent tissue layer in front of the pupil and iris

I. Bony mass at the base of the skull about 1″ (2.54 cm) behind the opening to the ear

J. Muscle and surrounding tissue behind the cornea that dilate and constrict the pupil

K. Transparent part of the eye through which images are focused on the retina

L. Connects the middle ear to the oropharynx

M. Small, rounded, fleshy bulge that lies immediately anterior to the ear canal

N. Cranial nerve that transmits visual information to the brain

O. Circular opening in the middle of the iris that admits light to the back of the eye

Multiple Choice

Read each item carefully and then select the one best response.

_____ **1.** As an EMT, your objective when treating patients with face and neck injuries is to:

A. prevent further injury.

B. manage any acute airway problems.

C. control bleeding.

D. all of the above.

_____ **2.** The head is divided into two parts: the cranium and the:

A. brain.

B. face.

C. skull.

D. medulla oblongata.

_____ **3.** The brain connects to the spinal cord through a large opening at the base of the skull known as the:

A. eustachian tube.

B. spinous process.

C. foramen magnum.

D. vertebral foramina.

_____ **4.** Approximately _____ of the nose is composed of bone. The remainder is composed of cartilage.

    A. nine tenths

    B. two thirds

    C. three quarters

    D. one third

_____ **5.** Motion of the mandible occurs at the:

    A. temporomandibular joint.

    B. mastoid process.

    C. chin.

    D. mandibular angle.

_____ **6.** You respond to a 71-year-old woman who is unresponsive. You try to get her to respond but have no success. Her airway is open, and she is breathing at a rate of 14 breaths/min. You know you can check a pulse on either side of the neck. You know that the jugular veins and several nerves run through the neck next to the trachea. What structure are you trying to locate to take a pulse?

    A. Hypothalamus

    B. Subclavian arteries

    C. Cricoid cartilage

    D. Carotid arteries

_____ **7.** The _____ connects the cricoid cartilage and thyroid cartilage.

    A. larynx

    B. cricoid membrane

    C. cricothyroid membrane

    D. thyroid membrane

_____ **8.** You respond to a 68-year-old man who was involved in a motor vehicle collision. He is unresponsive, and as you approach you notice he is not breathing. He was unrestrained and has massive facial injuries. When you check his airway, it is obstructed. Which of the following is NOT likely to cause an upper airway obstruction in a patient with facial trauma?

    A. Heavy bleeding

    B. Loosened teeth or dentures

    C. Soft-tissue swelling

    D. Inflamed tonsils

_____ **9.** You are dispatched to a residential neighborhood for a 6-year-old girl who was bitten by the family pet. The mother meets you at the door with the girl, who is crying uncontrollably and has blood covering the right side of her head. You look at the child and notice that her lower right ear has been completely avulsed. You control the bleeding with direct pressure and bandage the injury. You follow the blood trail back to where the incident occurred and find the avulsed part. How do you manage the avulsed tissue?

    A. Wrap the skin in a moist, sterile dressing; place it in a plastic bag; and keep it cool.

    B. Place the skin in a plastic "biohazard" bag and dispose of it properly.

    C. Place the skin in a plastic bag filled with ice and transport it to the ED.

    D. Leave it at the scene to be disposed of later.

_____ **10.** The nasal cavity is divided into two chambers by the:

    A. frontal sinus.

    B. middle turbinate.

    C. zygoma.

    D. nasal septum.

_____ 11. You are called to the home of a 48-year-old woman who has a history of high blood pressure and now has a major nose bleed. She is alert and oriented and converses freely with you. Her respirations and pulse are within normal limits. Her blood pressure is 194/108 mm Hg. You have been able to rule out trauma. How would you manage the nose bleed?

    A. Apply a sterile dressing.

    B. Pinch the nostrils together.

    C. Put the patient in a supine position.

    D. Have the patient hold ice in her mouth.

_____ 12. The middle ear is connected to the nasal cavity by the:

    A. frontal sinus.

    B. zygomatic process.

    C. eustachian tube.

    D. superior trachea.

_____ 13. Which of the following is NOT a sign or symptom of a laryngeal injury?

    A. Hoarsness

    B. Difficulty breathing

    C. Subcutaneous emphysema

    D. Wheezing

_____ 14. Which of the following is NOT a sign of a possible facial fracture?

    A. Bleeding in the mouth

    B. Absent or loose teeth

    C. Bleeding from the forehead

    D. Loose and/or moveable bone fragments

_____ 15. The presence of air in the soft tissues of the neck that produces a crackling sensation is called:

    A. the "Rice Krispy" effect.

    B. a pneumothorax.

    C. rales.

    D. subcutaneous emphysema.

_____ 16. Which of the following statements is NOT true regarding the treatment of bleeding from a neck injury?

    A. Apply firm pressure to the carotid artery to reduce the amount of bleeding.

    B. Apply pressure to the bleeding site using a gloved fingertip.

    C. Apply a sterile occlusive dressing.

    D. Use gauze to secure the dressing in place.

_____ 17. What is the main purpose of eye blinking?

    A. Clean the eye

    B. Prevent eye muscle atrophy

    C. Natural reflex to bright light

    D. Refocus the eye

_____ 18. When flushing an eye with saline to remove a foreign object, it is important to remember to:

    A. flush from the outside of the eye in toward the nose.

    B. flush from the top of the eye toward the bottom.

    C. flush from the nose side of the eye toward the outside.

    D. flush only along the bottom of the eye.

_____ 19. When stabilizing a large foreign object in the eye, you should first cover the eye with a moist dressing, then:

    A. irrigate the eye with saline.

    B. surround the object with a doughnut-shaped collar made from gauze.

    C. apply tape around the object and then secure the tape to the forehead.

    D. place an ice pack over the eye to reduce swelling.

_____   **20.** When a patient has a chemical burn to the eye, you should irrigate the eye for at least 5 minutes; however, if the burn was caused by an alkali or strong acid, you should irrigate for:

    A. 10 minutes.

    B. 15 minutes.

    C. 20 minutes.

    D. 25 minutes.

True/False

If you believe the statement to be more true than false, write the letter "T" in the space provided. If you believe the statement to be more false than true, write the letter "F."

_____   **1.** Injuries to the face often lead to airway problems.

_____   **2.** Care for facial injuries begins with standard precautions and the ABCs.

_____   **3.** Exposed eye or brain injuries are covered with a dry dressing.

_____   **4.** Clear fluid in the outer ear is normal.

_____   **5.** Any crushing injury of the upper part of the neck likely involves the larynx or the trachea.

_____   **6.** Soft-tissue injuries to the face are common.

_____   **7.** The opening that the spinal cord leaves the head through is called the occiput.

_____   **8.** The muscle that allows movement of the head is the temporomandibular.

_____   **9.** Standard precautions for assessing face and throat injuries should include eye and oral protection.

_____   **10.** The airway of choice with facial injuries is the nasopharyngeal.

_____   **11.** Stabilization and maintenance of an airway can be difficult in patients with facial injuries.

_____   **12.** Asymmetrical eyes could possibly indicate a brain injury.

_____   **13.** Gentle irrigation will usually wash out foreign material stuck in the cornea.

_____   **14.** Retinal injuries caused by exposure to extreme bright light are generally painful and result in permanent damage.

_____   **15.** You should never exert pressure on or manipulate an injured eye in any way.

_____   **16.** Bleeding into the anterior chamber of the eye is commonly called conjunctivitis.

_____   **17.** When dealing with an injured eye, you should always remove contact lenses before treatment.

_____   **18.** Open injuries to the larynx can occur as the result of a stabbing.

_____   **19.** Broken teeth and lacerations to the tongue cause minimal bleeding and are not concerning.

_____   **20.** Oxygen and airway management are important for all patients with face and neck injuries.

Fill-in-the-Blank

Read each item carefully and then complete the statement by filling in the missing words.

1. Pulsations in the neck are felt in the _____ vessels.

2. The _____ vertebrae are in the neck.

3. The _____ regions of the cranium are located on the lateral portion of the head.

4. The _____ connects the oropharynx and the larynx with the main air passages of the lungs.

5. The rings of the trachea are made of _____.

6. The Adam's apple is more prominent in _____ than in _____.

7. The _____ _____ is a large opening at the base of the skull.

8. Blunt trauma that causes fractures to the orbit are commonly called a(n) _____ _____.

9. Trauma to the face and skull that results in the posterior wall of the nasal cavity becoming unstable is caused by

_____ _____ _____.

10. When dealing with an avulsed tooth, handle it by its _____ and not by the _____.

11. A(n) _____ _____ results when an open vein sucks air into it and travels to the heart.

Labeling
Label the following diagrams with the correct terms.

1. The Face

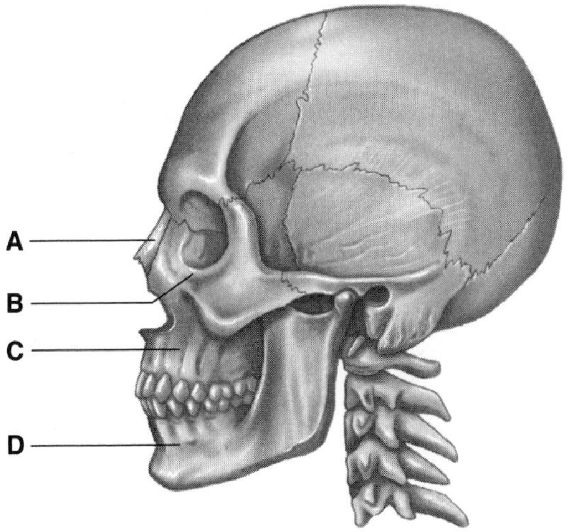

A. _____

B. _____

C. _____

D. _____

2. The Larynx

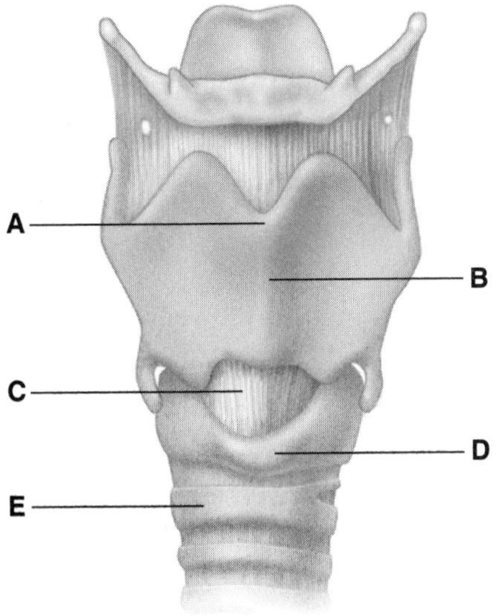

A. _____

B. _____

C. _____

D. _____

E. _____

3. The Eye

A. _____

B. _____

C. _____

D. _____

E. _____

F. _____

G. _____

H. _____

I. _____

J. _____

K. _____

L. _____

M. _____

N. _____

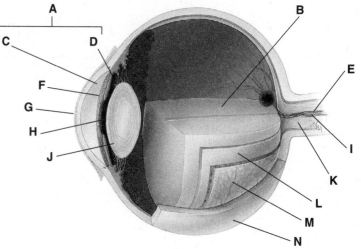

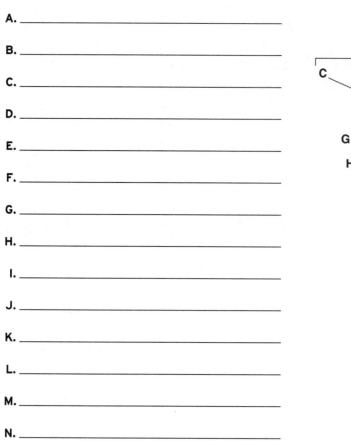

4. The Ear

A. _____

B. _____

C. _____

D. _____

E. _____

F. _____

G. _____

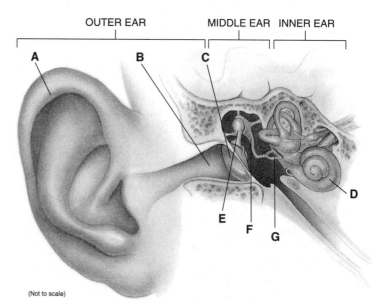

(Not to scale)

Crossword Puzzle

The following crossword puzzle is an activity provided to reinforce correct spelling and understanding of medical terminology associated with emergency care and the EMT. Use the clues in the column to complete the puzzle.

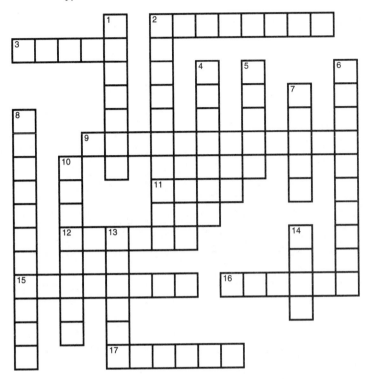

Across

2. The ear canal is known as the _____ auditory canal.
3. The circular opening in the middle of the iris that admits light to the back of the eye
9. A characteristic crackling sensation felt on palpation of the skin is known as _____ emphysema.
11. The muscle and surrounding tissue behind the cornea that dilate and constrict the pupil, regulating the amount of light that enters the eye
12. The light-sensitive area of the eye where images are projected
15. The _____ membrane is the eardrum, which lies between the external and middle ear.
16. The transparent tissue layer in front of the pupil and iris of the eye
17. The tough, fibrous, white portion of the eye that protects the more delicate inner structures

Down

1. A(n) _____ fracture is a fracture of the orbit or of the bones that support the floor of the orbit.
2. The _____ tube is a branch of the internal auditory canal that connects the middle ear to the oropharynx.
4. The _____ process is the prominent bony mass at the base of the skull about 1″ (2.5 cm) posterior to the external opening of the ear.
5. The external visible part of the ear
6. Naturally occurring uneven pupil size
7. The eyeball
8. The delicate membrane that lines the eyelids and covers the exposed surface of the eye
10. The _____ glands produce fluids to keep the eye moist.
13. The small, rounded, fleshy bulge that lies immediately anterior to the ear canal
14. The transparent part of the eye through which images are focused on the retina

Critical Thinking

Short Answer

Complete this section with short written answers using the space provided.

1. Describe bleeding-control methods for facial injuries.

_____

_____

2. Describe bleeding-control methods for lacerations to veins or arteries in the neck.

_____

_____

3. Explain the physical exam process for evaluation of the eye.

_____

_____

4. List three important guidelines to use when treating an eye laceration.

_____

_____

5. List five eye indications that suggest a closed head injury.

_____

_____

Ambulance Calls

The following case scenarios provide an opportunity to explore the concerns associated with patient management and to enhance critical-thinking skills. Read each scenario and answer each question to the best of your ability.

1. You are dispatched to assist a small child who was attacked by his family's dog. The dog bit the child's face and neck repeatedly, then grabbed him by the neck and shook him violently. The mother found the boy "making funny breathing sounds" and called for help. She has removed the dog from the area.

How would you best manage this patient?

_____

_____

_____

2. You are dispatched to a 37-year-old man with a large laceration to the right side of his neck. Bleeding is dark and heavy. He is alert, but weak.

How would you best manage this patient?

_____

_____

_____

3. You are dispatched to a Little League baseball game to assist an assault victim. Apparently, emotions were running high when two parents began to argue. You arrive to find a 40-year-old man with a bloody nose.

How would you best manage this patient?

_____

_____

_____

Skills

Skill Drill

Skill Drill 25-1: Removing a Foreign Object from Under the Upper Eyelid
Test your knowledge of this skill by filling in the correct words in the photo captions.

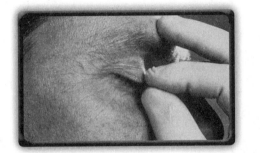

1. Have the patient look _____,
grasp the upper _____, and
gently pull the _____ away
from the eye.

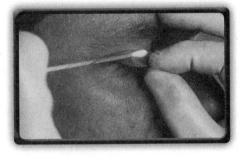

2. Place a cotton-tipped applicator on the
_____ surface of the
_____ lid.

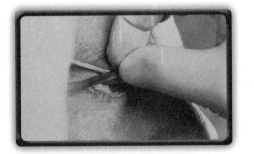

3. Pull the lid _____ and
_____, folding it back over
the applicator.

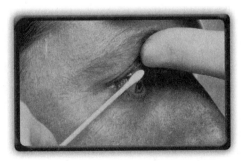

4. Gently remove the foreign object
from the eyelid with a moistened,
_____, cotton-tipped
applicator.

Skill Drill 25-2: Stabilizing a Foreign Object Impaled in the Eye
Test your knowledge of this skill by placing the photos below in the correct order. Number the first step with a "1," the second step with a "2," etc.

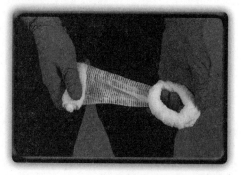

_____ Remove the gauze from you hand and wrap the remainder of the gauze roll radially around the ring that you have created.

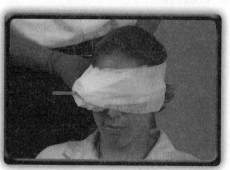

_____ Place the dressing over the eye and impaled object to hold the impaled object in place, and then secure it with a roller bandage.

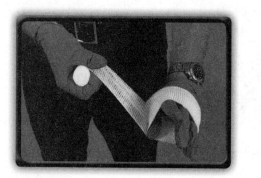

_____ To prepare a doughnut ring, wrap a 2″ (5-cm) roll around your fingers and thumb seven or eight times. Adjust the diameter by spreading your fingers or squeezing them together.

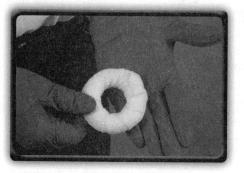

_____ Work around the entire ring to form a doughnut.

Assessment Review

Answer the following questions pertaining to the assessment of the types of emergencies discussed in this chapter.

_____ 1. You have responded to an automobile collision and find a 21-year-old man who has massive facial trauma. He is bleeding heavily and is unconscious. The first thing that you do in your treatment of this patient is to:

    A. take c-spine precautions.

    B. open the airway.

    C. assess his breathing.

    D. take standard precautions.

_____ 2. For the patient described above (question 1), how often would you reassess the patient's vitals during your ongoing assessment?

    A. Every 3 minutes

    B. Every 5 minutes

    C. Every 10 minutes

    D. Every 15 minutes

_____ 3. You have a patient who has severe epistaxis. You have been able to rule out trauma. How would you position this patient to help control the bleeding?

    A. Supine

    B. Prone

    C. Sitting leaning back

    D. Sitting leaning forward

_____ 4. You have a patient who has had a tooth knocked out. You find the tooth. How would you transport it to the hospital?

    A. In saline

    B. In dextrose

    C. In ice

    D. In a dry sterile dressing

_____ 5. You respond to a child who has placed a pebble in his ear. He is complaining that his ear hurts. You should:

    A. remove the pebble with a cotton-tipped applicator.

    B. have the child try and shake the pebble out.

    C. leave the pebble in the ear and transport.

    D. not load the patient, because this is not an emergency.

Emergency Care Summary

Fill in the following chart pertaining to the management of the types of emergencies discussed in this chapter.

Note: While the steps below are widely accepted, be sure to consult and follow your local protocol.

Ear Injuries

Place a soft, padded dressing between the ear and the scalp. If the ear is avulsed, wrap it in a(n) _____, sterile dressing and place in a plastic bag. Keep the avulsed tissue _____ and transport to the hospital with the patient. Leave any foreign object within the ear for the physician to remove. Note any clear fluid coming from the ear.

Facial Fractures

Remove and save loose teeth or _____ fragments from the mouth and transport them with you. Remove any loose dentures or dental bridges to protect against _____ obstruction. Maintain an open airway.

Injuries to the Neck

1. Apply _____ pressure to the bleeding site using a gloved fingertip if necessary to control bleeding.
2. Apply a sterile _____ _____ to ensure that air does not enter a vein or artery.
3. Use _____ _____ to secure a dressing in place.
4. Wrap the _____ around and under the patient's _____.

Head and Spine Injuries

General Knowledge

Matching

Match each of the items in the left column to the appropriate definition in the right column.

_____ 1. Distraction

_____ 2. Subluxation

_____ 3. Subdural hematoma

_____ 4. Retrograde amnesia

_____ 5. Concussion

_____ 6. Anterograde amnesia

_____ 7. Cerebral edema

_____ 8. Connecting nerves

_____ 9. Intervertebral disk

_____ 10. Meninges

A. Temporary loss of the brain's ability to function without actual physical damage

B. Swelling of the brain

C. Inability to remember events after an injury

D. The action of pulling the spine along its length

E. A partial or incomplete dislocation

F. Three distinct layers of tissue that surround and protect the brain and spinal cord

G. Inability to remember events leading up to a head injury

H. Accumulation of blood beneath the dura mater but outside the brain

I. Located in the brain and spinal cord, these connect the motor and sensory nerves within the skull and spinal canal.

J. Cushion that lies between the vertebrae

Multiple Choice

Read each item carefully and then select the one best response.

_____ 1. Which of the following is NOT part of the central nervous system?

   A. The brain

   B. The spinal cord

   C. Cerebrospinal fluid

   D. Cranial nerves

_____ 2. The nervous system is divided into the central nervous system and the:

   A. autonomic nervous system.

   B. peripheral nervous system.

   C. sympathetic nervous system.

   D. somatic nervous system.

_____ 3. The brain is divided into the cerebrum, the cerebellum, and the:

   A. foramen magnum.

   B. meninges.

   C. brain stem.

   D. spinal column.

_____ 4. Injury to the head and neck may indicate injury to the:

   A. thoracic spine.

   B. lumbar spine.

   C. cervical spine.

   D. sacral spine.

_____   **5.** The _____ is composed of three layers of tissue that suspend the brain and spinal cord within the skull and spinal canal.

    A. meninges

    B. dura mater

    C. pia mater

    D. arachnoid space

_____   **6.** The skull is divided into the cranium and the:

    A. occipital.

    B. face.

    C. parietal.

    D. foramen magnum.

_____   **7.** Peripheral nerves include the:

    A. connecting nerves.

    B. sensory nerves.

    C. motor nerves.

    D. all of the above.

_____   **8.** Which of the following is NOT a function of cerebrospinal fluid?

    A. Acts as a shock absorber

    B. Bathes the brain and spinal cord

    C. Buffers the brain and spinal cord from injury

    D. Provides continuous oxygen to the brain

_____   **9.** The autonomic nervous system is composed of the sympathetic nervous system and the:

    A. peripheral nervous system.

    B. central nervous system.

    C. parasympathetic nervous system.

    D. somatic nervous system.

_____   **10.** The most prominent and the most easily palpable spinous process is at the _____ cervical vertebra at the base of the neck.

    A. 7th

    B. 6th

    C. 5th

    D. 4th

_____   **11.** You respond to a 14-year-old boy who fell out of a tree at a local park. He is unresponsive. His airway is open and respirations are 16 breaths/min and regular. His pulse is strong and regular. Distal pulses are present. You manage the c-spine. Who should you ask for help in determining how the injury happened?

    A. First responders

    B. Family members

    C. Bystanders

    D. All of the above

_____   **12.** Emergency medical care of a patient with a possible spinal injury begins with:

    A. opening the airway.

    B. assessing level of consciousness.

    C. summoning law enforcement.

    D. standard precautions.

_____ 13. The _____ is a tunnel running the length of the spine, which encloses and protects the spinal cord.

    A. foramen magnum

    B. spinal canal

    C. foramen foramina

    D. meninges

_____ 14. Once the head and neck are manually stabilized, you should assess for:

    A. pulse.

    B. motor function.

    C. sensation.

    D. all of the above.

_____ 15. You are called to a motor vehicle collision where a 27-year-old woman has a bump on her head. You immediately begin manual stabilization of the head. Her airway is open and respirations are within normal limits. Her pulse is a little fast but strong and regular. Distal pulses are present. You can release manual stabilization when:

    A. the patient's head and torso are in line.

    B. the patient is secured to a backboard with the head immobilized.

    C. the rigid cervical collar is in place.

    D. the patient arrives at the hospital.

_____ 16. The ideal procedure for moving a patient from the ground to the backboard is the:

    A. four-person log roll.

    B. lateral slide.

    C. four-person lift.

    D. push-and-pull maneuver.

_____ 17. You respond to a motor vehicle collision with a 29-year-old woman who struck the rearview mirror and has serious bleeding from the scalp. Her airway is open and respirations are normal. The pulse is a little rapid but strong and regular. Distal pulses are present, and there is no deformity to the skull. Most bleeding from the scalp can be controlled by:

    A. direct pressure.

    B. elevation.

    C. pressure point.

    D. tourniquet.

_____ 18. Exceptions to using a short spinal extrication device include all of the following EXCEPT:

    A. you or the patient is in danger.

    B. the patient is conscious and complaining of lumbar pain.

    C. you need to gain immediate access to other patients.

    D. the patient's injuries justify immediate removal.

_____ 19. Neck rigidity, bloody cerebrospinal fluid, and headache are associated with what kind of bleeding in the brain?

    A. Epidural hematoma

    B. Subdural hematoma

    C. Intracerebral hematoma

    D. Subarachnoid hemorrhage

_____ 20. A _____ is a temporary loss or alteration of a part or all of the brain's abilities to function without actual physical damage to the brain.

    A. contusion

    B. concussion

    C. hematoma

    D. subdural hematoma

_____ **21.** Which of the following is NOT a symptom of a concussion?

    A. Dizziness

    B. Weakness

    C. Muscle tremors

    D. Visual changes

_____ **22.** Intracranial bleeding outside of the dura mater and under the skull is known as a(n):

    A. concussion.

    B. intracerebral hemorrhage.

    C. subdural hematoma.

    D. epidural hematoma.

_____ **23.** In supine patients with a head injury, the head should be elevated _____ to help reduce intracranial pressure.

    A. 10°

    B. 20°

    C. 30°

    D. 40°

_____ **24.** _____ is the most reliable sign of a head injury.

    A. Vomiting

    B. Decreased level of consciousness

    C. Seizures

    D. Numbness and tingling in extremities

_____ **25.** Hyperventilation should be used with caution in head injury patients and only be attempted when _____ is/are available.

    A. pulse oximetry

    B. capnography

    C. air medical services

    D. noninvasive blood pressure monitoring

_____ **26.** Common causes of head injuries include all of the following EXCEPT:

    A. falls.

    B. motor vehicle collisions.

    C. seizure activity.

    D. sports injuries.

_____ **27.** Assessment of mental status is accomplished through the use of the mnemonic:

    A. SAMPLE.

    B. OPQRST.

    C. AVPU.

    D. AEIOU-TIPS.

_____ **28.** You respond to a 38-year-old man who fell while rock climbing. He is unconscious with an open airway. The respiration and pulse rates are within normal limits. His distal pulses are intact. You check his pupils and find that they are unequal. You know this could be a sign of:

    A. increased intracranial pressure.

    B. hypoxia.

    C. seizure activity.

    D. chronic hypertension.

_____ **29.** Which of the following is NOT part of Cushing's triad?

    A. Increased blood pressure

    B. Decreased pulse rate

    C. Decreased pulse oximetry

    D. Irregular respirations

_____ 30. How many EMTs are required to immobilize a standing patient?

    A. Two

    B. Three

    C. Four

    D. Five

_____ 31. A cervical collar should be applied to a patient with a possible spinal injury based on:

    A. the mechanism of injury.

    B. the history.

    C. signs and symptoms.

    D. all of the above.

_____ 32. Helmets must be removed in all of the following cases EXCEPT:

    A. cardiac arrest.

    B. when the helmet allows for excessive movement.

    C. when there are no impending airway or breathing problems.

    D. when a shield cannot be removed for access to the airway.

_____ 33. Your BEST choice of action for a child involved in a motor vehicle collision and found in his or her car seat is to:

    A. immobilize the child in the car seat.

    B. rule out spinal injury and place the child with a parent.

    C. pad the sides of car seat but leave space to allow for lateral movement.

    D. move the child to a pediatric immobilization device.

True/False

If you believe the statement to be more true than false, write the letter "T" in the space provided. If you believe the statement to be more false than true, write the letter "F."

_____ 1. A distracted spine has been moved laterally.

_____ 2. If a sensory nerve in the reflex arc detects an irritating stimulus, it will bypass the motor nerve and send a message directly to the brain.

_____ 3. Voluntary activities are those actions we perform unconsciously.

_____ 4. The autonomic nervous system is composed of the sympathetic nervous system and the parasympathetic nervous system.

_____ 5. The parasympathetic nervous system reacts to stress with the fight-or-flight response whenever it is confronted with a threatening situation.

_____ 6. All patients with suspected head and/or spine injuries should have their head realigned to an in-line, neutral position.

_____ 7. When assessing a patient for possible spinal injury, you should begin with a head-to-toe physical examination.

_____ 8. Your ideal procedure for moving a patient from the ground to a backboard is the four-person log roll.

_____ 9. You should not try to put a patient on a short board if they are in danger.

_____ 10. To properly measure a cervical collar, use the manufacturer's specifications.

Fill-in-the-Blank

Read each item carefully and then complete the statement by filling in the missing words.

1. The _____ nerves carry information to the muscles.

2. The dura mater, arachnoid, and pia mater are layers of _____ within the skull and spinal canal.

3. The brain and spinal cord are part of the _____ nervous system.

4. The peripheral nervous system has _____ pairs of spinal nerves.

5. The _____ nerves pass through holes in the skull and transmit sensations directly to the brain.

6. Vertebrae are separated by cushions called _____ _____.

7. The skull has two large structures of bone, the _____ and the _____.

8. The _____ and _____ are the inner two layers of the meninges and are much thinner than the dura mater.

9. The _____ nervous system reacts to stress.

10. The _____ nervous system causes the body to relax.

11. A(n) _____ _____ involves bleeding within the brain tissue itself.

12. A(n) _____ is far more serious than a concussion because it involves physical injury to the brain tissue.

13. When immobilizing a small child, _____ may need to be added to maintain an in-line, neutral position.

14. Upon completion of spinal immobilization, reassessment of _____, _____, and _____ function in each extremity is necessary.

15. In a patient with a suspected head injury, you should use the _____ method for opening the airway.

Labeling

Label the following diagrams with the correct terms.

1. Brain

A. _____

B. _____

C. _____

D. _____

E. _____

F. _____

G. _____

H. _____

I. _____

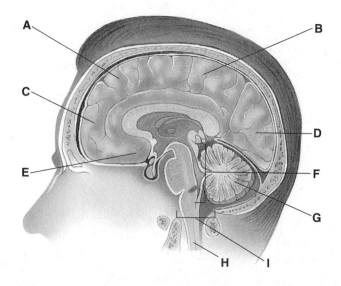

2. Connecting Nerves in the Spinal Cord

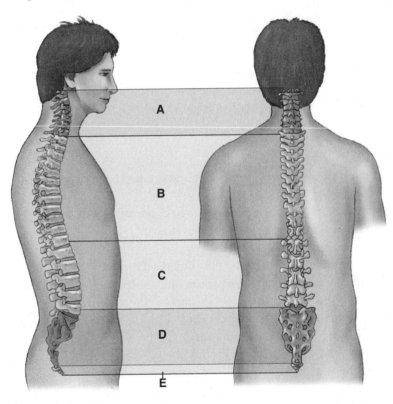

A. _____

B. _____

C. _____

D. _____

3. Spinal Column

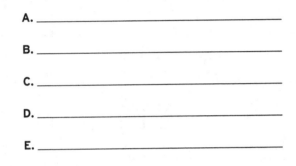

A. _____

B. _____

C. _____

D. _____

E. _____

Crossword Puzzle

The following crossword puzzle is an activity provided to reinforce correct spelling and understanding of medical terminology associated with emergency care and the EMT. Use the clues in the column to complete the puzzle.

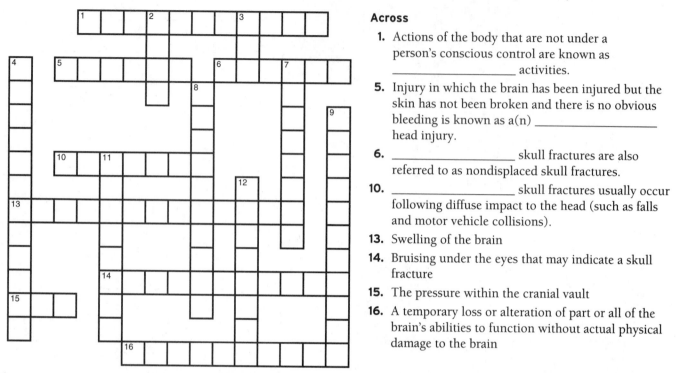

Across

1. Actions of the body that are not under a person's conscious control are known as _____ activities.

5. Injury in which the brain has been injured but the skin has not been broken and there is no obvious bleeding is known as a(n) _____ head injury.

6. _____ skull fractures are also referred to as nondisplaced skull fractures.

10. _____ skull fractures usually occur following diffuse impact to the head (such as falls and motor vehicle collisions).

13. Swelling of the brain

14. Bruising under the eyes that may indicate a skull fracture

15. The pressure within the cranial vault

16. A temporary loss or alteration of part or all of the brain's abilities to function without actual physical damage to the brain

Down

2. Injury to the head often caused by a penetrating object in which there may be bleeding and exposed brain tissue is known as a(n) _____ head injury.

3. A traumatic insult to the brain capable of producing physical, intellectual, emotional, social, and vocational changes

4. Bleeding into the subarachnoid space, where the cerebrospinal fluid circulates, is known as a(n) _____ hemorrhage.

7. A(n) _____ hematoma is an accumulation of blood between the skull and the dura mater.

8. The _____ log roll is the recommended procedure for moving a patient with a suspected spinal injury from the ground to a long backboard.

9. Bruising behind an ear over the mastoid process that may indicate a skull fracture

11. An accumulation of blood beneath the dura mater but outside the brain is known as a(n) _____ hematoma.

12. Three distinct layers of tissue that surround and protect the brain and the spinal cord within the skull and the spinal canal

Critical Thinking

Short Answer

Complete this section with short written answers using the space provided.

1. List the 10 mechanisms of injury where you are likely to encounter a head injury.

_____

_____

2. List the reasons for not placing the head and/or spine injury patient's head into a neutral in-line position.

_____

_____

3. What is the difference between a primary brain injury and a secondary brain injury?

_____

_____

4. List at least 10 signs and symptoms of a head injury.

_____

_____

5. List the three general principles for treating a head injury.

_____

_____

6. List the seven questions to ask yourself when deciding whether to remove a helmet.

_____

_____

Ambulance Calls

The following case scenarios provide an opportunity to explore the concerns associated with patient management and to enhance critical-thinking skills. Read each scenario and answer each question to the best of your ability.

1. You are dispatched to a bicycle-versus-car collision. The driver of the car is uninjured, but the bicyclist is reported as "severely injured." You arrive to find the patient lying in the street unconscious and with an apparent head injury. The patient was not wearing a helmet when she was struck by the car. Witnesses say she was launched into the windshield and then landed in the road.

   How would you best manage this patient?

   _____

   _____

   _____

2. You are dispatched to assist a "young child fallen." You arrive to find a frantic parent who tells you her daughter was playing on the family's trampoline in the backyard. She was bouncing very high and accidentally launched herself off the trampoline, landing face down onto a concrete pad in the neighbor's yard. She responds to painful stimuli and has snoring respirations.

   How would you best manage this patient?

   _____

   _____

   _____

3. You are dispatched to a motor vehicle collision with major damage to the patient compartment. Your patient, an 18-month-old boy, is still in his car seat in the center of the back seat. He responds appropriately, and there is no damage to his seat. He has no visible injuries, but a front seat passenger was killed.

   How would you best manage this patient?

   _____

   _____

   _____

Skills

Skill Drills

Skill Drill 26-1: Performing Manual In-Line Stabilization
Test your knowledge of this skill by filling in the correct words in the photo captions.

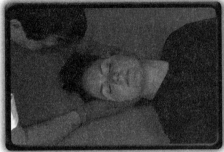
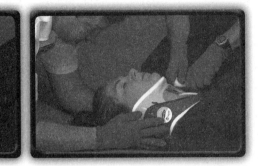
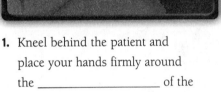

1. Kneel behind the patient and place your hands firmly around the _____ of the _____ on either _____.

2. Support the lower jaw with your _____ and _____ fingers, and the head with your _____. Gently lift the head into a(n) _____, _____ position, aligned with the torso. Do not _____ the head or neck excessively, forcefully, or rapidly.

3. Continue to _____ the head manually while your partner places a rigid _____ _____ around the neck. Maintain _____ _____ until you have completely secured the patient to a backboard.

Skill Drill 26-2: Immobilizing a Patient to a Long Backboard
Test your knowledge of this skill by placing the photos below in the correct order. Number the first step with a "1," the second step with a "2," etc.

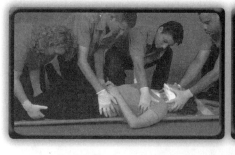

_____ Center the patient on the board.

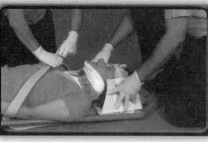

_____ Secure the upper torso first.

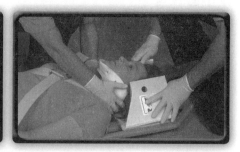

_____ Begin to secure the patient's head using a commercial immobilization device or rolled towels.

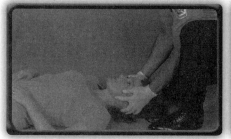

_____ Apply and maintain cervical motion restriction. Assess distal functions in all extremities.

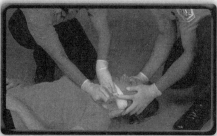

_____ Apply a cervical collar.

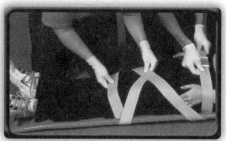

_____ Secure the pelvis and upper legs.

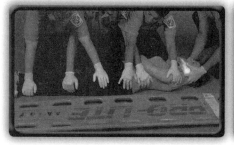

_____ Rescuers kneel on one side of the patient and place hands on the far side of the patient.

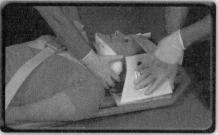

_____ Place tape across the patient's forehead to secure the immobilization device.

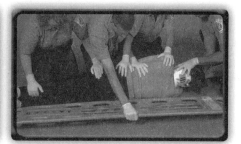

_____ On command, rescuers roll the patient toward themselves, quickly examine the back, slide the backboard under the patient, and roll the patient onto the board.

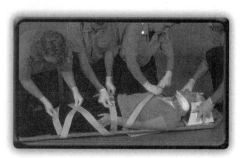

_____ Check all straps and readjust as needed. Reassess distal functions in all extremities.

Skill Drill 26-4: Immobilizing a Patient Found in a Standing Position
Test your knowledge of this skill by filling in the correct words in the photo captions.

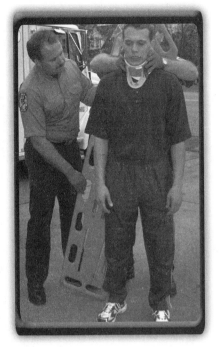

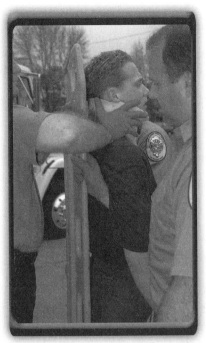

1. While _____ stabilizing the head
and neck, apply a(n) _____
_____. Position the board
_____ the patient.

2. Position EMTs at _____ and
_____ the patient. Side EMTs
reach under the patient's _____
and grasp _____ at or slightly
above _____ level.

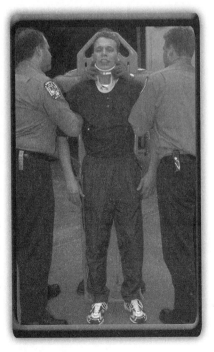

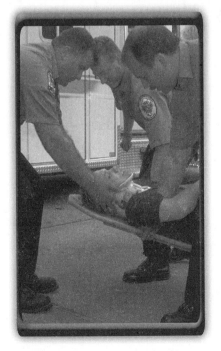

3. Prepare to lower the patient to the
_____.

4. On command, _____
the backboard to the ground as a unit
under the direction of the EMT at the
_____.

Skill Drill 26-5: Application of a Cervical Collar
Test your knowledge of this skill by filling in the correct words in the photo captions.

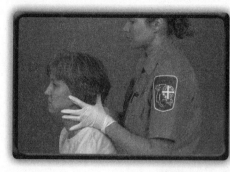

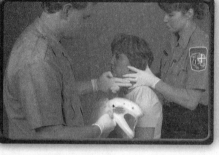

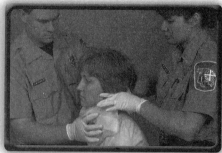

1. Apply in-line _____
_____.

2. Measure the proper
_____
_____.

3. Place the _____
_____ first.

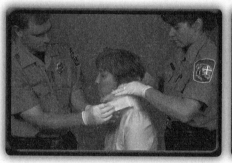

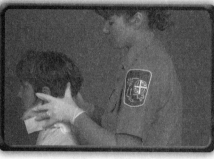

4. _____ the
collar around the neck and
_____ the collar.

5. Ensure proper _____
and maintain _____,
_____ motion
restriction until the patient is secured
to a(n) _____.

Assessment Review

Answer the following questions pertaining to the assessment of the types of emergencies discussed in this chapter.

_____ 1. You respond to a patient who was assaulted and is unconscious. Upon reaching his side, you check his airway and it is open. The breathing is at 18 breaths/min and regular. Pulse is strong and regular with distal pulses present. You want to administer oxygen. At what rate would you give it?

    A. 2 L/min

    B. 6 L/min

    C. 10 L/min

    D. 15 L/min

_____ 2. You and your partner have determined that you need to put the patient above (question 1) in full immobilization. When can your partner release manual stabilization of the head?

    A. When the cervical collar is applied

    B. When the torso is secured to the board

    C. When the patient is completely secured to the board

    D. When you arrive at the hospital

_____ 3. You decide to put the patient on a long backboard and will use the log-roll technique to accomplish the task. When do you check the patient's back?

    A. After securing the patient to the board

    B. As the patient is rolled onto his or her side

    C. Before any movement is attempted

    D. When you move the patient to the hospital bed

_____ 4. If you respond to a patient who is in a sitting position and stable, how would you immobilize them?

    A. Lay the patient down and perform the log-roll technique.

    B. Use a scoop stretcher.

    C. Use a short board.

    D. Have the patient lay down on your backboard.

_____ 5. You respond to a motorcycle accident. You decide that you need to remove the rider's helmet. What is the minimum number of people required to remove the helmet?

    A. Two

    B. Three

    C. Four

    D. Five

Emergency Care Summary

Fill in the following chart pertaining to the management of the types of emergencies discussed in this chapter.

Note: While the following steps are widely accepted, be sure to consult and follow your local protocol.

General Management of Head Injuries

1. Establish and maintain a(n) _____ airway. Provide high-flow _____ oxygen and provide

   _____ assistance, if needed.

2. Control _____. Do not apply pressure to an open or _____ skull injury. Begin

   _____ resuscitation, if necessary.

3. Assess the patient's baseline level of _____, and continuously monitor it.

4. Assess and treat other injuries.

5. Anticipate and manage _____ to prevent aspiration.

6. Be prepared for _____ and changes in the patient's condition.

7. Transport the patient promptly and with extreme care.

General Management of Spine Injuries

1. Open and maintain a patent airway with the _____ maneuver.

2. Hold the head still in a(n) _____, in-line position.

3. Consider inserting a(n) _____ airway.

4. Have a(n) _____ unit available.

5. Provide high-flow oxygen.

6. Continuously monitor the patient's airway.

7. Perform manual, in-line stabilization to protect the _____ spine.

8. Prepare the patient for transport according to patient's _____.

9. Transport to the appropriate _____ _____.

Chest Injuries

General Knowledge

Matching

Match each of the items in the left column to the appropriate definition in the right column.

_____ 1. Thoracic cage

_____ 2. Diaphragm

_____ 3. Exhalation

_____ 4. Inhalation

_____ 5. Aorta

_____ 6. Closed chest injury

_____ 7. Hemoptysis

_____ 8. Pericardium

_____ 9. Open chest injury

_____ 10. Tachypnea

_____ 11. Mediastinum

A. Chest rises

B. Chest

C. Center cavity of the thorax

D. Separates the chest from the abdomen

E. Major artery in the chest

F. Penetrating wound

G. Rapid respirations

H. Unusually blunt trauma

I. Coughing up blood

J. Sac around the heart

K. Chest falls

Multiple Choice

Read each item carefully and then select the one best response.

_____ 1. Air is supplied to the lungs via the:

   A. esophagus.

   B. trachea.

   C. nares.

   D. oropharnyx.

_____ 2. The _____ separates the thoracic cavity from the abdominal cavity.

   A. diaphragm

   B. mediastinum

   C. xyphoid process

   D. inferior border of the ribs

_____ 3. On inhalation, which of the following does NOT occur?

   A. The intercostal muscles contract, elevating the rib cage.

   B. The diaphragm contracts.

   C. The pressure inside the chest increases.

   D. Air enters through the nose and mouth.

_____ 4. You respond to the local rodeo arena for a bull rider. The scene is safe, and the patient is lying in the middle of the arena unconscious. His airway is open, and he is breathing at 20 breaths/min. His pulse is 128 beats/min and blood pressure is 110/64 mm Hg. There is no obvious bleeding. Bystanders tell you he was thrown into the air and landed on the bull's head. He was not wearing a vest. Which of the following is NOT indicated in blunt trauma to the chest?

   A. Bruising of the lungs and heart

   B. Fracture of whole areas of the chest wall

   C. Damage to the aorta

   D. Dissection of the carotid arteries

_____ 5. You respond to a motor vehicle collision and find a 29-year-old woman who is complaining of chest pain. Her chest struck the steering wheel. Her airway is open, she is breathing at 24 breaths/min, and she is coughing up blood. Her pulse is 130 beats/min, rapid and weak, and her blood pressure is 90/58 mm Hg. You notice cyanosis around the lips and note that her fingers are also blue. When you expose the chest, she tells you it hurts and points to a bruised spot. Which of the following is a symptom?

    A. Cyanosis around the lips or fingertips

    B. Rapid, weak pulse

    C. Hemoptysis

    D. Pain at the site of injury

_____ 6. Which of the following is NOT a sign or symptom of a chest injury?

    A. Bruising of the chest wall

    B. Crepitus with palpation of the chest

    C. Clear and equal breath sounds

    D. Unequal expansion of the chest wall

_____ 7. You respond to an 18-year-old man who has been assaulted with a baseball bat. He was hit in the chest. He is unresponsive, apneic, and pulseless. This condition is most likely related to:

    A. commotio cordis.

    B. cardiac tamponade.

    C. pneumothorax.

    D. traumatic asphyxia.

_____ 8. Paradoxical motion of the chest refers to:

    A. rib fractures that move with the chest wall during breathing.

    B. one segment of the chest wall moving opposite the remainder of the chest.

    C. unequal expansion of the chest wall.

    D. one segment of the chest wall moving out on inspiration and in on exhalation.

_____ 9. A _____ results when an injury allows air to enter through a hole in the chest wall or the surface of the lung as the patient attempts to breathe, causing the lung on that side to collapse.

    A. tension pneumothorax

    B. hemothorax

    C. hemopneumothorax

    D. pneumothorax

_____ 10. A sucking chest wound should be treated with:

    A. a standard dressing.

    B. taping down the chest.

    C. an occlusive dressing.

    D. a sandbag over the wound.

_____ 11. You respond to a 20-year-old man who was playing basketball and suddenly developed chest pain and respiratory difficulty. He is alert and oriented and complaining of chest pain. He is breathing at 24 breaths/min. His pulse is 140 beats/min and blood pressure is 160/90 mm Hg. Upon listening to the chest, you notice diminished breath sounds on the left side. This patient is most likely suffering from a(n):

    A. spontaneous pneumothorax.

    B. hemothorax.

    C. tension pneumothorax.

    D. open pneuomothorax.

_____ 12. Distended jugular veins, a narrowing pulse pressure, and muffled heart sounds are seen in which of the following conditions?

    A. Tension pneumothorax

    B. Cardiac tamponade

    C. Traumatic asphyxia

    D. Commotio cordis

_____ **13.** Common signs and symptoms of tension pneumothorax include all the following EXCEPT:

    A. increasing respiratory distress.

    B. distended neck veins.

    C. high blood pressure.

    D. tracheal deviation away from the injured site.

_____ **14.** Which of the following statements regarding hemothorax is correct?

    A. It can only be treated by a surgeon.

    B. It results from a collection of air in the pleural space.

    C. Breath sounds tend to be equal.

    D. It is not typically associated with shock.

_____ **15.** A _____ is the result of blunt chest trauma and is associated with an irregular pulse and sometimes dangerous cardiac rhythms.

    A. cardiac tamponade

    B. pulmonary contusion

    C. myocardial contusion

    D. traumatic asphyxia

_____ **16.** A patient with blunt trauma who is holding the lateral side of his chest and has rapid and shallow respirations is most likely suffering from:

    A. rib fractures.

    B. a sternal fracture.

    C. a pneumothorax.

    D. a pulmonary contusion.

_____ **17.** Traumatic asphyxia:

    A. is bruising of the lung.

    B. occurs when three or more adjacent ribs are fractured in two or more places.

    C. is a sudden, severe compression of the chest.

    D. results from the pericardial sac filling with blood.

_____ **18.** Which of the following would NOT give you a low pulse oximetry reading?

    A. Damaged heart

    B. Decrease in circulating red blood cells from bleeding

    C. Pulmonary contusion

    D. Carbon monoxide poisoning

_____ **19.** Which of the following is NOT a pertinent negative to note during your assessment of a patient with chest trauma?

    A. No heart murmurs

    B. No associated shortness of breath

    C. No rapid breathing

    D. No areas of deformity

_____ **20.** Large blood vessels in the chest that can result in massive hemorrhaging include all of the following EXCEPT:

    A. the pulmonary arteries.

    B. the femoral arteries.

    C. the aorta.

    D. the four main pulmonary veins.

True/False

If you believe the statement to be more true than false, write the letter "T" in the space provided. If you believe the statement to be more false than true, write the letter "F."

_____   **1.** Dyspnea is difficulty with breathing.

_____   **2.** Tachypnea is slow respirations.

_____   **3.** Distended neck veins may be a sign of a tension pneumothorax.

_____   **4.** Rib fractures are especially common in children.

_____   **5.** Narrowing pulse pressure is related to spontaneous pneumothorax.

_____   **6.** Laceration of the large blood vessels in the chest can cause minimal hemorrhage.

_____   **7.** The thoracic cage extends from the lower end of the neck to the umbilicus.

_____   **8.** Patients with spinal cord injuries at C3 or above can lose their ability to breathe.

_____   **9.** A flutter valve is a three-way valve that allows air to leave the chest cavity.

_____   **10.** Open chest injury is caused by penetrating trauma.

_____   **11.** It is considered acceptable to remain on scene with a seriously injured patient to facilitate splinting of an extremity fracture.

_____   **12.** Because patients with chest injury have so many risks of mortality, they should be reassessed every 10 minutes.

_____   **13.** You should control external bleeding with direct pressure and a bulky dressing.

_____   **14.** A rapid, weak pulse and low blood pressure are the principle signs of hypovolemic shock.

_____   **15.** The right lung contains two lobes, and the left lung contains three lobes.

Fill-in-the-Blank

Read each item carefully and then complete the statement by filling in the missing words.

1. The esophagus is located in the _____ of the chest.

2. During inhalation, the pressure in the chest _____.

3. In the anterior chest, ribs connect to the _____.

4. The trachea divides into the right and left main stem _____.

5. The _____ nerves supply the diaphragm.

6. Contents of the chest are protected by the _____.

7. The chest extends from the lower end of the neck to the _____.

8. _____ line the area between the lungs and chest wall.

9. The largest vessel located in the chest is the _____.

10. During inhalation, the diaphragm _____.

11. _____ is the body's ability to move air in and out of the chest and lung tissue.

12. The intercostals muscles are innervated from spinal nerves originating in the cervical regions of _____ and _____.

13. _____ _____ is the amount of air in mL that is moved into or out of the lungs during a

single breath.

14. The _____ _____ may drop as the brain becomes starved for oxygen and overloaded

with carbon dioxide and other waste products.

15. A patient may find it easier and less painful to breathe if a flail segment is _____.

Labeling

Label the following diagrams with the correct terms.

1. Anterior Aspect of the Chest

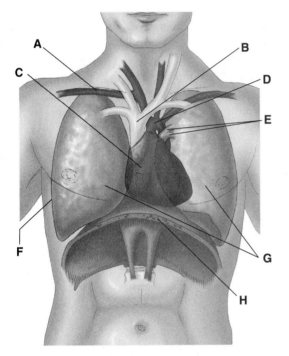

A. _____

B. _____

C. _____

D. _____

E. _____

F. _____

G. _____

H. _____

2. Pneumothorax

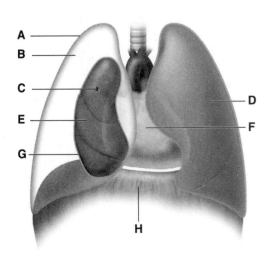

A. _____

B. _____

C. _____

D. _____

E. _____

F. _____

G. _____

H. _____

Crossword Puzzle

The following crossword puzzle is an activity provided to reinforce correct spelling and understanding of medical terminology associated with emergency care and the EMT. Use the clues in the column to complete the puzzle.

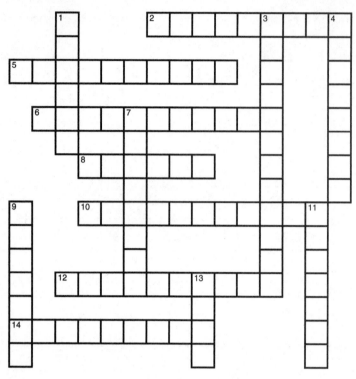

Across

2. Rapid respirations

5. A bruise of the heart muscle is known as a(n) _____ contusion.

6. The fibrous sac that surrounds the heart

8. A(n) _____ pneumothorax is any pneumothorax that is free from significant physiologic changes and does not cause drastic changes in the vital signs of the patient.

10. A(n) _____ pneumothorax occurs when a weak area on the lung ruptures in the absence of major injury, allowing air to leak into the pleural space.

12. A collection of blood in the pleural cavity

14. A(n) _____ dressing is made of Vaseline-impregnated gauze, aluminum foil, or plastic that protects a wound from air and bacteria.

Down

1. A(n) _____ chest injury is usually caused by blunt trauma.

3. An accumulation of air or gas in the pleural cavity

4. Traumatic _____ is a pattern of injuries seen after a severe force is applied to the chest, forcing blood from the great vessels back into the head and neck.

7. _____ cordis is a blunt chest injury caused by a sudden, direct blow to the chest that occurs only during the critical portion of a person's heartbeat.

9. A(n) _____ pneumothorax is an accumulation of air or gas in the pleural cavity that progressively increases pressure in the chest that interferes with cardiac function with potentially fatal results.

11. A(n) _____ chest wound is a chest wall wound through which air passes during inspiration and expiration, creating a sucking sound.

13. A(n) _____ chest injury is an injury in which the chest wall is penetrated by a fractured rib or by an external object.

Critical Thinking

Short Answer

Complete this section with short written answers using the space provided.

1. List the signs and symptoms associated with a chest injury.

_____

_____

2. Describe the two methods for sealing a sucking chest wound.

_____

_____

3. Describe the method(s) for immobilizing a flail chest wall segment.

_____

_____

4. Define *traumatic asphyxia* and describe its signs.

_____

_____

5. List the "deadly dozen" chest injuries.

_____

_____

Ambulance Calls

The following case scenarios provide an opportunity to explore the concerns associated with patient management and to enhance critical-thinking skills. Read each scenario and answer each question to the best of your ability.

1. You are dispatched to an area horse ranch for an injury to a rider. You arrive to find that a horse has kicked one of the riders in the chest. The patient is having significant difficulty breathing and appears to be in extreme pain.

   How would you best manage this patient?

   _____

   _____

   _____

2. You are dispatched for a man trapped under a car. As you travel to the location, the dispatcher informs you that your patient is now free, but is experiencing significant chest and mid-back pain.

   How would you best manage this patient?

   _____

   _____

   _____

3. You are dispatched to a lumberyard where a 27-year-old man was crushed by a piece of heavy equipment. Coworkers pulled the equipment off the patient. He presents with distended neck veins, cyanosis, and bloodshot eyes.

   How would you best manage this patient?

   _____

   _____

   _____

Skills

Assessment Review

Answer the following questions pertaining to the assessment of the types of emergencies discussed in this chapter.

_____ 1. You respond to an accidental shooting of a 37-year-old man. During the primary assessment, you find his airway to be open. His breathing is labored at 24 breaths/min. His pulse is rapid and weak. Upon exposing the chest you find a sucking chest wound. You should:

    A. take a blood pressure reading.

    B. cover the wound.

    C. continue your assessment.

    D. transport the patient immediately.

_____ 2. You respond to a 17-year-old girl who was hit in the chest with a lawn dart. Upon arrival, she is conscious and able to converse with you. Her airway is open, but her breathing is becoming progressively more difficult. Her pulse is rapid and weak. You can palpate a radial pulse. Upon examining the chest, you find that she has a penetrating injury to the chest and that there is a sucking sound as she breathes. How do you manage this wound?

    A. Apply oxygen by nasal cannula.

    B. Stabilize the c-spine.

    C. Use a 4″ × 4″ gauze pad.

    D. Use an occlusive dressing.

_____ 3. When bandaging an open chest wound, what is the minimum number of sides that have to be taped down?

    A. One

    B. Two

    C. Three

    D. Four

_____ 4. Dispatch sends you to a farm on the edge of town. A 57-year-old man was kicked in the chest by a horse. He walked into his house and collapsed. He is alert and oriented. His breathing is labored at 20 breaths/min, pulse is rapid and regular, and you are able to palpate a radial pulse. Upon examination of his chest, you notice paradoxical movement on the right chest wall. You should:

    A. take spinal precautions.

    B. put the patient in a position of comfort.

    C. provide oxygen by nasal cannula.

    D. stabilize the flail segment.

_____ 5. A 16-year-old boy walks into a pipe gate that hits him in the ribs on the left side. Upon your arrival, he is alert and oriented. His breathing is shallow at 22 breaths/min. His pulse is regular and strong. You palpate a radial pulse. You are able to rule out spinal trauma. What position do you transport him in?

    A. Position of comfort

    B. Supine

    C. Prone

    D. Recovery

Emergency Care Summary

Fill in the following chart pertaining to the management of the types of emergencies discussed in this chapter.

Note: While the following steps are widely accepted, be sure to consult and follow your local protocol.

General Management of Chest Injuries

Managing life threats to the patient's _____ is the primary concern with any traumatic emergency. The MOI that caused the chest injury may also have caused a(n) _____ injury or other fracture, and these must be managed at the appropriate time following local protocols. _____ difficulties are often present with chest injuries, as are injuries involving bleeding. With all chest injuries, once crew safety has been established, management of airway, breathing, and circulatory problems is a priority. For all of the chest injuries described in Chapter 27, begin with the following steps:

1. Ensure scene safety.

2. Determine the _____.

3. Consider _____ _____.

4. Open, clear, and maintain the patient's airway.

5. Inspect, palpate, and _____ the chest.

6. Administer high concentration oxygen via a nonrebreathing mask or bag-mask device, as appropriate.

7. Control bleeding, and treat for _____.

8. Transport to the appropriate treatment facility.

Abdominal and Genitourinary Injuries

General Knowledge

Matching

Match each of the items in the left column to the appropriate definition in the right column.

_____ 1. Closed abdominal injury

_____ 2. Evisceration

_____ 3. Flank

_____ 4. Guarding

_____ 5. Hollow organs

_____ 6. Kehr sign

_____ 7. Open abdominal injury

_____ 8. Peritoneal cavity

_____ 9. Solid organs

A. Contracting stomach muscles to minimize pain

B. Liver, pancreas, spleen

C. Left shoulder pain caused by blood in the peritoneal cavity

D. Injury where there is a break in the skin or mucous membrane

E. Soft-tissue damage inside the body, but the skin remains intact

F. Posterior region below the margin of the lower rib cage

G. Abdominal cavity

H. Stomach, small intestine, ureters

I. Displacement of organs outside the body

Multiple Choice

Read each item carefully and then select the one best response.

_____ 1. All of the following systems contain organs that make up the contents of the abdominal cavity EXCEPT:

A. the digestive system.

B. the urinary system.

C. the genitourinary system.

D. the limbic system.

_____ 2. Which of the following is NOT a hollow organ of the abdomen?

A. Stomach

B. Liver

C. Bladder

D. Ureters

_____ 3. Which of the following is NOT a solid organ of the abdomen?

A. Liver

B. Spleen

C. Gallbladder

D. Pancreas

_____ 4. The first signs of peritonitis include all of the following EXCEPT:

A. severe abdominal pain.

B. tenderness.

C. muscular spasm.

D. nausea.

_____ 5. Late signs of peritonitis may include:

A. a soft abdomen.

B. nausea.

C. normal bowel sounds.

D. diarrhea.

_____ **6.** _____ takes place in the solid organs.
- **A.** Digestion
- **B.** Excretion
- **C.** Energy production
- **D.** Absorption

_____ **7.** Because solid organs have a rich supply of blood, any injury can result in major:
- **A.** hemorrhaging.
- **B.** damage.
- **C.** pain.
- **D.** guarding.

_____ **8.** You are dispatched to a motor vehicle collision. You see a 25-year-old woman who was restrained but is complaining of abdominal pain. She is alert and oriented. The patient's airway is open, and she is breathing normally. Her pulse is regular but weak and rapid. She has a radial pulse. You inspect the abdomen for possible bleeding. You would expect to see all of the following EXCEPT:
- **A.** pain or tenderness.
- **B.** rigidity.
- **C.** urticaria.
- **D.** distention.

_____ **9.** Air in the abdominal cavity can cause all of the following EXCEPT:
- **A.** pain.
- **B.** diarrhea.
- **C.** infection.
- **D.** tissue ischemia and infarction.

_____ **10.** The abdomen is divided into four:
- **A.** quadrants.
- **B.** planes.
- **C.** sections.
- **D.** angles.

_____ **11.** The largest organ in the abdomen is the:
- **A.** liver.
- **B.** spleen.
- **C.** pancreas.
- **D.** kidneys.

_____ **12.** Open abdominal injuries are also known as:
- **A.** blunt injuries.
- **B.** eviscerations.
- **C.** penetrating injuries.
- **D.** peritoneal injuries.

_____ **13.** Blunt abdominal injuries may result from:
- **A.** a stab wound.
- **B.** seatbelts.
- **C.** a gunshot wound.
- **D.** an impaled object.

_____ **14.** The major complaint of patients with abdominal injury is:
- **A.** pain.
- **B.** tachycardia.
- **C.** rigidity.
- **D.** swelling.

_____ **15.** The most common sign of significant abdominal injury is:

    A. pain.

    B. tachycardia.

    C. rigidity.

    D. distention.

_____ **16.** Late signs of abdominal injury include all of the following EXCEPT:

    A. distention.

    B. increased blood pressure.

    C. change in mental status.

    D. pale, cool, moist skin.

_____ **17.** Your primary concern when dealing with an unresponsive patient with an open abdominal injury is:

    A. covering the wound with a moist dressing.

    B. maintaining the airway.

    C. controlling the bleeding.

    D. monitoring vital signs.

_____ **18.** You respond to an 18-year-old high school football player who was hit in the right flank with a helmet several hours ago. He is complaining of pain in the area. He is alert and oriented. His airway is open, and his respirations are within normal limits. His pulse is rapid and regular. He has a radial pulse. He tells you that he is noticing blood in his urine. Based on this information, the patient is likely to have an injury to the:

    A. liver.

    B. kidney.

    C. gallbladder.

    D. appendix.

_____ **19.** When performing a history on a patient with abdominal trauma, which of the following questions would be appropriate regarding trauma?

    A. Is there any blood in your stool?

    B. Does your pain go anywhere?

    C. Do you have any nausea, vomiting, or diarrhea?

    D. All of the above.

_____ **20.** When used alone, diagonal shoulder safety belts can cause all of the following EXCEPT:

    A. a bruised chest.

    B. a lacerated liver.

    C. decapitation.

    D. a ruptured appendix.

_____ **21.** You are dispatched to a motor vehicle collision. Your patient is a 42-year-old restrained woman. The air bag did deploy, and the woman has abrasions on her face. She is complaining of pain to both her chest and abdomen. Her airway is open and respirations are within normal limits. Her pulse is a little rapid but strong and regular. She has distal pulses. In assessing this patient, which of the following statements is NOT true?

    A. Bowel sounds can be difficult to hear in the field.

    B. Palpation is typically performed first with light touch.

    C. If light touch elicits pain, perform deep palpation to assess further injury.

    D. If you find an entry wound, you should always assess for an exit wound.

_____ **22.** Patients with open abdominal injuries often complain of:

    A. pain.

    B. nausea.

    C. vomiting.

    D. dyspnea.

_____ **23.** You are called to the local bar where a fight has taken place. The police department tells you that you have a 36-year-old man who has been stabbed twice in the abdomen. Upon your arrival, the patient is alert and oriented. His airway is open. His respirations are at 24 breaths/min; pulse is rapid, regular, and weak. He has distal pulses. With the penetrating trauma, you should assume that the object:

    A. has penetrated the peritoneum.

    B. has entered the abdominal cavity.

    C. has possibly injured one or more organs.

    D. all of the above.

_____ **24.** When treating a patient with an evisceration, you should:

    A. attempt to replace the abdominal contents.

    B. cover the protruding organs with a dry, sterile dressing.

    C. cover the protruding organs with moist, adherent dressings.

    D. cover the protruding contents with moist, sterile gauze compresses.

_____ **25.** The solid organs of the urinary system include the:

    A. kidneys.

    B. ureters.

    C. bladder.

    D. urethra.

_____ **26.** All of the following male genitalia lie outside the pelvic cavity EXCEPT the:

    A. urethra.

    B. penis.

    C. seminal vesicles.

    D. testes.

_____ **27.** Suspect kidney damage if the patient has a history or physical evidence of all of the following EXCEPT:

    A. an abrasion, laceration, or contusion in the flank.

    B. a penetrating wound in the region of the lower rib cage or the upper abdomen.

    C. fractures on either side of the lower rib cage.

    D. a hematoma in the umbilical region.

_____ **28.** Signs of injury to the kidney may include any of the following EXCEPT:

    A. bruises or lacerations on the overlying skin.

    B. shock.

    C. increased urgency of urination.

    D. hematuria.

_____ **29.** Suspect a possible injury of the urinary bladder in all of the following findings EXCEPT:

    A. bruising to the left upper quadrant.

    B. blood at the urethral opening.

    C. blood at the tip of the penis or a stain on the patient's underwear.

    D. physical signs of trauma on the lower abdomen, pelvis, or perineum.

_____ **30.** When treating a patient with an amputation of the penile shaft, your top priority is:

    A. locating the amputated part.

    B. controlling bleeding.

    C. keeping the remaining tissue dry.

    D. delaying transport until bleeding is controlled.

_____ **31.** In any case of trauma to a female patient, you should always determine if the patient:

    A. is on birth control.

    B. is pregnant.

    C. is currently menstruating.

    D. has a history of ovarian cysts.

_____ **32.** In cases of sexual assault, which of the following is true?

    A. You should always examine the genitalia for any sign of injury.

    B. Advise the patient not to wash, urinate, or defecate.

    C. In addition to recording the facts, it is important to include your personal thoughts.

    D. You should use plastic bags when collecting items such as clothes.

True/False

If you believe the statement to be more true than false, write the letter "T" in the space provided. If you believe the statement to be more false than true, write the letter "F."

_____ **1.** Hollow organs will bleed profusely if injured.

_____ **2.** One of the most common signs of an abdominal injury is an elevated pulse rate.

_____ **3.** Patients with abdominal injuries should be kept supine with the head elevated.

_____ **4.** Peritoneal irritation is in response to hollow organ injury.

_____ **5.** Eviscerated organs should be covered with a dry dressing.

_____ **6.** Injuries to the kidneys usually occur in isolation.

_____ **7.** Peritonitis is an inflammation of the peritoneum.

_____ **8.** The abdomen is divided into two quadrants.

_____ **9.** Small children can be injured by air bags.

_____ **10.** Patients with peritonitis will want to lie still with their legs drawn up.

Fill-in-the-Blank

Read each item carefully and then complete the statement by filling in the missing words.

1. Severe bleeding may occur with injury to _____ organs.

2. The _____ system is responsible for filtering waste.

3. Kidneys are located in the _____ space.

4. A penetrating wound that reaches the kidneys almost always involves _____ _____.

5. When ruptured, the organs of the abdominal cavity can spill their contents into the peritoneal cavity, causing an intense

   inflammatory reaction called _____.

6. Blood may irritate the _____ _____ and cause the patient to report abdominal pain.

7. Closed abdominal injuries are also known as _____ _____.

8. Open abdominal injuries are also known as _____ _____.

9. Another name for the right and left upper quadrants is _____.

10. An open wound that allows internal organs or fat to protrude through the wound is called _____.

Labeling

Label the following diagrams with the correct terms.

1. Hollow Organs

A. _____

B. _____

C. _____

D. _____

E. _____

F. _____

G. _____

H. _____

I. _____

J. _____

K. _____

2. Solid Organs

A. _____

B. _____

C. _____

D. _____

E. _____

F. _____

G. _____

H. _____

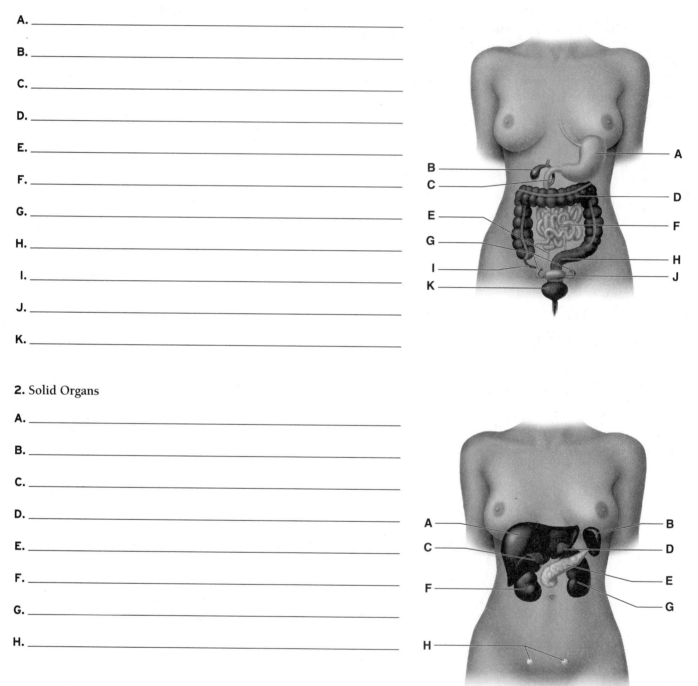

Crossword Puzzle

The following crossword puzzle is an activity provided to reinforce correct spelling and understanding of medical terminology associated with emergency care and the EMT. Use the clues in the column to complete the puzzle.

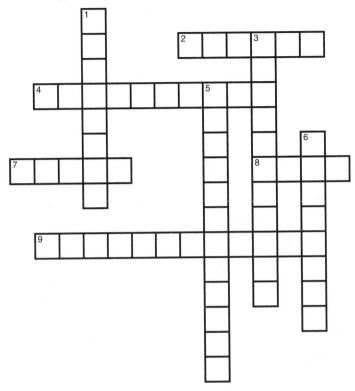

Across

2. In a(n) _____ abdominal injury, there is soft-tissue damage inside the body but the skin remains intact.

4. The abdominal cavity is known as the _____ cavity.

7. The posterior region below the margin of the lower rib cage

8. In a(n) _____ abdominal injury, there is a break in the surface of the skin or mucous membrane, exposing deeper tissue to potential contamination.

9. Structures through which materials pass, such as the stomach, small intestines, large intestines, ureters, and bladder

Down

1. Contracting the stomach muscles to minimize the pain of abdominal movement

3. Solid masses of tissue where much of the chemical work of the body takes place

5. The displacement of organs outside of the body

6. Left shoulder pain caused by blood in the peritoneal cavity

Critical Thinking

Short Answer

Complete this section with short written answers using the space provided.

1. List the hollow organs of the abdomen and urinary system.

_____

_____

2. List the solid organs of the abdomen and urinary system.

_____

_____

3. List the signs and symptoms of an abdominal injury.

_____

_____

4. List the steps to care for an open abdominal injury.

_____

_____

5. List the steps to care for an open abdominal wound with exposed organs.

_____

_____

6. List the major history or physical findings associated with possible kidney damage.

_____

_____

Ambulance Calls

The following case scenarios provide an opportunity to explore the concerns associated with patient management and to enhance critical-thinking skills. Read each scenario and answer each question to the best of your ability.

1. You are dispatched to a local bar where your patient, a 26-year-old man, was involved in an altercation. He has several superficial lacerations to his arms, and a knife is impaled in his right upper quadrant. He is lying supine on the floor. He is alert. The bar patrons tell you that he did not fall, but that they helped him to the floor.

How would you best manage this patient?

_____

_____

_____

2. You are dispatched to assist police with a mentally ill patient who has threatened harm to himself and others. Police officers found the man running around his home with a knife and blood all over his lower body. The man tells you "the voices" told him to cut off his penis.

How would you best manage this patient?

_____

_____

_____

3. You are dispatched to a construction site, where a man has fallen onto a piece of rebar. You arrive to find a man sitting on the ground with his legs drawn toward his chest. He tells you that he fell from a ladder onto a piece of rebar. He tells you, "Something's sticking out of me." As you visualize his abdomen, you can clearly see a portion of his bowel on the outside of his body.

How would you best manage this patient?

_____

_____

_____

Skills

Assessment Review

Answer the following questions pertaining to the assessment of the types of emergencies discussed in this chapter.

_____ 1. If you are treating a patient with an abdominal evisceration, you should use a(n):

    A. moist, sterile dressing.

    B. dry, sterile dressing.

    C. adhesive dressing.

    D. triangular bandage.

_____ 2. You have a male patient who has no immediate life threat, but does have bleeding genitalia. You should bandage with a(n):

    A. dry dressing.

    B. moist dressing.

    C. occlusive dressing.

    D. adhesive dressing.

_____ 3. You have a patient with suspected kidney injury but no spinal injury. How should he be positioned?

    A. Supine

    B. Prone

    C. Lateral recumbent

    D. Position of comfort

_____ 4. Your patient has his penis caught in his zipper. What do you need to do to relieve pressure?

    A. Pull the pants off the patient.

    B. Force the zipper open.

    C. Remove the foreskin.

    D. Cut the zipper out of the pants.

_____ 5. Whenever possible, you should always provide the sexual assault patient with:

    A. a police escort.

    B. rape crisis intervention.

    C. an attendant of the same gender.

    D. the name of the assailant.

Emergency Care Summary

Fill in the following chart pertaining to the management of the types of emergencies discussed in this chapter.

Note: While the steps below are widely accepted, be sure to consult and follow your local protocol.

Abdominal Trauma

Blunt Abdominal Injuries

Log roll the patient to a(n) _____ position on a backboard. If the patient vomits, turn him or her to one side and clear the mouth and throat of vomitus. Monitor the patient's vital signs for any indication of _____. If shock is present, administer high-flow supplemental oxygen via a nonrebreathing mask and treat for shock. Keep the patient _____. Provide prompt transport to the emergency department.

Penetrating Abdominal Injuries

The injuries from penetrating trauma may not be so obvious. Large amounts of _____ _____ may not be present, yet there can be significant blood loss internally. Accurate assessment of a penetrating injury takes place in the _____ _____. Prehospital treatment consists of controlling any external bleeding, immobilizing the patient on a long spine board, treating for shock, and transporting the patient to the appropriate specialty center. If the penetrating object is still in place (impaled), stabilize the object in place.

Abdominal Evisceration

Never attempt to replace protruding organs. Cover the exposed organs with a(n) _____, sterile dressing. If local protocol allows, cover the sterile dressing with a(n) _____ dressing. Maintain body temperature, treat for shock, and transport to the highest level trauma center available.

Genitourinary Trauma

Kidney Injuries

Damage to the kidneys may not be obvious on inspection of the patient. You may or may not see bruises or lacerations on the overlying skin. You will see signs of shock if the injury is associated with significant blood loss. Another sign of kidney damage is _____ in the urine (hematuria). Treat shock and associated injuries in the appropriate manner. Provide prompt transport to the hospital, monitoring the patient's vital signs carefully en route.

Urinary Bladder Injuries

Suspect a possible injury of the urinary bladder if you see blood at the _____ opening or physical signs of trauma on the lower abdomen, pelvis, or _____. There may be blood at the tip of the penis or a stain on the patient's underwear. The presence of associated injuries or of shock will dictate the urgency of transport. In most instances, provide prompt transport, and monitor the patient's vital signs en route.

Genitalia Injuries

Soft-tissue injuries to the external genitalia should be treated like any other soft-tissue injury once all life threats have been assessed and managed. Female patients with external genitalia trauma should be questioned about the possibility of _____. Use only external dressings, never place anything into the _____.

Trauma to the abdomen or genitourinary area may produce injury to the female patient's uterus, _____ _____, and ovaries. Treat for shock because injuries to these organs may be hidden.

Rectal Bleeding

Rectal bleeding can be significant and lead to shock. Place dressings in the crease between the _____ to manage bleeding. Contact medical control to determine the need for transport.

Sexual Assault

Follow local protocol for crime scene management and _____ preservation. If available, an EMT of the same sex as the patient should perform the assessment and treatment. Advise the patient not to change clothes, _____, drink, or eat. Maintain patient privacy at all times. Sexual assault victims may have serious multisystem trauma. Assessment and treatment should consist of managing life-threatening injuries. Do not examine the genitalia unless obvious bleeding must be managed.

Orthopaedic Injuries

General Knowledge

Matching

Match each of the items in the left column to the appropriate definition in the right column.

_____ **1.** Striated

_____ **2.** Tendons

_____ **3.** Smooth

_____ **4.** Joint

_____ **5.** Ligaments

_____ **6.** Closed fracture

_____ **7.** Point tenderness

_____ **8.** Displaced fracture

_____ **9.** Articular cartilage

_____ **10.** Open fracture

_____ **11.** Traction

A. Any injury that makes the limb appear in an unnatural position

B. Any fracture in which the skin has not been broken

C. A thin layer of cartilage, covering the articular surface of bones in synovial joints

D. Involuntary muscle

E. Any break in the bone in which the overlying skin has been damaged as well

F. Hold joints together

G. Skeletal muscle

H. The act of exerting a pulling force on a structure

I. Where two bones contact

J. Attach muscle to bone

K. Tenderness sharply located at the site of an injury

Multiple Choice

Read each item carefully and then select the one best response.

_____ **1.** Blood in the urine is known as:

    A. hematuria.

    B. hemotysis.

    C. hematocrit.

    D. hemoglobin.

_____ **2.** Smooth muscle is found in the:

    A. back.

    B. blood vessels.

    C. heart.

    D. all of the above.

_____ **3.** The bones in the skeleton produce _____ in the bone marrow.

    A. blood cells

    B. minerals

    C. electrolytes

    D. hormones

_____ **4.** _____ are held together in a tough fibrous structure known as a capsule.

    A. Tendons

    B. Joints

    C. Ligaments

    D. Bones

_____ **5.** Joints are bathed and lubricated by _____ fluid.
  A. cartilaginous
  B. articular
  C. synovial
  D. cerebrospinal

_____ **6.** A _____ is a disruption of a joint in which the bone ends are no longer in contact.
  A. torn ligament
  B. dislocation
  C. fracture dislocation
  D. sprain

_____ **7.** A _____ is an injury to the ligaments, the articular capsule, the synovial membrane, and the tendons crossing the joint.
  A. dislocation
  B. strain
  C. sprain
  D. torn ligament

_____ **8.** A _____ is a stretching or tearing of the muscle.
  A. strain
  B. sprain
  C. torn ligament
  D. split

_____ **9.** The zone of injury includes the:
  A. adjacent nerves.
  B. adjacent blood vessels.
  C. surrounding soft tissue.
  D. all of the above.

_____ **10.** A(n) _____ fractures the bone at the point of impact.
  A. direct blow
  B. indirect force
  C. twisting force
  D. high-energy injury

_____ **11.** A(n) _____ may cause a fracture or dislocation at a distant point.
  A. direct blow
  B. indirect force
  C. twisting force
  D. high-energy injury

_____ **12.** When caring for patients who have fallen, you must identify the _____ and the mechanism of injury so that you will not overlook associated injuries.
  A. site of injury
  B. height of fall
  C. point of contact
  D. twisting forces

_____ **13.** _____ produce severe damage to the skeleton, surrounding soft tissues, and vital internal organs.
  A. Direct blows
  B. Indirect forces
  C. Twisting forces
  D. High-energy injuries

_____ **14.** Regardless of the extent and severity of the damage to the skin, you should treat any injury that breaks the skin as a possible:

   A. closed fracture.

   B. open fracture.

   C. nondisplaced fracture.

   D. displaced fracture.

_____ **15.** A(n) _____ is also known as a hairline fracture.

   A. closed fracture

   B. open fracture

   C. nondisplaced fracture

   D. displaced fracture

_____ **16.** A(n) _____ produces actual deformity, or distortion, of the limb by shortening, rotating, or angulating it.

   A. closed fracture

   B. open fracture

   C. nondisplaced fracture

   D. displaced fracture

_____ **17.** You respond to a 19-year-old woman who was kicked in the leg by a horse. She is alert and oriented. Respirations are 20 breaths/min, regular and unlabored. Pulse is 110 beats/min and regular. Distal pulses are present. She has point tenderness at the site of the injury. You should compare the limb to:

   A. the opposite uninjured limb.

   B. one of your limbs or one of your partner's limbs.

   C. an injury chart.

   D. none of the above.

_____ **18.** _____ is the most reliable indicator of an underlying fracture.

   A. Crepitus

   B. Deformity

   C. Point tenderness

   D. Absence of distal pulse

_____ **19.** A(n) _____ fracture occurs in a growth section of a child's bone, which may prematurely stop growth if not properly treated.

   A. greenstick

   B. comminuted

   C. pathologic

   D. epiphyseal

_____ **20.** A(n) _____ fracture is an incomplete fracture that passes only partway through the shaft of a bone but may still cause severe angulation.

   A. greenstick

   B. comminuted

   C. pathologic

   D. epiphyseal

_____ **21.** You are called to the local assisted living facility where a 94-year-old man has fallen. He is alert and oriented and denies passing out. His respirations are 18 breaths/min and regular. Pulse is 106 beats/min, regular, and strong. Distal pulses are present. He states that he was walking, heard a pop, and fell to the floor. You suspect a(n) _____ fracture.

   A. greenstick

   B. comminuted

   C. pathologic

   D. epiphyseal

_____ **22.** A(n) _____ fracture is a fracture in which the bone is broken into two or more fragments.
  A. greenstick
  B. comminuted
  C. pathologic
  D. epiphyseal

_____ **23.** Your 24-year-old patient fell off a balance beam and landed on his arm. He is complaining of pain in the upper arm, and there is obvious swelling. You know that swelling is a sign of:
  A. bleeding.
  B. laceration.
  C. a locked joint.
  D. compartment syndrome.

_____ **24.** Fractures are almost always associated with _____ of the surrounding soft tissue.
  A. laceration
  B. crepitus
  C. ecchymosis
  D. swelling

_____ **25.** Signs and symptoms of a dislocated joint include all of the following EXCEPT:
  A. marked deformity.
  B. tenderness or palpation.
  C. locked joint.
  D. ecchymosis.

_____ **26.** Signs and symptoms of sprains include all of the following EXCEPT:
  A. point tenderness.
  B. pain preventing the patient from moving or using the limb normally.
  C. marked deformity.
  D. instability of the joint indicated by increased motion.

_____ **27.** Which of the following is not considered one of the "6 Ps" of the musculoskeletal assessment?
  A. Pain
  B. Pulselessness
  C. Pressure
  D. Peristalsis

_____ **28.** Which of the following statements about compartment syndrome is FALSE?
  A. It occurs 6 to 12 hours after an injury.
  B. It most commonly occurs with a fractured femur.
  C. It is usually a result of excessive bleeding, a severely crushed extremity, or the rapid return of blood to an ischemic limb.
  D. It is characterized by pain that is out of proportion to the injury.

_____ **29.** Always check neurovascular function:
  A. after any manipulation of the limb.
  B. before applying a splint.
  C. after applying a splint.
  D. all of the above.

_____ **30.** You respond to a 19-year-old woman who was involved in a motor vehicle collision. She is alert and oriented. Her airway is open, and respirations are 18 breaths/min and unlabored. Pulse is 94 beats/min and is strong and regular. Distal pulses are present. Her upper arm has obvious deformity. You splint the upper arm. You know that splinting will do all of the following EXCEPT:

   A. prevent the need for surgery.

   B. reduce shock.

   C. minimize compromised circulation.

   D. reduce pain.

_____ **31.** In-line _____ is the act of exerting a pulling force on a body structure in the direction of its normal alignment.

   A. stabilization

   B. immobilization

   C. traction

   D. direction

_____ **32.** Which of the following is a basic type of splint?

   A. Rigid

   B. Formable

   C. Traction

   D. All of the above

_____ **33.** Which of the following should you NOT use a traction splint for?

   A. Injuries of the pelvis

   B. An isolated femur fracture

   C. Partial amputation or avulsions with bone separation

   D. Lower leg or ankle injury

_____ **34.** While transporting a patient, you continue to recheck the splint you applied. You know that improperly applying a splint can cause all of the following EXCEPT:

   A. increase of distal circulation if the splint is too tight.

   B. delay in transport of a patient with a life-threatening injury.

   C. aggravation of the distal circulation.

   D. compression of nerves, tissues, and blood vessels.

_____ **35.** The _____ is one of the most commonly fractured bones in the body.

   A. scapula

   B. clavicle

   C. humerus

   D. radius

_____ **36.** What joint is frequently separated during football and hockey when a player falls and lands on the point of the shoulder?

   A. Glenohumeral joint

   B. Acromioclavicular joint

   C. Sternoclavicular joint

   D. None of the above

_____ **37.** Signs and symptoms associated with hip dislocation include all of the following EXCEPT:

   A. severe pain in the hip.

   B. lateral and posterior aspects of the hip region will be tender on palpation.

   C. being able to palpate the femoral head deep within the muscles of the buttock.

   D. decreased resistance to any movement of the joint.

_____ **38.** There is often a significant amount of blood loss, as much as _____ mL, after a fracture of the shaft of the femur.

    A. 100 to 250

    B. 250 to 500

    C. 500 to 1,000

    D. 100 to 1,500

_____ **39.** The knee is especially susceptible to _____ injuries, which occur when abnormal bending or twisting forces are applied to the joint.

    A. tendon

    B. ligament

    C. dislocation

    D. fracture-dislocation

_____ **40.** Signs and symptoms of knee ligament injury include:

    A. swelling.

    B. point tenderness.

    C. joint effusion.

    D. all of the above.

_____ **41.** Although substantial ligament damage always occurs with a knee dislocation, the more urgent injury is to the _____ artery, which is often lacerated or compressed by the displaced tibia.

    A. tibial

    B. femoral

    C. popliteal

    D. dorsalis pedis

_____ **42.** Because of local tenderness and swelling, it is easy to confuse a nondisplaced or minimally displaced fracture at the knee with a:

    A. tendon injury.

    B. ligament injury.

    C. dislocation.

    D. fracture-dislocation.

_____ **43.** Fracture of the tibia and fibula are often associated with _____ as a result of the distorted positions of the limb following injury.

    A. vascular injury

    B. muscular injury

    C. tendon injury

    D. ligament injury

_____ **44.** The _____ is one of the most commonly injured joints.

    A. knee

    B. elbow

    C. ankle

    D. hip

_____ **45.** Which of the following statements regarding the treatment of an amputation is FALSE?

    A. You should sever any partial amputation, because this will aid in the reattachment process.

    B. In some areas, wrapping the amputated part in a dry, sterile dressing is appropriate.

    C. In some areas, wrapping the amputated part in dressings moistened with sterile saline is appropriate.

    D. After wrapping the amputated part, place it in a plastic bag.

True/False

If you believe the statement to be more true than false, write the letter "T" in the space provided. If you believe the statement to be more false than true, write the letter "F."

_____ 1. All extremity injuries should be splinted before moving a patient unless the patient's life is in immediate danger.

_____ 2. Splinting reduces pain and prevents the motion of bone fragments.

_____ 3. You should use traction to reduce a fracture and force all bone fragments back into alignment.

_____ 4. When applying traction, the direction of pull is always along the axis of the limb.

_____ 5. Cover wounds with a dry, sterile dressing before applying a splint.

_____ 6. When splinting a fracture, you should be careful to immobilize only the joint above the injury site.

_____ 7. One of the steps of the neurologic examination is to palpate the pulse distal to the point of injury.

_____ 8. Assessment of neurovascular function should be repeated every 5 to 10 minutes until the patient arrives at the hospital.

_____ 9. A patient's ability to sense light touch in the fingers and toes distal to the injury site is a good indication that the nerve supply is intact.

_____ 10. If the hand or foot is involved in the injury, you should check motor function.

Fill-in-the-Blank

Read each item carefully and then complete the statement by filling in the missing words.

1. The _____ is the most frequently fractured tarsal bone.

2. Bone marrow produces _____ _____.

3. The humerus connects with the radius and ulna to form the _____ elbow joint.

4. The _____ is one of the most commonly fractured bones in the body.

5. Always carefully assess the _____ _____ _____ to try to determine the amount of kinetic energy that an injured limb has absorbed.

6. Penetrating injury should alert you to the possibility of a(n) _____ _____.

7. The _____ _____ is the most important nerve in the lower extremity; it controls the activity of muscles in the thigh and below the knee.

8. _____ _____ are used to splint the bony pelvis to reduce hemorrhage from bone ends, venous disruption, and pain.

9. A grating or grinding sensation known as _____ can be felt and sometimes even heard when fractured bone ends rub together.

10. A dislocated joint sometimes will spontaneously _____, or return to its normal position.

11. If you suspect that a patient has compartment syndrome, splint the affected limb, keeping it at the level of the heart, and provide immediate transport, checking _____ _____ frequently during transport.

Labeling

Label the following diagrams with the correct terms.

1. Pectoral Girdle

A. _____

B. _____

C. _____

D. _____

E. _____

F. _____

G. _____

H. _____

I. _____

J. _____

K. _____

L. _____

M. _____

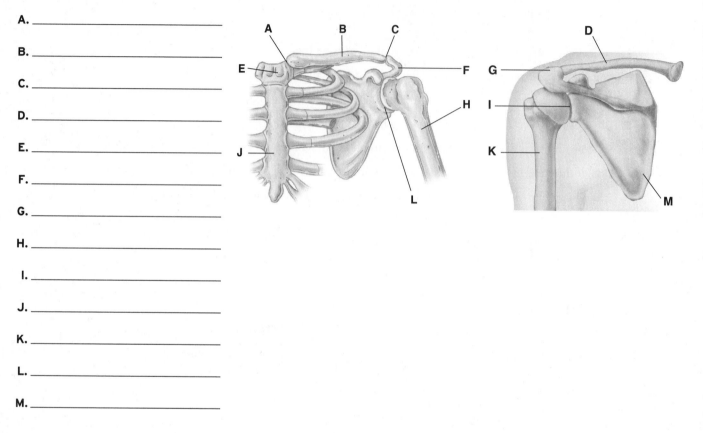

2. Anatomy of the Wrist and Hand

A. _____

B. _____

C. _____

D. _____

E. _____

F. _____

G. _____

H. _____

I. _____

J. _____

K. _____

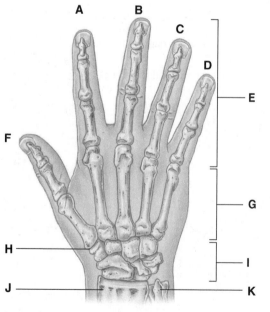

3. Bones of the Thigh, Leg, and Foot

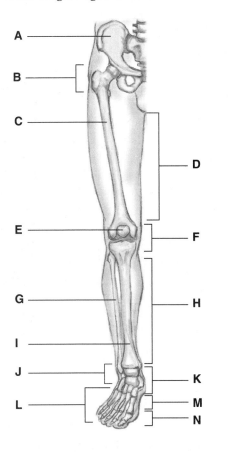

A. _____

B. _____

C. _____

D. _____

E. _____

F. _____

G. _____

H. _____

I. _____

J. _____

K. _____

L. _____

M. _____

N. _____

Crossword Puzzle

The following crossword puzzle is an activity provided to reinforce correct spelling and understanding of medical terminology associated with emergency care and the EMT. Use the clues in the column to complete the puzzle.

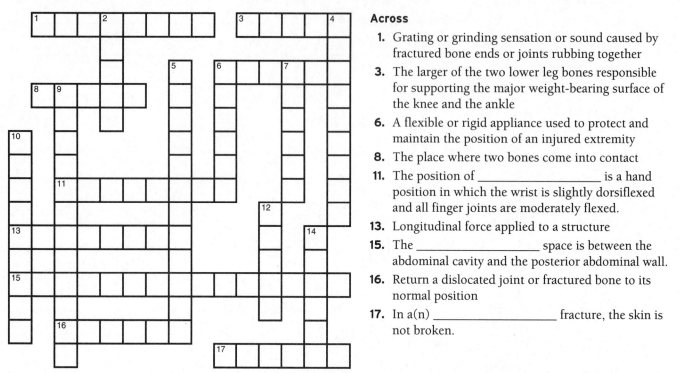

Across

1. Grating or grinding sensation or sound caused by fractured bone ends or joints rubbing together
3. The larger of the two lower leg bones responsible for supporting the major weight-bearing surface of the knee and the ankle
6. A flexible or rigid appliance used to protect and maintain the position of an injured extremity
8. The place where two bones come into contact
11. The position of _____ is a hand position in which the wrist is slightly dorsiflexed and all finger joints are moderately flexed.
13. Longitudinal force applied to a structure
15. The _____ space is between the abdominal cavity and the posterior abdominal wall.
16. Return a dislocated joint or fractured bone to its normal position
17. In a(n) _____ fracture, the skin is not broken.

Down

2. _____ tenderness is sharply localized at the site of the injury, found by gently palpating along the bone.
4. _____ cartilage is a pearly layer of specialized cartilage covering the articular surfaces of bones in synovial joints.
5. The major nerve to the lower extremities
6. A joint injury involving damage to supporting ligaments, and sometimes partial or temporary dislocation of bone ends
7. The zone of _____ is the area of potentially damaged soft tissue, adjacent nerves, and blood vessels surrounding an injury to a bone or a joint.
9. Any break in a bone in which the overlying skin has been damaged
10. Blood in the urine
12. A bandage or material that helps to support the weight of an injured upper extremity
14. A bandage that passes around the chest to secure an injured arm to the chest

Critical Thinking

Short Answer

Complete this section with short written answers using the space provided.

1. List the four types of forces that may cause injury to a limb.

_____

_____

2. List five of the signs associated with a possible fracture.

_____

_____

3. List the four items to check when assessing neurovascular function.

_____

_____

4. List the general principles of splinting.

_____

_____

5. What are the three goals of in-line traction?

_____

_____

Ambulance Calls

The following case scenarios provide an opportunity to explore the concerns associated with patient management and to enhance critical-thinking skills. Read each scenario and answer each question to the best of your ability.

1. You are dispatched to care for a 17-year-old boy who jumped from the top of a three-story home into a pool. He landed directly on his feet just short of the pool. He is now complaining of low back pain and numbness and tingling of his legs.

   How would you best manage this patient?

   _____

   _____

   _____

2. You are called to a local park where an 11-year-old girl fell off the parallel bars onto her right elbow. She is cradling the arm to her chest. She has obvious swelling and deformity in the area. She has good pulse, motor, and sensation at the wrist. ABCs are normal.

   How would you best manage this patient?

   _____

   _____

   _____

3. You are dispatched to an attempted suicide at the local prison. The inmate attempted to kill himself by strangling himself with an electrical cord. When you arrive he is cyanotic and not breathing.

   How would you best manage this patient?

   _____

   _____

   _____

Skills

Skill Drills

Skill Drill 29-1: Assessing Neurovascular Status
Test your knowledge of this skill by filling in the correct words in the photo captions.

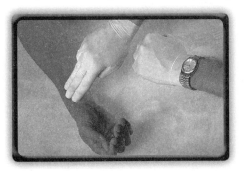

1. Palpate the _____ pulse in the upper extremity.

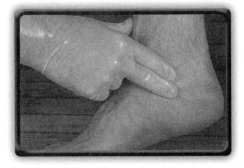

2. Palpate the _____ _____ and dorsalis pedis pulse in the lower extremity.

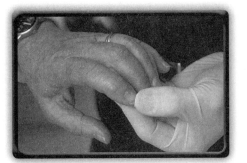

3. Assess capillary refill by blanching a fingernail or _____.

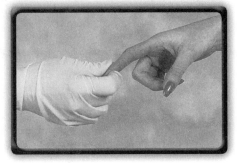

4. Assess sensation on the flesh near the _____ of the _____ finger and thumb, as well as the little finger.

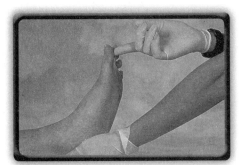

5. On the foot, first check sensation on the flesh near the _____ of the _____ _____.

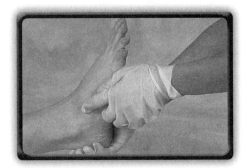

6. Also check foot sensation on the _____ _____ of the foot.

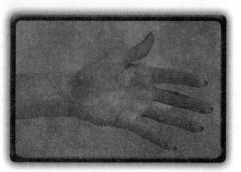

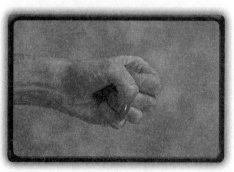

7. For an upper extremity injury, evaluate motor function by asking the patient to _____ the hand. (Perform motor tests only if the hand or foot is not _____. _____ a test if it causes pain.)

8. Also ask the patient to _____ a(n) _____.

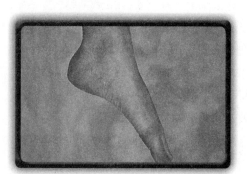

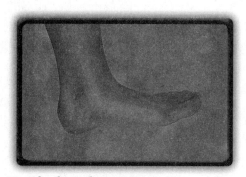

9. For a lower extremity injury, ask the patient to _____ the foot.

10. Also have the patient _____ the foot and _____ the toes.

Skill Drill 29-3: Applying a Rigid Splint
Test your knowledge of this skill by filling in the correct words in the photo captions.

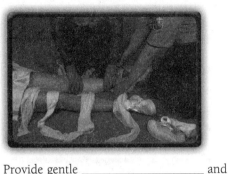

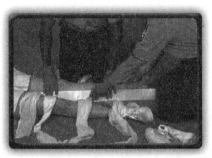

1. Provide gentle _____ and
_____ _____
for the limb.

2. Place the splint _____
or _____ the limb.
_____ between the limb
and the splint as needed to ensure even
pressure and contact.

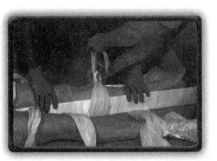

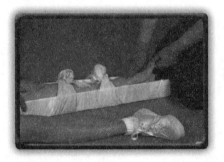

3. Secure the splint to the limb with
_____.

4. Assess and record _____
_____ function.

Skill Drill 29-6: Applying a Vacuum Splint
Test your knowledge of this skill by filling in the correct words in the photo captions.

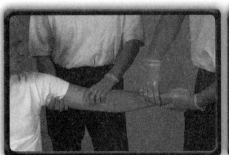

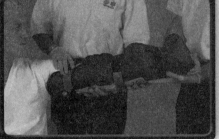

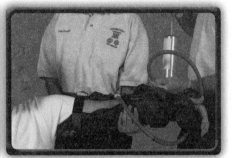

1. Your partner _____
and _____ the
injury.

2. Place the splint, and
_____ it around
the limb.

3. _____ the
air out of the splint through
the _____
_____, and then
_____ the valve.

Skill Drill 29-7: Applying a Hare Traction Splint
Test your knowledge of this skill by placing the photos below in the correct order. Number the first step with a "1," the second step with a "2," etc.

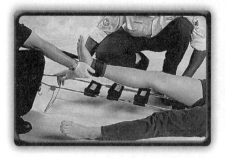

_____ Slide the splint into position under the injured limb.

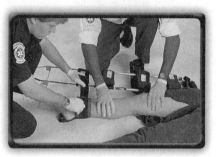

_____ Support the injured limb as your partner fastens the ankle hitch about the foot and ankle.

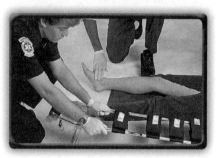

_____ Expose the injured limb and check pulse and motor and sensory function. Place the splint beside the uninjured limb, adjust the splint to proper length, and prepare the straps.

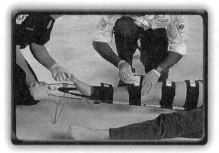

_____ Secure and check support straps. Assess pulse and motor and sensory functions.

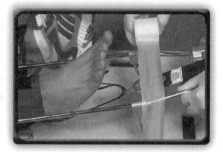

_____ Secure the patient and splint to the backboard in a way that will prevent movement of the splint during patient movement and transport.

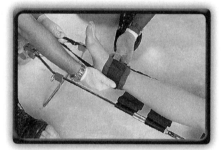

_____ Connect the loops of the ankle hitch to the end of the splint as your partner continues to maintain traction. Carefully tighten the ratchet to the point that the splint holds adequate traction.

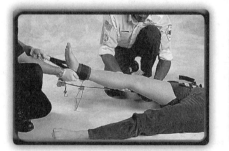

_____ Continue to support the limb as your partner applies gentle in-line traction to the ankle hitch and foot.

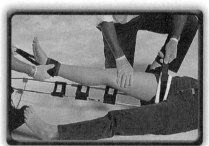

_____ Pad the groin and fasten the ischial strap.

Skill Drill 29-10: Splinting the Hand and Wrist
Test your knowledge of this skill by filling in the correct words in the photo captions.

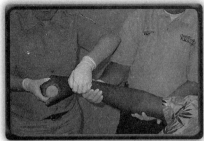

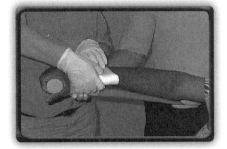

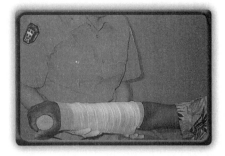

1. Support the injured limb and move the hand into the _____ of _____. Place a soft _____ _____ in the palm.

2. Apply a(n) _____ _____ splint on the _____ side with fingers _____.

3. Secure the splint with a(n) _____ _____.

Assessment Review

Answer the following questions pertaining to the assessment of the types of emergencies discussed in this chapter.

_____ 1. You respond to a motorcycle accident for a 41-year-old man who is unconscious. He has obvious deformity to both lower legs and is bleeding moderately from an open fracture. His airway is open, and he is making gurgling noises. Pulse is rapid and weak. Distal pulses are very weak. Your first priority with this patient is to:
   A. control bleeding.
   B. apply splints.
   C. maintain an airway.
   D. apply a pneumatic antishock garment.

_____ 2. You have loaded the patient in the question above and are on the way to the hospital. You have secured the airway and immobilized the fractures. How often should you reassess his vital signs?
   A. Every 3 minutes
   B. Every 5 minutes
   C. Every 10 minutes
   D. Every 15 minutes

_____ 3. You are called to a 16-year-old girl who was injured in a basketball game. She is alert and oriented. Her airway is open, and respirations are within normal limits. Her pulse is strong and regular. Distal pulses are present. She states that she felt her ankle pop and immediately became nauseated. You decide to assess neurovascular status. When would you not perform the motor test?
   A. When you get a pain response
   B. When the patient walks away
   C. When you feel a distal pulse
   D. When the patient feels your touch

_____ **4.** You are called to the local junior high school where a 12-year-old boy fell and hurt his wrist. There is obvious deformity. He is alert and oriented. Respirations and pulse are within normal limits. Distal pulse is present. It is important to remember to:

    A. use a zippered air splint.

    B. splint in a position of function.

    C. splint the wrist only.

    D. completely cover the wrist and hand.

_____ **5.** When you have applied a traction splint, the last thing that you do is:

    A. check pulse, motor, and sensation.

    B. release traction if the pulse disappears.

    C. apply elasticized straps.

    D. secure the patient to a backboard.

Environmental Emergencies

General Knowledge

Matching

Match each of the items in the left column to the appropriate definition in the right column.

_____ **1.** Conduction

_____ **2.** Air embolism

_____ **3.** Evaporation

_____ **4.** Hyperthermia

_____ **5.** Diving reflex

_____ **6.** Core temperature

_____ **7.** Convection

_____ **8.** Laryngospasm

_____ **9.** Turgor

_____ **10.** Radiation

_____ **11.** Hypothermia

_____ **12.** Ambient temperature

_____ **13.** Heat cramps

_____ **14.** Drowning

_____ **15.** Hymenoptera

A. Slowing of pulse rate caused by sudden immersion in cold water

B. Ability of the skin to resist deformation

C. Severe constriction of the larynx and vocal cords

D. Death from suffocation after submersion in water

E. Heat loss resulting from standing in a cold room

F. Bees, wasps, ants, and yellow jackets

G. Condition when body temperature decreases

H. Condition caused by air bubbles in the blood vessels

I. Heat loss that occurs from helicopter rotor blade downwash

J. Heat loss resulting from sitting on snow

K. Heat loss resulting from sweating

L. Painful muscle spasms that occur after vigorous exercise

M. Temperature of the surrounding environment

N. Temperature of the central part of the body

O. Core temperature greater than 101°F (38.3°C)

Multiple Choice

Read each item carefully and then select the one best response.

_____ **1.** _____ causes body heat to be lost as warm air in the lungs is exhaled into the atmosphere and cooler air is inhaled.

    A. Convection

    B. Conduction

    C. Radiation

    D. Respiration

_____ **2.** Evaporation, the conversion of a liquid to a gas, is a process that requires:

    A. energy.

    B. circulating air.

    C. a warmer ambient temperature.

    D. high humidity.

_____ **3.** The rate and amount of heat loss by the body can be modified by all of the following EXCEPT:

    A. increasing heat production.

    B. moving to an area where heat loss is decreased.

    C. wearing insulated clothing.

    D. increasing fluid intake.

_____ **4.** The characteristic appearance of blue lips and/or fingertips seen in hypothermia is the result of:
  A. lack of oxygen in venous blood.
  B. frostbite.
  C. blood vessels constricting.
  D. bruising.

_____ **5.** Signs and symptoms of severe systemic hypothermia include all of the following EXCEPT:
  A. weak pulse.
  B. coma.
  C. shivering.
  D. very slow respirations.

_____ **6.** Hypothermia is more common among all of the following EXCEPT:
  A. older individuals.
  B. long-distance athletes.
  C. infants and children.
  D. those who are already ill.

_____ **7.** To assess a patient's general temperature, pull back your glove and place the back of your hand on the patient's:
  A. abdomen, underneath the clothing.
  B. forehead.
  C. forearm, on the inside of the wrist.
  D. neck, at the area where you check the carotid pulse.

_____ **8.** Never assume that a(n) _____, pulseless patient is dead.
  A. apneic
  B. cyanotic
  C. cold
  D. hyperthermic

_____ **9.** Management of hypothermia in the field consists of all of the following EXCEPT:
  A. applying heat packs to the groin, axillary, and cervical regions.
  B. removing wet clothing.
  C. preventing further heat loss.
  D. massaging the cold extremities.

_____ **10.** All of the following conditions refer to when exposed parts of the body become very cold, but not frozen, EXCEPT:
  A. frostnip.
  B. trench foot.
  C. immersion foot.
  D. frostbite.

_____ **11.** When the body is exposed to more heat energy than it loses, _____ result(s).
  A. hyperthermia
  B. heat cramps
  C. heat exhaustion
  D. heatstroke

_____ **12.** Contributing factors to the development of heat illnesses include all of the following EXCEPT:
  A. high air temperature.
  B. vigorous exercise.
  C. high humidity.
  D. increased fluid intake.

_____ **13.** It is important to remain hydrated while on duty. Drink at least _____ of water per day, and more when exertion or heat is involved.

    A. 8 glasses

    B. 1 liter

    C. 2 liters

    D. 3 liters

_____ **14.** Which of the following statements about heat cramps is FALSE?

    A. They only occur when it is hot outdoors.

    B. They may be seen in well-conditioned athletes.

    C. The exact cause of heat cramps is not well understood.

    D. Dehydration may play a role in the development of heat cramps.

_____ **15.** Signs and symptoms of heat exhaustion and associated hypovolemia include all of the following EXCEPT:

    A. cold, clammy skin with ashen pallor.

    B. dizziness, weakness, or faintness.

    C. normal vital signs.

    D. normal thirst.

_____ **16.** Most spinal injuries in diving incidents affect the:

    A. cervical spine.

    B. thoracic spine.

    C. lumbar spine.

    D. sacrum/coccyx.

_____ **17.** Often, the first sign of heatstroke is:

    A. a change in behavior.

    B. an increase in pulse rate.

    C. an increase in respirations.

    D. hot, dry, flushed skin.

_____ **18.** The least common but most serious illness caused by heat exposure, occurring when the body is subjected to more heat than it can handle and normal mechanisms for getting rid of the excess heat are overwhelmed, is:

    A. hyperthermia.

    B. heat cramps.

    C. heat exhaustion.

    D. heatstroke.

_____ **19.** _____ is the body's reaction to an irritation of water entering the lower respiratory tract.

    A. Bronchoconstriction

    B. Laryngospasm

    C. Esophageal spasms

    D. Swelling in the oropharynx

_____ **20.** Treatment of drowning and/or near drowning begins with:

    A. opening the airway.

    B. ventilation with 100% oxygen via bag-mask device.

    C. suctioning the lungs to remove the water.

    D. rescue and removal from the water.

_____ **21.** In a diving emergency, _____ occurs when bubbles of gas, especially nitrogen, obstruct the blood vessels.

    A. compression sickness

    B. decompression sickness

    C. pulmonary sickness

    D. nitrogen toxicity

_____ **22.** If the near drowning victim has evidence of upper airway obstruction by foreign matter, which of the following would NOT be considered a method for clearing it?

    A. Remove the obstruction manually.

    B. Apply suction.

    C. Place the patient in the recovery position to allow drainage.

    D. Use abdominal thrusts.

_____ **23.** You should never give up on resuscitating a cold-water drowning victim because:

    A. when the patient is submerged in water colder than body temperature, heat is maintained in the body.

    B. the resulting hypothermia can protect vital organs from the lack of oxygen.

    C. the resulting hypothermia raises the metabolic rate.

    D. all of the above.

_____ **24.** The three phases of a dive, in the order they occur, are:

    A. ascent, descent, and bottom.

    B. descent, bottom, and ascent.

    C. orientation, bottom, and ascent.

    D. descent, orientation, and ascent.

_____ **25.** Areas usually affected by descent problems include:

    A. the lungs.

    B. the skin.

    C. the joints.

    D. vision.

_____ **26.** Potential problems associated with rupture of the lungs include all of the following EXCEPT:

    A. air emboli.

    B. pneumomediastinum.

    C. pneumothorax.

    D. hemopneumothorax.

_____ **27.** The organs most severely affected by air embolism are the:

    A. brain and spinal cord.

    B. brain and heart.

    C. heart and lungs.

    D. brain and lungs.

_____ **28.** Black widow spiders may be found in:

    A. New Hampshire.

    B. woodpiles.

    C. Georgia.

    D. all of the above.

_____ **29.** Coral snake venom is a powerful toxin that causes _____ of the nervous system.

    A. paralysis

    B. hyperactivity

    C. hypoactivity

    D. hemiparesis

_____ **30.** Rocky Mountain spotted fever and Lyme disease are both spread through the tick's:

    A. saliva.

    B. blood.

    C. hormones.

    D. excrement.

_____ **31.** Signs of envenomation by a pit viper include all of the following EXCEPT:

    A. swelling.

    B. chest pain.

    C. ecchymosis.

    D. severe burning pain at the site of the injury.

_____ **32.** Removal of a tick should be accomplished by:

    A. suffocating it with gasoline.

    B. burning it with a lighted match to cause it to release its grip.

    C. using fine tweezers to pull it straight out of the skin.

    D. suffocating it with Vaseline.

_____ **33.** Which of the following statements regarding the brown recluse spider is FALSE?

    A. It is larger than the black widow spider.

    B. It lives mostly in the southern and central parts of the country.

    C. Venom is not neurotoxic.

    D. Bites rarely cause systemic signs and symptoms.

_____ **34.** Treatment of a snake bite from a pit viper includes:

    A. calming the patient.

    B. providing BLS as needed if the patient shows no sign of envenomation.

    C. marking the skin with a pen over the swollen area to note whether swelling is spreading.

    D. all of the above.

Questions 35–39 are derived from the following scenario: At 1400 in July, the weather is 105°F (41°C) and very humid. You have been called for a "man down" at the park. As you arrive, you recognize him as an alcoholic who has been a "frequent flyer" with your service. It looks like he had been sitting under a tree when he fell over, unconscious.

_____ **35.** As you assess the patient, he has cold, clammy skin and a dry tongue. You suspect that:

    A. he is well-hydrated.

    B. he has suffered heat exhaustion.

    C. he is hypothermic.

    D. he has heatstroke.

_____ **36.** As you look closer, you note that he is shivering and his respirations are 20 breaths/min. You begin to have a stronger suspicion that he is now getting:

    A. hyperthermic.

    B. hypothermic.

    C. drunk.

    D. heatstroke.

_____ **37.** The direct transfer of heat from his body to the cold ground is called:

    A. conduction.

    B. convection.

    C. radiation.

    D. evaporation.

_____ **38.** You pull back on your glove and place the back of your hand on his skin at the abdomen, and the skin feels cool. Again, you suspect:

    A. hyperthermia.

    B. hypothermia.

    C. that he is drunk.

    D. heatstroke.

_____ **39.** How will you treat this patient?
   A. Prevent conduction heat loss.
   B. Prevent convection heat loss.
   C. Remove the patient from the environment.
   D. All of the above.

_____ **40.** Small infants have a poor ability to thermoregulate and are unable to shiver to control heat loss until about the age of:
   A. 4 to 6 months.
   B. 6 to 12 months.
   C. 12 to 18 months.
   D. 18 to 24 months.

_____ **41.** Most heat stroke cases occur when the temperature is around _____ and the humidity is 80%.
   A. 80°F (27°C)
   B. 90°F (32°)
   C. 100°F (38°C)
   D. 110°F (43°C)

True/False

If you believe the statement to be more true than false, write the letter "T" in the space provided. If you believe the statement to be more false than true, write the letter "F."

_____ **1.** Normal body temperature is 98.6°F (37.0°C).

_____ **2.** To assess the skin temperature in a patient experiencing a generalized cold emergency, you should feel the patient's skin.

_____ **3.** Mild hypothermia occurs when the core temperature drops to 85°F (29°C).

_____ **4.** The body's most efficient heat-regulating mechanisms are sweating and dilation of skin blood vessels.

_____ **5.** People who are at greatest risk for heat illnesses are the elderly and children.

_____ **6.** The strongest stimulus for breathing is an elevation of oxygen in the blood.

_____ **7.** Immediate bradycardia after jumping in cold water is called the diving reflex.

_____ **8.** Ice should be promptly applied to any insect sting or snake bite with swelling.

_____ **9.** The most common type of pit viper is the copperhead.

_____ **10.** Cottonmouths are known for aggressive behavior.

_____ **11.** Ticks should be removed by firmly grasping them with tweezers while rotating them counterclockwise.

_____ **12.** The pain of coelenterate stings may respond to flushing with cold water.

_____ **13.** If you are unsure as to whether a hypothermic patient has a pulse present, palpate the carotid artery for 15 to 20 seconds.

_____ **14.** The goal with the patient with moderate-to-severe hypothermia is to prevent further heat loss.

_____ **15.** After a lightning strike you should practice reverse triage.

_____ **16.** Extremes in temperature and humidity are needed to produce hot or cold injuries.

_____ **17.** When approaching a water rescue scene, it is better to drive through moving water than through stagnant water.

_____ **18.** Potential safety hazards in the environment can include wet grass, mud, or icy streets.

_____ **19.** Long-sleeved shirts and long pants are considered dangerous for EMS responders in extreme heat and are not necessary because they provide only minimal protection from exposure.

Fill-in-the-Blank

Read each item carefully and then complete the statement by filling in the missing words.

1. Do not attempt to actively rewarm patients who have _____ to _____ hypothermia, because they are prone to developing arrhythmias unless handled very carefully.

2. Most significant diving injuries occur during _____.

3. When treating a patient with frostbite, never attempt _____ if there is any chance that the part may freeze again before the patient reaches the hospital.

4. A patient at an altitude above 10,000′ (3,048 m) with shortness of breath and cough with pink sputum is likely to be suffering from _____ _____ _____.

5. _____, a common effect of hypothermia, is the body's attempt to maintain heat.

6. Whenever a person dives or jumps into very cold water, the _____ _____ may cause immediate bradycardia.

7. _____ is the transfer of heat by radiant energy.

8. Mild hypothermia occurs when the core temperature is between _____ and _____.

9. The _____ and _____ systems are the most commonly injured during a lightning strike.

10. _____ is the third most common cause of death from isolated environmental phenomena.

11. _____ is a serum containing antibodies that counteracts venom.

12. _____ (bees, wasps, ants, and yellow jackets) stings are painful but are not medical emergencies unless the patient is allergic to the venom.

13. Most snake bites occur between _____ and _____, when the animals are active.

14. In the United States, the most common form of pit viper is the _____.

15. _____ are eight-legged arachnids with a venom glad and stinger at the end of their tail.

16. Tick bites occur most commonly during the _____ months.

17. One-third of patients with Lyme disease will have a _____ rash.

18. To treat a sting from a jellyfish, pour _____ _____ on the affected area.

19. Coelenterates are responsible for more _____ than any other marine animals.

20. Toxins from the spines of urchins and stingrays are _____ _____.

Crossword Puzzle

The following crossword puzzle is an activity provided to reinforce correct spelling and understanding of medical terminology associated with emergency care and the EMT. Use the clues in the column to complete the puzzle.

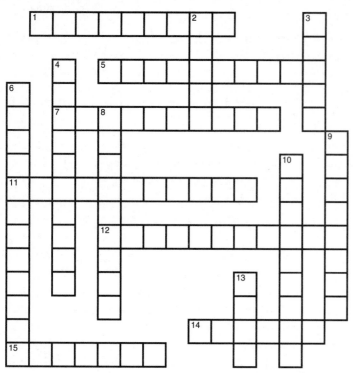

Across

1. _____ injuries are caused by the difference between the surrounding atmospheric pressure and the total gas pressure in various tissues, fluids, and cavities of the body.
5. The loss of heat by direct contact
7. Painful muscle spasms usually associated with vigorous activity in a hot environment
11. The loss of body heat as warm air in the lungs is exhaled into the atmosphere and cooler air is inhaled
12. Conversion of water or another fluid from a liquid to a gas
14. The ability of the skin to resist deformation
15. The temperature of the surrounding environment is known as the _____ temperature.

Down

2. A system that delivers air to the mouth and lungs at various atmospheric pressures, increasing with the depth of the dive
3. Common name for decompression sickness
4. With heat _____, the body loses significant amounts of fluid and electrolytes because of heavy sweating.
6. A condition in which the body core temperature rises to 101°F (38°C) or more
8. A serum that counteracts the effect of venom from an animal or insect
9. The process of experiencing respiratory impairment from submersion or immersion in liquid
10. The transfer of heat to colder objects in the environment by radiant energy
13. The _____ temperature is the temperature of the central part of the body.

Critical Thinking

Short Answer

Complete this section with short written answers using the space provided.

1. What are three ways to modify heat loss? Give an example of each.

   _____

   _____

2. What are the steps in treating heatstroke?

   _____

   _____

3. What is an air embolism and how does it occur?

   _____

   _____

4. For what diving emergencies are hyperbaric chambers used?

   _____

   _____

5. How should a frostbitten foot be treated?

   _____

   _____

6. What are four "Do Nots" in relation to local cold injuries?

   _____

   _____

7. What treatments for a snake bite assist with slowing and monitoring the spread of venom?

   _____

   _____

8. What are the two most common poisonous spiders in the United States and how do their bites differ?

   _____

   _____

Ambulance Calls

The following case scenarios provide an opportunity to explore the concerns associated with patient management and to enhance critical-thinking skills. Read each scenario and answer each question to the best of your ability.

1. You are called to the local airport for a 52-year-old man who is the pilot of his own aircraft. He tells you he is having severe abdominal pain and joint pain. History reveals that the patient is returning from a dive trip off the coast. He says he has had "the bends" before and this feels similar.

How would you best manage this patient?

_____

_____

_____

2. You are dispatched to a long-term care facility for an Alzheimer's patient with an "unknown problem." You arrive to find several staff members who greet you at the front door. They explain that the patient wandered out the back exit door of the Alzheimer's unit when the nurse was on her other rounds. They aren't sure how this happened, because each patient wears a necklace that triggers an alarm if the patient leaves this specialized wing of the facility. They found the man outside in the snow, and he has possibly been outdoors for 45 minutes.

How would you best manage this patient?

_____

_____

_____

3. You are dispatched to an unconscious female at a local beauty spa locally known for its "body wraps." You arrive to find a conscious, yet confused, 17-year-old girl. A friend tells you that the patient has been using over-the-counter "water pills" and laxative agents, along with strenuous exercise, to lose weight for the prom. She tells you that her friend is otherwise healthy, but she complained of feeling dizzy prior to undergoing the spa treatment.

How would you best manage this patient?

_____

_____

_____

Skills

Skill Drills

Skill Drill 30-1: Treating for Heat Exhaustion
Test your knowledge of this skill by filling in the correct words in the photo captions.

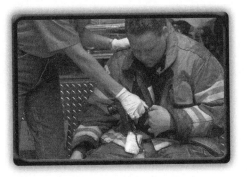

1. Move the patient to a(n) _____ _____. Remove extra _____.

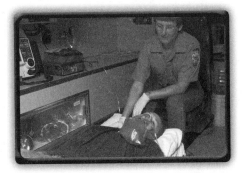

2. Give _____. Place the patient in a(n) _____ position, elevate the _____, and fan the patient.

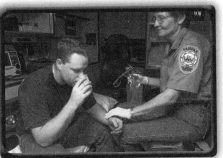

3. If the patient is fully alert, give _____ by mouth.

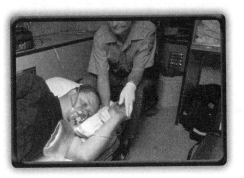

4. If _____ develops, secure and transport the patient on his or her side.

Skill Drill 30-2: Stabilizing a Suspected Spinal Injury in the Water
Test your knowledge of this skill by placing the photos below in the correct order. Number the first step with a "1," the second step with a "2," etc.

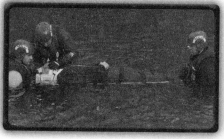

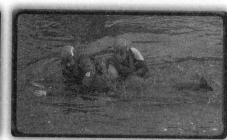

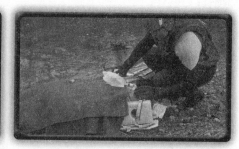

_____ Secure the patient to the backboard.

_____ Turn the patient to a supine position by rotating the entire upper half of the body as a single unit.

_____ Cover the patient with a blanket and apply oxygen if breathing. Begin CPR if breathing and pulse are absent.

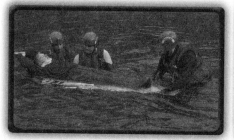

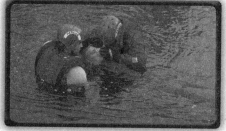

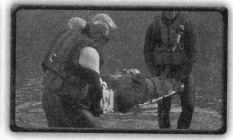

_____ Float a buoyant backboard under the patient.

_____ As soon as the patient is turned, begin artificial ventilation using the mouth-to-mouth method or a pocket mask.

_____ Remove the patient from the water.

Assessment Review

Answer the following questions pertaining to the assessment of the types of emergencies discussed in this chapter.

_____ 1. Most frostbitten parts are:

    A. soft and moist.

    B. hard and waxy.

    C. soft and waxy.

    D. hard and moist.

_____ 2. If a patient has a cold skin temperature, he or she likely is:

    A. hypothermic.

    B. hyperthermic.

    C. hypovolemic.

    D. hypoglycemic.

_____ 3. If a patient has a hot skin temperature, he or she likely is:

    A. hypothermic.

    B. hyperthermic.

    C. hypoglycemic.

    D. hypervolemic

_____ 4. When treating multiple victims of lightning strikes, who should you concentrate your efforts on first?

    A. Conscious patients

    B. Unconscious patients in respiratory or cardiac arrest

    C. All unconscious patients

    D. None of the above

_____ 5. What is the best method of inactivating a jellyfish sting?

    A. Urinating on it

    B. Flushing the site with cold water

    C. Applying vinegar

    D. Applying an ice pack

Emergency Care Summary

Fill in the following chart pertaining to the management of the types of emergencies discussed in this chapter.
Note: While the steps below are widely accepted, be sure to consult and follow your local protocol.

Cold Exposure Emergency

1. Establish and maintain a patent airway. Provide oxygen. Monitor for _____ and protect against aspiration.

2. Carefully move the patient to a protected environment. Remove any _____ clothing. Place dry

_____ over and under the patient.

3. Handle the patient gently to avoid further injury. With severe _____, careful handling of the patient is

necessary to prevent cardiac arrest; rough handling can cause ventricular fibrillation.

4. If the hypothermia is mild, begin _____ _____.

5. If the hypothermia is moderate or severe, prevent further heat loss and follow local protocols.

Diving Injuries

1. Remove the patient from the water.

2. Begin CPR if pulse and breathing are absent.

3. If pulse and breathing are present, administer _____.

4. Place the patient in a(n) _____ _____ _____ position with the head

_____.

5. Provide prompt transport to the nearest _____ facility for treatment.

Spider Bites

1. Provide basic life support for respiratory distress.

2. Apply _____ to the bite area and clean the wound with soap and water.

3. Transport the patient and, if possible, the spider to the hospital.

Snake Bites

1. Calm the patient and minimize movement.

2. Clean the bite area gently with soap and water or a mild _____. Do not apply _____.

3. Transport the patient and, if possible, the snake to the emergency department.

4. Notify the emergency department that you are bringing in a snake bite victim.

Obstetrics and Neonatal Care

General Knowledge

Matching

Match each of the items in the left column to the appropriate definition in the right column.

_____ **1.** Cervix

_____ **2.** Crowning

_____ **3.** Placenta

_____ **4.** Amniotic sac

_____ **5.** Fetus

_____ **6.** Birth canal

_____ **7.** Primigravida

_____ **8.** Umbilical cord

_____ **9.** Lightening

_____ **10.** Breech presentation

_____ **11.** Limb presentation

_____ **12.** Multigravida

_____ **13.** Nuchal cord

_____ **14.** Presentation

_____ **15.** Miscarriage

A. An umbilical cord that is wrapped around the infant's neck

B. A fluid-filled, baglike membrane inside the uterus that grows around the developing fetus

C. Appearance of the infant's head at the vaginal opening during labor

D. The neck of the uterus

E. Connects mother and infant

F. Sensation felt by a pregnant patient when the fetus positions itself for delivery

G. The part of the infant that appears first

H. The vagina and lower part of the uterus

I. A woman who has had previous pregnancies

J. Spontaneous abortion

K. Delivery in which the presenting part is a single arm, leg, or foot

L. Tissue that develops on the wall of the uterus and is connected to the fetus

M. First pregnancy

N. The developing, unborn infant

O. Delivery in which the buttocks come out first

Multiple Choice

Read each item carefully and then select the one best response.

_____ **1.** Which of the following is NOT true regarding delivery with a nuchal cord?

    A. Gently slip the cord over the infant's head or shoulder.

    B. Clamp the cord and cut it before delivering the infant.

    C. Clamp the cord, then suction the airway before cutting the cord.

    D. Clamp the cord and cut it, then gently unwind it from around the neck if wrapped around more than once.

_____ **2.** Which of the following refers to greenish or foul-smelling amniotic fluid?

    A. Nuchal rigidity

    B. Meconium staining

    C. Placenta previa

    D. Bloody show

_____ **3.** Which of the following is NOT performed immediately following delivery of the infant?

    A. Wrap the infant in a towel and place it on one side with head lowered.

    B. Be sure the head is covered and keep the neck in a neutral position.

    C. Use a sterile gauze pad to wipe the infant's mouth, then suction again.

    D. Obtain an Apgar score.

_____ 4. You may help control bleeding by massaging the _____ after delivery of the placenta.
   A. perineum
   B. fundus
   C. lower back
   D. inner thighs

_____ 5. The Apgar score should be calculated at _____ minutes after birth.
   A. 1 and 5
   B. 3 and 7
   C. 2 and 10
   D. 4 and 8

_____ 6. Once the infant is delivered, feel for a brachial pulse or the pulsations in the umbilical cord. If the pulse rate is below _____ beats/min, begin assisted ventilations.
   A. 60
   B. 80
   C. 100
   D. 120

_____ 7. When assisting ventilations in a newborn with a bag-mask device, the rate is _____ breaths/min.
   A. 20 to 30
   B. 30 to 50
   C. 35 to 45
   D. 40 to 60

_____ 8. When performing CPR on a newborn, a compression to ventilation ratio of 3:1 should be used; this will yield a total of _____ "actions" per minute.
   A. 90
   B. 100
   C. 110
   D. 120

_____ 9. You cannot successfully deliver a _____ presentation in the field.
   A. limb
   B. breech
   C. vertex
   D. cephalic

_____ 10. Which of the following is NOT performed when caring for a mother with a prolapsed cord?
   A. Clamp and cut the cord.
   B. Provide high-flow oxygen and rapid transport.
   C. Use your fingers to physically hold the infant's head off the cord.
   D. Position the mother to keep the weight of the infant off the cord.

_____ 11. When handling a delivery involving a drug- or alcohol-addicted mother, your first concern should be for:
   A. the mother's airway.
   B. your personal safety.
   C. the infant's airway.
   D. the need for CPR for the infant.

_____ **12.** Which of the following is NOT a stage of labor?

    A. Rupture of amniotic fluid

    B. Expulsion of the baby

    C. Delivery of the placenta

    D. Dilation of the cervix

_____ **13.** The first stage of labor begins with the onset of contractions and ends when:

    A. the infant is born.

    B. the cervix is fully dilated.

    C. the water breaks.

    D. the placenta is delivered.

_____ **14.** Which of the following is NOT a sign of the beginning of labor?

    A. Bloody show

    B. Contractions of the uterus

    C. Crowning

    D. Rupture of the amniotic sac

_____ **15.** The second stage of labor begins when the cervix is fully dilated and ends when:

    A. the infant is born.

    B. the water breaks.

    C. the placenta delivers.

    D. the uterus stops contracting.

_____ **16.** The third stage of labor begins with the birth of the infant and ends with the:

    A. release of milk from the breasts.

    B. cessation of uterine contractions.

    C. delivery of the placenta.

    D. cutting of the umbilical cord.

_____ **17.** The difference between preeclampsia and eclampsia is the onset of:

    A. seeing spots.

    B. seizures.

    C. swelling in the hands and feet.

    D. headaches.

_____ **18.** You should consider the possibility of a(n) _____ in women who have missed a menstrual cycle and complain of a sudden stabbing and usually unilateral pain in the lower abdomen.

    A. PID

    B. ectopic pregnancy

    C. miscarriage

    D. placenta abruptio

_____ **19.** Which of the following is NOT a reason for delivery of the fetus at the scene?

    A. Delivery can be expected within a few minutes.

    B. There is a natural disaster.

    C. There is severe inclement weather.

    D. The amniotic sac has ruptured.

_____ **20.** Which of the following statements regarding pregnancy is true?

    A. A patient in the third trimester is at a decreased risk for aspiration.

    B. As the pregnancy continues, the patient will experience slower and deeper breathing.

    C. By the 20th week of pregnancy, the uterus is at or above the belly button.

    D. Maternal blood volume increases up to 10% by the end of pregnancy.

_____ **21.** Low blood pressure resulting from compression of the inferior vena cava by the weight of the fetus when the mother is supine is called:

  A. pregnancy-induced hypertension.

  B. placenta previa.

  C. placenta abruptio.

  D. supine hypotensive syndrome.

_____ **22.** _____ is a situation in which the umbilical cord comes out of the vagina before the infant.

  A. Eclampsia

  B. Placenta previa

  C. Abruptio placenta

  D. Prolapsed cord

_____ **23.** Premature separation of the placenta from the wall of the uterus is known as:

  A. eclampsia.

  B. placenta previa.

  C. placenta abruptio.

  D. prolapsed cord.

_____ **24.** _____ is a condition in which the placenta develops over and covers the cervix.

  A. Eclampsia

  B. Placenta previa

  C. Placenta abruptio

  D. Prolapsed cord

_____ **25.** _____ is heralded by the onset of convulsions, or seizures, resulting from severe hypertension in the pregnant woman.

  A. Eclampsia

  B. Placenta previa

  C. Placenta abruptio

  D. Supine hypotensive syndrome

_____ **26.** Which of the following is NOT considered a possible effect to the fetus when the mother is a known substance abuser?

  A. Low birth weight

  B. Spina bifida

  C. Prematurity

  D. Severe respiratory depression

Questions 27–31 are derived from the following scenario: You have been dispatched to the side of a highway where a woman is reported to be delivering a baby. As you approach the vehicle, you see her lying down in the back seat.

_____ **27.** Which of the following signs tell you that the birth is imminent?

  A. Her water has not broken.

  B. Her contractions are 3 to 6 minutes apart.

  C. She is a primigravida.

  D. The infant is crowning.

_____ **28.** If the baby is crowning and the amniotic sac has not yet ruptured, you should:

  A. leave it in place and wait for ALS.

  B. puncture the sac only after ordered to do so by medical control.

  C. puncture the sac, allow the fluid to drain, and leave the sac in place.

  D. puncture the sac away from the head and then push the sac away from the infant's face.

_____ **29.** As you perform a visual exam, you note crowning. This means that:

    A. the baby is making a crowing-type of sound.

    B. the baby cannot be visualized.

    C. you can visualize the baby's head.

    D. the father is excited and needs care.

_____ **30.** Once the infant's head has been delivered:

    A. suction the infant's nose, and then the mouth.

    B. apply oxygen over the mother's vagina.

    C. suction the infant's mouth, then the nose.

    D. apply a nasal cannula at 3 L/min to the infant.

_____ **31.** Concerning the delivery of the placenta, which of the following are emergency situations?

    A. More than 30 minutes have elapsed and the placenta has not delivered.

    B. There is more than 500 mL of bleeding before delivery of the placenta.

    C. There is significant bleeding after delivery of the placenta.

    D. All of the above.

_____ **32.** Ovulation occurs approximately _____ before menstruation.

    A. 1 week

    B. 2 weeks

    C. 3 weeks

    D. 4 weeks

_____ **33.** Fertilization usually occurs when the egg is inside the:

    A. ovary.

    B. uterus.

    C. fallopian tube.

    D. endometrium.

_____ **34.** Which of the following statements is FALSE?

    A. Gestational diabetes will clear up in most women after delivery.

    B. The leading cause of abruptio placenta is an ectopic pregnancy.

    C. As pregnancy progresses, the uterus enlarges and rises out of the pelvis.

    D. Some cultures may not permit male EMTs to examine a female patient.

_____ **35.** The "P" in Apgar stands for:

    A. perfusion

    B. pulse

    C. pupils

    D. position

_____ **36.** Which of the following statements regarding multiple gestations is FALSE?

    A. You should consider the possibility of twins when the first infant is small and the mother's abdomen remains fairly large after the birth.

    B. You should record the time of birth on each twin separately.

    C. There is only one placenta with the birth of twins.

    D. The second baby will usually be born within 45 minutes of the first.

_____ **37.** An infant delivered before _____ weeks is considered premature.

    A. 36

    B. 37

    C. 38

    D. 39

_____ **38.** All of the following are correct regarding postterm pregnancy EXCEPT:

    A. infants can be larger, sometimes weighing 10 pounds (4.5 kg) or more.

    B. there is an increased risk of meconium aspiration.

    C. postterm is considered past 2 weeks gestation.

    D. ultrasounds are not accurate at determining due dates.

_____ **39.** A patient presents with a sudden onset of shortness of breath three days following a delivery. What is likely underlying cause of this condition?

    A. Pulmonary hypertension

    B. Pulmonary inflammation

    C. Pulmonary embolism

    D. Pulmonary fibrosis

_____ **40.** After delivery, if the infant does not begin breathing after _____ seconds, you should begin resuscitation efforts.

    A. 5 to 10

    B. 10 to 15

    C. 15 to 20

    D. 20 to 25

True/False

If you believe the statement to be more true than false, write the letter "T" in the space provided. If you believe the statement to be more false than true, write the letter "F."

_____ **1.** The small mucous plug from the cervix that is discharged from the vagina, often at the beginning of labor, is called a bloody show.

_____ **2.** Crowning occurs when the baby's head obstructs the birth canal, preventing normal delivery.

_____ **3.** Labor begins with the rupture of the amniotic sac and ends with the delivery of the baby's head.

_____ **4.** A woman who is having her first baby is called a multigravida.

_____ **5.** Once labor has begun, it can be slowed by holding the patient's legs together.

_____ **6.** Delivery of the buttocks before the baby's head is called a breech delivery.

_____ **7.** Massaging the abdomen after delivery helps to control bleeding.

_____ **8.** The placenta and cord should be properly disposed of in a biohazard container after delivery.

_____ **9.** The umbilical cord may be gently pulled to aid in delivery of the placenta.

_____ **10.** A limb presentation occurs when the baby's arm, leg, or foot is emerging from the vagina first.

_____ **11.** Multiple births may have more than one placenta.

_____ **12.** Pregnant teenagers may not know that they are pregnant.

_____ **13.** After delivery of the head, suction the nose first.

_____ **14.** Abuse during pregnancy increases the chance of miscarriage, premature delivery, and low birth weight.

_____ **15.** If called to deliver an infant who may have died in the uterus, you could notice skin blisters and dark discoloration to the infant.

_____ **16.** Most premature infants have vernix on their skin when delivered.

_____ **17.** Excessive bleeding after birth is usually caused by the muscles of the uterus not fully contracting.

Fill-in-the-Blank

Read each item carefully and then complete the statement by filling in the missing words.

1. After delivery, the _____, or afterbirth, separates from the uterus and is delivered.

2. The umbilical cord contains two _____ and one _____.

3. The amniotic sac contains about _____ to _____ mL of amniotic fluid, which helps to insulate and protect the floating fetus as it develops.

4. A full-term pregnancy is from _____ to _____ weeks, counting from the first day of the last menstrual cycle.

5. By the end of pregnancy, the pregnant patient's heart rate increases up to 20%, or about _____ beats more per minute.

6. There is a high potential of exposure due to _____ _____ released during childbirth.

7. The leading cause of maternal death in the first trimester is internal hemorrhage into the abdomen following rupture of a(n) _____ _____.

8. In serious trauma, the only chance to save the infant is to adequately _____ the mother.

9. During the delivery, be careful that you do not poke your fingers into the infant's eyes or into the two soft spots, called _____, on the head.

10. _____ _____ is a developmental defect in which a portion of the spinal cord protrudes outside the vertebrae.

11. Passage of the fetus and placenta before 20 weeks is called _____.

12. Preterm or false labor is commonly referred to as _____ _____ contractions.

13. The _____ _____ carries oxygenated blood from the woman to the heart of the fetus.

14. The _____ is the area of skin between the vagina and the anus.

15. Due to hormonal changes that cause joints in the musculoskeletal system to "loosen," a pregnant patient has a greater risk of _____.

Fill-in-the-Table

Fill in the missing parts of the table.

Apgar Scoring System			
Area of Activity	**Score**		
	2	1	0
Appearance			
Pulse			
Grimace or irritability			
Activity or muscle tone			
Respiration			

Labeling

Label the following diagram with the correct terms.

1. Anatomic Structures of the Pregnant Woman

A. _____

B. _____

C. _____

D. _____

E. _____

F. _____

G. _____

H. _____

I. _____

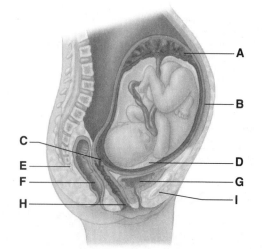

Crossword Puzzle

The following crossword puzzle is an activity provided to reinforce correct spelling and understanding of medical terminology associated with emergency care and the EMT. Use the clues in the column to complete the puzzle.

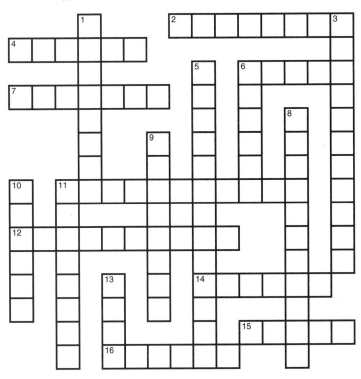

Across

2. The appearance of the infant's head at the vaginal opening during labor
4. _____ presentation is a delivery in which the buttocks come out first.
6. The developing, unborn infant inside the uterus
7. _____ pregnancy develops outside the uterus, typically in a fallopian tube.
11. The fluid-filled, baglike membrane in which the fetus develops
12. The vagina and cervix
14. Narrowest portion of the uterus that opens into the vagina
15. The scoring system for assessing the status of a newborn is known as the _____ score.
16. _____ show is a small amount of blood at the vagina that appears at the beginning of labor.

Down

1. A dark green material in the amniotic fluid that can indicate distress or disease in the newborn
3. _____ diabetes can develop during pregnancy in women who did not have diabetes before pregnancy.
5. The conduit connecting mother to infant via the placenta
6. The dome-shaped top of the uterus
8. The passage of the fetus and placenta before 20 weeks
9. _____ of the umbilical cord is a situation in which the umbilical cord comes out of the vagina before the infant.
10. The fertilized egg that is the early stages of a fetus
11. _____ placenta is a premature separation of the placenta from the wall of the uterus.
13. _____ presentation is a delivery in which the presenting part is a single arm, leg, or foot.

Critical Thinking

Multiple Choice

Read each item carefully and then select the one best response.
Determine the Apgar score for each of the following scenarios.

_____ 1. You assess an infant after delivery and note that the child has a loud cry and withdraws to pain. The heart rate is 94 beats/min, the extremities are cyanotic, respirations are rapid, and the infant strongly resists your attempts to straighten the knees.
   A. 2
   B. 10
   C. 8
   D. 4

_____ **2.** You arrive at the scene of a home delivery. Upon entering the scene, the father appears upset and hands you a limp baby. The child has a weak cry, is completely cyanotic, and has a pulse of 70 beats/min. Respirations are slow.

    A. 3

    B. 9

    C. 2

    D. 7

_____ **3.** You arrive on scene to assist another crew with a delivery. Upon your arrival, the crew on scene informs you that the delivery has already taken place and that you are going to be responsible for care of the infant. As you approach, you hear a very loud cry. The infant appears completely pink and moves his foot away when you flick the sole of his foot. The pulse is 120 beats/min and respirations are rapid. The infant has great muscle tone and resists your attempt to straighten the hips.

    A. 6

    B. 10

    C. 1

    D. 8

Short Answer

Complete this section with short written answers using the space provided.

1. What are some possible causes of vaginal hemorrhage in early and late pregnancy?

_____

_____

2. In what position should pregnant patients who are not delivering be transported and why?

_____

_____

3. List three signs that indicate the beginning of labor.

_____

_____

4. When determining whether delivery is imminent and whether there are complications, what questions should you ask the patient?

_____

_____

5. Once the baby's head emerges, what actions should be taken to prevent too rapid a delivery?

_____

_____

6. Why is it important to avoid pushing on the fontanelles?

_____

_____

7. How can you help decrease perineal tearing?

_____

_____

8. What are the two situations in which an EMT may insert his or her fingers into a patient's vagina?

_____

_____

9. What are three fetal effects of maternal drug or alcohol addiction?

_____

_____

10. List five signs/symptoms associated with preeclampsia.

_____

_____

_____

Ambulance Calls

The following case scenarios provide an opportunity to explore the concerns associated with patient management and to enhance critical-thinking skills. Read each scenario and answer each question to the best of your ability.

1. You are dispatched to a grocery store for an "unknown medical problem." You arrive to find a 20-year-old woman who is in her 32nd week of pregnancy. She tells you that this is her first pregnancy and she had made an appointment to see her obstetrician later that day because she was not feeling well. She's been experiencing a headache, swelling in her hands and feet, and transient problems with her vision. She states that she suddenly felt lightheaded and had to sit down. She appears unhurt.

How would you best manage this patient?

_____

_____

_____

2. You are enjoying a quiet lunch at the fire station when you hear the back doorbell ring. As you look out the window, you see a young woman running away from the building. You open the door to call to her and when you look down you see something bundled in a wet sheet. It's a newborn; she's wet with amniotic fluid, and she's not breathing very well.

How would you best manage this patient?

_____

_____

_____

3. You are on the scene with a 32-year-old woman who is 38 weeks pregnant. Delivery is imminent. As the infant starts to crown, you notice that the amniotic sac is still intact.

How would you best manage this patient?

_____

_____

_____

Skills

Skill Drill

Test your knowledge of this skill by placing the photos below in the correct order. Number the first step with a "1," the second step with a "2," etc.

Skill Drill 31-1: Delivering the Baby

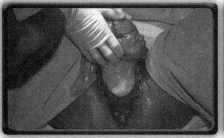 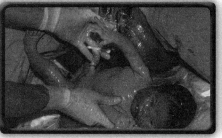 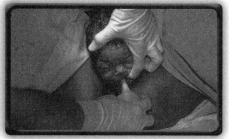

_____ Support the head and upper body as the lower shoulder delivers, guiding the head up if needed.

_____ Place the umbilical cord clamps 2″ to 4″ (5 to 10 cm) apart, and cut between them.

_____ Support the bony parts of the head with your hands as it emerges. Suction fluid from the mouth, then nostrils.

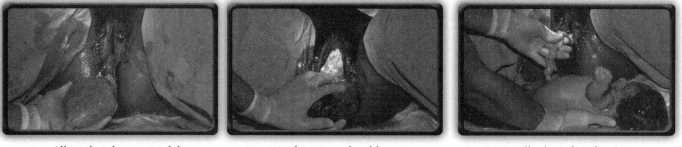

_____ Allow the placenta to deliver itself. Do not pull on the cord to speed delivery.

_____ As the upper shoulder appears, guide the head down slightly, if needed, to deliver the shoulder.

_____ Handle the infant firmly but gently, keeping the neck in neutral position to maintain the airway. Keep the infant approximately at the level of the vagina until the umbilical cord is cut.

Assessment Review

Answer the following questions pertaining to the assessment of the types of emergencies discussed in this chapter.

_____ **1.** During delivery, after the head has been delivered and the shoulder appears:

   A. guide the head down slightly, to deliver the shoulder.

   B. apply a nasal cannula to the infant.

   C. guide the head up slightly, to deliver the shoulder.

   D. pull gently.

_____ **2.** When giving chest compressions to an infant:

   A. use the hands-encircling technique or the two-finger technique.

   B. press the palm of your hand over the sternum, compressing 1″ to 1 1/2″ (2.5 to 3 cm) deep.

   C. compress at a rate of 60 to 80 times a minute.

   D. compress the sternum one quarter the depth of the chest.

_____ **3.** Which of the following would NOT be a typical question to ask when taking a history on a woman in labor?

   A. Are you having a boy or a girl?

   B. When is your due date?

   C. Did your physician mention the possibility of any complications?

   D. Is this your first pregnancy?

_____ **4.** Once the infant is completely delivered, you should:

   A. dry and wrap the infant in a blanket.

   B. keep the infant at the level of the vagina until the umbilical cord is cut.

   C. use sterile gauze and wipe out the infant's mouth.

   D. all of the above.

_____ **5.** When cutting the umbilical cord:

   A. place the clamps 7″ to 10″ (18 to 25 cm) apart.

   B. place the clamps 2″ to 4″ (5 to 10 cm) apart.

   C. tie the cord with shoelaces if you don't have any clamps.

   D. tie the cord with string if you don't have any clamps.

Emergency Care Summary

Fill in the following chart pertaining to the management of the types of emergencies discussed in this chapter.

Note: While the steps below are widely accepted, be sure to consult and follow your local protocol.

General Management of Obstetric Emergencies

Managing life threats to the patient's ABCs are primary concerns with any obstetric emergency. Avoid tunnel vision. Complete a(n) _____ scan, remaining alert for signs and symptoms of _____. Manage as per local protocol. Request additional resources if delivery is imminent or has occurred. Provide high-concentration oxygen.

Delivery Complications

Nuchal Cord

When the _____ _____ is wrapped around the infant's neck, it is called a nuchal cord. If it is wound tightly it will strangle the infant, so it must be removed. Attempt to slip the cord over the infant's head or shoulder. If you are unable to slip the cord over the head or shoulder, you will need to clamp the cord in _____ places about 2" (5 cm) apart, if possible, and cut the cord between the clamps. After cutting the cord, you can unwrap it and continue with the delivery as usual.

Spontaneous Abortion (Miscarriage)

If the delivery is occurring before the _____ week of gestation, be prepared to treat the patient for bleeding and shock. Place a sterile pad/dressing on the _____. Collect any expelled tissue to take to the hospital, but never pull tissue out of the vagina. Transport immediately, continually monitoring the patient's ABCs while assessing for signs of shock.

Multiple Gestation

The procedure for delivering multiple infants is the same as that for a single newborn. If you suspect more than one infant, _____ _____ should be called for immediately. Record the time of birth for each infant separately, making sure to label them for identification after the delivery process is over. At 1- and 5-minute intervals, assess and record the _____ score for each infant.

Postterm Pregnancy

Pregnancies lasting more than 42 weeks can lead to problems with the mother and infant. Infants can be larger, leading to a more difficult delivery and injury to the infant. _____ aspiration risk increases, as does infection and _____ birth. Respiratory and _____ functions may be affected, so be prepared to resuscitate the infant.

SPECIAL PATIENT POPULATIONS

Pediatric Emergencies

General Knowledge

Matching

Match each of the items in the left column to the appropriate definition in the right column.

_____	**1.** Adolescents	**A.** Sign of increased work of breathing
_____	**2.** Blanching	**B.** Optimal neutral head position for uninjured airway management
_____	**3.** Infancy	**C.** 12 to 18 years of age
_____	**4.** Grunting	**D.** Failure to provide life necessities
_____	**5.** Neglect	**E.** Infant to 3 years of age
_____	**6.** Pediatrics	**F.** First year of life
_____	**7.** Pertussis	**G.** Medical practice devoted to care of the young
_____	**8.** Preschool-age	**H.** 3 to 6 years of age
_____	**9.** Sniffing position	**I.** Turning white
_____	**10.** Toddler	**J.** Paroxysmal cough that ends in a whooping inspiration

Multiple Choice

Read each item carefully and then select the one best response.

_____ **1.** Making eye contact, recognizing caregivers, and following a bright light with their eyes are initially noticed in what age group?

    A. 0 to 2 months

    B. 2 to 6 months

    C. 6 to 12 months

    D. 12 to 18 months

_____ **2.** Saying their first word, sitting without support, and teething are initially noticed in what age group?

    A. 0 to 2 months

    B. 2 to 6 months

    C. 6 to 12 months

    D. 12 to 18 months

_____ **3.** Which of the following is NOT initially seen in children 12 to 18 months old?

    A. Speak four to six words

    B. Know the major body parts

    C. Can open doors

    D. Understand cause and effect

_____ **4.** Toilet training is typically mastered at what age level?

    A. 6 to 12 months

    B. 12 to 18 months

    C. Preschool-age

    D. School-age

_____ **5.** Which of the following is FALSE regarding the pediatric airway?

    A. The trachea is larger in diameter and shorter in length.

    B. The glottis opening is higher and positioned more anterior.

    C. The neck appears to be nonexistent.

    D. The lungs are smaller.

_____ **6.** Breath sounds in the pediatric population are more easily heard because:

    A. their chest walls are thinner.

    B. the size of their lungs amplifies the sounds.

    C. the chest cavity is small in proportion to the rest of the body.

    D. children typically have upper airway problems.

_____ **7.** An infant's heart can beat as many as _____ times or more per minute if the body needs to compensate for injury or illness.

    A. 110

    B. 120

    C. 140

    D. 160

_____ **8.** Which of the following is NOT a common cause of altered mental status in pediatric patients?

    A. Drug and alcohol ingestion

    B. Hypertension

    C. Seizure

    D. Hypoglycemia

_____ **9.** A fracture of the femur is rare and is a major source of _____ in the pediatric population.

    A. infection

    B. growth abnormalities

    C. blood loss

    D. nerve damage

_____ **10.** When you assess a pediatric patient, it is best to place _____ on the patient's chest to feel the rise and fall of the chest wall.

    A. the left hand

    B. the right hand

    C. both hands

    D. the stethoscope

_____ **11.** Tachycardia in pediatric patients may be an indication of all of the following EXCEPT:

    A. hypothermia.

    B. hypoxia.

    C. fever.

    D. pain.

_____ **12.** When assessing capillary refill in pediatric patients, the color should return after:

    A. 1 second.

    B. 2 seconds.

    C. 3 seconds.

    D. 4 seconds.

_____ **13.** Pupillary response in pediatric patients may be abnormal in the presence of all of the following EXCEPT:

    A. anxiety.

    B. hypoxia.

    C. brain injury.

    D. drugs.

_____ **14.** When obtaining information from the family regarding the pediatric patient's history, which of the following is NOT an appropriate inquiry?

  A. Does the child have any rashes?

  B. What has been the child's recent activity level?

  C. Has there been any vomiting or diarrhea?

  D. What types of toys does the child play with?

_____ **15.** When examining the head of a pediatric patient, which of the following statements is FALSE?

  A. You should look for bruising, swelling, and hematomas.

  B. Significant blood loss can come from the scalp.

  C. A bulging fontanelle suggests dehydration.

  D. The head is larger in proportion to the rest of the body.

_____ **16.** In pediatric patients, guarding of the abdomen suggests:

  A. diarrhea.

  B. nausea.

  C. infection.

  D. dehydration.

_____ **17.** Which of the following is NOT a sign of increased work of breathing in pediatric patients?

  A. Nasal flaring

  B. Grunting

  C. Equal chest expansion

  D. Retractions

_____ **18.** Which of the following is NOT an infection that can cause an airway obstruction in pediatric patients?

  A. Pneumonia

  B. Asthma

  C. Croup

  D. Epiglottitis

_____ **19.** Signs and symptoms of a lower airway obstruction in pediatric patients include:

  A. stridor.

  B. friction rub.

  C. drooling.

  D. wheezing.

_____ **20.** Exposure to cold air, infection, and emotional stress are all triggers of:

  A. pneumonia.

  B. asthma.

  C. bronchiolitis.

  D. epiglottitis.

_____ **21.** Which of the following statements regarding pediatric asthma is FALSE?

  A. Use strong, forceful breaths when ventilating to get air past the obstruction.

  B. The wheezing may be so loud that you can hear it without a stethoscope.

  C. The patient may be in the tripod position.

  D. A bronchodilator via a metered-dose inhaler may be helpful.

_____ **22.** All of the following are signs associated with pneumonia in pediatric patients EXCEPT:

  A. bradycardia.

  B. grunting.

  C. nasal flaring.

  D. hypothermia.

_____ **23.** Bronchiolitis usually occurs during the first _____ of life.

    A. 2 years

    B. 3 years

    C. 4 years

    D. 6 years

_____ **24.** Which of the following is NOT a common cause of shock in pediatric patients?

    A. Diseases of the heart

    B. Severe infection

    C. Dehydration

    D. Renal failure

_____ **25.** Signs of shock in children include all of the following EXCEPT:

    A. altered mental status.

    B. poor capillary refill.

    C. hypertension.

    D. tachycardia.

_____ **26.** A pediatric patient with hives, wheezing, increased work of breathing, and hypoperfusion is likely suffering from:

    A. pneumonia.

    B. bronchiolitis.

    C. asthma.

    D. anaphylaxis.

_____ **27.** Which of the following is appropriate when treating pediatric patients with seizures?

    A. Clear the mouth with suction.

    B. Provide 100% oxygen.

    C. Consider placing the patient in the recovery position.

    D. All of the above.

_____ **28.** Which of the following populations is at the greatest risk for contracting meningitis?

    A. Females

    B. Children who have had head trauma

    C. Children with preexisting heart conditions

    D. Children of parents with a history of meningitis

_____ **29.** A pediatric patient with a fever, pain on palpation of the right lower quadrant, and rebound tenderness is likely to be suffering from:

    A. cholecystitis.

    B. gastroenteritis.

    C. appendicitis.

    D. constipation.

_____ **30.** Which of the following is NOT a question you would ask if you suspected a poisoning emergency?

    A. Did the substance have an odor?

    B. Are there any changes in behavior or level of consciousness?

    C. What is the substance involved?

    D. Was there any choking or coughing after the exposure?

_____ **31.** Activated charcoal is not indicated for pediatric patients who have ingested a(n):

    A. acid.

    B. alkali.

    C. petroleum product.

    D. all of the above.

_____ **32.** Which of the following is not a sign of severe dehydration in pediatric patients?

  A. Bulging fontanelles

  B. Very dry lips and gums

  C. Eyes look sunken

  D. Sleepiness

_____ **33.** Young children can compensate for fluid losses by:

  A. decreasing blood flow to the brain and heart.

  B. decreasing blood flow to the extremities.

  C. increasing blood flow to the extremities.

  D. increasing blood flow to the gastrointestinal tract.

_____ **34.** All of the following are common causes of a fever in pediatric patients EXCEPT:

  A. infection.

  B. status epilepticus.

  C. drug ingestion.

  D. cholecystitis.

_____ **35.** A pediatric patient involved in a drowning emergency may present with:

  A. cerebral edema.

  B. hypoglycemia.

  C. abdominal distention.

  D. chest pain.

_____ **36.** Head and neck injuries are common after high-speed collisions in all of the following contact sports EXCEPT:

  A. wrestling.

  B. football.

  C. lacrosse.

  D. basketball.

_____ **37.** All children with abdominal injuries should be monitored for signs and symptoms of:

  A. pain.

  B. shock.

  C. hypothermia.

  D. nausea.

_____ **38.** Which of the following is NOT a common exposure when dealing with pediatric burns?

  A. Scalding water in a bathtub

  B. Electrocution from poor wiring

  C. Hot items on a stove

  D. Cleaning solvents

_____ **39.** How many triage categories are there in the JumpSTART system?

  A. Three

  B. Four

  C. Five

  D. Six

_____ **40.** Which of the following is NOT a known risk factor for SIDS?

  A. Mother younger than 20 years old

  B. Mother smoked during pregnancy

  C. Gestational diabetes

  D. Low birth weight

_____ **41.** When you are performing a scene assessment at an incident involving SIDS, you should focus your attention on all of the following EXCEPT:

    A. signs of illness, including medication, humidifiers, and thermometers.

    B. the general condition of the house.

    C. the site where the infant was discovered.

    D. the temperature of the room.

_____ **42.** Incidents involving the death of a child pose extra stress on EMS workers. Which of the following is NOT a sign of posttraumatic stress?

    A. Cold intolerance

    B. Nightmares

    C. Difficult sleeping

    D. Loss of appetite

True/False

If you believe the statement to be more true than false, write the letter "T" in the space provided. If you believe the statement to be more false than true, write the letter "F."

_____ **1.** You should avoid letting the parent or caregiver hold an infant during your assessment.

_____ **2.** Toddlers have a hard time describing or localizing pain because they do not have the verbal ability to be precise.

_____ **3.** It is considered acceptable to lie to a preschool-age child because they will not be able to understand their true medical condition.

_____ **4.** Adolescence is a time for experimentation and risk-taking behaviors.

_____ **5.** Some of the risks that adolescents take can ultimately facilitate development and judgment.

_____ **6.** Congenital cardiovascular problems are the leading cause of cardiopulmonary arrest in the pediatric population.

_____ **7.** Sprains are uncommon in the pediatric population.

_____ **8.** Infants and young children should be kept warm during a transport or when the patient is exposed to assess or reassess an injury.

_____ **9.** Bradypnea usually indicates that the pediatric patient's condition is improving.

_____ **10.** Pediatric patients weighing less than 27 kg (60 lb) should be transported by car seat.

_____ **11.** Blood pressure is usually not assessed in pediatric patients younger than 4 years.

_____ **12.** A prolonged asthma attack that is unrelieved may progress to a condition known as status asthmaticus.

_____ **13.** An oropharyngeal airway should be used for pediatric patients who are unconscious and in possible respiratory failure.

_____ **14.** Blow-by oxygen is as effective as a face mask or nasal cannula for delivering oxygen to a pediatric patient.

_____ **15.** A rectal temperature is the most accurate for infants to toddlers.

_____ **16.** At around 8 to 10 years of age, children no longer require padding underneath the torso to create a neutral position.

_____ **17.** Extremity injuries in the pediatric population are managed much differently than extremity injuries in adults.

_____ **18.** EMTs in all states must report all cases of suspected abuse, even if the emergency department fails to do so.

_____ **19.** Do not examine the genitalia of a young child unless there is evidence of bleeding or there is an injury that must be treated.

_____ **20.** You should use a euphemism such as "passed away" when informing the family of a pediatric death to lessen their emotional pain.

Fill-in-the-Blank

Read each item carefully and then complete the statement by filling in the missing words.

1. Children not only have a higher metabolic rate, but also a higher _____ _____, which is twice that of an adult.

2. Breathing requires the use of the _____ muscles and diaphragm.

3. _____ _____ occurs when the pediatric patient has exhausted all compensatory mechanisms and waste products begin to collect.

4. Located on the front (anterior) and back (posterior) portions of the head are soft spots, the _____.

5. The _____ _____ _____ is a structured assessment tool that allows you to rapidly form a general impression of the pediatric patient's condition without touching him or her.

6. Always position the airway in a neutral _____ _____.

7. Car seats are designed to be either _____ or _____; they cannot be mounted sideways on a bench seat.

8. A child in respiratory distress or possible respiratory failure needs supplemental _____.

9. _____ is an infection of the soft tissue in the area above the vocal cords.

10. _____ _____ are recommended to relieve a severe airway obstruction in an unconscious pediatric patient.

11. _____ is an acute spasm of the smaller air passages.

12. Inserting a(n) _____ _____ in a responsive patient may cause a spasm of the larynx and result in vomiting.

13. _____ is a congenital condition in which the patient lacks one or more of the normal clotting factors of blood.

14. _____ is common in pediatric patients and if left untreated can lead to peritonitis or shock.

15. _____ is the second most common cause of unintentional death among children in the United States.

16. In pediatric patients, chest injuries are usually the result of _____ _____, rather than penetrating trauma.

17. One common problem following burn injuries in children is _____.

18. _____ is refusal or failure on the part of the caregiver to provide life necessities.

Crossword Puzzle

The following crossword puzzle is an activity provided to reinforce correct spelling and understanding of medical terminology associated with emergency care and the EMT. Use the clues in the column to complete the puzzle.

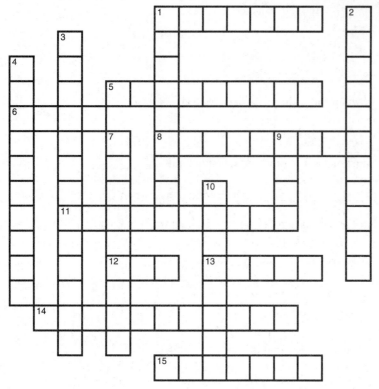

Across

1. The period following infancy until 3 years of age
5. Children between 6 to 12 years of age
6. An event that causes unresponsiveness, cyanosis, and apnea in an infant, who then resumes breathing with stimulation
8. An acute infectious disease characterized by a catarrhal stage, followed by a paroxysmal cough that ends in a whooping inspiration. Also called whooping cough.
11. A specialized medical practice devoted to the care of the young
12. A structured assessment tool that allows you to rapidly form a general impression of the infant or child without touching him or her; consists of assessing appearance, work of breathing, and circulation to the skin
13. The external openings of the nostrils
14. A(n) _____ tonic-clonic seizure features rhythmic back-and-forth motion of an extremity and body stiffness.
15. Refusal or failure on the part of the caregiver to provide life necessities

Down

1. Increased respiratory rate
2. Children between 12 to 18 years of age
3. Pulses that are closest to the core part of the body where the vital organs are located
4. _____ syndrome is seen in abused infants and children.
7. Slow respiratory rate; ominous sign in a child that indicates impending respiratory arrest
9. Death of an infant or young child that remains unexplained after a complete autopsy
10. An "uh" sound heard during exhalation, reflecting the child's attempt to keep the alveoli open

Critical Thinking

Short Answer

Complete this section with short written answers using the space provided.

1. What does each letter in the mnemonic TICLS mean?

_____

_____

2. What are the signs of increased work of breathing in a pediatric patient, and what do they mean?

_____

_____

3. List the indications for immediate transport of a pediatric patient.

_____

_____

4. What tool is used to determine the appropriate blood pressure for a pediatric patient between 1 and 10 years of age?

_____

_____

5. When assessing for circulation, what are the specific areas to focus on, and what questions should you ask yourself?

_____

_____

Ambulance Calls

The following case scenarios provide an opportunity to explore the concerns associated with patient management and to enhance critical-thinking skills. Read each scenario and answer each question to the best of your ability.

1. You are dispatched to the residence of a toddler who has a history of fever and who is now unresponsive. You arrive to find a 13-year-old babysitter who tells you that she is not sure what is wrong with the 2-year-old boy. She tells you that he started "shaking all over" and she didn't know what to do. He is currently responsive to painful stimuli and warm to the touch.

How would you best manage this patient?

_____

_____

_____

2. You are dispatched to the residence of a 3-year-old child with a history of lung problems. The child, a very small boy, is cyanotic and lethargic. He is pain responsive. He has copious mucous secretions in his airway. The grandmother, who was sitting with the child, is hysterical.

How would you best manage this patient?

_____

_____

_____

3. You are called to a residence for a 2-year-old child with difficulty breathing. The little girl has stridor and expiratory wheezes, as well as intercostal retractions. She is very upset by your arrival and clings to her mother. Her breathing worsens with agitation. Her mother tells you that she is currently taking medication for an upper respiratory infection and has spent much of her life in and out of hospitals with respiratory problems.

How would you best manage this patient?

_____

_____

_____

4. It's 0530, and you are dispatched to the home of a 6-month-old girl who is not breathing. You arrive to find a crying, young mother holding a lifeless baby. The infant is not breathing, is cold to the touch, and appears to have dependent lividity.

How would you best manage this patient?

_____

_____

_____

Skills

Skill Drills

Skill Drill 32-1: Positioning the Airway in a Pediatric Patient
Test your knowledge of this skill by filling in the correct words in the photo captions.

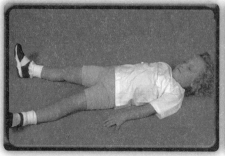 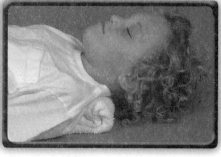 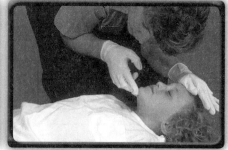

1. Position the pediatric patient on a(n) _____ surface.

2. Place a(n) _____ towel about _____-inch(es) thick under the _____ and _____.

3. _____ the forehead to limit _____ and use the head tilt–chin lift maneuver to open the airway.

Skill Drill 32-2: Inserting an Oropharyngeal Airway in a Pediatric Patient
Test your knowledge of this skill by filling in the correct words in the photo captions.

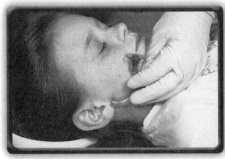
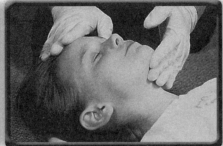
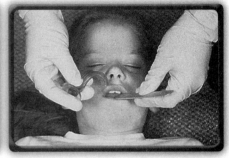

1. Determine the appropriately _____ airway. Confirm the correct size _____, by placing it next to the patient's _____.

2. Position the pediatric patient's _____ with the appropriate method.

3. Open the mouth. Insert the airway until the _____ rests against the _____. _____ the airway.

Skill Drill 32-3: Inserting a Nasopharyngeal Airway in a Pediatric Patient
Test your knowledge of this skill by filling in the correct words in the photo captions.

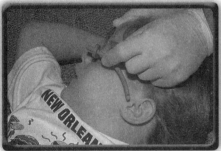
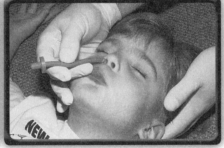
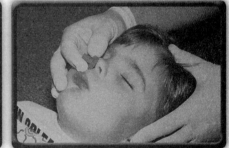

1. Determine the correct airway size by comparing its _____ to the opening of the _____ (naris). Place the airway next to the pediatric patient's _____ to confirm correct _____. _____ the airway.

2. _____ the airway. Insert the _____ into the right naris with the bevel pointing toward the _____.

3. Carefully move the tip forward until the _____ rests against the _____ of the nostril. Reassess the _____.

Skill Drill 32-4: One-Rescuer Bag-Mask Device Ventilation on a Pediatric Patient
Test your knowledge of this skill by placing the photos below in the correct order. Number the first step with a "1," the second step with a "2," etc.

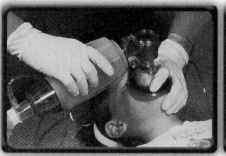

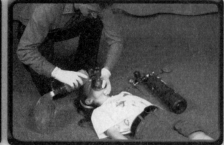

_____ Hold the mask on the patient's face with a one-handed head tilt–chin lift technique (E-C grip). Ensure a good mask–face seal while maintaining the airway.

_____ Assess effectiveness of ventilation by watching bilateral rise and fall of the chest.

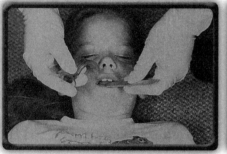

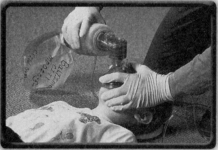

_____ Open the airway and insert the appropriate airway adjunct.

_____ Squeeze the bag using the correct ventilation rate of 12 to 20 breaths/min. Allow adequate time for exhalation.

Skill Drill 32-6: Immobilizing a Patient in a Car Seat
Test your knowledge of this skill by filling in the correct words in the photo captions.

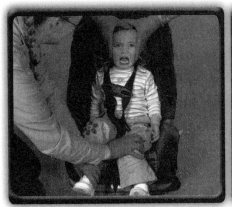

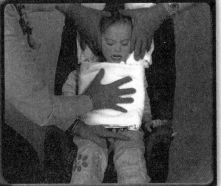

1. Carefully _____ the patient's head in a(n) _____ position.

2. Place an appropriately sized _____ collar on the patient if available. Otherwise, place rolled _____ or padding alongside the patient.

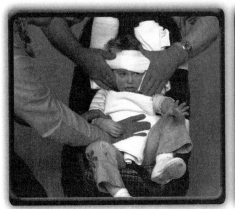

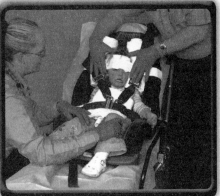

3. Carefully secure the _____, using tape to keep it in place.

4. Secure the car seat to the _____.

Skill Drill 32-7: Immobilizing a Patient Out of a Car Seat
Test your knowledge of this skill by placing the photos below in the correct order. Number the first step with a "1," the second step with a "2," etc.

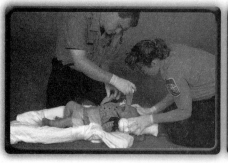

_____ Secure the head to the board.

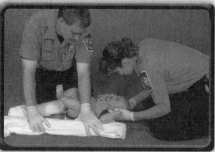

_____ Slide the patient onto the board.

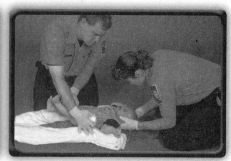

_____ Place a towel under the back, from the shoulders to the hips, to ensure neutral head position.

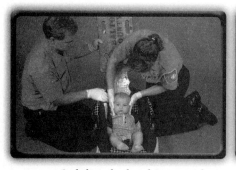

_____ Stabilize the head in neutral position.

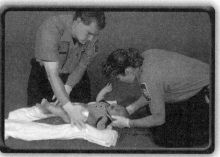

_____ Secure the torso first; pad any voids.

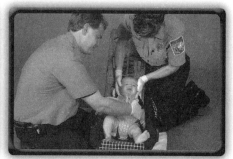

_____ Place an immobilization device between the patient and the surface he or she is resting on.

SPECIAL PATIENT POPULATIONS
Geriatric Emergencies

General Knowledge

Matching

Match each of the items in the left column to the appropriate definition in the right column.

_____ 1. Aneurysm	**A.** Forward curling of the back
_____ 2. Cataract	**B.** Fluid in the abdomen
_____ 3. Delirium	**C.** Clouding of the lens of the eye
_____ 4. Dementia	**D.** Reduced bone mass leading to fractures after minimal trauma
_____ 5. Syncope	**E.** Abnormal blood-filled dilation of a blood vessel
_____ 6. Dyspnea	**F.** Difficulty breathing
_____ 7. Osteoporosis	**G.** Inability to focus, think logically, or maintain attention
_____ 8. Polypharmacy	**H.** Use of multiple medications
_____ 9. Kyphosis	**I.** Slow onset of progressive disorientation
_____ 10. Ascites	**J.** Fainting

Multiple Choice

Read each item carefully and then select the one best response.

_____ 1. Which of the following is NOT one of the leading causes of death in the older population?

    A. Heart disease

    B. Diabetes

    C. AIDS

    D. Cancer

_____ 2. Geriatric patients present as a special problem for caregivers because:

    A. the classic presentation of disease is often altered.

    B. geriatric patients tend not to understand their underlying conditions.

    C. their medications are rather difficult to learn.

    D. the typical diseases of the geriatric population are uncommon.

_____ 3. Stereotyping of elderly people that often leads to discrimination is called:

    A. geritism.

    B. geriographics.

    C. oldism.

    D. ageism.

_____ 4. Which of the following is NOT a common stereotype regarding geriatrics?

    A. Most elderly people have dementia.

    B. Elderly people are hard of hearing.

    C. Geriatric patients are likely to die on an EMS call.

    D. Elderly people are immobile.

_____   **5.** Which of the following is generally NOT acceptable when interviewing an older patient?

    A. Do not initiate eye contact, because many geriatric patients might find this disrespectful.

    B. Speak slowly and distinctly.

    C. Give the patient time to respond unless the condition appears urgent.

    D. Explain what you are doing before you do it.

_____   **6.** Which of the following is NOT considered a common condition of the elderly?

    A. Hypertension

    B. Sinusitis

    C. Gastroenteritis

    D. Arthritis

_____   **7.** Geriatric patients are commonly found living in all of the following locations EXCEPT:

    A. their homes.

    B. nursing homes.

    C. skilled nursing facilities.

    D. churches.

_____   **8.** You are responding to the dementia unit at a nursing home for respiratory distress. When you arrive, you notice that the patient is experiencing mild dyspnea and has an altered mental status. What can you do to help determine if the patient's altered mental status is appropriate for her underlying dementia?

    A. As long as the patient is alert and able to answer most questions there is no need to determine if this is normal behavior.

    B. Ask the patient's roommate if this is normal behavior for the patient.

    C. Find a staff member who can explain the patient's underlying mental status to you.

    D. Because the patient already has dementia, there is no need to investigate this further.

_____   **9.** Anatomic changes that occur as a person ages predisposes geriatric patients to:

    A. airway problems.

    B. fungal infections.

    C. communicable diseases.

    D. mental status changes.

_____   **10.** Which of the following statements regarding geriatrics is FALSE?

    A. Chronic mental status impairment is a normal process of aging.

    B. Multiple disease processes and complaints can make assessment complicated.

    C. Communication may be more complicated with an older adult.

    D. You should find and account for all patient medications.

_____   **11.** The last meal is particularly important in a patient with:

    A. hypertension.

    B. myocardial infarction.

    C. COPD.

    D. diabetes.

_____   **12.** The heart rate should be in the normal adult rage for a geriatric patient but can be altered by medications such as:

    A. insulin.

    B. beta-blockers.

    C. alpha-blockers.

    D. aspirin.

_____ **13.** Which of the following is NOT considered a typical intervention when treating an elderly patient?

  A. Oxygenation

  B. Administration of glucose

  C. Immobilization

  D. Psychological support

_____ **14.** The "E" of the GEMS diamond stands for:

  A. environmental assessment.

  B. events leading to the incident.

  C. extrication of the patient.

  D. emergency assessment.

_____ **15.** The alveoli in an older patient's lung tissue can become enlarged and less elastic, making it:

  A. easier to inhale air.

  B. harder to inhale air.

  C. easier to exhale air.

  D. harder to exhale air.

_____ **16.** _____ is the leading cause of death from infection in Americans older than age 65 years.

  A. Chronic bronchitis

  B. Pneumonia

  C. Endocarditis

  D. Influenza

_____ **17.** A patient with leg pain who complains of sudden shortness of breath, tachycardia, fever, chest pain, and a feeling of impending doom is likely experiencing a(n):

  A. pulmonary embolism.

  B. pneumonia.

  C. myocardial infarction.

  D. aortic aneurysm.

_____ **18.** Geriatric patients are at risk for _____, an accumulation of fatty material in the arteries.

  A. vasculitis

  B. arteriosclerosis

  C. atherosclerosis

  D. varicose veins

_____ **19.** A drop in blood pressure with a change in position is referred to as:

  A. orthostatic hypotension.

  B. metastatic hypotension.

  C. malignant hypotension.

  D. psychogenic hypotension.

_____ **20.** Which of the following is NOT considered a risk factor for geriatric patients to develop heart failure?

  A. Hypertension

  B. Coronary artery disease

  C. Atrial fibrillation

  D. Palpitations

_____ **21.** All of the following are true of delirium EXCEPT:

    A. it may have metabolic causes.

    B. the patient may be hypoglycemic.

    C. it develops slowly over a period of years.

    D. the memory remains mostly intact.

_____ **22.** An 82-year-old woman has slurred speech, weakness on the left side of her body, visual disturbances, and a headache. This patient is likely to be suffering from a:

    A. myocardial infarction.

    B. stroke.

    C. diabetic emergency.

    D. spinal cord injury.

_____ **23.** The brain decreases in terms of _____ and volume as a person ages.

    A. length

    B. width

    C. size

    D. weight

_____ **24.** Older people develop an inability to differentiate colors and have:

    A. increased sensitivity to light.

    B. decreased eye movement.

    C. decreased daytime vision.

    D. decreased night vision.

_____ **25.** _____ and long-term exposure to loud noises are the main factors that contribute to hearing loss.

    A. Heredity

    B. Injury

    C. Infection

    D. Medications

_____ **26.** Which of the following statements regarding dementia is FALSE?

    A. Patients may have anxiety about going to the hospital.

    B. Some patients are confused and angry.

    C. There may be a decreased ability to communicate.

    D. Due to memory loss, they are able to adapt easily to changes in their daily routine.

_____ **27.** Which of the following statements about changes to the gastrointestinal system is correct?

    A. Gastric secretions are reduced as a person ages.

    B. Dental loss is not a normal result of the aging process.

    C. Blood flow to the liver is increased as a person ages.

    D. Gastric motility increases and results in an increase in gastric emptying.

_____ **28.** All of the following are common specific gastrointestinal problems in the elderly EXCEPT:

    A. ulcerative colitis.

    B. diverticulitis.

    C. peptic ulcer disease.

    D. gallbladder disease.

_____ **29.** A patient with an abdominal aortic aneurysm most commonly complains of abdominal pain that radiates to the:

    A. chest.

    B. lower legs.

    C. back.

    D. shoulders.

_____ **30.** Changes to the kidney and genitourinary tract in elderly patients can cause all of the following EXCEPT:

    A. urinary incontinence.

    B. urinary retention.

    C. an increased response to sodium deficiency.

    D. enlargement of the prostate.

_____ **31.** A patient experiencing weight gain, fatigue, cold intolerance, drier skin and hair, and a slower heart rate could be suffering from:

    A. hyperglycemia.

    B. ketosis.

    C. hyperthyroidism.

    D. hypothyroidism.

_____ **32.** Which of the following is NOT a factor that affects the development of osteoporosis?

    A. Hypertension

    B. Smoking

    C. Level of activity

    D. Alcohol consumption

_____ **33.** _____ is a progressive disease of the joints that destroys cartilage and leads to joint spurs and stiffness.

    A. Osteoporosis

    B. Osteosarcoma

    C. Osteoarthritis

    D. Osteoplegia

_____ **34.** All of the following are considered to be reasons for medication noncompliance EXCEPT:

    A. financial challenges.

    B. patient disagrees with the diagnosis.

    C. impaired cognitive ability.

    D. inability to open pill bottles.

_____ **35.** Which of the following statements regarding depression is true?

    A. Treatment typically involves medication, because counseling typically does not work.

    B. Older adults in skilled nursing facilities are less likely to develop depression.

    C. It generally does not interfere with ability to function in the elderly.

    D. It is diagnosed three times more commonly in women than in men.

_____ **36.** Elderly pedestrians struck by a vehicle commonly suffer injuries to the:

    A. chest.

    B. abdomen.

    C. extremities.

    D. back.

_____ **37.** All of the following are common predisposing events that can lead to suicide in the elderly EXCEPT:

    A. death of a loved one.

    B. hallucinations.

    C. alcohol abuse.

    D. physical illness.

_____ **38.** Elderly people are more likely to experience burns because of:

    A. altered mental status.

    B. inattention.

    C. compromised neurologic status.

    D. all of the above.

_____ **39.** Signs and symptoms of possible abuse include all of the following EXCEPT:

    A. chronic pain with no medical explanation.

    B. no history of repeated visits to the emergency department or clinic.

    C. depression or lack of energy.

    D. self-destructive behavior.

_____ **40.** Because the brain tissue shrinks with age, older patients are more likely to sustain:

    A. basilar skull fractures.

    B. depressed skull fractures.

    C. open head injuries.

    D. closed head injuries.

_____ **41.** The most important piece of information to establish immediately when responding to a skilled nursing facility is determining:

    A. when someone last saw the patient.

    B. which nurse is overseeing patient care.

    C. what is wrong with the patient.

    D. how often this patient is transported to the hospital.

_____ **42.** MRSA is commonly found on which of the following?

    A. Decubitus ulcers

    B. Feeding tubes

    C. Indwelling catheters

    D. All of the above

_____ **43.** In most states, for a DNR to be considered valid it must have been signed within the last:

    A. 12 months.

    B. 18 months.

    C. 24 months.

    D. DNRs are valid regardless of the timeframe.

_____ **44.** Burns in elderly abuse typically result from which of the following?

    A. Cigarettes

    B. Matches

    C. Hot liquids

    D. All of the above

_____ **45.** Clues that might indicate elderly abuse would include all of the following EXCEPT:

    A. bruises on the buttocks and lower back.

    B. weight gain.

    C. wounds in various stages of healing.

    D. lack of hygiene.

True/False

If you believe the statement to be more true than false, write the letter "T" in the space provided. If you believe the statement to be more false than true, write the letter "F."

_____ **1.** Some elderly people may not take all of their medications to save money.

_____ **2.** Your first words to the patient and the attitude behind them can gain or lose a patient's trust.

_____ **3.** Hip fractures are less likely to occur when the patient has osteoporosis.

_____ **4.** Chest pain, shortness of breath, and an altered mental status should always be considered serious.

_____ **5.** More responsive nerve stimulation may lower the heart rate and the strength of heart contractions.

_____ **6.** Multiple disease processes and multiple and/or vague complaints can make assessment complicated.

_____ **7.** The "S" in the GEMS diamond stands for social assessment.

_____ **8.** Loss of mechanisms to protect the upper airway include increased cough and gag reflexes.

_____ **9.** Changes in the cardiovascular performance of a geriatric patient are the direct consequence of aging.

_____ **10.** Respiratory rates in an elderly patient with chest pain tend to be lower.

_____ **11.** The treatment goal of a stroke is to salvage as much brain tissue as possible.

_____ **12.** Glaucoma, macular degeneration, and retinal detachment can all cause vision problems in the geriatric patient.

_____ **13.** Taste can be diminished in an older patient due to a decrease in the number of taste buds.

_____ **14.** Neuropathy is a dysfunction of the central nervous system.

_____ **15.** Irritation of the lining of the stomach or ulcers can cause forceful vomiting that tears the esophagus.

_____ **16.** Inflammation of the gallbladder will present with left upper quadrant pain and fever.

_____ **17.** The blood glucose level will be greater than 500 mg/dL in DKA.

_____ **18.** Pneumonia and urinary tract infections are common in patients who are bedridden.

_____ **19.** Decreased liver function makes it easier for the liver to detoxify the blood.

_____ **20.** Most elderly suicides occur in people who have recently been diagnosed with depression.

_____ **21.** There is a lower mortality from penetrating trauma in older adults.

_____ **22.** Many elderly patients take blood-thinning medications that can help correct internal bleeding.

_____ **23.** Broken bones are common in the geriatric population and should be splinted in a manner appropriate to the injury.

_____ **24.** Most indoor hypothermia deaths involve geriatric patients.

_____ **25.** A "health care power of attorney" is an advance directive that is exercised by a person who has been authorized by the patient to make medical decisions for the patient.

Fill-in-the-Blank

Read each item carefully and then complete the statement by filling in the missing words.

1. Using the patient's _____ shows respect and helps the patient to focus on your questions.

2. Hip fractures are more likely to occur when bones are weakened by _____ or infection.

3. _____ is a useful therapy for many geriatric problems, including vague complaints of weakness or dizziness.

4. _____ is an inflammation/infection of the lung from bacterial, viral, or fungal causes.

5. The core body temperature should be assessed to determine the presence of a(n) _____.

6. _____ refers to stiffening of the blood vessel wall.

7. Severe blood loss can occur when a(n) _____ bursts.

8. With _____ heart failure, fluid backs up into the lungs.

9. _____ is the gradual hearing loss that occurs as we age.

10. An older person may have a decreased sense of _____ and _____ perception from the loss of end nerve fibers.

11. _____ is a condition in which small pouches protrude from the colon.

12. _____ _____ form when a patient is lying or sitting in the same position for a long time.

13. As you get older, the brain shrinks, leading to higher risk of _____ _____ following head trauma.

14. _____ _____ may help determine if a loss of consciousness occurred before an accident.

15. Dentures may cause a(n) _____ _____ in a trauma patient.

16. When assessing the abdomen, remember that elderly patients have a _____ _____ _____ and may not show signs of rigidity in abdominal trauma.

17. Patients with _____ will require padding in order to keep the patient supine.

18. In addition to hip fractures, elderly people with osteoporosis are at risk for _____ fractures.

19. _____ _____ are facilities that serve patients who need 24-hour care; they are sometimes a step down from a hospital.

20. _____ _____ are specific legal papers that direct relatives and caregivers about what kinds of medical treatment may by given to patients who cannot speak for themselves.

Fill-in-the-Table

Fill in the missing parts of the table.

Categories of Elder Abuse	
Physical	• _____ • _____ • _____ • _____ • _____
Psychological	• _____ • _____ • _____ • _____
Financial	• _____ • _____

Crossword Puzzle

The following crossword puzzle is an activity provided to reinforce correct spelling and understanding of medical terminology associated with emergency care and the EMT. Use the clues in the column to complete the puzzle.

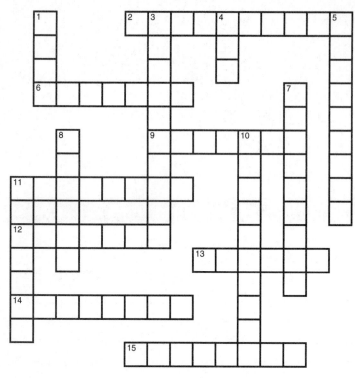

Across

2. The assessment and treatment of disease in someone who is 65 years or older

6. Fluid in the abdomen

9. _____ directives are written documentation that specify medical treatment for a competent patient should the patient become unable to make decisions.

11. A sudden change in mental status marked by the inability to focus, think logically, and maintain attention

12. A fainting spell or transient loss of consciousness, often caused by an interruption of blood flow to the brain

13. _____ ulcer disease is an abrasion of the stomach or small intestine.

14. A pulmonary _____ is a condition that causes a sudden blockage of the pulmonary artery by a venous clot.

15. An enlargement of a part of an artery, resulting from weakening of the arterial wall

Down

1. A bacterium that causes infections in different parts of the body and is often resistant to commonly used antibiotics

3. Any action on the part of an older person's family member, caregiver, or other associated person that takes advantage of the older person

4. A condition in which the walls of the aorta in the abdomen weaken and blood leaks into the layers of the vessel, causing it to bulge.

5. Respiratory _____ virus is highly contagious and causes an infection of the upper and lower respiratory system.

7. An inflammation/infection of the lung from a bacterial, viral, or fungal cause

8. Black, tarry stools

10. A group of conditions in which the nerves leaving the spinal cord are damaged, resulting in distortion of signals to or from the brain

11. Shortness of breath or difficulty breathing

Critical Thinking

Short Answer

Complete this section with short written answers using the space provided.

1. List the six most common conditions found in the elderly patient.

_____

_____

2. What are the types of nerves affected in neuropathy, and what are the associated symptoms?

_____

_____

3. What are the differences between hyperosmolar hyperglycemic nonketotic coma (HHND) and diabetic ketoacidosis (DKA)?

_____

_____

4. List at least five informational items that may be important in assessing possible elder abuse.

_____

_____

5. Briefly describe the three possible causes of syncope in the elderly patient.

_____

_____

Ambulance Calls

The following case scenarios provide an opportunity to explore the concerns associated with patient management and to enhance critical-thinking skills. Read each scenario and answer each question to the best of your ability.

1. It is 0300, and you are dispatched to a long-term care facility for a geriatric woman with an "unknown emergency." You arrive to find no staff around, but you hear someone crying for help. You follow the voice and find an older woman lying on the floor holding her right hip. Her bed is made and the side rails are up. When a staff member finally appears, you ask how long she's been lying there. They respond, "We don't know. How are we supposed to know that? We don't have enough help around here."

   How would you best manage this patient?

   _____

   _____

   _____

2. You are dispatched to the home of a 65-year-old woman who is complaining of severe back pain. She tells you that she tried to pick up the lawnmower when she "heard a pop and felt a crack in her back." She is experiencing intense pain in her lower back and feels some numbness in her legs.

   How would you best manage this patient?

   _____

   _____

   _____

3. You are dispatched to a private residence for a woman who has fallen. She tells you that she tripped over her granddaughter's toys and fell onto the hardwood floor. She tried to get up several times but couldn't. She denies any head, neck, or back pain, or loss of consciousness. Her only complaint is pain in her right hip.

   How would you best manage this patient?

   _____

   _____

   _____

4. It is early evening, and you are dispatched to the parking lot of a popular shopping mall. Over the past several hours, local weather conditions have consisted of a combination of freezing rain and snow, making for very icy road conditions. Your patient is an older woman who has fallen and now complains of back pain and shortness of breath. She has severe kyphosis and will not tolerate traditional methods of spinal immobilization.

   How would you best manage this patient?

   _____

   _____

   _____

Fill-in-the-Patient Care Report

Read the incident scenario and then complete the following patient care report (PCR).

You are dispatched at 0843 to an unknown medical emergency at 222 Orchid Lane. You note the incident number as 011727 and immediately mark your unit as responding with the dispatcher. The dispatcher informs you that the fire department was also dispatched to assist you.

You arrive 6 minutes later to find an older woman who greets you at the front door. She tells you her 78-year-old husband is lying on the bathroom floor, and he's too heavy for her to lift. As you enter the small bathroom, you notice a large man on the floor with a laceration and hematoma on his forehead.

"I was on the toilet and must have fallen, but I don't remember exactly what happened," the patient tells you.

You immediately maintain cervical spine stabilization as the fire department personnel arrive on scene. Your partner grabs the necessary immobilization equipment as you interview the patient.

The patient continues to tell you that he does not remember what happened, but states that his head hurts.

"I heard a loud 'thud' in the bathroom and came in to find him on the floor," the wife states. "He was awake when I came in, but I saw the blood and called 9-1-1."

You ask, "Are you having any other pain?"

"No, I feel OK other than my head," says the patient. The patient rates his pain as a 4 out of 10 and denies radiation. The patient also denies neck pain.

You inquire about dizziness, sweating, chest pain, shortness of breath, nausea, or vomiting, all of which the patient denies.

Your partner arrives along with the fire personnel with the immobilization equipment. While they immobilize the patient, you apply 15 L/min of oxygen via nonrebreathing mask at 0851 and place a bandage on the patient's forehead to control the bleeding.

After the patient is immobilized, you complete a rapid head-to-toe scan of the patient and find no other deformities/abnormalities other than a hematoma and a 3-cm (1.2″) laceration noted to the patient's right forehead with minor bleeding, now controlled.

Your partner obtains vital signs 2 minutes after the patient is immobilized and finds the following: pulse, 86 beats/min; respirations, 20 breaths/min; blood pressure, 110/68 mm Hg; pulse oximetry, 98%.

The patient tells you that he is allergic to aspirin and that he takes metoprolol, Lisinopril, Actos, metformin, Zocor, Celebrex, allopurinol, Lasix, K-dur, Plavix, and a multivitamin. You're able to decipher much of the history from the medications, but ask the patient to confirm. The patient tells you that he had a heart attack several years ago in which a stent was placed; he has congestive heart failure, hypertension, diabetes, arthritis, gout, and high cholesterol.

The fire personnel package the patient onto the litter and take the patient to the unit with your partner. The patient tells you that he wants to go to Mercy Hospital down the road. Because this is the closest trauma facility, you are happy to accommodate the patient's wishes.

You depart the scene at 0902 and reassess vital signs and physical exam. The vital signs are as follows: pulse, 84 beats/min; respirations, 18 breaths/min; blood pressure, 116/76 mm Hg; pulse oximetry, 100%. The patient's status remains stable through the transport, although he continues to complain about his head pain.

You arrive at Mercy Hospital 6 minutes later. The patient states that his head still hurts, but that he otherwise feels fine. He states that his pain is still 4/10.

You bring the patient to room 4 and give your report to the nurse. You state that it appears the patient had a syncopal episode and bumped his head; however, he's been stable throughout your care.

You replace the supplies while your partner cleans the unit. The unit is back in service at 0915.

Fill-in-the-Patient Care Report

EMS Patient Care Report (PCR)					
Date:	Incident No.:		Nature of Call:		Location:
Dispatched:	En Route:	At Scene:	Transport:	At Hospital:	In Service:
Patient Information					
Age: Sex: Weight (in kg [lb]):			Allergies: Medications: Past Medical History: Chief Complaint:		
Vital Signs					
Time:	BP:		Pulse:	Respirations:	Sao_2:
Time:	BP:		Pulse:	Respirations:	Sao_2:
Time:	BP:		Pulse:	Respirations:	Sao_2:
EMS Treatment (circle all that apply)					
Oxygen @ ___ L/min via (circle one): NC NRM Bag-Mask Device		Assisted Ventilation		Airway Adjunct	CPR
Defibrillation	Bleeding Control		Bandaging	Splinting	Other Shock Treatment
Narrative					

Patients With Special Challenges

General Knowledge

Matching

Match each of the items in the left column to the appropriate definition in the right column.

_____ **1.** Cerebral palsy

_____ **2.** Colostomy

_____ **3.** Developmental disability

_____ **4.** Down syndrome

_____ **5.** Ileostomy

_____ **6.** Obesity

_____ **7.** Sensorineural deafness

_____ **8.** Shunts

_____ **9.** Spina bifida

_____ **10.** Tracheostomy tube

A. A surgical opening between the small intestine and the outside of the body

B. A portion of the spinal cord that protrudes outside of the vertebrae

C. A group of disorders characterized by poorly controlled body movement

D. An excessive amount of body fat

E. A plastic tube placed in a stoma

F. Insufficient development of the brain

G. Damage to the inner ear resulting in a permanent lack of hearing

H. A surgical opening between the colon and the outside of the body

I. Tubes that drain fluid from the brain or other parts of the body

J. Round head with a flat occiput and slanted, wide-set eyes

Multiple Choice

Read each item carefully and then select the best response.

_____ **1.** Which of the following is NOT considered a potential cause of a developmental disability?

    A. Genetic factors

    B. Complications at birth

    C. Folic acid deficiency

    D. Malnutrition

_____ **2.** Which of the following statements is FALSE regarding patients with autism?

    A. They fail to use or understand nonverbal communication.

    B. They will talk with normal tone and speech patterns.

    C. They may have extreme difficulty with complex tasks that require many steps.

    D. They have difficulty making eye-to-eye contact.

_____ **3.** All of the following are associated with Down syndrome EXCEPT:

    A. a small face.

    B. short, wide hands.

    C. a protruding tongue.

    D. narrow-set eyes.

_____ **4.** Down syndrome patients are at an increased risk for medical complications. Which of the following is NOT one of those potential complications?

    A. Respiratory complications

    B. Cardiovascular complications

    C. Gastrointestinal complications

    D. Endocrine complications

_____ **5.** Which of the following is true regarding airway management of patients with Down syndrome?

    A. Patients often have large tongues.

    B. Patients have large oral and nasal cavities.

    C. Mask ventilation is relatively easy to achieve.

    D. Use the head tilt–chin lift maneuver to open the airway.

_____ **6.** When caring for a patient with a previous head injury, you should:

    A. speak in a loud, commanding tone.

    B. expect the patient to be able to walk.

    C. watch the patient for signs of anxiety.

    D. never consider restraining the patient.

_____ **7.** Which of the following is NOT a possible cause of visual impairment?

    A. Disease

    B. Injury

    C. Congenital defect

    D. Regeneration of the eyeball, optic nerve, or nerve pathway

_____ **8.** When caring for a patient with a visual impairment, which of the following is NOT appropriate?

    A. Identify noises

    B. Always transport the patient's service dog

    C. Describe the situation and surroundings

    D. Tell the patient what is happening

_____ **9.** Conductive hearing loss can be caused by:

    A. advanced age.

    B. damage to the inner ear.

    C. nerve damage.

    D. a perforated eardrum.

_____ **10.** Which of the following is NOT considered a clue that your patient might be hearing impaired?

    A. Slurred speech

    B. Presence of hearing aids

    C. Poor pronunciation of words

    D. Failure to respond to your questions

_____ **11.** All of the following are possible causes of cerebral palsy EXCEPT:

    A. maternal preeclampsia.

    B. damage to the developing fetal brain in utero.

    C. traumatic brain injury at birth.

    D. postpartum infection.

_____ **12.** Cerebral palsy is associated with all of the following conditions EXCEPT:

    A. epilepsy.

    B. cardiovascular complications.

    C. difficulty communicating.

    D. mental retardation.

_____ **13.** Which of the following statements is FALSE regarding the care of a patient with cerebral palsy?

    A. Do not assume these patients are mentally disabled.

    B. Limbs are often underdeveloped and are prone to injury.

    C. Walkers or wheelchairs should not be taken in the ambulance.

    D. Be prepared to care for a seizure if one occurs.

_____ **14.** Patients with spina bifida will have:

    A. partial or full paralysis of the lower extremities.

    B. multiple cardiovascular problems.

    C. daily episodes of neck pain.

    D. a tendency to resist sitting.

_____ **15.** When suctioning a tracheostomy tube, be sure not to suction for longer than:

    A. 5 seconds.

    B. 10 seconds.

    C. 15 seconds.

    D. 20 seconds.

_____ **16.** If a patient's mechanical ventilator malfunctions, you should remove the patient from the ventilator and:

    A. place the patient on a nasal cannula.

    B. place the patient on a nonrebreathing mask.

    C. begin ventilations with a bag-mask device.

    D. contact medical control.

_____ **17.** An apnea monitor is indicated in all of the following situations EXCEPT:

    A. premature birth.

    B. severe gastroesophageal reflux.

    C. family history of SIDS.

    D. asthma.

_____ **18.** Which of the following is NOT a risk factor associated with the implantation of a left ventricular assist device?

    A. Excessive bleeding

    B. Acute heart failure

    C. Renal failure

    D. Stroke

_____ **19.** Central venous catheters are located in all of the following areas EXCEPT:

    A. the upper arm.

    B. the lower leg.

    C. the chest.

    D. the clavicle.

_____ **20.** Patients with gastric tubes who have difficulty breathing should be transported sitting or lying on the:

    A. left side, with the head elevated 30°.

    B. right side, with the head elevated 30°.

    C. right side, with the head elevated 45°.

    D. left side, with the head elevated 45°.

_____ **21.** A ventricular atrium shunt drains excess fluid from the ventricles of the brain into the:

    A. right atrium of the heart.

    B. left atrium of the heart.

    C. right ventricle of the heart.

    D. left ventricle of the heart.

_____ **22.** Services offered by home care agencies include all of the following EXCEPT:

    A. providing personal hygiene.

    B. wound care.

    C. taking the patient to restaurants.

    D. yard maintenance.

_____ **23.** All of the following are diseases or conditions that are associated with patients receiving hospice EXCEPT:

    A. AIDS.

    B. end-stage Alzheimer disease.

    C. cancer.

    D. pneumonia.

_____ **24.** Which of the following is NOT a disease prevention strategy that people living in poverty are lacking?

    A. Vaccinations

    B. Nutrition

    C. Exercise

    D. Dental care

_____ **25.** The term *obese* is used when someone is _____ over his or her ideal body weight.

    A. 10% to 20%

    B. 20% to 30%

    C. 30% to 40%

    D. 40% to 50%

True/False

If you believe the statement to be more true than false, write the letter "T" in the space provided. If you believe the statement to be more false than true, write the letter "F."

_____ **1.** It is important to make sure you are at eye level when communicating with patients.

_____ **2.** Visually impaired patients can be guided, pulled, or pushed to help them move.

_____ **3.** Some patients with paralysis will have normal sensation.

_____ **4.** In severe or morbid obesity, the person is 11 to 34 kg (25 to 75 lb) over his or her ideal weight.

_____ **5.** Tracheostomy tubes are prone to obstruction from mucus plugs and saliva.

_____ **6.** You can estimate the size of a suction catheter for a tracheostomy tube by doubling the inner diameter of the tracheostomy tube.

_____ **7.** Patients with tracheostomies breathe through their mouth and nose.

_____ **8.** You should never place defibrillator paddles or pacing patches directly over an implanted defibrillation device.

_____ **9.** Patients who have a gastric tube in place may still be at increased risk of aspiration.

_____ **10.** Interaction with the caregiver of a child or adult with special needs will be an important part of the patient assessment process.

Fill-in-the-Blank

Read each item carefully and then complete the statement by filling in the missing word.

1. _____ is a pervasive developmental disorder characterized by impairment of social interaction.

2. You may allow a patient with a visual impairment to rest his or her hand on your _____, because this may help with balance and security while moving.

3. _____ _____ can be either external or internal, depending on the type of hearing damage.

4. The two most common forms of hearing loss are _____ deafness and _____ hearing loss.

5. _____ _____ is a term for a group of disorders characterized by poorly controlled body movement.

6. To reduce the occurrence of spina bifida, pregnant women are advised to take _____ _____.

7. A(n) _____ _____ _____ _____ is a special piece of medical equipment that takes over the function of either one or both heart ventricles.

8. _____ are tubes that extend from the brain to the abdomen to drain excess cerebrospinal fluid.

9. If you encounter a patient with a colostomy or ileostomy bag, assess for signs of _____ if the patient has been complaining of diarrhea or vomiting.

10. Comfort care, or _____ _____, improves the patient's quality of life before the patient dies.

Fill-in-the-Table

Complete the missing information to the right of the mnemonic.

DOPE Mnemonic	
D	
O	
P	
E	

Crossword Puzzle

The following crossword puzzle is an activity provided to reinforce correct spelling and understanding of medical terminology associated with emergency care and the EMT. Use the clues in the column to complete the puzzle.

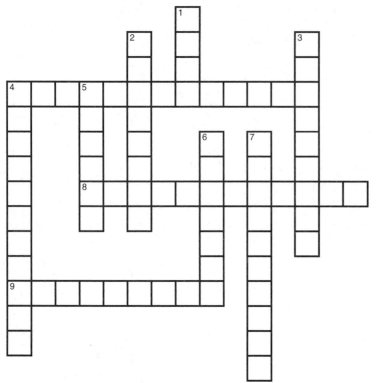

Across

4. _____ deafness is a permanent lack of hearing caused by a lesion or damage of the inner ear.

8. A(n) _____ tube is a plastic tube placed within the tracheostomy site.

9. A surgical procedure to create an opening between the small intestine and the surface of the body

Down

1. _____ syndrome is a genetic chromosomal defect that can occur during fetal development and that results in mental retardation.

2. _____ palsy is a term for a group of disorders characterized by poorly controlled body movement.

3. A surgical procedure to establish an opening between the colon and the surface of the body

4. A developmental defect in which a portion of the spinal cord or meninges may protrude outside of the vertebrae

5. Tubes that drain fluid from the brain to another part of the body outside of the brain

6. A condition in which a person has an excessive amount of body fat

7. Insufficient development of the brain, resulting in some level of dysfunction or impairment, is known as developmental _____.

Critical Thinking

Short Answer

Complete this section with short written answers using the space provided.

1. List at least four helpful hints for working with patients with hearing impairments.

_____

_____

2. Describe the various troubleshooting methods for a hearing aid malfunction.

_____

_____

3. List the four types of hearing aids.

_____

_____

4. List at least eight helpful tips to use when moving a morbidly obese patient.

_____

_____

5. List six questions you should ask when caring for a patient with an implanted pacemaker.

_____

_____

Ambulance Calls

The following case scenarios provide an opportunity to explore the concerns associated with patient management and to enhance critical-thinking skills. Read each scenario and answer each question to the best of your ability.

1. You respond to a nursing home for a 75-year-old man whose internal defibrillator continues to fire. When you arrive on scene, you find the patient being assisted by the nursing staff. The patient is pale with an altered mental status. You notice he "jumps" every few minutes.

How would you best manage this patient?

_____

_____

_____

2. You are dispatched to a residence for a 12-year-old girl having a seizure. When you arrive on scene you are met at the door by the patient's mother. The mother tells you her daughter has Down syndrome and is prone to seizures. She states that her daughter has had two "tonic-clonic seizures" today. When you walk into the room, you see the patient lying on the floor in what appears to be a postictal state. The patient is being attended by other family members.

How would you best manage this patient?

_____

_____

_____

Skills

Assessment Review

Answer the following questions pertaining to the assessment of the types of emergencies discussed in this chapter.

_____ 1. When treating a patient with autism, remember that the patient:

    A. will be able to describe his or her underlying condition to you.

    B. will speak in a clear, inflected voice.

    C. is not likely to maintain eye contact with you.

    D. will be able to follow most of your commands without difficulty.

_____ 2. What sign found at a scene might indicate that your patient is visually impaired?

    A. No carpet

    B. Animals

    C. No stairs

    D. A cane

_____ 3. What can be done for a patient with a tracheostomy who needs oxygen when you do not have a proper tracheostomy mask?

    A. Immediately assist ventilations with a bag-mask device.

    B. Place a nasal cannula on the patient.

    C. Place a face mask over the patient's mouth.

    D. Place a face mask over the stoma.

_____ 4. Which of the following is NOT a sign of infection at a colostomy site?

    A. Tenderness

    B. Bleeding

    C. Warm skin

    D. Redness

Lifting and Moving Patients

General Knowledge

Matching

Match each of the items in the left column to the appropriate definition in the right column.

_____ **1.** Extremity lift

_____ **2.** Flexible stretcher

_____ **3.** Stair chair

_____ **4.** Basket stretcher

_____ **5.** Scoop stretcher

_____ **6.** Backboard

_____ **7.** Direct ground lift

_____ **8.** Portable stretcher

_____ **9.** Wheeled ambulance stretcher

_____ **10.** Bariatrics

A. Separates into two or four pieces

B. Tubular framed stretcher with rigid fabric stretched across it

C. Used for patients who are supine or sitting without an extremity or spinal injury

D. Specifically designed stretcher that can be rolled along the ground

E. Commonly used in technical and water rescues; Stokes litter

F. Used for patients who are found lying supine with no suspected spinal injury

G. Concerned with management of obesity

H. Used to carry patients up and down stairs

I. Spine board or longboard

J. Can be folded or rolled up

Multiple Choice

Read each item carefully and then select the one best response.

_____ **1.** _____ safety depends on the use of proper lifting techniques and maintaining a proper hold when lifting or carrying a patient.

    A. Your

    B. Your team's

    C. The patient's

    D. All of the above

_____ **2.** You should perform an urgent move in all of the following situations EXCEPT:

    A. if a patient has an altered level of consciousness.

    B. if the patient is complaining of neck pain.

    C. in extreme weather conditions.

    D. if a patient has inadequate ventilation or shock.

_____ **3.** You may injure your back if you lift:

    A. with your back curved.

    B. with your back straight, but bent significantly forward at the hips.

    C. with the shoulder girdle anterior to the pelvis.

    D. all of the above.

_____ **4.** When lifting, you should:

    A. spread your legs past shoulder width.

    B. lift a patient while reaching far in front of your torso.

    C. keep the weight that you are lifting as close to your body as possible.

    D. use your back muscles by bending at the waist.

_____ **5.** Which of the follow statements is FALSE regarding proper lifting?

   A. Avoid twisting.

   B. Bend at the waist.

   C. Keep the weight close to your body.

   D. Bend at the knees.

_____ **6.** In lifting with the palm down, the weight is supported by the _____ rather than the palm.

   A. fingers

   B. forearm

   C. lower back

   D. wrist

_____ **7.** When you must carry a patient up or down a flight of stairs or other significant incline, use a _____ if possible.

   A. backboard

   B. stair chair

   C. stretcher

   D. short spine board

_____ **8.** Because of the weight distribution on backboards and stretchers, the stronger EMTs should be at the:

   A. head.

   B. foot.

   C. side.

   D. front corner.

_____ **9.** A backboard is a device that provides support to patients who you suspect have:

   A. hip injuries.

   B. pelvic injuries.

   C. spinal injuries.

   D. all of the above.

_____ **10.** Before any lifting is initiated, the team leader should do all of the following EXCEPT:

   A. give a command of execution.

   B. indicate where each team member is to be located.

   C. rapidly describe the sequence of steps that will be performed.

   D. give a brief overview of the stages.

_____ **11.** Special _____ are usually required to move any patient who weighs more than 350 pounds (159 kg) to an ambulance.

   A. techniques

   B. equipment

   C. resources

   D. all of the above

_____ **12.** Which of the follow statements is FALSE regarding the use of a stair chair?

   A. Keep your back in a locked-in position.

   B. Lean back to help distribute the weight.

   C. Keep the patient's weight and your arms as close to your body as possible.

   D. Flex at the hips, not at the waist.

_____ **13.** When you use a body drag to move a patient:

   A. your back should always be locked and straight.

   B. you should encourage twisting so that the vertebrae can flex during the move.

   C. consider hyperextending to gain more leverage.

   D. drag the patient by the ankles.

_____ **14.** When pulling a patient, you should do all of the following EXCEPT:

    A. extend your arms no more than about 15″ to 20″ (38 to 50 cm).

    B. reposition your feet so that the force of pull will be balanced equally.

    C. when you can pull no farther, lean forward another 15″ to 20″ (38 to 50 cm).

    D. pull the patient by slowly flexing your arms.

_____ **15.** When log rolling a patient, you should do all of the following EXCEPT:

    A. kneel as close to the patient's side as possible.

    B. lean solely from the hips.

    C. reach as far as possible to maintain stability.

    D. use your shoulder muscles to help with the roll.

_____ **16.** If the weight you are pushing is lower than your waist, you should push from:

    A. the waist.

    B. a kneeling position.

    C. the shoulder.

    D. a squatting position.

_____ **17.** If you are alone and must remove an unconscious patient from a car, you should first move the patient's:

    A. legs.

    B. head.

    C. torso.

    D. pelvis.

_____ **18.** Situations in which you should use an emergency move include all of the following EXCEPT:

    A. when fire, explosives, or hazardous materials are present.

    B. when the patient feels like he or she might pass out.

    C. when you are unable to gain access to others in a vehicle who need lifesaving care.

    D. when you are unable to protect the patient from other hazards.

_____ **19.** You can move a patient on his or her back along the floor or ground by using all of the following methods EXCEPT:

    A. pulling on the patient's clothing in the neck and shoulder area.

    B. placing the patient on a blanket, coat, or other item that can be pulled.

    C. pulling the patient by the legs if they are the most accessible part.

    D. placing your arms under the patient's shoulders and through the armpits, and while grasping the patient's arms, dragging the patient backward.

_____ **20.** The _____ is both the mechanical weight-bearing base of the spinal column and the fused central posterior section of the pelvic girdle.

    A. lumbar spine

    B. sacrum

    C. coccyx

    D. ileum

_____ **21.** Which of the following is NOT an indication for use of the rapid extrication technique?

    A. The patient is in severe pain.

    B. The patient's condition cannot be properly assessed before being removed from the car.

    C. The patient blocks access to another seriously injured patient.

    D. The vehicle or the scene is unsafe.

_____ **22.** To avoid the strain of unnecessary lifting and carrying, you should use _____ or assist an able patient to the stretcher whenever possible.

    A. the direct ground lift

    B. the extremity lift

    C. the draw sheet method

    D. a scoop stretcher

_____ **23.** You should use a rigid _____, often called a Stokes litter, to carry a patient across uneven terrain from a remote location that is inaccessible by ambulance or other vehicle.

    A. basket stretcher

    B. scoop stretcher

    C. molded backboard

    D. flotation device

_____ **24.** You should not attempt to lift a patient who weighs more than _____ without at least four rescuers.

    A. 220 lbs (100 kg)

    B. 230 lbs (104 kg)

    C. 240 lbs (109 kg)

    D. 250 lbs (113 kg)

_____ **25.** Which of the following is FALSE regarding the lifting and moving of geriatric patients?

    A. Many geriatric patients have great fear when being transported.

    B. Most patients will be able to lie supine on a backboard without problems.

    C. Geriatric patients tend to have brittle bones.

    D. Some patients may require you to use towels and blankets to assist with immobilization.

_____ **26.** Bariatrics is:

    A. the branch of medicine concerned with the elderly.

    B. the branch of medicine concerned with the obese.

    C. the branch of medicine concerned with infants.

    D. the method used to assess blood pressure.

Questions 27–30 are derived from the following scenario: You have been called to the scene of a high-speed motor vehicle collision involving two compact cars. The first vehicle was a roll-over, ejecting the driver. The second vehicle contained both a driver and a front-seat passenger who cannot be reached because the door is up against a building.

_____ **27.** What device will you use to put the roll-over victim onto the wheeled ambulance stretcher?

    A. Extremity lift

    B. Scoop stretcher

    C. Short backboard

    D. Backboard

_____ **28.** For the passenger in the second vehicle, you may need to perform a(n) _____ on the driver in order to reach the patient.

    A. extremity lift

    B. emergency move

    C. short backboard

    D. You should do nothing different; treat each patient the same.

_____ **29.** Which of the following is an advantage of the diamond carry?

    A. It uses an even number of people (less likely to drop).

    B. It can be done with one person, freeing up others for patient care.

    C. The patient can be slid along the ground.

    D. It provides the best means of spinal immobilization.

_____ **30.** You'll likely use the _____ to transfer the patient from your stretcher to the hospital bed.

    A. diamond carry

    B. scoop stretcher

    C. portable stretcher

    D. draw sheet method

True/False

If you believe the statement to be more true than false, write the letter "T" in the space provided. If you believe the statement to be more false than true, write the letter "F."

_____ 1. A portable stretcher is typically a lightweight folding device that does not have the undercarriage and wheels of a true ambulance stretcher.

_____ 2. The term "power lift" refers to a posture that is safe and helpful for EMTs when they are lifting.

_____ 3. If you find that lifting a patient is a strain, try to move the patient to the ambulance as quickly as possible to minimize the possibility of back injury.

_____ 4. The use of adjunct devices and equipment, such as sheets and blankets, may make the job of lifting and moving a patient more difficult.

_____ 5. One-person techniques for moving patients should be used only when immediate patient movement is necessary due to a life-threatening hazard and only one EMT is available.

_____ 6. A scoop stretcher may be used alone for a standard immobilization of a patient with a spinal injury.

_____ 7. When carrying a patient down stairs or on an incline, make sure the stretcher is carried with the head end first.

_____ 8. The rapid extrication technique is the preferred technique to use on all sitting patients with possible spinal injuries.

_____ 9. It is unprofessional for you to discuss and plan a lift at the scene in front of the patient.

_____ 10. Bariatrics is a new field of medicine that deals with the care of the obese.

_____ 11. A minimum of five personnel should be present when restraining a combative patient.

_____ 12. An isolette is used to transport neonatal patients.

_____ 13. The flexible stretcher is the most comfortable of all of the various lifting devices.

_____ 14. Pneumatic stretchers were developed to increase patient comfort on the road.

_____ 15. The most important feature of the bariatric stretcher is the increased weight-lifting capacity.

Fill-in-the-Blank

Read each item carefully and then complete the statement by filling in the missing words.

1. To avoid injury to you, the patient, or your partners, you will have to learn how to lift and carry the patient

   properly, using proper _____ _____ and a power grip.

2. The key rule of lifting is to always keep the back in a straight, _____ position and to lift

   without twisting.

3. The safest and most powerful way to lift, lifting by extending the properly placed flexed legs, is called a(n)

   _____ _____.

4. The arm and hand have their greatest lifting strength when facing _____ up.

5. Be sure to pick up and carry the backboard with your back in the _____ position.

6. You should not attempt to lift a patient who weighs more than _____ pounds with fewer than

   four rescuers, regardless of individual strength.

7. During a body drag where you and your partner are on each side of the patient, you will have to alter the usual pulling technique to prevent pulling _____ and producing adverse lateral leverage against your lower back.

8. When you are rolling the wheeled ambulance stretcher, your back should be _____, straight, and untwisted.

9. Be careful that you do not push or pull from a(n) _____ position.

10. Remember to always consider whether there is an option that will cause _____ _____ to you and the other EMTs.

11. The manual support and immobilization that you provide when using the rapid extrication technique produce a greater risk of _____ _____.

12. The _____ _____ _____ is used for patients with no suspected spinal injury who are found lying supine on the ground.

13. The _____ _____ may be especially helpful when the patient is in a very narrow space or when there is not enough room for the patient and a team of EMTs to stand side by side.

14. The mattress on a stretcher must be _____ _____ so that it does not absorb any type of potentially infectious material, including water, blood, or other body fluid.

15. A(n) _____ _____ may be used for patients who have been struck by a motor vehicle.

Crossword Puzzle

The following crossword puzzle is an activity provided to reinforce correct spelling and understanding of medical terminology associated with emergency care and the EMT. Use the clues in the column to complete the puzzle.

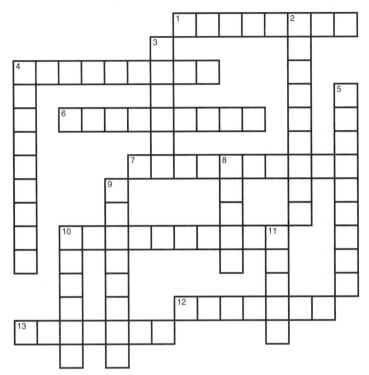

Across

1. A(n) _____ stretcher is a rigid carrying device when secured around a patient but can be folded or rolled when not in use.

4. A lifting technique in which the EMT's back is held upright, with legs bent, and the patient is lifted when the EMT straightens the legs to raise the upper body and arms

6. A(n) _____ lift is used for patients who are supine or in a sitting position with no suspected extremity or spinal injuries.

7. A lightweight folding device that is used to carry a conscious, seated patient up or down stairs

10. A branch of medicine concerned with the management (prevention or control) of obesity and allied diseases

12. The _____ carry technique involves one EMT at the head end of the stretcher or backboard, one at the foot end, and one at each side of the patient; all are able to face forward as they walk.

13. A(n) _____ ambulance stretcher is a specially designed stretcher to be rolled along the ground.

Down

2. A device used to provide support to a patient who is suspected of having a hip, pelvic, spinal, or lower extremity injury

3. The _____ ground lift is used for patients who are found lying supine on the ground with no suspected spinal injury.

4. A technique in which the litter or backboard is gripped by inserting each hand under the handle with the palm facing up and the thumb extended

5. In a(n) _____ move, the patient is dragged or pulled from a dangerous scene before assessment and care are provided.

8. A(n) _____ extrication technique is used to move a patient from a sitting position inside a vehicle to supine on a backboard in less than 1 minute.

9. A(n) _____ stretcher features a strong rectangular tubular metal frame with rigid fabric stretched across it.

10. A(n) _____ stretcher is commonly used in technical and water rescues.

11. A(n) _____ stretcher is designed to be split into two or four sections that can be fitted around a patient who is lying on the ground or other relatively flat surface.

Critical Thinking

Short Answer

Complete this section with short written answers using the space provided.

1. List the one-rescuer drags, carries, and lifts.

_____

_____

2. List the situations where the rapid extrication technique is used.

_____

_____

3. List three guidelines for loading the stretcher into the ambulance.

_____

_____

4. List five guidelines for carrying a patient on a stretcher.

_____

_____

5. Identify the key rule of lifting.

_____

_____

Ambulance Calls

The following case scenarios provide an opportunity to explore the concerns associated with patient management and to enhance critical-thinking skills. Read each scenario and answer each question to the best of your ability.

1. You are dispatched to a construction site for a 26-year-old man who fell into a ravine. He is approximately 35′ (11 m) down a rocky ledge. He is alert with an unstable pelvis and weak radial pulses. You have all the help you need from the construction crew and the volunteer fire department.

   How would you best manage this patient?

   _____

   _____

   _____

2. You are dispatched to an "unknown medical problem" at a local residence. You are met at the door by the wife of the patient who tells you that her husband is in the bathroom and is not acting right. You find the 350-pound (159-kg) patient lying in the bathroom, stuck between the toilet and the wall. He is not breathing and has no pulse.

   How would you best manage this patient?

   _____

   _____

   _____

3. You are dispatched to "difficulty breathing" at a nearby apartment complex. The patient's apartment is located on the top floor of a three-story building, is accessed through an exterior entryway, and no elevators are available. Your patient is morbidly obese and cannot walk.

   How would you best manage this patient?

   _____

   _____

   _____

Skills

Skill Drill

Skill Drill 35-1: Performing the Power Lift

Test your knowledge of this skill by filling in the correct words in the photo captions.

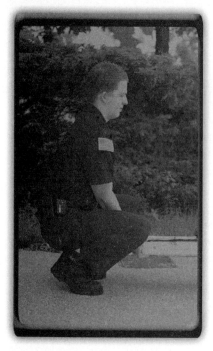

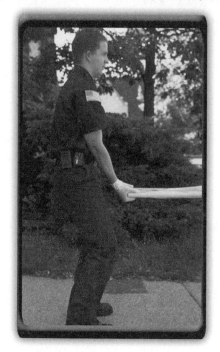

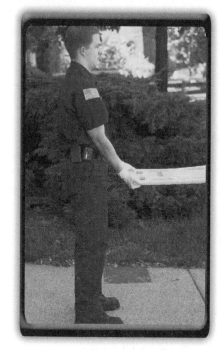

1. Lock your back into a(n) _____ curve. _____ and bend your legs. Grasp the backboard, palms up and just in front of you. _____ and _____ the weight between your arms.

2. Position your feet, _____ the object, and _____ weight.

3. Lift by _____ your legs, keeping your back locked in.

Skill Drill 35-2: Performing the Diamond Carry
Test your knowledge of this skill by placing the photos below in the correct order. Number the first step with a "1," the second step with a "2," etc.

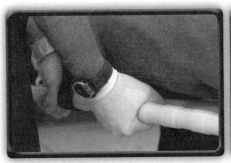 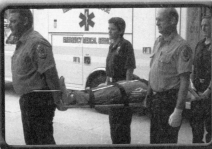 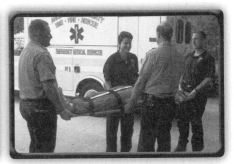

_____ The EMTs at the side each turn the head-end hand palm down and release the other hand.

_____ The EMTs at the side turn toward the foot end. The EMT at the foot turns to face forward.

_____ Position yourselves facing the patient.

Skill Drill 35-3: Performing the One-Handed Carrying Technique
Test your knowledge of this skill by filling in the correct words in the photo captions.

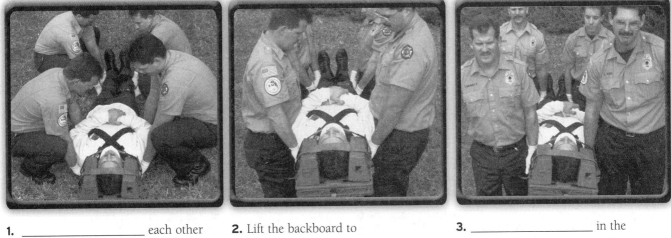

1. _____ each other and use both _____.

2. Lift the backboard to
_____
_____.

3. _____ in the direction you will walk, and _____ to using one hand.

Skill Drill 35-6: Performing the Rapid Extrication Technique
Test your knowledge of this skill by placing the photos below in the correct order. Number the first step with a "1," the second step with a "2," etc.

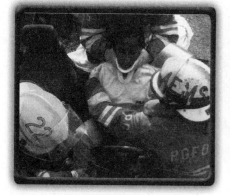

_____ The second EMT supports the torso. The third EMT frees the patient's legs from the pedals and moves the legs together, without moving the pelvis or spine.

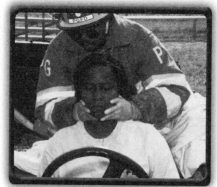

_____ The first EMT provides in-line manual support of the head and cervical spine.

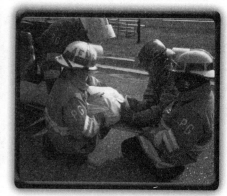

_____ The third EMT exits the vehicle, moves to the backboard opposite the second EMT, and they continue to slide the patient until the patient is fully on the board.

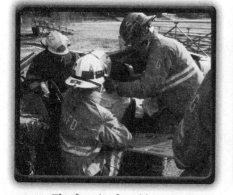

_____ The first (or fourth) EMT places the backboard on the seat against patient's buttocks.

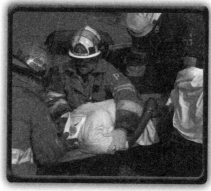

_____ The third EMT moves to an effective position for sliding the patient. The second and the third EMTs slide the patient along the backboard in coordinated, 8" to 12" (20- to 30-cm) moves until the patient's hips rest on the backboard.

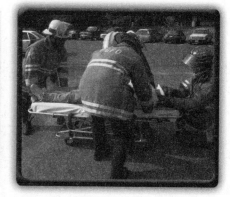

_____ The first (or fourth) EMT continues to stabilize the head and neck while the second EMT and the third EMT carry the patient away from the vehicle and onto the prepared stretcher.

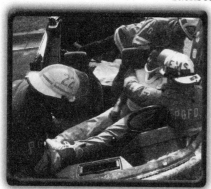

_____ The second EMT and the third EMT rotate the patient as a unit in several short, coordinated moves. The first EMT (relieved by the fourth EMT or a bystander as needed) supports the patient's head and neck during rotation (and later steps).

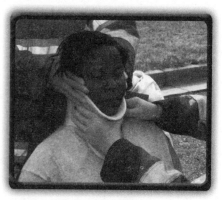

_____ The second EMT gives commands, applies a cervical collar, and performs the primary assessment.

Skill Drill 35-8: Extremity Lift
Test your knowledge of this skill by filling in the correct words in the photo captions.

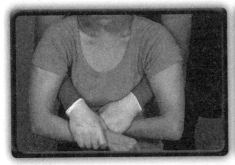 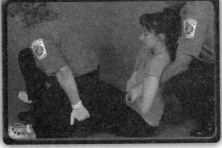 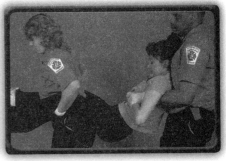

1. The patient's hands are _____ over the chest. The first EMT grasps patient's wrists or _____ and pulls the patient to a(n) _____ position.

2. The second EMT moves to a position between the patient's _____, facing in the _____ direction as the patient, and places his or her hands under the _____.

3. Both EMTs rise to a _____ position. On _____, both lift and begin to move.

Skill Drill 35-9: Direct Carry
Test your knowledge of this skill by filling in the correct words in the photo captions.

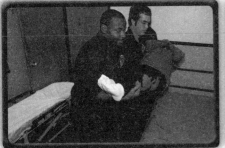 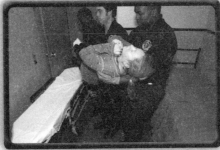 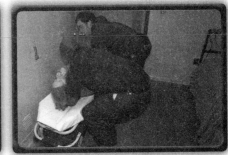

1. Place the stretcher _____ to the bed with the patient's _____ facing the head of the stretcher. Secure the _____ to prevent movement. Face the patient while standing between the _____ and the _____. Slide one arm under the patient's _____ and cup the patient's _____. Your partner should slide his or her hand under the patient's _____ and lift slightly. You should then slide your other arm under the patient's _____, and your partner should place both arms underneath the patient's _____ and _____.

2. Lift the patient in a smooth, _____ fashion. Slowly walk the patient around, and position him or her over the _____.

3. Slowly and _____ lower the patient onto the stretcher.

Skill Drill 35-10: Using a Scoop Stretcher
Test your knowledge of this skill by filling in the correct words in the photo captions.

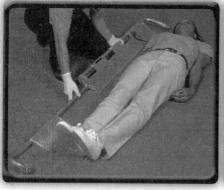

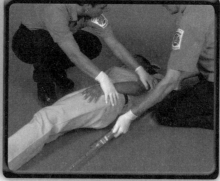

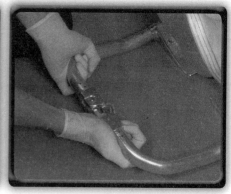

1. Adjust the _____ of the _____.

2. _____ the patient slightly and _____ the stretcher into place, one side at a time.

3. _____ the stretcher ends together, avoiding _____ the patient.

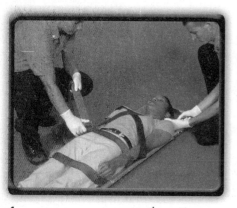

4. _____ the patient to the scoop stretcher, and _____ it to the stretcher.

Transport Operations

General Knowledge

Matching

Match each of the items in the left column to the appropriate definition in the right column.

_____ **1.** Medivac
_____ **2.** Emergency mode
_____ **3.** Spotter
_____ **4.** Sterilization
_____ **5.** Ambulance
_____ **6.** Cleaning
_____ **7.** Disinfection

A. The use of lights and sirens
B. The killing of pathogenic agents by direct application of chemicals
C. The process of removing dirt, dust, blood, or other visible contaminants
D. Medical evacuation of a patient by helicopter
E. A person who assists a driver in backing up an ambulance
F. Specialized vehicle for treating and transporting sick and injured patients
G. Removes microbial contamination

Multiple Choice

Read each item carefully and then select the one best response.

_____ **1.** Ambulances today are designed according to strict government regulations based on _____ standards.
  A. local
  B. state
  C. national
  D. individual

_____ **2.** Features of the modern ambulance include all of the following EXCEPT:
  A. a self-contained breathing apparatus.
  B. a patient compartment.
  C. two-way radio communication.
  D. a driver's compartment.

_____ **3.** The first thing you do each day when you arrive at work is to make sure all equipment and supplies are functioning and in their assigned place. This is the _____ phase of transport operations.
  A. preparation
  B. dispatch
  C. arrival at scene
  D. transport

_____ **4.** The type _____ ambulance is a standard van with a forward-control integral cab body.
  A. I
  B. II
  C. III
  D. IV

_____ **5.** Which of the following items are needed to care for life-threatening conditions?
  A. Equipment for airway management
  B. Equipment for artificial ventilation
  C. Oxygen-delivery devices
  D. All of the above

_____ **6.** Oropharyngeal airways can be used for:
  A. adults.
  B. children.
  C. infants.
  D. all of the above.

_____ **7.** When attached to oxygen supply with the oxygen reservoir in place, a bag-mask device is able to supply almost _____ oxygen.
  A. 100%
  B. 95%
  C. 90%
  D. 85%

_____ **8.** Oxygen masks, with and without nonrebreathing bags, should be transparent, disposable, and available in sizes for:
  A. adults.
  B. children.
  C. infants.
  D. all of the above.

_____ **9.** Basic wound care supplies include all of the following EXCEPT:
  A. sterile sheets.
  B. an OB kit.
  C. an assortment of adhesive bandages.
  D. large safety pins.

_____ **10.** Your supervisor approaches you and tells you he wants you to make up jump kits for each ambulance. He has told you that he will leave it up to you as to what goes into the kit. You would want to include everything that you might need within the first _____ minutes of arrival at the patient's side.
  A. 2
  B. 3
  C. 4
  D. 5

_____ **11.** Deceleration straps over the shoulders prevent the patient from continuing to move _____ in case the ambulance suddenly slows or stops.
  A. forward
  B. backward
  C. laterally
  D. down

_____ **12.** The ambulance inspection should include checks of:
  A. fuel level.
  B. brake fluid.
  C. wheels and tires.
  D. all of the above.

_____ **13.** You are hired at the local EMS service. During your orientation, you are given a tour of the station and the ambulances you will be riding on. Your duties include station cleanup and checking the unit for mechanical problems. You should also check all medical equipment and supplies:
  A. after every call.
  B. after every emergency transport.
  C. every 12 hours.
  D. every day.

_____ **14.** For every emergency request, the dispatcher should gather and record all of the following EXCEPT:

    A. the nature of the call.

    B. the patient's location.

    C. medications that the patient is currently taking.

    D. the number of patients and possible severity of their condition.

_____ **15.** During the _____ phase, the team should review dispatch information and assign specific initial duties and scene management tasks to each team member.

    A. preparation

    B. dispatch

    C. en route

    D. transport

_____ **16.** Basic requirements for the driver to operate an ambulance safely include:

    A. physical fitness.

    B. emotional fitness.

    C. proper attitude.

    D. all of the above.

_____ **17.** The _____ phase may be the most dangerous part of the call.

    A. preparation

    B. en route

    C. transport

    D. on scene

_____ **18.** To operate an emergency vehicle safely, you must know how it responds to _____ under various conditions.

    A. steering

    B. braking

    C. acceleration

    D. all of the above

_____ **19.** You must always drive:

    A. offensively.

    B. defensively.

    C. under the speed limit.

    D. all of the above.

_____ **20.** When driving with lights and siren, you are _____ drivers to yield the right-of-way.

    A. requesting

    B. demanding

    C. offering

    D. none of the above

_____ **21.** Vehicle size and _____ will greatly influence braking and stopping distances.

    A. length

    B. height

    C. weight

    D. width

_____ **22.** When on an emergency call, before proceeding past a stopped school bus with its lights flashing you should stop before reaching the bus and wait for the driver to:

    A. make sure the children are safe.

    B. close the bus door.

    C. turn off the warning lights.

    D. all of the above.

_____ **23.** The _____ is probably the most overused piece of equipment on an ambulance.

    A. stethoscope

    B. siren

    C. cardiac monitor

    D. stretcher

_____ **24.** The _____ is the most visible, effective warning device for clearing traffic in front of the vehicle.

    A. front light bar

    B. rear light bar

    C. high-beam flasher unit

    D. standard headlight

_____ **25.** If you are involved in a motor vehicle collision while operating an emergency vehicle and are found to be at fault, you may be charged:

    A. civilly.

    B. criminally.

    C. both civilly and criminally.

    D. neither civilly nor criminally.

_____ **26.** _____ crashes are the most common and usually the most serious type of collision in which ambulances are involved.

    A. T-bone

    B. Intersection

    C. Lateral

    D. Rollover

_____ **27.** You respond to a multiple-vehicle collision. You and your partner are reviewing dispatch information en route to the scene. You will be at a major intersection of two state highways. As you approach the scene, you review the guidelines for sizing up the scene. The guidelines include:

    A. looking for safety hazards.

    B. evaluating the need for additional units or other assistance.

    C. evaluating the need to stabilize the spine.

    D. all of the above.

_____ **28.** The main objectives in directing traffic include:

    A. warning other drivers.

    B. preventing additional crashes.

    C. keeping vehicles moving in an orderly fashion.

    D. all of the above.

_____ **29.** Transferring the patient to a receiving staff member occurs during the _____ phase.

    A. arrival

    B. transport

    C. delivery

    D. postrun

_____ **30.** Cleaning the vehicle inside and out, refueling the vehicle, disposing of contaminated waste, and replacing equipment and supplies all are accomplished during the _____ phase.

    A. preparation

    B. transport

    C. delivery

    D. postrun

_____ **31.** You have called for an air ambulance. While your partner is monitoring the patient, he tells you to go set up a landing zone for the helicopter. When clearing a landing site for an approaching helicopter, look for:

    A. loose debris.

    B. electric or telephone wires.

    C. poles.

    D. all of the above.

True/False

If you believe the statement to be more true than false, write the letter "T" in the space provided. If you believe the statement to be more false than true, write the letter "F."

_____ **1.** Equipment and supplies should be placed in the unit according to their relative importance and frequency of use.

_____ **2.** A CPR board is a pocket-sized reminder that the EMT carries to help recall CPR procedures.

_____ **3.** Having the ability to exchange equipment between units or between your unit and the emergency department decreases the time that you and your unit must stay at the hospital.

_____ **4.** The en route or response phase of the emergency call is the least dangerous for the EMT.

_____ **5.** When the siren is on, you can speed up and assume that you have the right-of-way.

_____ **6.** Use the "4-second rule" to help you maintain a safe following distance.

_____ **7.** Always approach a helicopter from the front.

_____ **8.** Fixed-wing air ambulances are generally used for short-haul patient transfers.

_____ **9.** A clear landing zone of 50′ by 50′ (15 m by 15 m) is recommended for EMS helicopters.

Fill-in-the-Blank

Read each item carefully and then complete the statement by filling in the missing words.

1. A(n) _____ _____ is a portable kit containing items that are used in the initial care of the patient.

2. The six-pointed star that identifies vehicles that meet federal specifications as licensed or certified ambulances is known as the _____ _____ _____.

3. For many decades after 1906, a(n) _____ was the vehicle that was most often used as an ambulance.

4. _____ _____ _____ respond initially to the scene with personnel and equipment to treat the sick and injured until an ambulance can arrive.

5. An ambulance call has _____ phases.

6. Devices should either be disposable or easy to clean and _____, which means to remove radiation, chemicals, or other hazardous materials.

7. Suction tubing must reach the patient's _____, regardless of the patient's position.

8. A(n) _____ _____ provides a firm surface under the patient's torso so that you can give effective chest compressions.

Labeling

Label the following diagrams with the correct terms.

1. Helicopter Hand Signals

A. _____

B. _____

C. _____

D. _____

E. _____

F. _____

Crossword Puzzle

The following crossword puzzle is an activity provided to reinforce correct spelling and understanding of medical terminology associated with emergency care and the EMT. Use the clues in the column to complete the puzzle.

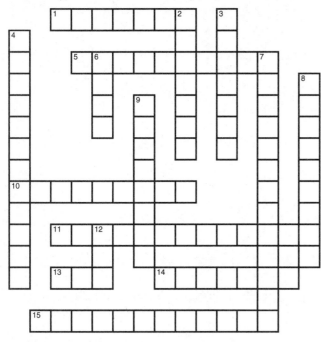

Across

1. Medical evacuation of a patient by helicopter
5. Areas of the road that are blocked from your sight by your own vehicle or mirrors
10. A specialized vehicle for treating and transporting sick and injured patients
11. To remove or neutralize radiation, chemicals, or other hazardous material from clothing, equipment, vehicles, and personnel
13. _____ ambulances are fixed-wing aircraft and helicopters that have been modified for medical care.
14. A portable kit containing items that are used in the initial care of the patient
15. The killing of pathogenic agents by direct application of chemicals

Down

2. Keeping a safe distance between your vehicle and other vehicles on any side of you is known as a(n) _____ of safety.
3. A person who assists a driver in backing up an ambulance to compensate for blind spots at the back of the vehicle
4. A condition in which the tires of a vehicle may be lifted off the road surface as water "piles up" under them, making the vehicle feel as though it is floating
6. The Star of _____ identifies vehicles that meet federal specifications as licensed or certified ambulances.
7. A process, such as heating, that removes microbial contamination
8. _____ disinfection is the killing of pathogenic agents by using potent means of disinfection.
9. The process of removing dirt, dust, blood, or other visible contaminants from a surface
12. A(n) _____ board provides a firm surface under the patient's torso.

Critical Thinking

Multiple Choice

Read each critical-thinking item carefully and then select the one best response.

Questions 1–5 are derived from the following scenario: You are requested out to County Road 93 for a vehicle collision at a rural area known for serious crashes. After driving with lights and sirens for nearly 20 minutes to reach the scene, you arrive at the intersection at the east end of the county. As you pull up, you see two pickup trucks crushed into a mass of twisted, smoking metal. A sheriff's deputy is shouting and waving you over to the passenger side door of one of the demolished trucks. You quickly look down all four roads leading to the scene and note that they are deserted as far as you can see.

_____ 1. Specifically regarding the transport of patients from this scene, you should immediately consider _____ before stepping out of the ambulance.

    A. scene safety

    B. parking 100′ (30 m) past the scene

    C. requesting a medical helicopter

    D. the risks versus benefits of using the siren

_____ 2. Which phase of an ambulance call does this scenario demonstrate?

    A. Fifth

    B. Fourth

    C. Third

    D. Second

_____ 3. Which of the following would you most likely NOT need for this incident?

    A. Jump kit

    B. Airway kit

    C. Extrication kit

    D. Obstetrics kit

_____ 4. How would you ensure the proper control of traffic around this scene?

    A. Put out flares in a pattern that leads other vehicles safely around the involved vehicles.

    B. Because the roads were deserted when you arrived, it is not a priority.

    C. Ask the law enforcement officer to control any traffic.

    D. Pull completely off the roadway and leave your red emergency lights flashing.

_____ 5. You end up transporting an unstable trauma patient from this scene. Assuming that the patient is breathing adequately, what should you be doing about every 5 minutes during the transport phase?

    A. Reassessing vital signs

    B. Providing an update to the receiving facility

    C. Checking your ETA with the navigational equipment

    D. Attempting to rendezvous with an ALS crew

Short Answer

Complete this section with short written answers using the space provided.

1. Describe the three basic ambulance designs.

_____

_____

2. List the phases of an ambulance call.

_____

_____

3. Define the term *siren syndrome.*

_____

_____

4. Describe the three basic principles that govern the use of warning lights and sirens.

_____

_____

5. List four guidelines for safe ambulance driving.

_____

_____

6. List the general considerations used for selecting a helicopter landing site.

_____

_____

Ambulance Calls

The following case scenarios provide an opportunity to explore the concerns associated with patient management and to enhance critical-thinking skills. Read each scenario and answer each question to the best of your ability.

1. You are cross-trained as a fire fighter, and your station has been dispatched to a working structure fire. As you near the scene, another call is dispatched for "an unknown medical emergency." You are the closest unit to the medical emergency.

How would you best manage this situation?

_____

_____

_____

2. Your department's coverage area is quite large, including ALS coverage for the entire county as well as surrounding areas out of state. You are dispatched to an unfamiliar address for "CPR in progress" and are working with a newly hired partner who is not familiar with your coverage area.

How would you best manage this situation?

_____

_____

_____

3. You are called to the scene of a motor vehicle collision. The car is situated in a curve and traffic is heavy. Police are not on the scene. Your patient is alert and looking around but is stuck in the vehicle due to traffic. You see blood smeared across her face, but it appears to be minimal.

How would you best manage this situation?

_____

_____

_____

Fill-in-the-Patient Care Report

Read the incident scenario and then complete the following patient care report (PCR).

It is just before dawn (0512 by the clock on the dashboard), and the darkness is broken only by the occasional burst of lightning in the clouds above, which briefly illuminates the heavy rainfall that has been coming down all night long. You are just about to tell your partner, Alejandro, that you are surprised by the absence of vehicle collisions tonight with the weather the way it is when the dispatch tones burst from the speakers.

"4-0-9, Central Dispatch, emergency call to Highway 12 and Nest Creek Road for a motor vehicle collision."

"4-0-9 copies," Alejandro responds as you start the truck. "En route to Highway 12 and Nest Creek."

"Station time, 0513."

You drive carefully through the torrential rain, the flashing strobes mounted above the cab reflecting off of the raindrops and reducing your visibility, turning what would normally be a 6-minute drive into 10. Thankfully, the heavy rain eases as you arrive on the scene, dissipating to a gentle shower. You park safely off the roadway, which has been shut down by the highway patrol, and approach the scene while Alejandro pulls the equipment from the back.

"We've got two drivers and two cars involved," a highway patrol officer wearing a plastic-covered, wide-brimmed hat says as you approach. "One's not injured but the other is bleeding pretty good from her nose. I think she hit the steering wheel."

You walk over to the small white car where the injured woman is still in the driver's seat and see that the highway patrol has chocked the wheels and disconnected the battery. You approach from the front, so the 41-year-old woman can see you directly out of the windshield, and Alejandro moves to the rear door.

"Ma'am," you say loudly through the windshield. "Keep looking straight ahead at me and do not move your head. My partner is going to get in the back of your car right now and hold your head steady."

As soon as Alejandro is holding the woman's head in a neutral, in-line position you set about applying a cervical collar and, finding no injuries other than a swollen (no longer bleeding) nose, you apply the vest-type extrication device and initiate high-flow oxygen therapy. Eight minutes after arriving on scene, and with the rain starting to fall harder again, you have the 90-kg (198-lb) patient secured to a long spine board and loaded into the back of the ambulance.

One minute after closing the back doors you have obtained a baseline set of vital signs, and Alejandro has pulled out onto the roadway and has started driving to the nearest emergency department, 14 minutes south. The patient's vital signs are: blood pressure, 142/100 mm Hg; pulse, 100 beats/min; respirations, 16 breaths/min and unlabored (but she cannot breathe through her nose); and SaO_2 of 98%.

"What is your blood pressure normally?" you ask while filling out the PCR.

"It's high," she says. "I'm supposed to take Lisinopril, but I always forget. I had something like a stroke when I was 36. They called it a TIA or something."

"Do you have any other medical issues or allergies?"

"No. But my nose and cheeks are killing me."

"Okay," you say, patting her arm. "I'm sorry about that, we'll be at the hospital in a few minutes, and they will be able to help with that."

You then pick up the radio and contact the hospital to provide a patient report and your ETA.

Three minutes before arriving at the emergency department, you get a second set of vital signs and find that they are the same as the first except that the patient's breathing has slowed by two breaths per minute as she relaxed. You and Alejandro unload the gurney from the ambulance and deliver the patient to the waiting staff of County Medical Center, where you provide a verbal report to the accepting nurse and properly turn over care.

A total of 45 minutes after the initial dispatch, you notify the dispatch center that you are available and ready for more calls.

EMS Patient Care Report (PCR)

Date:	Incident No.:	Nature of Call:		Location:

Dispatched:	En Route:	At Scene:	Transport:	At Hospital:	In Service:

Patient Information

Age:	Allergies:
Sex:	Medications:
Weight (in kg [lb]):	Past Medical History:
	Chief Complaint:

Vital Signs

Time:	BP:	Pulse:	Respirations:	Sao$_2$:
Time:	BP:	Pulse:	Respirations:	Sao$_2$:
Time:	BP:	Pulse:	Respirations:	Sao$_2$:

EMS Treatment
(circle all that apply)

Oxygen @ ___ L/min via (circle one): 　NC　　NRM　　Bag-Mask Device	Assisted Ventilation	Airway Adjunct	CPR
Defibrillation	Bleeding Control	Bandaging	Splinting	Other Shock Treatment

Narrative

Vehicle Extrication and Special Rescue

General Knowledge

Matching

Match each of the items in the left column to the appropriate definition in the right column.

_____ 1. Extrication	**A.** Access requiring no special tools and training
_____ 2. Simple access	**B.** Individual who has overall command of the scene in the field
_____ 3. Hazardous material	**C.** Area where individuals can be exposed to sharp objects and hazardous materials
_____ 4. Access	**D.** Access requiring special tools and training
_____ 5. Incident commander	**E.** Removal from entrapment or a dangerous situation or position
_____ 6. SWAT	**F.** Gaining entry to an enclosed area to reach a patient
_____ 7. Complex access	**G.** Fire in a house, apartment building, or other building
_____ 8. Disentanglement	**H.** The removal of the motor vehicle from around the patient
_____ 9. Technical rescue group	**I.** Individuals trained to respond to special rescue situations
_____ 10. Structure fire	**J.** Special weapons and tactic team
_____ 11. SCBA	**K.** Self-contained breathing apparatus
_____ 12. Danger zone	**L.** Toxic, poisonous, radioactive, flammable, or explosive

Multiple Choice

Read each item carefully and then select the one best response.

_____ 1. During all phases of rescue, your primary concern is:
   A. extrication.
   B. safety.
   C. patient care.
   D. rapid transport.

_____ 2. When you arrive at the scene where there is a potential for hazardous materials exposure:
   A. turn off your warning light.
   B. do not waste time waiting for the scene to be marked and protected.
   C. park your unit downhill of the scene.
   D. park your unit uphill of the scene.

_____ 3. _____ is the ability to recognize any possible issues once you arrive on the scene and to act proactively to avoid a negative impact.
   A. Situational awareness
   B. Situational consciousness
   C. Situational alertness
   D. Situational disregard

4. Controlling traffic at a scene is typically the responsibility of:

   A. a fire fighter.

   B. law enforcement.

   C. the rescue group.

   D. EMS personnel.

5. During a 360° walk-around at an accident scene, you should look for all of the following EXCEPT:

   A. the mechanism of injury.

   B. leaking fuels or fluids.

   C. trapped or ejected patients.

   D. the amount of air left in the tires.

6. You should communicate with members of _____ throughout the extrication process.

   A. law enforcement

   B. the media

   C. the rescue team

   D. the insurance company

7. If there are downed power lines near a vehicle involved in a crash, you should:

   A. attempt to move the power lines yourself.

   B. touch the power lines with an object to see if there is active electricity.

   C. have the patient slowly exit the vehicle.

   D. have the patient remain in the vehicle.

8. _____ is responsible for properly securing and stabilizing the vehicle and providing a safe entrance and access to the patient.

   A. Law enforcement

   B. The rescue team

   C. The EMS service

   D. The HazMat unit

9. Prior to attempting to gain access into a vehicle, the parking brake should be on and the _____ should be disconnected.

   A. radio

   B. battery

   C. hydraulics

   D. brake lines

10. Lighting at a scene, establishing a tool and equipment area, and marking for a helicopter landing all fall under:

   A. logistic operations.

   B. EMS operations.

   C. support operations.

   D. law enforcement.

11. When removing an injured patient from a vehicle due to an environmental threat or the need to perform CPR, it is best to use the _____ technique.

   A. rapid extrication

   B. KED board

   C. upright chest compression

   D. intermediate extrication

12. When attempting simple access into a vehicle, you should:

   A. use complex tools.

   B. try opening the doors using the door handles first.

   C. break the windows initially.

   D. make sure that all the windows are rolled up.

_____ **13.** Which of the following is NOT considered a specialized rescue situation?

  A. Cave rescue

  B. Dive rescue

  C. Truck rescue

  D. Mine rescue

_____ **14.** When arriving at the scene of a cave-in or trench collapse, response vehicles should be parked at least _____ away from the scene.

  A. 50′ (15 m)

  B. 150′ (46 m)

  C. 250′ (76 m)

  D. 500′ (152 m)

_____ **15.** Which of the following statements regarding tactical emergency medical support is FALSE?

  A. Some incidents pose an increased risk to EMS.

  B. Once you have checked in at the command post, you are free to roam the area looking for ways to help.

  C. Lights and sirens should be turned off when nearing the scene.

  D. Planning measures and working with the incident commander will reduce the potential for chaos.

True/False

If you believe the statement to be more true than false, write the letter "T" in the space provided. If you believe the statement to be more false than true, write the letter "F."

_____ **1.** At a fire scene, you must ensure that your ambulance will not block or hinder other arriving equipment.

_____ **2.** Ambulances are not typically summoned to search and rescue scenes.

_____ **3.** When you arrive at the site of a technical rescue, you should identify the stable location to which the technical rescue team will bring the patient.

_____ **4.** Following the termination of a rescue incident, all equipment used at the scene must be checked before being reloaded onto the apparatus.

_____ **5.** White-water rescue, structural collapse, and mountain-climbing rescue require specialized rescue teams.

_____ **6.** Regardless of the external environment conditions, you should remain on scene to complete your assessment and treatment of someone involved in a rescue situation.

_____ **7.** Securing an injured arm to the body is generally considered to be acceptable until the patient is fully extricated.

_____ **8.** When determining a rescue plan, your input will be essential so that the patient's injuries will be considered during the rescue process.

_____ **9.** The rescue team is responsible for dictating the way in which medical care, packaging, and transport of the patient will be performed.

_____ **10.** Rescue personnel should coordinate with you to determine the best route for removing the patient from the vehicle.

_____ **11.** It is generally uncommon for EMTs to be in the vehicle with a patient during the disentanglement process.

_____ **12.** Providing medical care to a patient who is trapped in a vehicle is principally the same as for any other patient.

_____ **13.** Simple access typically involves breaking glass.

_____ **14.** When there are multiple patients, you should locate and rapidly triage each patient to determine who needs urgent care.

_____ **15.** A vehicle on its side is typically not a danger to you as long as the vehicle is not swaying.

_____ **16.** Air bags can be located in the steering wheel, doors, or seats.

_____ **17.** There are five phases to the extrication process.

Fill-in-the-Blank

Read each item carefully and then complete the statement by filling in the missing words.

1. In addition to posing a threat to you and others at the scene, _____ _____ may pose a threat to a much larger area and population.

2. You must always be _____ and _____ prepared for any incident that requires rescue or extrication.

3. _____ is the term used when a person is caught within a closed area with no way out or who has a limb or other body part trapped.

4. When you arrive at a rescue scene, you should position your vehicle in a(n) _____ location.

5. _____ is the ongoing process of information gathering and scene evaluation to determine measures for managing an emergency.

6. Use _____ _____ to warn oncoming vehicles of your presence.

7. _____ _____ are responsible for providing immediate assessment and treatment of injured people at rescue scenes.

8. Extinguishing fires, preventing additional ignition, and removing any spilled fuel is primarily the responsibility of _____ _____.

9. The rescue team will set up a(n) _____ _____ that is off-limits to bystanders to protect their safety.

10. No matter what the fuel source of a crashed vehicle is, one common practice remains the same—the need to disconnect the _____.

11. You should not attempt to gain access into a vehicle until you are sure that it has been _____.

12. All EMS personnel should wear proper _____ _____ while in the working area.

13. The _____ _____ should provide you with the entrance you need to gain access to the patient.

14. _____ among team members and clear leadership are essential to safe, efficient provision of proper emergency care.

15. A lack of identifiable _____ at the scene hinders the rescue effort and patient care.

16. You and the patient should be covered with a thick, _____ _____ or _____ for protection from broken glass during disentanglement.

17. Cave rescue, confined space rescue, and search and rescue are all considered to be _____ _____ situations.

18. You should consider using a(n) _____ _____ _____ if the patient will need to be transported an extensive distance.

19. Unless otherwise instructed, only the _____ _____ should communicate any news or progress of a search and rescue to a victim's family.

20. _____ is usually the cause of secondary collapse in a trench collapse.

21. At no time should medical personnel enter a trench deeper than _____ _____ without proper shoring in place.

22. In most areas, an ambulance is dispatched with the fire department to any _____ _____.

Crossword Puzzle

The following crossword puzzle is an activity provided to reinforce correct spelling and understanding of medical terminology associated with emergency care and the EMT. Use the clues in the column to complete the puzzle.

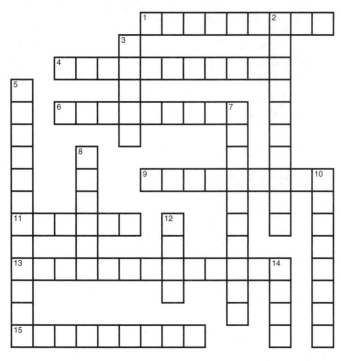

Across

1. The incident _____ has overall command of the incident in the field.
4. Removal of a patient from entrapment or a dangerous situation or position
6. A fire in a house, apartment building, office, school, plant, warehouse, or other building is known as a(n) _____ fire.
9. Any substances that are toxic, poisonous, radioactive, flammable, or explosive and cause injury or death with exposure are _____ materials.
11. Gaining entry to an enclosed area and reaching a patient
13. Complicated entry that requires special tools and training and includes breaking windows or using other force
15. A technical rescue _____ requires special technical skills and equipment in one of many specialized rescue areas.

Down

2. An area where individuals can be exposed to hazards such as sharp metal edges, broken glass, toxic substances, lethal rays, or ignition or explosion of hazardous materials
3. A team of individuals from one or more departments in a region who are trained and on call for certain types of technical rescue is known as a technical rescue _____.
5. Access that is easily achieved without the use of tools or force
7. To be caught (trapped) within a vehicle, room, or container with no way out or to have a limb or other body part trapped
8. The ongoing process of information gathering and scene evaluation to determine appropriate strategies and tactics to manage an emergency
10. An area of protection providing safety from the danger zone (hot zone)
12. A specialized law enforcement tactical unit
14. Respirator with independent air supply used by fire fighters to enter toxic and otherwise dangerous atmospheres

Critical Thinking

Short Answer

Complete this section with short written answers using the space provided.

1. Explain the individual responsibilities of EMS, fire fighters, law enforcement, and rescue teams at a rescue scene.

_____

_____

2. List the questions you and your team should consider whenever you need to determine the exact location and position of a patient.

_____

_____

3. List the steps for assessing and caring for a patient who is entrapped once access has been gained.

_____

_____

4. List the 10 phases of extrication.

_____

_____

5. Explain the proper technique for patient removal once the patient is disentangled from a vehicle.

_____

_____

Ambulance Calls

The following case scenarios provide an opportunity to explore the concerns associated with patient management and to enhance critical-thinking skills. Read each scenario and answer each question to the best of your ability.

1. You are dispatched to "chest pain" by a third-party caller. No one answers the front door when you knock, and the door is locked. You hear a dog barking inside. The dispatcher informs you that the call was placed by the man's wife, who is not on the premises. She told the dispatcher that her husband called her cellular phone complaining of chest pain and that he has recently been released from the hospital.

How would you best manage this situation?

_____

_____

_____

2. It is spring, and the water runoff from melting snow has caused the local viaduct to swell with cold, fast-moving waters. You are off duty when you hear a tone out for "small boy swept away by flood waters." You arrive to the scene before your department's on-duty responders. You see a boy of approximately 13 years who is clinging to life in the middle of the channel, holding onto a trapped log. His mother is hysterical and screaming for you to "jump in and get him." You have no safety equipment available.

How would you best manage this patient?

_____

_____

_____

3. You are dispatched to a chemical spill where a train car derailed. The patient is the engineer; he was injured when he went to the back of the train to survey the damage. He is lying beside the tracks. From your vantage point at the staging area, he appears to be breathing. HazMat team members are suiting up to go in and retrieve the patient. They will decontaminate him before bringing him to the staging area.

How would you best manage this patient?

_____

_____

_____

General Knowledge

Matching

Match each of the items in the left column to the appropriate definition in the right column.

_____ **1.** Carboys
_____ **2.** Cold zone
_____ **3.** Control zone
_____ **4.** Danger zone
_____ **5.** Decontamination

_____ **6.** Demobilization
_____ **7.** Disaster
_____ **8.** Hot zone
_____ **9.** Intermodal tanks

_____ **10.** Placards

_____ **11.** Primary triage
_____ **12.** Secondary containment
_____ **13.** Secondary triage
_____ **14.** Span of control
_____ **15.** Warm zone

A. Shipping and storage vessels that may or may not be pressurized
B. Areas designated as hot, warm, and cold
C. Patient sorting used to rapidly categorize patients
D. Patient sorting used in the treatment sector; involves retriage of patients
E. Removing or neutralizing hazardous materials from patients and equipment
F. Controlling spills when main containment vessel fails
G. Required on all four sides of vehicles transporting hazardous materials
H. Glass, plastic, or steel containers ranging in volume from 5 to 15 gallons
I. Area surrounding hazardous materials spill/incident that is directly dangerous
J. Area where you can be exposed to toxic substances, lethal rays, or explosion
K. Area located between hot zone and cold zone
L. Widespread event that disrupts community resources and function
M. The supervisor-to-worker ratio
N. Safe area at a hazardous materials incident
O. Responders return to their facilities when work at a disaster is completed.

Multiple Choice

Read each item carefully and then select the one best response.

_____ **1.** Major incidents require the involvement and coordination of all the following EXCEPT:
   A. multiple jurisdictions.
   B. local and national media.
   C. functional agencies.
   D. emergency response disciplines.

_____ **2.** Which of the following is NOT part of NIMS standardization?
   A. Personnel training
   B. Resource classification
   C. Terminology
   D. Funding

_____ **3.** In the incident command system, organizational divisions may include sections, branches, divisions, and:
   A. groups.
   B. teams.
   C. platoons.
   D. squads.

4. Which of the following is NOT considered a function of the finance section in the ICS?

A. Time unit

B. Procurement unit

C. Cost unit

D. Logistics unit

5. Which of the following statements regarding the function of the public information officer is true?

A. Positions headquarters away from the incident

B. Is not responsible for the safety of the media

C. Monitors the scene for conditions that may be unsafe

D. Relays information and concerns among the command and general staff

6. What is one of the three main questions used during the scene size-up at a potential MCI?

A. Is my ambulance stocked for an MCI?

B. Where am I?

C. What resources do I need?

D. How long will it take to get help here?

7. Which of the following is considered a priority when determining "what needs to be done" during the scene size-up?

A. Rescue operations

B. Incident stabilization

C. Notifying hospitals

D. Establishing operations

8. Once you have performed a good scene size-up, _____ should be established by the most senior official.

A. operations

B. communications

C. command

D. rescue

9. The primary duty of the triage division is to:

A. begin basic treatment.

B. establish zones for categorized patients.

C. communicate with the treatment division.

D. ensure that every patient receives a primary assessment.

10. Documenting and tracking of transporting vehicles, transported patients, and facility destinations is the responsibility of the:

A. operations supervisor.

B. transportation supervisor.

C. logistics supervisor.

D. triage supervisor.

11. Which of the following is NOT a sign of stress a rehabilitation supervisor is responsible for recognizing?

A. Fatigue

B. Headache

C. Complete collapse

D. Altered thinking patterns

12. Which of the following definitions of MCI is correct?

A. Any call that involves three or more patients

B. Any situation that meets the demand of equipment or personnel

C. Any incident that does not require mutual aid response

D. Any call that has at least one motor vehicle involved

_____ **13.** Triaged patients are primarily divided into how many categories?

    A. Two

    B. Four

    C. Six

    D. Eight

_____ **14.** Delayed patients would be identified by using the color:

    A. black.

    B. red.

    C. yellow.

    D. green.

_____ **15.** Immediate patients would be identified by using the color:

    A. black.

    B. red.

    C. yellow.

    D. green.

_____ **16.** Minimal patients are the third priority and are identified using the color:

    A. black.

    B. red.

    C. yellow.

    D. green.

_____ **17.** Patients who are dead or whose injuries are so severe that they have, at best, a minimal change of survival, are categorized using what color?

    A. Black

    B. Grey

    C. White

    D. Brown

_____ **18.** Facilities, food, lighting, and medical equipment are the responsibility of the:

    A. operations section.

    B. planning section.

    C. logistics section.

    D. finance section.

_____ **19.** When using the START triage system, a patient who is breathing faster than 30 breaths/min is triaged as:

    A. immediate.

    B. delayed.

    C. minimal.

    D. expectant.

_____ **20.** "If you can hear my voice and are able to walk…" is said to immediately identify patients categorized as:

    A. immediate.

    B. delayed.

    C. minimal.

    D. expectant.

_____ **21.** A pediatric patient who is breathing 12 breaths/min would be categorized as:

    A. immediate.

    B. delayed.

    C. minimal.

    D. expectant.

_____ **22.** You are at the scene on a hazardous materials incident when your partner slips and falls, injuring his leg. He is alert and responds appropriately to your questions. His respirations are 20 breaths/min, and he has a radial pulse. What triage category does your partner fall into?

    A. Immediate

    B. Delayed

    C. Minimal

    D. Expectant

_____ **23.** Clues that you may be dealing with a hazardous material include all of the following EXCEPT:

    A. dead grass.

    B. animals near the scene.

    C. discolored pavement.

    D. visible vapors or puddles.

_____ **24.** Rail tank cars, intermodal tanks, and highway cargo tank are all considered:

    A. oversize storage containers.

    B. gross storage containers.

    C. mass storage containers.

    D. bulk storage containers.

_____ **25.** Soap flakes, sodium hydroxide pellets, and food-grade materials are sometimes found in:

    A. bags.

    B. carboys.

    C. drums.

    D. cylinders.

_____ **26.** The US Department of Transportation (DOT) uses all of the following for hazardous identification EXCEPT:

    A. placards.

    B. labels.

    C. signals.

    D. markings.

_____ **27.** Some materials are so hazardous that shipping any amount of them requires a placard. Which of the following is NOT considered to be one of those hazards?

    A. Poison gases

    B. Low-level radioactive substances

    C. Water-reactive solids

    D. Explosives

_____ **28.** Which of the following statements regarding MSDS is FALSE?

    A. They are no longer required by law to be provided to the consumer.

    B. They provide basic information about the chemical makeup of a substance.

    C. They list the potential hazards associated with a substance.

    D. They list appropriate first aid in the event of an exposure.

_____ **29.** Control zones at HazMat incidents are labeled as:

    A. hot.

    B. warm.

    C. cold.

    D. all of the above.

_____ **30.** Nonencapsulated protective clothing, eye protection, and a breathing device that contains an air supply fall into what level of personal protective equipment?

    A. Level A

    B. Level B

    C. Level C

    D. Level D

True/False

If you believe the statement to be more true than false, write the letter "T" in the space provided. If you believe the statement to be more false than true, write the letter "F."

_____   **1.** The most challenging situations you can be called to are disasters and mass casualty incidents.

_____   **2.** The individuals who will participate in the many tasks in an MCI or a disaster should use the ICS.

_____   **3.** The purpose of the response plan is to designate the support agencies in several kinds of MCI.

_____   **4.** Safety priorities include your life, then your patient's, and then your partner's.

_____   **5.** A key role of the transportation supervisor is to communicate with the area hospitals to determine where to transport patients.

_____   **6.** The staging supervisor should be established near the scene.

_____   **7.** The morgue should be out of view of the living patients and other responders.

_____   **8.** A way of tracking and accounting for patients is to issue only 20 to 25 triage tags at a time with a scorecard.

_____   **9.** Infants and children not developed enough to walk or follow commands should be taken as soon as possible to the triage sector for immediate secondary triage.

_____   **10.** When you approach a hazardous scene, you should stay downhill and upwind.

_____   **11.** The farther you are from the incident when you notice a problem, the safer you will be.

_____   **12.** The nature of the chemical dictates the construction of the storage drum.

_____   **13.** The DOT system requires that all chemical shipments be marked with placards and labels.

_____   **14.** Some substances are not hazardous but can become highly toxic when mixed with another substance.

_____   **15.** If you are treating a patient who was partially decontaminated, you will not need to wear additional protective clothing.

Fill-in-the-Blank

Read each item carefully and then complete the statement by filling in the missing words.

1. Two important underlying principles of the NIMS are _____ and _____.

2. One of the organizing principles of the ICS is limiting the _____ _____ _____ of any one individual.

3. A(n) _____ command system is one in which one person is in charge, even if multiple agencies respond.

4. The _____ section solves problems as they arise during the MCI.

5. _____ involves the decisions made and basic planning done before an incident occurs.

6. The _____ _____ is ultimately in charge of counting and prioritizing patients.

7. _____ _____ ensure that secondary triage of patients is performed.

8. The main information needed on a triage tag is a unique _____ and a triage _____.

9. The _____ and type of _____ are two good indicators of the possible presence of a hazardous material.

10. Containers of material are divided into two categories: _____ and _____

storage containers.

11. _____ _____ may be constructed of plastic, paper, or plastic-lined paper.

12. _____ _____ are established at a HazMat incident based on the chemical and physical

properties of the released material and the environmental factors.

13. The _____ _____ is where personnel and equipment transition into and out of the

hot zone.

14. Anyone who leaves a hot zone must pass through the _____ area.

15. A(n) _____ _____ is shipped to a facility, where it is stored and used, and then

returned to the shipper for refilling.

Fill-in-the-Table

Fill in the missing parts of the table.

Triage Priorities	
Triage Category	**Typical Injuries**
Red tag: first priority (immediate) Patients who need immediate care and transport Treat these patients first, and transport as soon as possible	• _____ • _____ • _____ • _____ • _____ • _____
Yellow tag: second priority (delayed) Patients whose treatment and transport can be temporarily delayed	• _____ • _____ • _____
Green tag: third priority, minimal (walking wounded) Patients who require minimal or no treatment and transport can be delayed until last	• _____ • _____
Black tag: fourth priority (expectant) Patients who are already dead or have little chance for survival; treat salvageable patients before treating these patients	• _____ • _____ • _____ • _____

Crossword Puzzle

The following crossword puzzle is an activity provided to reinforce correct spelling and understanding of medical terminology associated with emergency care and the EMT. Use the clues in the column to complete the puzzle.

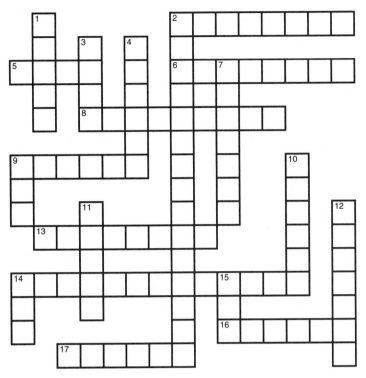

Across

2. A widespread event that disrupts community resources and functions, in turn threatening public safety, citizens' lives, and property

5. A system designed to enable governments and private sector and nongovernmental organizations to effectively and efficiently prepare for, prevent, respond to, and recover from domestic incidents

6. A safe area at a hazardous materials incident for the agencies involved in the operations

8. _____ containment is an engineered method to control spilled or released product if the main containment vessel fails.

9. In incident command, the _____ supervisor works with area medical examiners, coroners, and law enforcement agencies to coordinate the disposition of dead victims.

13. The area located between the hot zone and the cold zone at a hazardous materials incident

14. A type of patient sorting used to rapidly categorize patients

16. In incident command, the _____ officer gives the "go ahead" to a plan or may stop an operation when rescuer safety is an issue.

17. An incident _____ plan states general objectives reflecting the overall strategy for managing an incident.

Down

1. The _____ information center is an area designated by the incident commander, or a designee, in which public information officers disseminate information about the incident.

2. The process of removing or neutralizing and properly disposing of hazardous materials from equipment, patients, and rescue personnel

3. A form containing information about chemical composition, physical and chemical properties, health and safety hazards, emergency response, and waste disposal of a specific material

4. In incident command, the _____ supervisor determines the type of equipment and resources needed for a situation involving extrication or special rescue.

7. In incident command, the _____ officer relays information, concerns, and requests among responding agencies.

9. An emergency situation involving three or more patients

10. The process of sorting patients based on the severity of injury and medical need to establish treatment and transportation priorities

11. Barrel-like containers used to store a wide variety of substances, including food-grade materials, corrosives, flammable liquids, and grease

12. Glass, plastic, or steel containers ranging in volume from 5 to 15 gallons

14. In incident command, the person who keeps the public informed and relates any information to the press

15. A system implemented to manage disasters and mass casualty incidents in which section chiefs report to the incident commander

Critical Thinking

Short Answer

Complete this section with short written answers using the space provided.

1. List the major components of the NIMS.

_____

_____

2. List the five factors included in mobilization and deployment.

_____

_____

3. What information should be communicated from the triage supervisor to the branch medical director?

_____

_____

4. Based on the HAZWOPER regulation, what are the competencies a first responder should be able to demonstrate at the awareness level?

_____

_____

5. What information is typically included on an MSDS?

_____

_____

Ambulance Calls

The following case scenarios provide an opportunity to explore the concerns associated with patient management and to enhance critical-thinking skills. Read each scenario and answer each question to the best of your ability.

1. You are dispatched to a multi-vehicle crash where you encounter three patients: a 4-year-old boy with bilateral femur fractures and absent radial pulse, a 27-year-old woman with a laceration to the head and a humerus fracture, and a 42-year-old man who is apneic and pulseless with an open skull fracture.

How should you triage these patients?

_____

_____

_____

2. Your response area contains a large portion of farming and other agricultural lands, including many orchards and vineyards. Right at shift change, there is a tone out for a "crop-duster accident" in a remote area of your jurisdiction. It appears that 15 to 30 agricultural workers were accidentally sprayed with pesticides and other chemicals from a crop-dusting plane. They are now experiencing a variety of signs and symptoms, including nausea, vomiting, and eye and upper airway irritation.

How would you best manage this situation?

_____

_____

_____

_____

3. You and your partner are enjoying an unusually uneventful evening at work when you receive a dispatch for "overturned semitruck." As you approach the scene, you see a semitractor trailer that has left the roadway and rolled down a steep embankment. You see the driver attempting to climb up to the roadway, where many passersby have stopped to see what has happened. He is vigorously coughing, and you can see a liquid dripping from the truck's tank.

How would you best manage this situation?

_____

_____

_____

_____

Assessment Review

Answer the following questions pertaining to the assessment of the types of emergencies discussed in this chapter.

_____ **1.** You are at the scene of a multi-vehicle incident involving eight people. Your partner has established command and is requesting additional resources as you begin to triage patients. You see patients in various areas as you visually inspect the scene. "If are any of you are able to walk to me, please do so," you state to the patients. Three of the eight people are able to walk to you. What category of triage do these patients initially fall into?

   A. Immediate

   B. Delayed

   C. Minimal

   D. Expectant

_____ **2.** As you continue moving through the scene, you come across two people in a vehicle. The first person has obvious bleeding from her forehead and is emotionally upset. She is slow to respond to your questions and cannot tell you what today's date is. When you ask her to show you "two fingers" she is able to, but with some delay. Her radial pulse is 106 beats/min, and her respirations are 22 breaths/min and nonlabored. What category of triage does this patient initially fall into?

   A. Immediate

   B. Delayed

   C. Minimal

   D. Expectant

_____ **3.** The next patient in the vehicle has an obvious open femur fracture. The patient is breathing at a rate of 32 breaths/min, but is completely alert, oriented, and able to follow commands without hesitation. The patient's radial pulse is 102 beats/min and weak. What category of triage does this patient initially fall into?

A. Immediate

B. Delayed

C. Minimal

D. Expectant

_____ **4.** Additional EMS have arrived on the scene, and you are being assisted by two other EMTs in the triage process. The last patient you encounter is a 7-year-old boy with neck and back pain. He is quite upset and keeps asking for his parents. His respirations are 38 breaths/min, and his radial pulse is 110 beats/min. What category of triage does this patient initially fall into?

A. Immediate

B. Delayed

C. Minimal

D. Expectant

Terrorism Response and Disaster Management

General Knowledge

Matching

Match each of the items in the left column to the appropriate definition in the right column.

_____ **1.** Mutagen

_____ **2.** Vesicants

_____ **3.** Disease vector

_____ **4.** Phosgene

_____ **5.** Neurotoxins

_____ **6.** Bacteria

_____ **7.** Volatility

_____ **8.** Cyanide

_____ **9.** Vapor hazard

_____ **10.** Lymph nodes

_____ **11.** Incubation

_____ **12.** Ricin

_____ **13.** Dissemination

_____ **14.** Radioactive material

_____ **15.** Viruses

A. Substance that emits radiation

B. Describes how long a chemical agent will stay on a surface before it evaporates

C. Period of time from exposure to onset of symptoms

D. Agent that enters the body through the respiratory tract

E. Animal that, once infected, spreads the disease to another animal

F. Agent that affects the body's ability to use oxygen

G. Germs that require a living host to multiply and survive

H. Means by which a terrorist will spread a disease

I. Neurotoxin derived from mash that is left from the castor bean

J. Biologic agents that are the most deadly substances known to humans

K. Microorganisms that reproduce by binary fission

L. Substance that mutates and damages the structures of DNA in the body's cells

M. Area of the lymphatic system where infection-fighting cells are housed

N. Pulmonary agent that is a product of combustion

O. Blister agents

Multiple Choice

Read each item carefully and then select the one best response.

_____ **1.** Examples of terrorist groups include:

   A. violent religious groups.

   B. extremist political groups.

   C. technology groups.

   D. all of the above.

_____ **2.** An example of a single-issue group is:

   A. antiabortion groups.

   B. separatist groups.

   C. Aum Shinrikyo.

   D. the KKK.

_____ **3.** When were chemical agents first introduced?

  A. Spanish-American War

  B. World War I

  C. World War II

  D. Korean War

_____ **4.** What does it mean when the US Department of Homeland Security Advisory System is at yellow?

  A. Severe risk of terrorist attack

  B. Significant risk of terrorist attack

  C. High risk of terrorist attack

  D. General risk of terrorist attack

_____ **5.** You are called to the scene of an unexplained explosion at the local shopping mall. The reports are that there are multiple injuries. You are the first unit to arrive on the scene. Your first responsibility is:

  A. to ensure scene safety.

  B. to set up the incident command system.

  C. to start triage.

  D. to request additional resources.

_____ **6.** In the previous scenario, you have been informed that there are numerous agencies responding with many different types of apparatus. They are approaching the scene from all directions and will be arriving shortly. You need to:

  A. set up a staging area.

  B. separate the different types of apparatus.

  C. let them continue as they are.

  D. have them come in from downwind.

_____ **7.** _____ agents can remain on a surface for long periods, usually longer than 24 hours.

  A. Volatile

  B. Persistent

  C. Secondary

  D. Vapor

_____ **8.** _____ is a brownish, yellowish oily substance that is generally considered very persistent.

  A. Lewisite

  B. Phosgene oxime

  C. Sulfur mustard

  D. Vesicant

_____ **9.** An example of a pulmonary agent is:

  A. chlorine.

  B. phosgene oxime.

  C. G agents.

  D. lewisite.

_____ **10.** The most lethal of all the nerve agents is:

  A. V agent.

  B. sarin.

  C. soman.

  D. tabun.

_____ **11.** What two medications do MARK 1 antidote kits contain?

    A. Atropine and 2-PAM chloride

    B. Atropine and epinephrine

    C. Epinephrine and 2-PAM chloride

    D. Lidocaine and atropine

_____ **12.** You are dispatched to a local farm where an unconscious 41-year-old man has been discovered. The patient's airway is open, but he has been vomiting. Respirations are within normal limits, and distal pulses are present. The patient has muscle twitches and has urinated on himself. There is a funny odor that seems to be coming from the patient's clothing. You would suspect:

    A. alcohol poisoning.

    B. organophosphate poisoning.

    C. drug overdose.

    D. respiratory agent.

_____ **13.** You are dispatched to a patient who is having respiratory problems. He is awake but is working so hard to breathe that he can't answer questions. His distal pulses are present and strong. There is an odor of almonds in the air. You would suspect:

    A. cyanide.

    B. sarin.

    C. soman.

    D. tabun.

_____ **14.** The period of time between the person becoming exposed to an agent and when symptoms begin is called:

    A. contagious.

    B. incubation.

    C. communicability.

    D. remission.

_____ **15.** Which of the following is NOT an example of a viral hemorrhagic fever?

    A. Ebola

    B. Rift Valley

    C. Yellow Fever

    D. Smallpox

_____ **16.** Which of the following statements regarding anthrax is FALSE?

    A. It enters the body through inhalation, cutaneous, and gastrointestinal routes.

    B. It is caused by a deadly bacterium that lies dormant in a spore.

    C. A vaccine is available to prevent anthrax infections.

    D. Pulmonary anthrax is associated with the lowest risk of death if left untreated.

_____ **17.** Bubonic plague infects the:

    A. respiratory system.

    B. circulatory system.

    C. lymphatic system.

    D. digestive system.

_____ **18.** The deadliest substances know to humans are:

   A. neurotoxins.

   B. hemotoxins.

   C. plagues.

   D. bacteria.

_____ **19.** The least toxic route for ricin is:

   A. oral.

   B. inhalation.

   C. injection.

   D. absorption.

_____ **20.** The EMS role in helping to determine a biologic event is to:

   A. administer medications.

   B. be aware of an unusual number of calls for unexplainable flu.

   C. quarantine infected individuals.

   D. set up field hospitals.

_____ **21.** The most powerful of all radiation is:

   A. alpha.

   B. neutron.

   C. beta.

   D. gamma.

_____ **22.** To protect yourself from radiation exposure, you should do all of the following EXCEPT:

   A. limit the time of exposure.

   B. increase distance between yourself and the source.

   C. use shielding.

   D. wear a mask to prevent respiratory exposure.

_____ **23.** Which organ is most susceptible to pressure changes during an explosion?

   A. Liver

   B. Lung

   C. Heart

   D. Kidney

True/False

If you believe the statement to be more true than false, write the letter "T" in the space provided. If you believe the statement to be more false than true, write the letter "F."

_____ 1. Atlanta's Centennial Park bombing during the 1996 Summer Olympics is an example of international terrorism.

_____ 2. WMDs are easy to obtain or create.

_____ 3. Most acts of terrorism occur after a warning is given to the general public.

_____ 4. Understanding and being aware of the current threat is only the beginning of responding safely.

_____ 5. Failure to park your ambulance in a safe location can place you and your partner in danger.

_____ 6. You should have all units responding to an explosion converge on the main entrance to the building.

_____ 7. Vapor hazards enter the body through the pores in the skin.

_____ 8. The primary route of exposure of vesicants is through inhalation.

_____ 9. Phosgene and phosgene oxime are two different classes of agents.

_____ 10. Tabun looks like baby oil.

_____ 11. Seizures are the most common symptom of nerve agent exposure.

_____ 12. Organophosphate is the basic ingredient in nerve agents.

_____ 13. Cyanide binds with the body's cells, preventing oxygen from being used.

_____ 14. When dealing with smallpox, gloves are all the standard precautions you need.

_____ 15. Outbreaks of the viral hemorrhagic fevers are extremely rare worldwide.

_____ 16. Pulmonary anthrax infections are associated with a 90% death rate if untreated.

_____ 17. Pneumonic plague is deadlier than bubonic plague.

_____ 18. Ricin is deadlier than botulinum.

_____ 19. Ingestion of ricin causes necrosis of the lungs.

_____ 20. Large containers called "life packs" are delivered during a biologic event.

_____ 21. The dirty bomb is an ineffective WMD.

_____ 22. Being exposed to a radiation source does not make a patient contaminated or radioactive.

_____ 23. Neurologic injuries and head trauma are the most common causes of death from blast injuries.

Fill-in-the Blank

Read each item carefully and then complete the statement by filling in the missing words.

1. The bombing of the Alfred P. Murrah Federal Building in Oklahoma City is an example of _____ _____.

2. Any agent designed to bring about mass death, casualties, and/or massive damage to property and infrastructure is a(n) _____ _____ _____ _____.

3. _____ _____ is when a nation has close ties with terrorist groups.

4. If there is a high risk of a terrorist attack, the Homeland Security Advisory system will be at threat level _____.

5. _____ occurs when you come into contact with a contaminated person who has not been decontaminated.

6. _____ _____ _____ is a term used to describe how the agent most effectively enters the body.

7. An agent that gives off very little or no vapor and enters the body through the skin is called a(n) _____ _____.

8. _____ _____ are among the most deadly chemicals developed.

9. _____ means that vapors are continuously released over a period of time.

10. _____ is the means by which a terrorist will spread the agent.

11. _____ is a germ that requires a living host to multiply and survive.

12. The group of viruses that cause the blood in the body to seep out from the tissues and blood vessels is called _____ _____ _____.

13. _____ is a deadly bacterium that lies dormant in a spore.

14. Buboes are formed when the _____ _____ become infected and grow.

15. The most potent neurotoxin is _____.

16. _____ _____ _____ are existing facilities that are established in a time of need for the mass distribution of antibiotics, antidotes, vaccinations, and other medical supplies.

17. Any device that is designed to disperse a radioactive device is called a(n) _____ _____ _____.

18. A(n) _____ _____ _____ results from being struck by flying debris, such as projectiles or secondary missiles, that have been set in motion by the explosion.

Crossword Puzzle

The following crossword puzzle is an activity provided to reinforce correct spelling and understanding of medical terminology associated with emergency care and the EMT. Use the clues in the column to complete the puzzle.

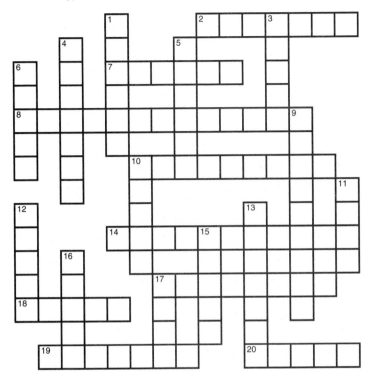

Across

2. A substance that mutates, damages, and changes the DNA in the body's cells
7. A clear, oily agent that has no odor and looks like baby oil
8. _____ terrorism is carried out by people in a country other than their own.
10. Name given to a bomb that is used as a radiologic dispersal device
14. An agent that enters the body through the respiratory tract
17. Microorganisms that reproduce by binary fission
18. A type of energy that is emitted from a strong radiologic source and require lead or several inches of concrete to prevent penetration
19. A disease caused by deadly bacteria that lies dormant in a spore
20. A highly volatile, colorless, and odorless nerve agent that turns from liquid to gas within seconds to minutes at room temperature

Down

1. An act in which the public safety community generally has no prior knowledge of the time, location, or nature of the attack
3. A type of energy that is the least harmful penetrating type of radiation and cannot travel fast or through most objects
4. A(n) _____ hazard gives off very little or no vapors; the skin is the primary route for this type of chemical to enter the body.
5. An animal that spreads a disease, once infected, to another animal is known as a disease _____.
6. Phosgene _____ is a blistering agent that has a rapid onset of symptoms and produces immediate, intense pain and discomfort on contact.
9. The _____ system is a passive circulatory system that transports a plasmalike liquid called lymph, a thin fluid that bathes the tissues of the body.
10. A natural process in which a material that is unstable attempts to stabilize itself by changing its structure
11. Small suitcase-sized nuclear weapons that were designed to destroy individual targets, such as important buildings, bridges, tunnels, and large ships
12. The process by which the temporary bond between the organophosphate and acetylcholinesterase undergoes hydrolysis, resulting in a permanent covalent bond
13. Early nerve agents that were developed by German scientists in the period after World War I and into World War II.
15. A neurotoxin derived from mash that is left from the castor bean
16. A nerve agent that has a fruity odor, as a result of the type of alcohol used in the agent
17. A type of energy that is emitted from a strong radiologic source and requires a layer of clothing to stop it

Critical Thinking

Short Answer

Complete this section with short written answers using the space provided.

1. What are the key questions you should ask yourself when dealing with WMDs?

   _____

   _____

2. List the four classes of chemical agents.

   _____

   _____

3. What things should you observe on every call to determine the potential for a terrorist attack?

   _____

   _____

4. List the signs of vesicant exposure to the skin.

   _____

   _____

5. What are some of the later signs and symptoms of chlorine inhalation?

   _____

   _____

6. What does the mnemonic SLUDGEM stand for?

   _____

   _____

7. What are the signs and symptoms of high doses of cyanide?

   _____

   _____

8. List the signs and symptoms of ricin ingestion.

   _____

   _____

9. List three places that radioactive waste may be found.

_____

_____

10. What should you use to best protect yourself from the effects of radiation?

_____

_____

Ambulance Calls

The following case scenarios provide an opportunity to explore the concerns associated with patient management and to enhance critical-thinking skills. Read each scenario and answer each question to the best of your ability.

1. You are dispatched to an explosion at a nearby shopping mall. No other information is available regarding the nature of the explosion, only that there are possibly upwards of five fatally wounded and 50 severely injured.

How would you best manage this situation?

_____

_____

_____

2. Your emergency system is suddenly inundated with numerous calls for people experiencing fever, chills, headache, muscle aches, nausea/vomiting, diarrhea, severe abdominal cramping, and GI bleeding. All of the patients attended a local indoor sporting event 6 hours earlier.

How would you best manage this situation?

_____

_____

_____

3. You are dispatched to treat numerous patients with known exposure to cyanide. This occurred in a neighboring jurisdiction, and they have requested your assistance. The local fire department has set up a decontamination area, and you are asked to transport patients to the nearest appropriate medical facility.

What are important considerations to note about cyanide exposure?

_____

_____

_____

Assessment Review

Answer the following questions pertaining to the assessment of the types of emergencies discussed in this chapter.

_____ 1. A patient complains of a high fever for the past few days and now has blisters on the face and extremities. This is most consistent with:

   A. viral hemorrhagic fever.

   B. bubonic plague.

   C. smallpox.

   D. anthrax.

_____ 2. A patient complains of a fever, headache, muscle pain, shortness of breath, and extreme lymph node pain and enlargement. This is most consistent with:

   A. viral hemorrhagic fever.

   B. bubonic plague.

   C. smallpox.

   D. anthrax.

_____ 3. A patient was exposed to a package containing an unknown powder. The patient now complains of 3 to 5 days of flulike symptoms, difficulty breathing, and fever. The patient is also showing signs of shock, pulmonary edema, and respiratory failure. This is most consistent with:

   A. viral hemorrhagic fever.

   B. bubonic plague.

   C. smallpox.

   D. anthrax.

_____ 4. A patient complains of a sudden onset of fever, weakness, muscle pain, headache, and sore throat. Signs of external and internal hemorrhaging are noted, along with vomiting. This is most consistent with:

   A. viral hemorrhagic fever.

   B. bubonic plague.

   C. smallpox.

   D. anthrax.

ALS Assist

General Knowledge

Matching

Match each of the items in the left column to the appropriate definition in the right column.

_____ 1. End-tidal carbon dioxide detector
_____ 2. Infiltration
_____ 3. Access port
_____ 4. Gauge
_____ 5. Phlebitis
_____ 6. Stylet
_____ 7. Laryngoscope
_____ 8. Arrhythmia
_____ 9. Catheter
_____ 10. Limb leads
_____ 11. Extubation
_____ 12. King LT
_____ 13. Combitube
_____ 14. Endotracheal intubation
_____ 15. Drip chamber

A. Plastic-coated wire that gives rigidity to endotracheal tubes
B. Inflammation of a vein
C. Placed on arms and legs
D. Flexible, hollow structure that delivers fluids
E. Removal of a tube after placement
F. Escape of fluid into surrounding tissue
G. Measure of interior diameter of catheter
H. Indicator that signals by color change
I. Instrument used to view vocal cords
J. Insertion of a tube through the vocal cords
K. Sealed hub on administration set
L. Fluid accumulates to keep tubing filled with fluid
M. Abnormal rhythm of the heart
N. Supraglottic airway
O. Multilumen airway, two balloons, two ventilation ports

Multiple Choice

Read each item carefully and then select the one best response.

_____ 1. The purpose of advanced airway management is to provide better protection and improve
_____ in patients by using a tube to create a direct channel to the trachea.
   A. respiration
   B. ventilation
   C. oxygenation
   D. patency

_____ 2. The upper airway includes all of the following EXCEPT the:
   A. nose.
   B. mouth.
   C. trachea.
   D. pharynx.

_____ 3. The _____ is located at the glottic opening and prevents food and liquid from entering the lower airway during swallowing.
   A. larynx
   B. vocal cords
   C. epiglottis
   D. carina

_____ **4.** After _____ minutes without oxygen, cells in the brain and nervous system may die.

    A. 2 to 3

    B. 3 to 5

    C. 4 to 6

    D. 5 to 8

_____ **5.** The first step in airway management is:

    A. suctioning.

    B. c-spine control.

    C. applying oxygen.

    D. opening the airway.

_____ **6.** _____ is a very effective way to control a patient's airway and has many advantages over other airway management techniques.

    A. An oropharyngeal adjunct

    B. Endotracheal intubation

    C. A nasopharyngeal adjunct

    D. A jaw thrust

_____ **7.** The purpose of a _____ is to sweep the tongue out of the way and to align the airway so that you can see the vocal cords and pass the ET tube through them.

    A. laryngoscope

    B. lighted stylet

    C. Magill forceps

    D. 10-mL syringe

_____ **8.** A good rule of thumb is to always have a(n) _____ ETT on hand; this size tube will fit most male or female adult patients.

    A. 6.5-mm

    B. 7.0-mm

    C. 7.5-mm

    D. 8.0-mm

_____ **9.** A plastic-coated wire called a _____ may be inserted into the ETT to add rigidity and shape to the tube.

    A. Murphy eye

    B. stylet

    C. pipe cleaner

    D. vallecula

_____ **10.** You will use the _____ to test for air leaks in the ETT before intubation.

    A. 10-mL syringe

    B. lighted stylet

    C. Murphy eye

    D. pilot balloon

_____ **11.** An intubation attempt should not take more than _____ seconds.

    A. 20

    B. 25

    C. 30

    D. 60

_____ **12.** A syringe with plunger and a bulb syringe are commonly used as:
  A. end-tidal carbon dioxide detectors.
  B. esophageal detector devices.
  C. a device to secure an endotracheal tube.
  D. a device to clear secretions from the endotracheal tube.

_____ **13.** Which of the following is NOT used as a secondary confirmation device for endotracheal tube placement?
  A. Capnography
  B. An esophageal detector device
  C. Pulse oximetry
  D. An end-tidal carbon dioxide detector

_____ **14.** Which of the following is NOT considered a complication of intubation?
  A. Left main-stem bronchus intubation
  B. Increased hypoxia from a delayed intubation attempt
  C. Esophageal intubation
  D. Laryngospasm

_____ **15.** Which of the following is NOT a benefit of using a multilumen airway?
  A. No mask seal is necessary.
  B. It requires a deeply comatose patient.
  C. It can be inserted blindly.
  D. It can be easily placed.

_____ **16.** Contraindications of multilumen airways include all of the following EXCEPT:
  A. patients with a gag reflex.
  B. children younger than 14 years.
  C. patients with known liver disease.
  D. patients who have ingested a caustic substance.

_____ **17.** Which of the following statements regarding the King LT airway is true?
  A. It can be used in patients shorter than 4′ (1.2 m).
  B. It does not protect from vomiting and aspiration.
  C. It can be placed in the trachea or the esophagus.
  D. It does not require a secondary confirmation device.

_____ **18.** Which of the following statements regarding the laryngeal mask airway is FALSE?
  A. It was originally developed for the operating room.
  B. It consists of two parts.
  C. The epiglottis is contained within the mask.
  D. The device comes in four sizes.

_____ **19.** When an IV solution is taken out of its protective sterile plastic bag, it must be used within:
  A. 12 hours.
  B. 24 hours.
  C. 36 hours.
  D. 48 hours.

_____ **20.** A microdrip administration set requires _____ drops to flow 1 mL.
    A. 15
    B. 30
    C. 45
    D. 60

_____ **21.** The gauge of a catheter refers to the:
    A. strength of the needle.
    B. length of the needle.
    C. diameter of the needle.
    D. use of the needle.

_____ **22.** Intraosseous IVs are generally started in the:
    A. external jugular.
    B. proximal tibia.
    C. hand.
    D. antecubital vein.

_____ **23.** Risk associated with starting an IV include all of the following EXCEPT:
    A. infiltration.
    B. phlebitis.
    C. occlusion.
    D. impaired blood clotting.

_____ **24.** An accumulation of blood in the tissues surrounding an IV site is called a:
    A. contusion.
    B. hematoma.
    C. bruise.
    D. rupture.

_____ **25.** The best administration set to use when giving fluids to a pediatric patient is the:
    A. macrodrip.
    B. microdrip.
    C. Volutrol.
    D. minidrip.

_____ **26.** Studies have indicated a 95% or better accuracy rate in the diagnosis of myocardial infarction with the use of a:
    A. 3-lead ECG.
    B. 4-lead ECG.
    C. 6-lead ECG.
    D. 12-lead ECG.

_____ **27.** In the normally functioning heart, the electrical impulse originates at the:
    A. AV node.
    B. SA node.
    C. internodal pathway.
    D. bundle of His.

_____ **28.** On the ECG paper, how many boxes equal 1 second?

   A. Five big boxes

   B. Five little boxes

   C. Two big boxes

   D. Two little boxes

_____ **29.** Tachycardia refers to a heart rate:

   A. below 60 beats/min.

   B. above 100 beats/min.

   C. above 60 beats/min.

   D. below 100 beats/min.

_____ **30.** Which leads have to be placed exactly?

   A. Positive leads

   B. Negative leads

   C. Chest leads

   D. Limb leads

True/False

If you believe the statement to be more true than false, write the letter "T" in the space provided. If you believe the statement to be more false than true, write the letter "F."

_____ **1.** Rapid defibrillation is the most effective treatment for ventricular fibrillation.

_____ **2.** The fastest pacer of the heart is the AV node.

_____ **3.** Bradycardia is a heart rate above 60 beats/min.

_____ **4.** The normal heart rate is between 60 and 100 beats/min.

_____ **5.** Many cardiac monitors are capable of reading a 12-lead ECG and indicating whether the patient may be having a STEMI.

_____ **6.** A STEMI is treatable by techniques that rapidly restore perfusion to the coronary arteries.

_____ **7.** The balloon cuff around the end of an ETT holds 25 mL of air.

_____ **8.** When a wire stylet is used, it should stick out 1/2″ (1.3 cm) beyond the tip of the ETT.

_____ **9.** ETTs come in three different sizes.

_____ **10.** A large-gauge IV catheter corresponds to a large diameter.

_____ **11.** An occlusion is the physical blockage of a vein.

_____ **12.** Fluid overload is not a problem with geriatric patients.

_____ **13.** If a hematoma develops when an IV catheter insertion is attempted, the procedure should stop.

_____ **14.** A 14-gauge catheter has a greater diameter than a 22-gauge catheter.

_____ **15.** Starting an external jugular IV requires a different technique than starting other IVs.

Fill-in-the-Blank

Read each item carefully and then complete the statement by filling in the missing words.

1. During _____, the diaphragm contracts.

2. _____ tubes should be used when intubating older children and adults.

3. A standard _____ adapter attaches to any ventilation device

4. The heart contains a network of specialized tissue that is capable of conducting electrical current through the heart; it is

   known as the _____ _____ _____.

5. _____ _____ is a rhythm in which the SA node acts as the pacemaker.

6. _____ _____ is a rapid, completely disorganized ventricular rhythm with chaotic

   characteristics.

7. _____ refers to the complete absence of any electrical cardiac activity.

8. _____ _____ are used specifically in 12-lead ECGs.

9. A(n) _____ _____ relieves gastric distention caused by air in the stomach from

   positive pressure ventilation.

10. _____ can be used in a breathing patient who is alert and able to follow commands and who may be

   suffering from congestive heart failure.

11. _____ _____ are a way to maintain an active IV site without having to run fluids

   through the vein.

12. An inflammation of the vein is called _____.

13. _____ _____ are best used for rapid fluid replacement.

14. _____ _____ occurs when part of the catheter is pinched against the needle and the

   needle slices through the catheter, creating a free-floating segment.

15. A(n) _____ _____ moves fluid from the IV bag into the patient's vascular system.

Labeling

1. ECG Rythms

Label the following ECGs with the correct rhythms.

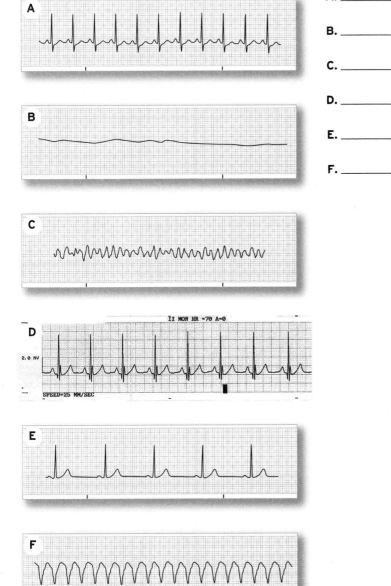

A. _____

B. _____

C. _____

D. _____

E. _____

F. _____

Crossword Puzzle

The following crossword puzzle is an activity provided to reinforce correct spelling and understanding of medical terminology associated with emergency care and the EMT. Use the clues in the column to complete the puzzle.

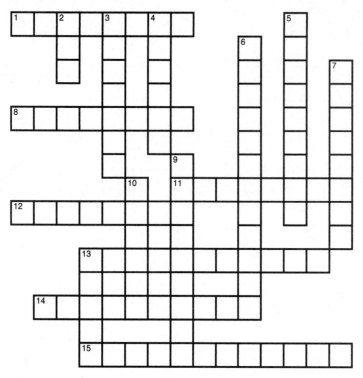

Across

1. The hard, sharpened plastic spike on the end of the administration set designed to pierce the sterile membrane of the intravenous bag is known as a(n) _____ spike.

8. _____ carbon dioxide detectors are plastic, disposable indicators that signal by color change when an endotracheal tube is in the proper place.

11. The complete absence of any electrical cardiac activity, appearing as a straight or almost straight line on an ECG strip

12. A flexible, hollow structure that drains or delivers fluids

13. Special types of intravenous apparatus, also called heparin caps and heparin locks

14. The leads that are used only with a 12-lead ECG and must be placed exactly

15. The escape of fluid into the surrounding tissue when the IV catheter is not in the vein

Down

2. An electronic tracing of the heart's electrical activity through leads

3. _____ monitoring is the act of viewing the electrical activity of the heart through the use of an ECG machine.

4. A(n) _____ sinus rhythm has consistent P waves, consistent P-R intervals, and a regular heart rate of between 60 and 100 beats/min.

5. Blockage, usually of a tubular structure such as a blood vessel

6. _____ catheters are rigid, boring catheters placed into a bone to provide intravenous fluids.

7. Another name for administration sets

9. A(n) _____ mask airway is an advanced airway device that is blindly inserted into the mouth to isolate the larynx for direct ventilation.

10. A plastic-coated wire that gives added rigidity and shape to the endotracheal tube

13. Elevation of the ST segment of the 12-lead ECG that is likely evidence that the patient is having a heart attack

Critical Thinking

Short Answer

Complete this section with short written answers using the space provided.

1. Trace the electrical pathway of the heart.

_____

_____

2. List the ECG tracing through the cardiac cycle.

_____

_____

3. List 10 possible complications associated with endotracheal intubation.

_____

_____

4. What are some examples of common local reactions when starting an IV?

_____

_____

5. List the common systemic complications associated with IV insertion.

_____

_____

Ambulance Calls

The following case scenarios provide an opportunity to explore the concerns associated with patient management and to enhance critical-thinking skills. Read each scenario and answer each question to the best of your ability.

1. You are dispatched to assist with a patient who is experiencing chest pain and dizziness. You notice another EMT on the scene assisting with the application of the ECG. As the paramedic's attention is focused on starting an IV, you see that the EMT has forgotten to attach one of the leads. The paramedic now begins assessing the patient's cardiac rhythm, but he appears confused by what he sees.

How would you best manage this situation?

_____

_____

_____

2. You are dispatched to a pulseless, apneic 45-year-old man. After assessing the patient, your partner decides to perform endotracheal intubation (a newly allowed skill by your medical program director). This is the first field intubation either you or your partner has attempted without supervision of a paramedic or physician on-scene. Your partner tells you that he "thinks" he passed through the cords. As you auscultate the chest, you do not hear breath sounds, but you do hear gurgling over the epigastrium.

How would you best manage this situation?

_____

_____

_____

3. You are in the patient compartment with your EMT partner who is taking care of a patient with congestive heart failure. Your partner has initiated IV therapy and is now giving a radio report to the receiving hospital. You notice the IV tubing is still running wide open and that nearly the entire liter of fluid has been administered over a few minutes. The patient states his shortness of breath is worsening.

How would you best manage this situation?

_____

_____

_____

Skills

Skill Drills

Skill Drill 40-1: Performing Orotracheal Intubation
Test your knowledge of this skill by placing the photos below in the correct order. Number the first step with a "1," the second step with a "2," etc.

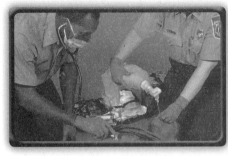

_____ Ventilate and confirm placement.

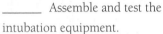

_____ Assemble and test the intubation equipment.

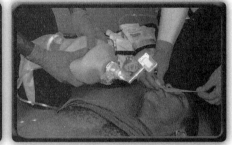

_____ Secure the tube. Note the depth of insertion. Reconfirm placement with every move.

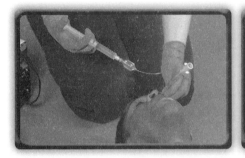

_____ Inflate the balloon cuff, and remove the syringe as your partner prepares to ventilate.

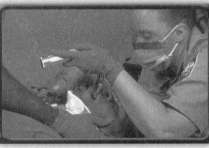

_____ For trauma patients, maintain the cervical spine in-line and neutral.

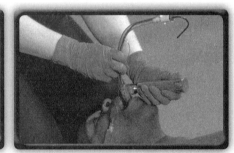

_____ Visualize the vocal cords and watch the ET tube pass between them. Remove the laryngoscope and stylet. Hold the tube carefully.

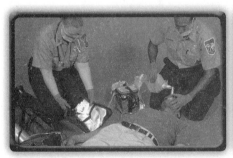

_____ Open and clear the airway. Insert an oral airway, and oxygenate with a bag-mask device.

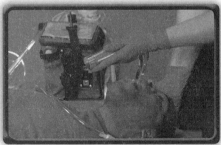

_____ Position the patient's head and remove the oral airway.

Skill Drill 40-2: Spiking the Bag
Test your knowledge of this skill by placing the photos below in the correct order. Number the first step with a "1," the second step with a "2," etc.

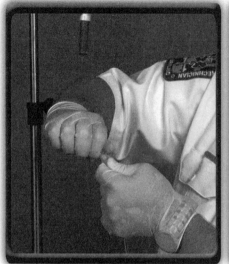 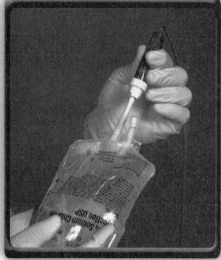 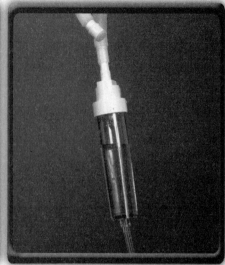

_____ Prime the line to remove air.

_____ Check the drip chamber. It should only be half filled. If the fluid level is too low, squeeze the chamber until it fills. If the drip chamber fills completely, invert the IV bag and squeeze the excess back into the bag.

_____ Slide the spike into the IV bag port.

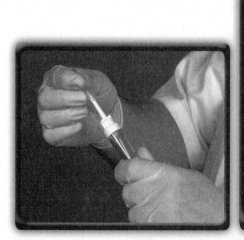 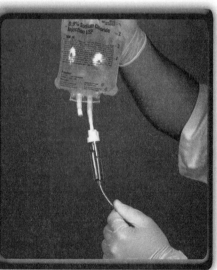

_____ Remove the pigtail from the port on the IV bag and the cover from the spike on the administration set.

_____ Prime the chamber.

Skill Drill 40-3: Starting an IV
Test your knowledge of this skill by placing the photos below in the correct order. Number the first step with a "1," the second step with a "2," etc.

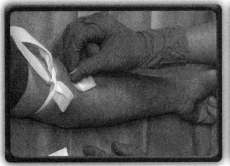

_____ Clean the area using aseptic technique.

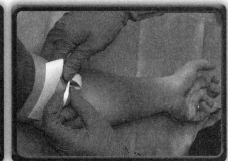

_____ Secure the catheter with tape or a commercial device. Secure IV tubing and adjust the flow rate.

_____ Apply the constricting band above the intended IV site.

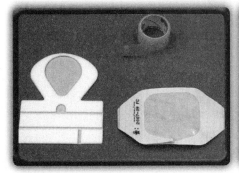

_____ Tear the tape before venipuncture, or have a commercial device available.

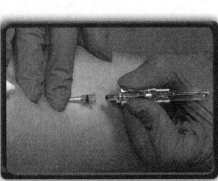

_____ Occlude the catheter to prevent blood leaking while removing the stylet.

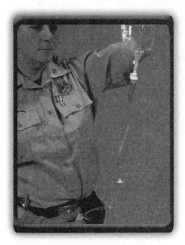

_____ Flush or "bleed" the tubing to remove any air bubbles by opening the roller clamp.

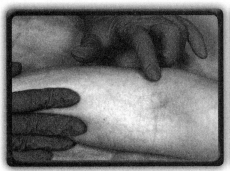

_____ Apply gloves before making contact with the patient. Palpate a suitable vein.

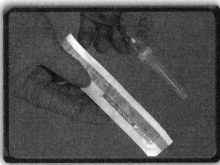

_____ Choose the appropriately sized catheter, and examine it for any imperfections.

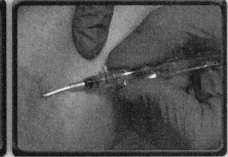

_____ Observe for "flashback" as blood enters the catheter.

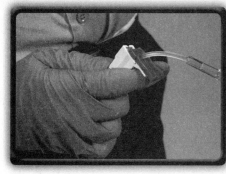

_____ Open the IV line to ensure fluid is flowing and the IV is patent. Observe for swelling and infiltration around the IV site.

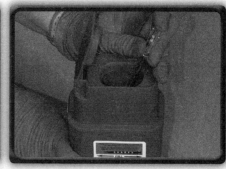

_____ Dispose of all sharps in the proper container.

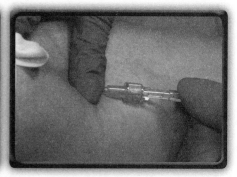

_____ Attach the prepared IV line.

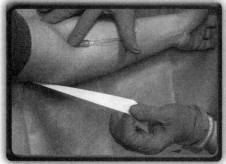

_____ Remove the constricting band.

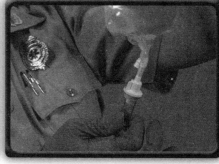

_____ Prepare the solution and tubing to be used. Fill the drip chamber halfway by squeezing it.

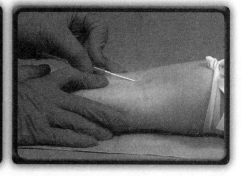

_____ Insert the catheter at an angle of approximately 45° with the bevel up while applying distal traction with the other hand.

Chapter 1: EMS Systems

General Knowledge

Matching

1. H (page 6)
2. F (page 8)
3. M (page 6)
4. G (page 6)
5. A (page 6)
6. K (page 16)
7. B (page 17)
8. C (page 5)
9. L (page 16)
10. E (page 17)
11. I (page 16)
12. D (page 16)
13. J (page 8)

Multiple Choice

1. B (page 7)
2. A (pages 16–17)
3. D (page 17)
4. C (page 17)
5. A (page 24)
6. C (page 16)
7. D (pages 16–17)
8. D (page 6)
9. A (page 6)
10. B (page 12)

True/False

1. F (page 6)
2. T (page 11)
3. F (page 17)
4. T (page 24)
5. T (page 20)
6. T (page 24)

Fill-in-the-Blank

1. Continuous quality improvement (page 17)
2. medical director (page 16)
3. automated external (page 12)
4. service (page 16)
5. access point (page 15)

Crossword Puzzle

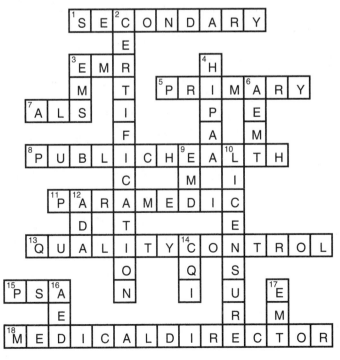

Critical Thinking

Short Answer

1. The EMT is one of the four levels of prehospital care. The EMT provides basic life support, including automated external defibrillation, use of airway adjuncts, and assisting patients with certain medications. (page 6)

2. The Department of Transportation (DOT) has developed a series of guidelines, curricula, funding sources, and assessment tools designed to develop and improve EMS in the United States. (page 9)

3. Keep vehicles and equipment ready for an emergency.

   Ensure the safety of yourself, your partner, the patient, and bystanders.

   Emergency vehicle operation.

   Be an on-scene leader.

   Perform an evaluation of the scene.

   Call for additional resources as needed.

   Gain patient access.

   Perform a patient assessment.

   Give emergency medical care to the patient while awaiting the arrival of additional medical resources.

   Only move patients when absolutely necessary to preserve life.

   Give emotional support to the patient, the patient's family, and other responders.

   Maintain continuity of care by working with other medical professionals.

   Resolve emergency incidents.

   Uphold medical and legal standards.

   Ensure and protect patient privacy.

   Give administrative support.

   Constantly continue your professional development.

   Cultivate and sustain community relations.

   Give back to the profession. (page 23)

4. Online medical direction is provided through radio or telephone connections between the EMT and the medical control facility. Off-line medical direction is provided through written protocols, training, and standing orders. (pages 16–17)

Ambulance Calls

1. You would decline the assistance of an ALS ambulance crew. ALS, or advanced life support, means that the crew would have a higher level of training and could perform more advanced patient care procedures than you or your partner. Because there were no injuries resulting from this motor vehicle collision, there would be no reason to summon advanced care.

2. Because none of the EMT-level airway skills were successful, it is critical to request or rendezvous with a provider capable of using advanced airway techniques. You would contact dispatch and arrange to have an ALS crew either meet you at the patient's location or load the patient and meet up with an ALS crew while en route to the hospital.

Chapter 2: Workforce Safety and Wellness

General Knowledge

Matching

1. D (page 70)
2. A (page 38)
3. C (page 35)

4. F (page 46)
5. B (page 45)
6. E (page 35)

7. M (page 33)
8. G (page 41)
9. L (page 64)

10. I (page 33)
11. J (page 36)
12. N (page 35)

13. H (page 53)
14. K (page 35)

Multiple Choice

1. C (page 55)
2. C (page 55)
3. A (page 55)
4. D (page 55)
5. B (page 55)
6. A (page 56)
7. D (page 56)
8. C (page 57)

9. B (page 57)
10. D (page 57)
11. D (page 57)
12. D (page 59)
13. D (page 60)
14. B (page 72)
15. D (page 45)
16. D (page 46)

17. B (page 46)
18. D (page 46)
19. A (page 48)
20. D (page 48)
21. D (page 46)
22. B (page 49)
23. C (page 46)
24. D (page 46)

25. D (page 47)
26. D (page 53)
27. B (pages 53–54)
28. C (page 62)
29. B (page 36)
30. D (pages 33–34)
31. A (page 40)
32. C (page 38)

33. D (pages 44–45)
34. D (pages 63–67)
35. B (page 42)
36. C (page 63)
37. D (page 71)

True/False

1. F (page 36)
2. F (page 38)

3. T (page 55)
4. F (page 35)

5. F (page 45)
6. T (pages 48–50)

Fill-in-the-Blank

1. well-being (page 33)
2. emotional stress (page 55)
3. heart disease (page 55)

4. hazardous (page 63)
5. handwashing (page 35)
6. concealment (page 70)

7. depression (page 55)
8. minor (page 62)

Crossword Puzzle

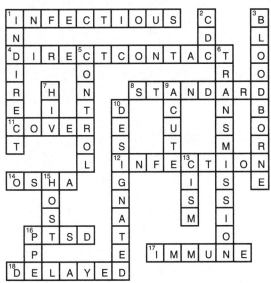

Critical Thinking

Multiple Choice

1. C (page 56)   **2.** D (page 48)   **3.** B (page 46)   **4.** D (page 47)   **5.** A (page 62)

Short Answer

1. Standard precautions are based on the assumption that every person is potentially infected or can spread an organism that could be transmitted in the health care setting. Therefore, you must apply infection-control procedures to reduce infection in patients and health care personnel. (page 35)

2. 1. Denial
   2. Anger/hostility
   3. Bargaining
   4. Depression
   5. Acceptance (page 55)

3. Irritability toward coworkers, family, and friends
   Inability to concentrate
   Difficulty sleeping, increased sleeping, or nightmares
   Anxiety; indecisiveness; guilt
   Loss of appetite (gastrointestinal disturbances)
   Loss of interest in sexual activities
   Isolation
   Loss of interest in work
   Increased use of alcohol
   Recreational drug use
   Physical symptoms such as chronic pain (headache, backache)
   Feelings of hopelessness (page 47)

4. Minimize or eliminate stressors.
   Change partners to avoid a negative or hostile personality.
   Change work hours.
   Change the work environment.

Cut back on overtime.
Change your attitude about the stressor.
Talk about your feelings with people you trust.
Seek professional counseling if needed.
Do not obsess over frustrating situations; focus on delivering high-quality care.
Try to adopt a more relaxed, philosophical outlook.
Expand your social support system apart from your coworkers.
Sustain friends and interests outside emergency services.
Minimize the physical response to stress by employing various techniques. (page 48)

5. 1. Use soap and water.
   2. Rub your hands together for at least 20 seconds to work up a lather.
   3. Rinse your hands using warm water.
   4. Dry your hands with a paper towel and use the paper towel to turn off the faucet. (page 36)

6. 1. Thin inner layer
   2. Thermal middle layer
   3. Outer layer (pages 67–68)

7. 1. Past history
   2. Posture
   3. Vocal activity
   4. Physical activity (page 71)

8. During procedures and patient care activities when contact of the EMT's clothing/exposed skin to blood, body fluids, secretions, excretions, or contaminated items is anticipated

Ambulance Calls

1. Continue to treat the patient appropriately, including c-spine stabilization and transport. Allowing the cut to bleed, as long as the bleeding is minimal, will help to wash/clean it out. Clean the wound with an alcohol gel, if available.

   Once patient care has been transferred at the receiving facility, immediately wash thoroughly with soap and water and report to your supervisor. Follow up with prompt medical attention.

2. As always, you should wear exam gloves and eye protection. Because this call is for a respiratory issue and the possibility of tuberculosis is high, you should also don a HEPA respirator and place a nonrebreathing mask on the patient. It is also very important that you pass the information about potential infection to the receiving facility staff in both your patient report while en route and again when you hand off care in the emergency department.

Fill-in-the-Patient Care Report

EMS Patient Care Report (PCR)			
Date: Today's Date	**Incident No.:** 2011-1234	**Nature of Call:** Overdose	**Location:** 7979 Fisher Blvd.
Dispatched: 0912	**En Route:** 0912	**At Scene:** 0926 **Transport:** 0947	**At Hospital:** 0952 **In Service:** 1005

Patient Information	
Age: 16 Years **Sex:** Female **Weight (in kg [lb]):** 48 kg (106 lb)	**Allergies:** None **Medications:** None **Past Medical History:** Attempted suicide 2 years ago—aspirin overdose **Chief Complaint:** Unresponsive/Overdose

Vital Signs				
Time: 0934	**BP:** 116/76	**Pulse:** 46	**Respirations:** 8 GTV	**Sao₂:** 96%
Time: 0947	**BP:** 114/74	**Pulse:** 38	**Respirations:** 8 GTV	**Sao₂:** 95%

EMS Treatment (circle all that apply)				
Oxygen @ 15 **L/min via (circle one):** NC (NRM) Bag-Mask Device	**Assisted Ventilation**	**Airway Adjunct**		**CPR**
Defibrillation	**Bleeding Control**	**Bandaging**	**Splinting**	**Other Shock Treatment**

Narrative
Dispatched for an overdose. Arrived on scene to find the patient, a 16-year-old girl, unresponsive on the bathroom floor with a hypodermic needle next to her. Although unresponsive, she had a patent airway and was breathing adequately. She was moved out to the living room to allow better access. The patient's mother advised that the patient had attempted suicide 2 years ago with an aspirin overdose and had recently been struggling with heroin use. According to law enforcement on scene, the patient had apparently been arguing with her mother prior to today's events. Vital signs indicated that she was initially stable, but I chose to start her on high-flow oxygen therapy due to the potential for respiratory compromise. The patient was moved to the gurney and placed in the ambulance. I immediately obtained a second set of vitals, which showed a slight decrease in cardiac activity and oxygen saturation, and I continued to monitor her while en route to the receiving hospital without incident. While en route, I called the report in to the hospital and upon turning care of the patient over to the emergency department, I gave a verbal report to the charge nurse. **End of Report**

Skills

Skill Drills

Skill Drill 2-2 Proper Glove Removal Technique

1. Partially remove the first glove by pinching at the **wrist**. Be careful to touch only the **outside** of the glove.

2. Remove the **second** glove by pinching the **exterior** with your partially gloved hand.

3. Pull the second glove inside-out toward the **fingertips**.

4. Grasp both gloves with your **free** hand, touching only the clean, **interior** surfaces. (page 38)

Chapter 3: Medical, Legal, and Ethical Issues

General Knowledge

Matching

1. H (page 91)
2. I (page 91)
3. G (page 84)
4. E (page 91)
5. L (page 90)
6. A (page 84)
7. D (page 79)
8. F (page 90)
9. B (page 80)
10. C (page 81)
11. M (page 80)
12. N (page 80)
13. J (page 90)
14. K (page 88)

Multiple Choice

1. C (page 87)
2. A (page 88)
3. D (page 90)
4. D (page 90)
5. C (page 91)
6. B (page 92)
7. D (page 83)
8. D (pages 91–93)
9. B (page 90)
10. A (page 85)
11. A (page 86)
12. D (page 86)
13. B (page 83)

True/False

1. T (page 90)
2. F (page 80)
3. T (page 80)
4. T (page 81)
5. F (page 85)

Fill-in-the-Blank

1. scope of practice (page 87)
2. standard of care (page 88)
3. duty to act (page 90)
4. negligence (page 90)
5. termination (page 91)
6. Expressed; implied (page 80)
7. assault; battery (page 91)
8. advance directive; DNR order (page 84)
9. refuse treatment (page 82)
10. special reporting (pages 93–94)

Crossword Puzzle

Across:
2. SLANDER
5. GOOD SAMARITAN
9. EXPRESSED
11. PHI
12. LIBEL
13. MORALITY
14. BATTERY
16. ETHICS
17. BIOETHICS

Down:
1. SCOPE
3. (DN...)
4. CONSENT
6. (DEO...)
7. ASSAULT
8. PROXI (PROXIMATE)
10. PR(ECEDENCE)
15. (CONSCIENCE)

Critical Thinking

Multiple Choice

1. B (page 80)
2. A (page 80)
3. A (page 80)
4. C (page 80)
5. B (page 83)
6. D (page 95)

Short Answer

1. If the minor is emancipated, a member of the armed services, married, a parent, or pregnant (page 81)
2. You must continue to care for the patient until the patient is transferred to another medical professional of equal or higher skill level, or another medical facility. (page 91)
3. 1. Obtain refusing party's signature on an official medical release form that acknowledges refusal.
   2. Obtain a signature from a witness of the refusal.
   3. Keep the refusal form with the incident report.
   4. Note the refusal on the incident report.
   5. Keep a department copy of the records for future reference. (page 83)
4. 1. If it wasn't documented, it did not happen.
   2. Incomplete or disorderly records equate to incomplete or inexpert medical care. (page 93)
5. 1. Inform medical control.
   2. Treat the patient as you would any patient.
   3. Take any steps necessary to preserve life.
   4. If saving the patient is not possible, take steps to make sure the organs remain viable. (page 87)

Ambulance Calls

1. This patient needs to be evaluated at the hospital. Her parents will likely feel a right to be informed of their child's medical conditions and medical care. Laws regarding reproductive rights of minors vary from state to state. Some states allow minors to make decisions regarding birth control, prenatal care, or pregnancy termination without consenting parents, whereas others do not. You must know your local laws. You will have to provide information regarding the pregnancy to other health care providers directly involved in her care, and you should explain that fact and the necessity of such to the patient. Be tactful. Don't unnecessarily break your patient's trust by immediately sharing this knowledge with her parents. Document carefully and consult medical control.
2. You have a duty to act regardless of your current off-duty status (some states/provider levels/paid status varies), and you did the right thing by stopping to help the child. Once you have initiated care, you must ensure that the child's parent(s) or legal guardian is notified. Although the grandfather is home, you now have another dilemma. The condition of the house/capability of the grandfather to care for the child while the mother is away is such that the question of neglect arises. You should speak with the grandfather and attempt to contact the mother of the child. If you believe that neglect or abuse of a child is occurring, you are legally required to intervene. You should document the condition of the house and notify medical control and/or child protective serves in accordance with your local protocols.
3. Assess the patient's mental status. If he is intoxicated or has an altered mental status, he is treated under implied consent. If he is alert and oriented, you may attempt to talk him into being treated by explaining what you feel is necessary and what may happen if he does not receive care. If he has an altered mental status, orders from medical control may be obtained to restrain the patient with the help of law enforcement and to transport him to the hospital.

Fill-in-the-Patient Care Report

EMS Patient Care Report (PCR)					
Date: Today's Date	**Incident No.:** 2010-555	**Nature of Call:** MCA		**Location:** Grand and Hopper	
Dispatched: 2115	**En Route:** 2116	**At Scene:** 2122	**Transport:** 2132	**At Hospital:** 2138	**In Service:** 2152

Patient Information	
Age: 24 Years **Sex:** Female **Weight (in kg [lb]):** 52 kg (114 lb)	**Allergies:** N/A **Medications:** N/A **Past Medical History:** N/A **Chief Complaint:** N/A

Vital Signs				
Time: 2127	**BP:** 90/54	**Pulse:** 100 Weak/Irreg	**Respirations:** 12	**Sao$_2$:** 94%
Time: N/A	**BP:** N/A	**Pulse:** N/A	**Respirations:** N/A	**Sao$_2$:** N/A
Time: N/A	**BP:** N/A	**Pulse:** N/A	**Respirations:** N/A	**Sao$_2$:** N/A

EMS Treatment
(circle all that apply)

Oxygen @ 15 L/min via (circle one): NC NRM (Bag-Mask Device)	(Assisted Ventilation)	(Airway Adjunct)	CPR
Defibrillation (Bleeding Control)	(Bandaging)	(Splinting)	Other Shock Treatment

Narrative

9-1-1 dispatch for a motorcycle vs. auto. Upon arrival, found the driver of the auto unhurt and the motorcycle operator unresponsive in the street. She was bleeding heavily from a forehead laceration and did not have a patent airway—snoring respirations observed. Appropriate c-spine precautions taken, OPA inserted, and provided assisted ventilations using bag-mask device with 15 L/min oxygen. Fire crew arrived on scene and assisted in bleeding control, obtaining vitals and immobilizing patient to long backboard. Once adequately immobilized, patient was moved to the stretcher and loaded into the ambulance for transport to the University Trauma Center. Reassessment not completed while en route due to continuation of assisted ventilations. Delivered patient to trauma center and provided verbal report and copy of this written report to the charge nurse.
End of Report

Chapter 4: Communications and Documentation

General Knowledge

Matching

1. M (page 127)
2. G (page 127)
3. J (page 127)
4. K (page 128)
5. H (page 128)
6. L (page 127)
7. I (page 127)
8. C (page 128)
9. A (page 127)
10. F (page 129)
11. E (page 129)
12. D (page 127)
13. B (page 112)

Multiple Choice

1. D (page 127)
2. A (page 127)
3. D (page 127)
4. B (page 128)
5. B (page 128)
6. D (pages 128–129)
7. C (page 129)
8. D (page 130)
9. B (page 131)
10. D (page 132)
11. A (page 134)
12. B (page 134)
13. D (page 134)
14. D (pages 131–133)
15. D (page 134)
16. A (page 134)
17. A (page 134)
18. D (page 108)
19. C (page 131)
20. D (page 135)
21. B (page 118)
22. D (page 107)
23. D (page 118)
24. D (page 109)
25. C (page 116)
26. D (page 114)
27. C (page 116)
28. A (page 117)
29. B (page 120)
30. D (page 119)
31. D (page 121)
32. A (page 119)
33. D (page 125)

True/False

1. T (page 127)
2. T (page 127)
3. F (page 108)
4. F (page 127)
5. T (page 127)
6. T (page 119)
7. F (page 128)
8. F (page 128)
9. F (page 117)
10. T (page 113)

Fill-in-the-Blank

1. patient care report (page 119)
2. transmitter; receiver (page 127)
3. dedicated line (page 127)
4. telemetry (page 128)
5. cell phones (page 128)
6. Pagers (page 131)
7. importance (page 131)
8. medical control (page 132)
9. slander (page 134)
10. medical control (page 134)
11. repeat (page 135)
12. standing orders (page 136)
13. eye contact (page 109)
14. honest (page 115)
15. interpreter (page 117)
16. minimum data set (page 119)
17. Competent (page 124)

Crossword Puzzle

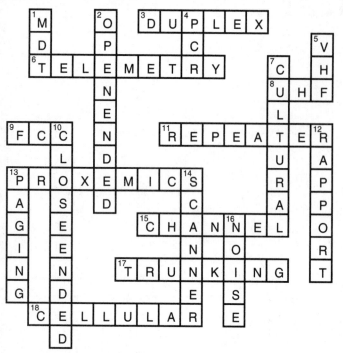

Critical Thinking

Multiple Choice

1. C (page 124)

2. D (page 124)

3. A (page 124)

4. D (page 123)

5. C (page 124)

Short Answer

1. **1.** Allocating specific radio frequencies for use by EMS providers

   2. Licensing base stations and assigning appropriate radio call signs for those stations

   3. Establishing licensing standards and operating specifications for radio equipment used by EMS providers

   4. Establishing limitations for transmitter power output

   5. Monitoring radio operations (page 130)

2. Health Insurance Portability and Accountability Act. It is a government regulation concerning patient privacy and confidentiality. (page 118)

3. **1.** Continuity of care

   2. Legal documentation

   3. Education

   4. Administrative information

   5. Essential research record

   6. Evaluation and continuous quality improvement (page 119)

4. **1.** Traditional, written form with check boxes and a narrative section

   2. Computerized, using electronic clipboard or similar device (page 121)

Ambulance Calls

1. Dispatch the closest ambulance for an emergency response. Call for assistance from the fire department and local law enforcement. Try to calm down the caller to obtain additional information. If the caller is still of no help, ask her to get someone else to the phone. Relay any additional information to the responding units.

2. You should determine whether anyone on scene can translate for you. (Children will often speak both English and Spanish.) If no one on scene can translate, you should contact a department translator. Every department should have a group of translators for different languages common to your community. (Ideally, you should speak languages commonly heard in your area.) If neither of these options is available, you should attempt as much nonverbal communication as possible, obtain baseline vital signs, and perform a primary assessment to determine the nature of the problem. If the patient appears to refuse your help, you are in a tough situation. You cannot leave without knowing what the medical emergency is (if any), and you cannot obtain an informed refusal if clear communication does not occur.

3. Attempt to locate any identification that he may have on his person. If this is not possible or you cannot locate any forms of identification, you should notify law enforcement officers. The child should undergo a medical examination to ensure that no injuries or other medical emergencies are present. Take care to communicate in a nonintimidating manner (taking care in level/tone of voice and posture) and attempt to establish trust with the patient.

Fill-in-the-Patient Care Report

EMS Patient Care Report (PCR)					
Date: Today's Date	**Incident No.:** 2011-8898		**Nature of Call:** Dirt bike crash/ Trauma	**Location:** 18553 Old Redwood Highway	
Dispatched: 1721	**En Route:** 1721	**At Scene:** 1728	**Transport:** 1735	**At Hospital:** 1741	**In Service:** 1800

Patient Information	
Age: 19 Years	**Allergies:** Unknown
Sex: Male	**Medications:** Unknown
Weight (kg [lb]): 73 kg (161 lb)	**Past Medical History:** Unknown
	Chief Complaint: Partial amputation of left foot

Vital Signs				
Time: 1736	**BP:** 104/66	**Pulse:** 102	**Respirations:** 18 Unlabored	**Sao$_2$:** 97%
Time: 1741	**BP:** 110/72	**Pulse:** 90	**Respirations:** 14 Unlabored	**Sao$_2$:** 99%

EMS Treatment (circle all that apply)				
Oxygen @ <u>15</u> L/min via (circle one): NC (NRM) Bag-Mask Device		Assisted Ventilation	Airway Adjunct	CPR
Defibrillation	(Bleeding Control)	(Bandaging)	(Splinting)	(Other Shock Treatment)

Narrative
Responded to 9-1-1 dispatch to a motocross park for a dirt bike crash. Arrived to find the patient, a 19-year-old man, lying supine on the ground and in obvious pain from near amputation of his left foot below the ankle. Patient had patent airway and adequate breathing, and I controlled the bleeding at the injury site with direct pressure. Patient was placed on high-flow oxygen therapy, secured to the backboard utilizing all appropriate spinal precautions, and loaded into ambulance. First set of vitals indicated possible onset of hypoperfusion, so I covered the patient with a blanket and elevated the foot end of the backboard. Called report to the receiving facility and obtained a second set of vitals, which showed improvement when compared to the first. Patient was transported without incident and appropriately turned over to the trauma center staff after I provided a complete verbal report. **End of Report**

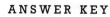

Chapter 5: The Human Body

General Knowledge

Matching

1. F (page 145)	**9.** M (page 167)	**17.** B (page 151)	**25.** B (page 153)	**33.** A (page 176)
2. K (page 168)	**10.** J (page 145)	**18.** A (page 149)	**26.** A (page 153)	**34.** C (pages 174–177)
3. D (page 143)	**11.** O (page 166)	**19.** B (page 151)	**27.** A (page 153)	**35.** E (page 177)
4. G (page 145)	**12.** B (page 145)	**20.** B (page 151)	**28.** C (page 153)	**36.** B (page 176)
5. E (page 144)	**13.** H (page 145)	**21.** A (page 150)	**29.** B (page 153)	**37.** F (page 174)
6. L (page 166)	**14.** N (page 166)	**22.** A (page 150)	**30.** C (page 163)	**38.** D (page 177)
7. A (page 145)	**15.** I (page 145)	**23.** A (page 153)	**31.** A (page 153)	
8. C (page 145)	**16.** B (page 151)	**24.** B (page 153)	**32.** C (page 163)	

Multiple Choice

1. B (page 145)	**3.** B (page 181)	**5.** D (page 166)	**7.** B (page 185)
2. C (page 145)	**4.** B (page 184)	**6.** D (page 181)	

True/False

1. F (page 166)	**3.** T (pages 150–151)	**5.** F (page 149)	**7.** F (page 169)
2. F (page 152)	**4.** F (page 164)	**6.** F (page 159)	

Fill-in-the-Blank

1. 7 (page 148)

2. mandible (page 148)

3. 5 (page 157)

4. Twelve (page 148)

5. 33 (page 148)

6. talus (page 151)

7. frontal; parietal; temporal; occipital (page 174)

8. interstitial (page 171)

9. ventilation (page 158)

10. V/Q (page 189)

Labeling

1. Directional Terms (page 144)
  A. Medial
  B. Lateral
  C. Midline
  D. Posterior (rear)
  E. Superior
  F. Anterior
  G. Proximal
  H. Distal
  I. Inferior

2. Anatomic Positions (page 146)
  A. Prone
  B. Supine
  C. Shock position (modified Trendelenburg's position)
  D. Fowler's position
  E. Recovery position

3. The Skull (page 148)
  A. Parietal bone
  B. Frontal bone
  C. Maxilla
  D. Temporal bone
  E. Nasal bones
  F. Zygomatic bone
  G. Maxillae
  H. Foramen magnum
  I. Occipital bone
  J. Mandible

4. The Spinal Column (page 149)

   A. Cerebrum

   B. Foramen magnum

   C. Brain stem

   D. Cerebellum

   E. Cervical nerves

   F. Cervical vertebrae

   G. Thoracic nerves

   H. Thoracic vertebrae

   I. Lumbar vertebrae

   J. Lumbosacral nerves

   K. Sacral vertebrae

   L. Coccygeal vertebrae

5. The Thorax (page 149)

   A. Jugular notch

   B. Manubrium

   C. Sternum

   D. Body

   E. Xiphoid process

   F. Anterior ribs

   G. Costal arch

6. The Shoulder Girdle (page 149)

   A. Sternoclavicular joint

   B. Clavicle

   C. Acromioclavicular (A/C) joint

   D. Humerus

   E. Sternum

   F. Scapula

   G. Glenohumeral (shoulder) joint

7. The Wrist and Hand (page 150)

   A. Index

   B. Long

   C. Ring

   D. Small

   E. Phalanges

   F. Thumb

   G. Metacarpals

   H. Carpometacarpal joint

   I. Carpals

   J. Radius

   K. Ulna

8. The Pelvis (page 150)

   A. Inferior vena cava

   B. Descending aorta

   C. Iliac crest

   D. Ilium

   E. Sacrum

   F. Pubis

   G. Acetabulum

   H. Pubic symphysis

   I. Ischial tuberosity

   J. Femoral artery

   K. Ischium

   L. Femoral vein

9. The Lower Extremity (page 151)

   A. Pelvis

   B. Femoral head

   C. Greater trochanter

   D. Hip

   E. Lesser trochanter

   F. Femur

   G. Thigh

   H. Patella (knee cap)

   I. Knee

   J. Fibula

   K. Leg

   L. Tibia (shin bone)

   M. Ankle

   N. Tarsals

   O. Foot

   P. Metatarsals

   Q. Phalanges

10. The Foot (page 151)

   A. Achilles tendon

   B. Medial malleolus

   C. Talus

   D. Navicular

   E. Medial cuneiform

   F. Phalanges

   G. Metatarsal

   H. Calcaneus

11. The Respiratory System (page 156)

   A. Upper airway

   B. Nasopharynx

   C. Nasal air passage

   D. Pharynx

   E. Oropharynx

   F. Mouth

   G. Epiglottis

   H. Larynx

   I. Trachea

   J. Apex of the lung

   K. Bronchioles

   L. Lower airway

   M. Carina

   N. Main bronchi

   O. Base of the lung

   P. Diaphragm

   Q. Alveoli

12. The Circulatory System (page 164)

   A. Tissue cells

   B. Systemic (body) capillaries

   C. Venule

   D. Arteriole

   E. Vein

   F. Aorta

   G. Artery

   H. Pulmonary (lung) capillaries

   I. Right atrium

   J. Heart

   K. Left atrium

   L. Right ventricle

   M. Left ventricle

13. Central and Peripheral Pulses (page 168)

   A. Superficial temporal

   B. External maxillary

   C. Carotid

   D. Brachial

   E. Ulnar

   F. Radial

   G. Femoral

   H. Posterior tibial

   I. Dorsalis pedis

14. The Brain (page 175)

   A. Cerebrum

   B. Brain stem

   C. Cerebellum

15. Anatomy of the Skin (page 178)

   A. Hair

   B. Pore

   C. Epidermis

   D. Germinal layer of epidermis

   E. Sebaceous gland

   F. Erector pillae muscle

   G. Dermis

   H. Nerve (sensory)

   I. Sweat gland

   J. Hair follicle

   K. Blood vessel

   L. Subcutaneous fat

   M. Fascia

   N. Subcutaneous tissue

   O. Muscle

16. The Male Reproductive System
(page 186)

A. Ureter

B. Urinary bladder

C. Vasa deferentia

D. Prostate gland

E. Pubic bone

F. Prostate gland

G. Urethra

H. Urethra

I. Epididymis

J. Testis

K. Penis

L. Glans penis

M. Scrotum

17. The Female Reproductive System
(page 187)

A. Uterine (fallopian) tube

B. Uterus

C. Ovary

D. Cervix

E. Vagina

Crossword Puzzle

Critical Thinking

Multiple Choice

1. C (page 151) **2.** A (page 148) **3.** A (page 180) **4.** A (page 147) **5.** B (page 147)

Short Answer

1. **1.** Plasma: A sticky, yellow fluid that carries the blood cells and nutrients

2. Red blood cells: Give blood its red color and carry oxygen

3. White blood cells: Play a role in the body's immune defense mechanism against infection

4. Platelets: Essential in the formation of blood clots (pages 169–170)

2. **1.** Cervical spine: 7 vertebrae

2. Thoracic spine: 12 vertebrae

3. Lumbar spine: 5 vertebrae

4. Sacrum: 5 vertebrae

5. Coccyx: 4 vertebrae (page 148)

3. **RUQ:** liver, gallbladder, large intestine, small intestine

LUQ: stomach, spleen, large intestine, small intestine

RLQ: large intestine, small intestine, appendix, ascending colon

LLQ: large intestine, small intestine (page 180)

4. **1.** Superior and inferior vena cava

2. Right atrium

3. Right ventricle

4. Pulmonary artery

5. Lungs

6. Pulmonary vein

7. Left atrium

8. Left ventricle

9. Aorta (page 164)

Ambulance Calls

1. Lacerated liver, gallbladder, small intestine, large intestine, pancreas, diaphragm, right lung if the pathway is up, right kidney depending on length of knife. You could also have involvement of the other four quadrants based on the direction of travel of the blade. The description would be a puncture wound or stab wound.

2. The mechanism of injury is significant in this scenario. Not only did the patient's vehicle impact a solid, stationary object, but there was also enough force to deform the steering wheel. This patient was not restrained, and the abrupt deceleration caused the driver's chest to impact the steering wheel with significant force. He could have numerous internal injuries, including pneumo- and/or hemothorax, cardiac or pulmonary contusions, and fractured ribs/sternum (not to mention spinal and head injuries). Immediate transport with full spinal precautions and high-flow oxygen is required.

3. Depending on the condition of the track, the rider's use of protective gear, and the speed and height of the fall, he may or may not have sustained significant injuries. Given his self-splinting, it can be assumed that he has (at minimum) fractures to the left humerus, radius and/or ulna, and clavicle. Treat and transport according to local protocols.

Fill-in-the-Patient Care Report

EMS Patient Care Report (PCR)					
Date: Today's date	**Incident No.:** 2011-0000		**Nature of Call:** Assault		**Location:** Alpha St. and 15th Ave.
Dispatched: 2312	**En Route:** 2312	**At Scene:** 2329	**Transport:** 2341	**At Hospital:** 2354	**In Service:** 0009
Patient Information					
Age: 38 Years			**Allergies:** Unknown		
Sex: Female			**Medications:** Unknown		
Weight (in kg [lb]): 52 kg (115 lb)			**Past Medical History:** Unknown		
			Chief Complaint: Generalized Pain		
Vital Signs					
Time: 2343	**BP:** 108/56	**Pulse:** 96	**Respirations:** 16 GTV/Labored		**Sao₂:** 96%
Time: 2349	**BP:** 104/54	**Pulse:** 104	**Respirations:** 18 Adequate Tidal Volume/Labored		**Sao₂:** 95%
EMS Treatment **(circle all that apply)**					
Oxygen @ 15 **L/min via (circle one):** NC NRM Bag-Mask Device			**Assisted Ventilation**	**Airway Adjunct:**	**CPR**
Defibrillation	**Bleeding Control**		**Bandaging**	(**Splinting**)	(**Other Shock Treatment**)
Narrative					

Dispatched to 9-1-1 scene for assault victim. Arrived to find 38-year-old woman lying on the sidewalk guarding her torso and moaning. Police officer on scene advised that patient was assaulted by several people. Confirmed airway, breathing, and adequate circulation. Properly secured patient to long backboard after initiating oxygen therapy via nonrebreathing mask. Once en route to the trauma center, baseline vitals were obtained, indicating possible onset of hypoperfusion. Patient found to have contusions to both upper extremities, left lateral chest, anterior of both lower extremities, as well as abdominal rigidity and guarding. Subsequent vitals indicated continuing trend of possible hypoperfusion. Treated patient for shock and contacted receiving facility to give verbal report. Arrived at the trauma center and properly transferred patient to their care, providing a full verbal report to attending physician. **End of Report**

Chapter 6: Life Span Development

General Knowledge

Matching

1. L (page 205)
2. J (page 204)
3. A (page 211)
4. E (page 205)
5. B (page 209)
6. N (page 206)
7. K (page 206)
8. C (page 208)
9. H (page 202)
10. I (page 206)
11. M (page 202)
12. D (page 202)
13. F (page 204)
14. G (page 208)

Multiple Choice

1. B (page 211)
2. C (page 206)
3. D (page 206)
4. A (page 211)
5. D (page 207)
6. C (page 201)
7. A (page 209)
8. C (page 209)
9. B (page 203)
10. C (page 210)
11. B (page 204)
12. C (page 210)
13. A (page 205)
14. D (page 208)
15. B (page 203)

True/False

1. F (page 212)
2. F (page 202)
3. T (page 205)
4. T (page 210)
5. F (page 211)
6. F (page 207)
7. F (page 205)
8. T (page 203)
9. T (page 202)
10. F (page 207)

Fill-in-the-Blank

1. Early; 40 (page 208)
2. 90; 150; 20; 30 (page 205)
3. life's goals (page 209)
4. well; clearly (page 211)
5. identity (page 207)
6. neonate; 8; 25 (page 202)
7. fragile; barotrauma (page 202)
8. 18; effect (page 206)
9. nutritional; older (page 211)
10. mental; terminal drop (page 212)

Crossword Puzzle

Critical Thinking

Multiple Choice

1. C (page 206)
2. A (page 206)
3. B (page 206)

Short Answer

1. As people age, the size of the airway increases and the surface area of the alveoli decreases. The natural elasticity of the lungs also decreases, forcing individuals to use the muscles between their ribs, called intercostal muscles, more to breathe. As the elasticity of the lungs decreases, the overall strength of the intercostal muscles and diaphragm also decreases. (page 210)
2. Conventional reasoning means that children are looking for approval from their peers and society. (page 206)
3. "Trust and mistrust" refers to a stage of development from birth to about 18 months of age that involves an infant's needs being met by his or her parents or caregivers. When caregivers and parents provide an organized, routine environment, the infant gains trust in those individuals. If the environment is not perceived as secure by the infant, a sense of mistrust will develop. (page 204)
4. Until about 5 years before death, most late-stage adults retain high brain function. In the 5 years preceding death, however, mental function is presumed to decline, a theory referred to as the terminal drop hypothesis. (page 212)
5. Neonate (0 to 1 month)

   Infant (1 month to 1 year)

   Toddler (1 to 3 years)

   Preschool age (3 to 6 years)

   School age (6 to 12 years)

   Adolescent (12 to 18 years)

   Early adult (19 to 40 years)

   Middle adult (41 to 60 years)

   Late adult (61 and older) (page 201)

Ambulance Calls

1. You should be concerned about intracranial bleeding with this patient, because he is at an age where brain shrinkage has likely occurred and the hematoma suggests that he hit his head after falling, which could have ruptured some of the bridging blood vessels.
2. The first thing you must keep in mind is that our daily experiences as EMTs can "color" our responses. This means that you can begin to see similarities between calls where none actually exist. It is very important to treat each call as a new and different situation and not to make assumptions without very clear reasons. In this particular situation, you should not try to speak to the child alone. Children between the ages of 10 and 18 months are at the pinnacle of the separation anxiety stage, and removing the child from the parents will likely cause her to become noncommunicative and very upset. In this situation, you should keep the child with her parents, and if you truly suspect some type of abuse, you should report it afterwards based on your local guidelines.
3. The best way to help this patient is to separate him from the other students before asking him about his injuries. Adolescents are very focused on their public image and are easily embarrassed. Falling off the stage in front of his peers would have embarrassed this teen enough, and publicly admitting to a subsequent injury would make it even worse for him.

Fill-in-the-Patient Care Report

EMS Patient Care Report (PCR)			
Date: Today's Date	**Incident No.:** 2011-9999	**Nature of Call:** Respiratory distress	**Location:** 16654 Geary Street
Dispatched: 0345	**En Route:** 0348	**At Scene:** 0359	**Transport:** 0410	**At Hospital:** 0417	**In Service:** 0435

Patient Information	
Age: 93 Years	**Allergies:** Penicillin
Sex: Female	**Medications:** Blood pressure
Weight (kg [lb]): 44 kg (97 lb)	**Past Medical History:** Three MIs
	Chief Complaint: Respiratory distress

Vital Signs				
Time: N/A	**BP:** N/A	**Pulse:** N/A	**Respirations:** N/A	**Sao$_2$:** 95%

EMS Treatment
(circle all that apply)

Oxygen @ 15 L/min via (circle one): NC NRM (Bag-Mask Device)	(Assisted Ventilation)	Airway Adjunct	CPR
Defibrillation	**Bleeding Control**	**Bandaging**	**Splinting**	**Other Shock Treatment**

Narrative

Dispatched on a 9-1-1 call for a respiratory distress patient. Arrived to find the patient, a 93-year-old woman, in the tripod position and clearly struggling to breathe. Just as patient contact was made, patient went into respiratory arrest and bag-mask ventilations were immediately initiated. Patient was moved to the gurney and loaded into the ambulance for transport. Due to ongoing interventions, no vital signs were obtained except for a consistent Sao$_2$ reading of 95% while en route to the receiving facility. Patient report to the receiving facility was relayed through the dispatch center, and ventilations were continued during entire transport. At the receiving facility, patient care was properly transferred to the facility staff and a full verbal report was provided. **End of Report**

Chapter 7: Principles of Pharmacology

General Knowledge

Matching

1. I (page 222)
2. J (page 222)
3. F (page 222)
4. G (page 232)
5. D (page 221)
6. H (page 222)
7. B (page 221)
8. C (page 221)
9. E (page 224)
10. A (page 226)

Multiple Choice

1. C (page 221)
2. A (page 234)
3. A (page 222)
4. A (page 223)
5. D (page 224)
6. D (page 225)
7. B (page 237)
8. D (page 236)
9. B (page 236)
10. A (page 234)
11. A, B, C (page 234)
12. C (pages 230–231)
13. C (page 233)
14. A (page 222)
15. B (page 233)
16. B (page 237)

True/False

1. F (page 237)
2. F (page 233)
3. F (page 235)
4. T (page 235)
5. F (page 234)
6. T (page 228)
7. F (page 236)
8. F (page 234)

Fill-in-the-Blank

1. Glucose (page 233)
2. Epinephrine (page 235)
3. sublingually (page 235)
4. intravenous injection (page 223)
5. solutions (page 225)
6. medication (page 221)

Crossword Puzzle

Critical Thinking

Multiple Choice

1. D (page 233)   **2.** D (page 234)   **3.** B (page 236)   **4.** A (page 233)   **5.** C (page 234)

Short Answer

1. **1.** intravenous
   2. intramuscular
   3. transcutaneous
   4. oral
   5. intraosseous
   6. inhalation
   7. sublingual
   8. subcutaneous
   9. per rectum
   10. intranasal (pages 223–224)

2. **1.** Obtain an order from medical control.
   2. Verify the proper patient, medication, and prescription.
   3. Verify the form, dose, and route.
   4. Check the expiration date and condition of medication.
   5. Reassess vital signs, especially heart rate and blood pressure, at least every 5 minutes or as the patient's condition changes.
   6. Document. (page 228)

3. Many drugs adsorb (stick to) activated charcoal, preventing the drugs from being absorbed by the body. It needs to be shaken because it is a suspension and should be given in a covered container with a straw. (pages 226, 232)

4. **1.** Secreted naturally by the adrenal glands
   2. Dilates lung passages
   3. Constricts blood vessels
   4. Increases heart rate and blood pressure (page 236)

5. By pressing it into the skin (page 236)

6. **1.** Headache
   2. Burning under the tongue
   3. Hypotension
   4. Nausea (page 231)

7. To aim the spray properly and ensure inhalation of all medication (page 238)

Ambulance Calls

1. This patient is in serious trouble. The history of the events combined with his level of consciousness, stridor, and hypotension are obvious signs of an anaphylactic reaction. You must immediately administer epinephrine in order to counteract the effects of the insect stings (ie, histamine release). If available, ALS providers should be requested. If not available, transport to the nearest appropriate facility should occur without delay. With the presence of multiple stings, this patient will likely need repeat doses of epinephrine as well as the administration of antihistamines, breathing treatments, and possibly advanced airway maneuvers. Your partner should apply high-flow oxygen and remove any remaining stingers in the neck or face by scraping them from the skin. Your prompt action is essential to patient survival.

2. This patient is suffering from hypoglycemia. Although this patient is confused, he is able to talk and swallow. Some states allow EMTs to perform blood glucose tests, and this would provide information regarding this patient's blood glucose level. If your local protocols do not allow for this skill, you can gather much information about this patient through his physical signs and medical history (all indicative of low blood sugar). You should administer (at least) one tube of oral glucose and reassess his mentation and vital signs. Provide treatment and transport according to local protocols.

3. Place patient in position of comfort.

   Give 100% oxygen via nonrebreathing mask.

   Check blood pressure!

   Check the expiration date on the nitroglycerin.

   Contact medical control for permission to assist patient with one nitroglycerin tablet, SL.

   Monitor vital signs.

   Provide rapid transport.

Fill-in-the-Patient Care Report

EMS Patient Care Report (PCR)			
Date: Today's Date	**Incident No.:** 2010-345	**Nature of Call:** Respiratory Distress	**Location:** Northern Park
Dispatched: N/A	**En Route:** N/A	**At Scene:** 1300	**Transport:** 1308	**At Hospital:** 1318	**In Service:** 1348

Patient Information	
Age: 38 Years	**Allergies:** Unknown
Sex: Female	**Medications:** Metered Dose Inhaler for Asthma
Weight (in kg [lb]): 45 kg (100 lb)	**Past Medical History:** Asthma
	Chief Complaint: Respiratory Distress

Vital Signs				
Time: 1308	**BP:** 142/98	**Pulse:** 110 Regular	**Respirations:** 28 Labored	**Sao$_2$:** 88%
Time: 1313	**BP:** 138/90	**Pulse:** 102 Regular	**Respirations:** 24 Labored	**Sao$_2$:** 92%
Time: 1318	**BP:** 132/88	**Pulse:** 96 Regular	**Respirations:** 20 GTV	**Sao$_2$:** 96%

EMS Treatment
(circle all that apply)

Oxygen @ 15 L/min via (circle one): NC (NRM) Bag-Mask Device	Assisted Ventilation	Airway Adjunct	CPR
Defibrillation	Bleeding Control	Bandaging	Splinting	Other Shock Treatment

Narrative

Summoned by civilian on scene for a respiratory distress. Arrived at patient's location to find a 38-year-old female on a park bench in the tripod position and struggling to breathe. Additionally I observed a bluish hue around the patient's mouth and fingernails and accessory muscle use in her neck. A bystander handed me a metered dose inhaler prescribed for asthma and told me that the patient had dropped it. The patient took the inhaler and inhaled one full puff of the device. The patient was then placed on high-concentration oxygen via nonrebreathing mask and prepared for transport. The patient was already beginning to show signs of improvement (bluish color fading, better tidal volume) as I obtained the first set of vitals and began transport to the emergency department. During transport, I was able to initiate reassessments, obtaining two more full sets of vital signs, which tended to show that the patient was improving as a result of the inhaler use and the oxygen therapy. While en route, I provided the receiving facility with a patient report and the transport was uneventful. Once at the emergency department, the patient was properly transferred to their care and a full verbal report was provided. **End of Report**

Skills

Skill Drill

Skill Drill 7-1: Oral Medication Administration

Take **standard** precautions. Prepare the appropriate amount of medication. Instruct the patient to **chew** (if appropriate) or swallow the medication with water, if administering a **pill** or **tablet**. (page 233)

Chapter 8: Patient Assessment

General Knowledge

Matching

1. P (page 258)	**8.** A (page 266)	**15.** K (page 262)	**22.** L (page 282)	**28.** B (page 281)
2. Q (page 272)	**9.** O (page 280)	**16.** C (page 269)	**23.** C (page 282)	**29.** J (page 282)
3. M (page 303)	**10.** R (page 273)	**17.** D (page 273)	**24.** E (page 282)	**30.** G (page 282)
4. T (page 272)	**11.** G (page 273)	**18.** J (page 273)	**25.** H (page 282)	**31.** A (page 281)
5. B (page 272)	**12.** E (page 262)	**19.** H (page 289)	**26.** K (page 282)	**32.** D (page 282)
6. S (page 253)	**13.** F (page 282)	**20.** N (page 303)	**27.** F (page 282)	
7. L (page 269)	**14.** I (page 270)	**21.** I (page 282)		

Multiple Choice

1. C (page 254)	**10.** C (page 262)	**19.** D (page 273)	**28.** B (page 268)	**37.** B (page 269)
2. A (page 255)	**11.** B (page 262)	**20.** C (page 274)	**29.** C (page 283)	**38.** A (page 270)
3. B (page 257)	**12.** B (page 266)	**21.** A (page 257)	**30.** B (page 284)	**39.** B (page 273)
4. C (page 257)	**13.** D (page 270)	**22.** C (page 262)	**31.** C (page 289)	**40.** C (page 270)
5. B (page 268)	**14.** A (page 270)	**23.** B (page 289)	**32.** D (page 296)	**41.** B (page 306)
6. A (page 289)	**15.** A (page 272)	**24.** C (page 264)	**33.** A (page 297)	**42.** A (page 253)
7. C (page 280)	**16.** C (page 270)	**25.** A (page 264)	**34.** B (page 301)	**43.** D (page 296)
8. B (page 259)	**17.** D (page 271)	**26.** D (page 266)	**35.** B (page 303)	**44.** A (page 287)
9. B (page 261)	**18.** D (pages 272–273)	**27.** A (page 265)	**36.** A (page 306)	**45.** C (page 286)

True/False

1. F (page 262)	**7.** F (page 303)	**13.** F (pages 264–265)	**19.** T (page 280)	**25.** F (page 285)
2. F (page 306)	**8.** F (page 304)	**14.** F (page 266)	**20.** F (page 282)	**26.** T (page 285)
3. T (page 301)	**9.** T (page 306)	**15.** T (page 266)	**21.** T (page 283)	**27.** T (page 286)
4. F (page 270)	**10.** T (page 256)	**16.** T (page 275)	**22.** T (page 284)	**28.** F (page 286)
5. T (page 261)	**11.** F (pages 261–262)	**17.** F (page 277)	**23.** F (page 284)	**29.** T (pages 291, 301)
6. T (page 291)	**12.** T (page 264)	**18.** T (page 278)	**24.** T (page 285)	**30.** T (page 302)

Fill-in-the-Blank

1. sign (page 253)
2. Standard precautions (pages 257–258)
3. incident command system (page 258)
4. Advanced life support (ALS) (page 258)
5. primary assessment (page 261)
6. general impression (page 261)
7. Perfusion (page 262)
8. Orientation (page 262)
9. constrict (page 264)
10. stridor (page 265)
11. jaw-thrust (page 265)
12. exhalation (page 266)
13. airway (page 266)
14. suction (page 267)
15. respiratory infection (page 267)
16. Nasal flaring (page 269)
17. CPR (page 270)
18. Tachycardia (page 272)
19. conjunctiva (page 272)
20. hypoperfusion (page 273)

21. diaphoretic (page 273)
22. two (page 274)
23. Airway (page 274)
24. 60; 90 (page 275)
25. Golden Period (page 277)
26. life threats (page 278)
27. History taking (page 280)
28. open-ended (page 280)

29. SAMPLE (page 281)
30. Pertinent negatives (page 282)
31. hypoxia (page 286)
32. Palpation (page 289)
33. Capnography (page 290)
34. Diastolic pressure (page 296)
35. neurologic (page 301)

Crossword Puzzle

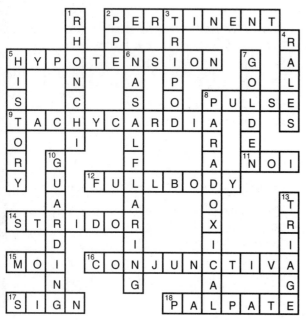

Critical Thinking

Short Answer

1. To identify and initiate treatment of immediate or potential life threats (page 261)
2. Age, sex, race, level of distress, and overall appearance (page 261)
3. **A**—Airway
   B—Breathing
   C—Circulation (page 261)
4. Orientation to person, place, time, and event. Person (name) evaluates long-term memory. Place and time evaluate intermediate-term memory. Event evaluates short-term memory. (pages 262–263)
5. 1. Does the patient appear to be choking?
   2. Is the respiratory rate too fast or too slow?
   3. Are the patient's respirations shallow or deep?

4. Is the patient cyanotic (blue)?
5. Do you hear abnormal sounds when listening to the lungs?
6. Is the patient moving air into and out of the lungs on both sides? (page 266)

6. **D**—Deformities
   C—Contusions
   A—Abrasions
   P—Punctures/penetrations
   B—Burns
   T—Tenderness
   L—Lacerations
   S—Swelling (page 289)

7. Mechanisms of injury
1. Pedestrian struck by a vehicle
2. Motor vehicle collisions
3. Assaults
4. Stabbings
5. Gunshot wounds

Natures of illness
1. Seizures
2. Heart attacks
3. Diabetic problems
4. Poisonings (page 257)

Ambulance Calls

1. Maintain cervical spine control and immediately manage the airway by suction and oxygen. Conduct a rapid survey and transport the patient to the nearest appropriate facility. This patient is a load-and-go based on his mechanism of injury, level of consciousness, and airway compromise. Damage to the vehicle indicates possible occult injuries.

2. This patient is having a very serious asthma attack. Accessory muscle use (nasal flaring, tracheal tugging, suprasternal and intercostal muscle retractions), work of breathing, wheezing, and one- to two-word responses all point to the seriousness of his attack. You should transport immediately, apply high-flow oxygen, and assist with metered-dose administration, according to your local protocols.

8. Pupils equal and round, regular in size, react to light (pages 264–265)

9. A sign is a condition that can be seen, heard, felt, smelled, or measured (objective). A symptom is something that the patient reports to you as a problem or feeling (subjective). (page 253)

10. 1. How many patients are there?
   2. What is the nature of their conditions?
   3. Who contacted EMS?
   4. Does the scene pose a threat to you, your patient, or others? (page 259)

3. Mechanism of injury is significant for this patient. Not only did he fall down a flight of wooden stairs, but he landed on a cement floor. His head injury is likely more significant than the bruising and laceration you can see. He could also have skull fractures, contusions, or intracranial bleeding. With any significant trauma to the head comes the likelihood for cervical spine fractures. You should also question the mechanism of his fall, because medical conditions can sometimes precipitate injuries. Full cervical spine precautions must be taken along with application of high-flow oxygen and prompt transport.

Skills

Skill Drills

Skill Drill 8-1: Rapid Scan
1. Assess the head. Have your partner maintain in-line stabilization if trauma is suspected.
2. Assess the neck.
3. Apply a cervical spinal immobilization device on trauma patients.
4. Assess the chest. Listen to breath sounds on both sides of the chest.
5. Assess the abdomen.
6. Assess the pelvis. If there is no pain, gently compress the pelvis downward and inward to look for tenderness and instability.
7. Assess all four extremities. Assess pulse and the motor and sensory function.
8. Assess the back. In trauma patients, roll the patient in one motion. (pages 276–277)

Skill Drill 8-3: Obtaining Blood Pressure by Auscultation
1. Follow standard precautions. Check for ports, central lines, mastectomy, and injury to the arm. If any are present, use the other arm. Apply the cuff snugly. The lower border of the cuff should be about 1" above the antecubital space.
2. Support the exposed arm at the level of the heart. Palpate the brachial artery.
3. Place the stethoscope over the brachial artery, and grasp the ball-pump and turn-valve.
4. Close the valve, and pump to 30 mm Hg above the point at which you stop hearing pulse sounds. Note the systolic and diastolic pressures as you let air escape slowly.
5. Open the valve, and quickly release remaining air. (pages 299–300)

Chapter 9: Airway Management

General Knowledge

Matching

1. C (page 324)
2. I (page 326)
3. H (page 322)
4. G (page 323)
5. K (page 326)
6. E (page 325)
7. A (page 323)
8. F (page 324)
9. L (page 319)
10. D (page 321)
11. J (page 326)
12. B (page 333)

Multiple Choice

1. D (page 327)
2. B (page 337)
3. B (page 331)
4. B (page 327)
5. A (page 324)
6. A (page 332)
7. C (page 339)
8. D (page 358)
9. C (page 359)
10. C (page 344)
11. A (page 354)
12. C (page 328)
13. D (page 331)
14. B (page 332)
15. C (page 346)

True/False

1. F (page 338)
2. T (page 352)
3. F (page 339)
4. F (page 347)
5. F (page 347)

Fill-in-the-Blank

1. mouth and nose (page 324)
2. higher (page 326)
3. 21; 78 (page 327)
4. carbon dioxide (page 324)
5. diaphragm; intercostal muscles (page 324)
6. Positive; Pressure (page 362)
7. hypoxia (page 326)

Labeling

1. **Upper and Lower Airways**
   - **A.** Upper airway
   - **B.** Nasopharynx
   - **C.** Nasal air passage
   - **D.** Pharynx
   - **E.** Oropharynx
   - **F.** Mouth
   - **G.** Epiglottis
   - **H.** Larynx
   - **I.** Trachea
   - **J.** Apex of the lung
   - **K.** Bronchioles
   - **L.** Lower airway
   - **M.** Carina
   - **N.** Main bronchus
   - **O.** Pulmonary capillaries
   - **P.** Base of the lung
   - **Q.** Diaphragm
   - **R.** Alveoli (page 320)

2. **Oral Cavity**
   - **A.** Hard palate
   - **B.** Soft palate
   - **C.** Entrance to auditory tube
   - **D.** Nasal cavity
   - **E.** Upper lip
   - **F.** Tongue
   - **G.** Nasopharynx
   - **H.** Gingiva
   - **I.** Uvula
   - **J.** Oropharynx
   - **K.** Epiglottis
   - **L.** Laryngopharynx
   - **M.** Hyoid bone (page 321)

3. **Thoracic Cavity**
   - **A.** Trachea
   - **B.** Vena cava
   - **C.** Aorta
   - **D.** Bronchus
   - **E.** Heart
   - **F.** Lung (page 323)

Crossword Puzzle

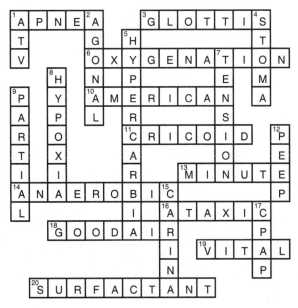

Critical Thinking

Multiple Choice

1. B (page 337)   **2.** D (page 343)   **3.** C (page 338)   **4.** D (page 359)   **5.** A (page 355)

Short Answer

1. **1.** restlessness
   2. tachycardia
   3. irritability
   4. anxiety
   5. apprehension (page 327)

2. Adults: 12 to 20 breaths/min
   Children: 15 to 30 breaths/min
   Infants: 25 to 50 breaths/min (page 332)

3. Give slow, gentle breaths. (page 365)

4. **1.** A peak flow rate of 100% oxygen at up to 40 L/min
   2. An inspiratory pressure safety release valve that opens at approximately 60 cm of water and vents any remaining volume to the atmosphere or stops the flow of oxygen
   3. An audible alarm that sounds whenever you exceed the relief valve pressure
   4. The ability to operate satisfactorily under normal and varying environmental conditions
   5. A trigger positioned so that both your hands can remain on the mask to provide an airtight seal while supporting and tilting the patient's head and keeping the jaw elevated (page 361)

5. **1.** Respiratory rate of less than 12 breaths/min or greater than 20 breaths/min

2. Accessory muscle use
3. Skin pulling in around the ribs during inspiration
4. Pale, cyanotic, or cool (clammy) skin
5. Irregular rhythm
6. Diminished, absent, or noisy breath sounds
7. Reduced flow of expired air at the nose and mouth
8. Unequal or inadequate chest expansion
9. Shallow depth (pages 331–332)

6. They are the secondary muscles of respiration. They are not used in normal breathing. They include:
   1. Sternocleidomastoid (neck) muscles
   2. Chest pectoralis major muscles
   3. Abdominal muscles (pages 324, 332)

7. When the patient has experienced severe trauma to the head or face (page 340)

8. **1.** Select the proper-size airway and apply a water-soluble lubricant.
   2. Place the airway in the larger nostril with the curvature following the curve of the floor of the nose.
   3. Advance the airway gently.
   4. Continue until the flange rests against the skin. (page 342)

9. Tonsil tips are best because they have a large diameter and do not collapse. In addition, they are curved, which allows easy, rapid placement. (pages 343–344)

10. 15 seconds (page 344)

Ambulance Calls

1. Maintain cervical spine stabilization. Immediately open the airway with the jaw-thrust maneuver. Suction to remove the obstruction. Assess the airway for breathing (rate, rhythm, quality) and provide oxygen via nonrebreathing mask or bag-mask device. Continue initial assessment, rapid extrication, and rapid transport.

2. You should reposition the head and attempt to reventilate the patient. If you are unsuccessful in your second attempt, you must take action to clear her airway. If you fail to clear her airway, she will likely go into cardiac arrest as well. Choking victims have been known to walk away from others without indicating that they are choking, and when this occurs in a restaurant setting many of these people will go into a bathroom. If you find a patient in a restroom who cannot be ventilated, they likely have a foreign body airway obstruction (FBAO), most often as a result of ingested food.

3. The most common cause of airway obstruction in an unconscious patient is the tongue. The patient's husband told you that he helped her to the ground without injury, so it is safe to place her in the recovery position. If you were unsure of the presence of trauma, this position would not be used. Instead, you would use the jaw-thrust maneuver to manage her airway. In either case, you must continually monitor her condition and be prepared for vomitus.

Fill-in-the-Patient Care Report

EMS Patient Care Report (PCR)			
Date: Today's Date	**Incident No.:** 2011-0000	**Nature of Call:** Possible overdose	**Location:** Market Street High School
Dispatched: 1530	**En Route:** 1530	**At Scene:** 1543	**Transport:** 1556	**At Hospital:** 1408	**In Service:** 1635

Patient Information	
Age: 14 Years	**Allergies:** Unknown
Sex: Female	**Medications:** Unknown
Weight (in kg [lb]): 50 kg (110 lb)	**Past Medical History:** Unknown
	Chief Complaint: Unresponsive

Vital Signs				
Time: 1545	**BP:** 124/86	**Pulse:** 112/regular	**Respirations:** 12 shallow/inadequate tidal volume	**Sao2:** 93%

EMS Treatment

(circle all that apply)

Oxygen @ 15 L/min via (circle one): NC NRM (Bag-Mask Device)	(Assisted Ventilation)	(Airway Adjunct: OPA)	CPR
Defibrillation	Bleeding Control	Bandaging	Splinting	Other Shock Treatment

Narrative

Responded to 9-1-1 call for possible drug overdose at Market Street High School. Arrived and was directed to an unresponsive 14-year-old girl on the floor of a restroom and was advised that patient had previous "troubles" with drugs, although no physical evidence was observed in the patient's immediate surroundings. Patient presented with no response to painful stimulus; cyanosis around lips and fingernails; and shallow, snoring respirations. Patient's respirations were immediately assisted with a bag-mask device and 100% oxygen, and she was loaded into the ambulance where a fire fighter rode along to assist. Vital signs, when compared to the baseline set, indicated that assisted ventilations and oxygen therapy were improving the patient's SaO₂ levels. While en route, receiving facility was updated with patient condition and on arrival she was transferred appropriately to the care of the ED staff and a full verbal report was provided to the charge RN. **End of Report**

Skills

Skill Drills

Skill Drill 9-2: Positioning the Unconscious Patient

1. Support the **head** while your partner straightens the patient's legs.
2. Have your partner place his or her **hand** on the patient's far **shoulder** and hip.
3. **Roll** the patient as a unit with the responder at the patient's **head** calling the count to begin the move.
4. **Open** and **assess** the patient's airway and **breathing** status. (page 336)

Skill Drill 9-3: Inserting an Oral Airway

1. Size the **airway** by measuring from the patient's **earlobe** to the corner of the **mouth**.
2. Open the patient's **mouth** with the **cross**-finger technique. Hold the **airway** upside down with your other hand. Insert the airway with the tip facing the **roof** of the mouth.
3. **Rotate** the airway **180°**. Insert the airway until the **flange** rests on the patient's lips and teeth. In this position, the airway will hold the **tongue** forward. (page 339)

Skill Drill 9-7: Placing an Oxygen Cylinder into Service

1. Using an oxygen **wrench**, turn the valve **counterclockwise** to slowly "crack" the cylinder.
2. Attach the regulator/flowmeter to the **valve** stem using the two pin-**indexing** holes and make sure that the **washer** is in place over the larger hole.
3. Align the **regulator** so that the pins fit snugly into the correct holes on the **valve** stem, and hand tighten the **regulator**.
4. Attach the **oxygen** connective tubing to the **flowmeter**. (page 350)

Skill Drill 9-8: Performing Mouth-to-Mask Ventilation

1. Once the patient's head is properly **positioned** and an airway **adjunct** is inserted, place the mask on the patient's face. **Seal** the mask to the face using both hands (EC **clamp**).
2. **Breathe** into the one-way valve until you note visible **chest** rise.
3. Remove your **mouth** and watch the patient's chest fall during **exhalation**. (page 357)

Chapter 10: Shock

General Knowledge

Matching

1. B (page 381)
2. G (page 381)
3. H (page 383)
4. C (page 383)
5. E (page 383)
6. A (page 387)
7. F (page 386)
8. I (page 388)
9. D (page 389)

Multiple Choice

1. A (page 381)
2. B (page 383)
3. D (page 383)
4. C (page 383)
5. D (page 383)
6. D (page 384)
7. D (page 385)
8. C (page 388)
9. B (page 386)
10. A (page 387)
11. D (pages 386–387)
12. A (page 387)
13. B (page 388)
14. A (page 388)
15. A (page 388)
16. A (page 384)
17. B (page 392)
18. C (page 395)
19. B (page 395)
20. B (page 388)

True/False

1. T (page 387)
2. F (page 395)
3. T (page 381)
4. F (page 381)
5. F (page 389)
6. T (page 398)
7. T (page 386)
8. F (page 381)
9. F (page 384)
10. F (page 389)

Fill-in-the-Blank

1. Hypoperfusion (page 381)
2. contraction (page 383)
3. tolerant (page 382)
4. perfusion (page 383)
5. heart; vessels; blood (page 382)
6. shock (hypoperfusion) (page 382)
7. Sphincters; contract; dilate (page 383)
8. Diastolic, systolic (page 383)
9. Blood (page 383)
10. involuntary (page 383)

Crossword Puzzle

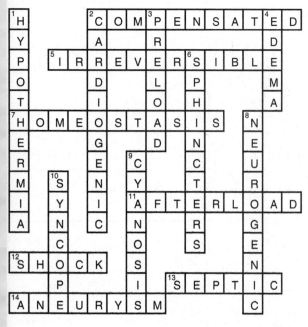

Critical Thinking

Multiple Choice

1. A (page 385)   **2.** C (page 387)   **3.** C (page 386)   **4.** B (page 389)   **5.** D (page 395)

Short Answer

1. Causes: allergic reaction (most severe form)

   Signs/Symptoms: Can develop within seconds; mild itching/rash; burning skin; vascular dilation; generalized edema; profound coma; rapid death

   Treatment: Manage airway. Assist ventilations. Administer high-flow oxygen. Determine cause. Assist with administration of epinephrine. Transport promptly. (page 396)

2. Causes: Inadequate heart function; disease of muscle tissue; impaired electrical system; disease or injury

   Signs/Symptoms: Chest pain; irregular pulse; weak pulse; low blood pressure; cyanosis (lips, under nails); cool, clammy skin; anxiety; rales; pulmonary edema

   Treatment: Position comfortably. Administer oxygen. Assist ventilations. Transport promptly. (page 396)

3. Causes: Loss of blood or fluid

   Signs/Symptoms: Rapid, weak pulse; low blood pressure; change in mental status; cyanosis (lips, under nails); cool, clammy skin; increased respiratory rate

   Treatment: Secure airway. Assist ventilations. Administer high-flow oxygen. Control external bleeding. Elevate legs. Keep warm. Transport promptly. (page 397)

4. Causes: Damaged cervical spine, which causes widespread blood vessel dilation

   Signs/Symptoms: Bradycardia (slow pulse); low blood pressure; signs of neck injury

   Treatment: Secure airway. Spinal stabilization. Assist ventilations. Administer high-flow oxygen. Preserve body heat. Transport promptly. (page 396)

5. Causes: Temporary, generalized vascular dilation; anxiety; bad news; sight of injury/blood; prospect of medical treatment; severe pain; illness; tiredness

   Signs/Symptoms: Rapid pulse; normal or low blood pressure

   Treatment: Determine duration of unconsciousness. Record initial vital signs and mental status. Suspect head injury if patient is confused or slow to regain consciousness. Transport promptly. (page 397)

6. Causes: Severe bacterial infection

   Signs/Symptoms: Warm skin; tachycardia; low blood pressure

   Treatment: Transport promptly. Administer oxygen en route. Provide full ventilatory support. Elevate legs. Keep patient warm. (page 396)

7. 1. Poor pump function

   2. Blood or fluid loss from blood vessels

   3. Poor vessel function (blood vessels dilate) (page 385)

8. Falling blood pressure; labored or irregular breathing; ashen, mottled, or cyanotic skin; thready or absent peripheral pulses; dull eyes or dilated pupils; and poor urinary output (page 389)

Ambulance Calls

1. When assessing the victim of a fall, you must take into consideration not only the patient's complaints and obvious injuries, but also the mechanism of injury, including the height of the fall, the surface on which he or she landed, the position in which he or she landed, and any medical and/or previous traumatic injuries that could exacerbate the injuries. This patient landed on a hard surface, most likely a wooden floor, and now presents with numbness and tingling of his lower body. These are all indicators of spinal cord injury. Assume spinal fractures are present; ensure that you assess pulse, motor, and sensation of all extremities prior to placing him in full spinal precautions; and reassess again after he is stabilized. Be alert for signs of neurogenic shock, which in this case would be an absence of sweating and normal, warm skin below the level of the suspected injury. Document your findings and continue this assessment en route to the hospital.

2. This patient is in shock and it seems to be related to an infectious organism (septic shock). In this case, although he has not lost blood volume through hemorrhage, his vessels or "container" has become too large, making his available blood volume inadequate. Immediate transport is required. The patient should be given high-flow oxygen.

3. Treat this patient for anaphylactic shock. Apply high-flow oxygen while inquiring if the patient has an EpiPen. Obtain orders and administer the EpiPen, if available. Monitor the patient's vital signs. Rapid transport is required.

Fill-in-the-Patient Care Report

EMS Patient Care Report (PCR)			
Date: Today's Date	**Incident No.:** 2010-123	**Nature of Call:** MCA	**Location:** Highway 62 at Exit 19

Dispatched: 0200	**En Route:** 0200	**At Scene:** 0205	**Transport:** 0213	**At Hospital:** 0218	**In Service:** 0233

Patient Information	
Age: 18 Years	**Allergies:** Unknown
Sex: Male	**Medications:** Unknown
Weight (in kg [lb]): 65 kg (143 lb)	**Past Medical History:** Unknown
	Chief Complaint: Not able to move legs.

Vital Signs				
Time: 0213	**BP:** 98/62	**Pulse:** 110/Weak	**Respirations:** 18/Shallow – Adequate Tidal Volume	**Sao$_2$:** 94% on O$_2$

EMS Treatment
(circle all that apply)

Oxygen @ 15 L/min via (circle one): NC **(NRM)** Bag-Mask Device	Assisted Ventilation	Airway Adjunct:	CPR
Defibrillation	Bleeding Control	Bandaging	**(Splinting)**	**(Other Shock Treatment)**

Narrative

Summoned by highway patrol for a motorcyclist down on Highway 62 at exit 19. Arrived to find an 18-year-old man supine on the highway, complaining of inability to move his legs and feeling "odd." Patient was alert, had a patent airway, and although his breathing was rapid and shallow it seemed to be producing adequate oxygenation. Initiated spinal stabilization and high-flow oxygen therapy via nonrebreathing mask prior to applying cervical collar and immobilizing patient to the long backboard. Once en route to the trauma center, I obtained vitals—showing hypotension; increased heart rate; rapid breathing; decreased O$_2$ sat with high-flow oxygen; and pale, cool, moist skin. Removed patient's clothing to check for injuries and found that his lower extremities were cooler than his torso and that the skin on his legs was dry. Immediately upgraded transport to lights and sirens, treated patient for shock, and called verbal report to the receiving facility. Arrived at the trauma center prior to obtaining second set of vitals, and the patient was properly transferred to their care. A full verbal report was provided. **End of Report**

Skills

Skill Drills

Skill Drill 10-1: Treating Shock

1. Keep the patient supine, open the airway, and check breathing and pulse.
2. Control obvious external bleeding. Apply a tourniquet, if necessary, to achieve rapid control of blood loss from extremities.
3. Splint the patient on a backboard. Splint any broken bones or joint injuries during transport.
4. Give high-flow oxygen if you have not already done so, and place blankets under and over the patient. (page 394)

Assessment Review

1. D (page 390) **2.** A (page 390) **3.** B (page 391) **4.** B (page 395) **5.** C (page 395)

Emergency Care Summary (pages 406–408)

Treating Cardiogenic Shock

This type of shock is a failure of the pump (heart) and is often the result of a myocardial infarction. Since the heart is no longer an effective pump, fluid backs up in the body and the lungs.

1. Assess **ABCs**. Patient will often have **rales** (fluid in the lungs).
2. Patient is often complaining of **chest** pain.
3. Administer high-flow oxygen via a **nonrebreathing mask**.
4. Place the patient in a **sitting** or semi-**sitting** position to assist breathing.
5. Do not administer **nitroglycerin** if blood pressure is low; contact medical control.
6. Keep the patient calm, request **ALS** if available, and transport promptly.
7. Keep alert for the need to assist **ventilation**, perform cardiopulmonary resuscitation, or **defibrillate**.

Treating Septic Shock

A systemic infection causes the blood vessels to become leaky and dilate, causing the container to enlarge. Patient requires complex management in the hospital.

1. Assess and manage **life threats** to the ABCs.
2. Administer high-flow oxygen.
3. Prevent **heat** loss.
4. **Transport** as promptly as possible.

Treating Anaphylactic Shock

Severe allergic reactions can rapidly progress to anaphylactic shock. The body's response to the allergen causes widespread vasodilation.

1. Request **ALS**.
2. Be prepared to assist the patient with their prescribed **epinephrine auto-injector**.
3. Oxygenate and ventilate the patient as necessary.
4. Prompt **transport** to the closest emergency department is essential.

Treating Hypovolemic Shock

This type of shock is caused by a loss of blood or body fluids. It should be suspected first whenever a patient presents with signs and symptoms of shock. Blood loss may be external or internal secondary to a traumatic injury. Body fluids can be lost due to burns, excessive vomiting, or diarrhea.

1. Management of a patient with hypovolemic shock focuses on preventing further **blood** or **fluid** loss.
2. Manage threats to the **ABCs**.
3. Control **external bleeding** with direct pressure, pressure dressings, and **tourniquets**.
4. **Internal** bleeding is difficult to manage. Splinting injured extremities may **slow** blood loss.
5. Place the patient on a **long backboard**. The **Trendelenburg's** or the shock position may be used to assist with perfusion.
6. High-flow oxygen should be administered to **all** hypovolemic patients.
7. Prompt transport to a **trauma** center is required. Do not delay transport.

Treating Respiratory Insufficiency

Patients in shock as a result of respiratory insufficiency require immediate airway maintenance and oxygen.

1. Clear **obstructions** and **suction** airway as required.
2. Give supplemental **oxygen** and assist ventilations if necessary.
3. **Transport** promptly.

Chapter 11: BLS Resuscitation

General Knowledge

Matching

1. G (page 422)
2. E (page 438)
3. C (page 413)
4. D (page 414)
5. A (page 414)
6. F (page 415)
7. J (page 428)
8. I (page 420)
9. B (page 420)
10. H (page 421)

Multiple Choice

1. D (page 413)
2. D (page 414)
3. B (page 414)
4. B (page 442)
5. A (page 417)
6. D (page 429)
7. D (pages 429)
8. D (page 436)
9. C (page 437)
10. D (page 417)
11. B (page 420)
12. C (page 424)
13. B (page 423)
14. A (page 421)
15. D (page 417)
16. A (page 419)
17. D (page 419)
18. B (page 430)
19. D (page 432)
20. C (page 432)
21. D (page 437)
22. B (page 438)
23. D (page 439)
24. C (page 437)

True/False

1. T (page 416)
2. F (page 417)
3. T (page 416)
4. F (page 421)
5. F (pages 422)
6. T (page 436)
7. T (pages 419)
8. F (page 424)
9. F (page 419)
10. T (pages 435)
11. F (page 435)
12. F (page 416)
13. F (page 419)
14. T (page 425–426)

Fill-in-the-Blank

1. 4; 6 (page 414)
2. barrier (page 422)
3. chest compressions (page 416)
4. pacemaker (page 416)
5. Advance directives (pages 436–437)
6. firm (page 417)
7. airway (page 419)
8. automated external defibrillator (page 415)
9. carotid (page 417)
10. mechanical piston device (page 429)

Crossword Puzzle

Critical Thinking

Short Answer

1. **1.** Rigor mortis, or stiffening of the body after death

2 Dependent lividity (livor mortis), a discoloration of the skin due to pooling of blood

3. Putrefaction or decomposition of the body

4. Evidence of nonsurvivable injury, such as decapitation (page 436)

2. **1.** Early access

2. Early CPR

3. Early defibrillation

4. Early advanced care (pages 414–415)

5. Integrated post-arrest care

3. **1.** Injury, both blunt and penetrating

2. Infections of the respiratory tract or another organ system

3. A foreign body airway obstruction

4. Near drowning

5. Electrocution

6. Poisoning or drug overdose

7. Sudden infant death syndrome (SIDS) (pages 429)

4. To perform the head tilt–chin lift maneuver, make sure the patient is supine. Place one hand on the patient's forehead and apply firm backward pressure with your palm to tilt the head back. Next, place the tips of your fingers of your other hand under the lower jaw near the bony part of the chin. Lift the chin upward, bringing the entire lower jaw with it, helping to tilt the head back. (page 420–421)

5. To perform the jaw-thrust maneuver, kneel above the patient's head. Place your fingers behind the angle of the lower jaw on both sides. Forcefully move the jaw forward. Use your thumbs to pull the patient's lower jaw down to allow breathing through the mouth and nose. (page 420–421)

6. Once you have determined that the patient is unresponsive, call for additional help. Ensure that the patient is on a firm, flat surface in a supine position. Place your hands in the proper position. Give 30 compressions at a rate of at least 100 beats/minute for an adult. Using a rhythmic motion, apply pressure vertically from your shoulders down through both arms to depress the sternum 1.5″ to 2″ (2.5 to 3.8 cm) in an adult, then rise up gently and fully. Count the compressions aloud. (page 419–420)

7. Rescuer one begins another cycle of CPR while rescuer two moves to the opposite side of the chest and moves into position to begin compressions. Rescuer one delivers two ventilations. Rescuer two begins compressing until 30 compressions have been completed. (page 426–427)

8. **Standing:** Stand behind the patient and wrap your arms around his or her abdomen. Make a fist with one hand, then grasp the fist with the other hand. Place the thumb side of the fist against the patient's abdomen between the umbilicus and the xiphoid process. Press your fist into the patient's abdomen in quick inward and upward thrusts until the object is expelled or the patient becomes unconscious.

Supine: Straddle the patient's legs. Place the heel of one hand against the patient's abdomen, just above the umbilicus, and the other hand on top of the first. Press your hands into the patient's abdomen in a series of quick inward and upward thrusts. (pages 439–440)

9. **Standing:** Stand behind the patient and wrap your arms under the armpits and around the patient's chest. Make a fist with one hand, then grasp the fist with the other hand. Place the thumb side of the fist against the patient's sternum. Press your fist into the patient's chest and perform backwards thrusts until the object is expelled or the patient becomes unconscious.

Supine: Kneel next to the patient. Place your hands as you would to deliver chest compressions. Deliver 30 slow chest thrusts, open the airway, and look in the mouth. If the object is visible, remove it. If not, continue the cycle of chest compressions and opening the airway. (pages 439–441)

10. **1.** Hold the infant face down, with the body resting on your forearm. Support the infant's jaw and face with your hand and keep the head lower than the body.

2. Deliver five back slaps between the shoulder blades, using the heel of your hand.

3. Turn the infant face up.

4. Give five quick chest thrusts on the sternum using two fingers. (pages 442–444)

Ambulance Calls

1. Question the family about the last time they spoke with her. Explain that she has been down too long for CPR to be effective. Comfort family members. Notify your dispatcher to alert the supervisor and either law enforcement, the coroner, or a funeral home according to local protocols.

2. With the FDA's approval of AEDs for home use, it will become more common to see them being used by the lay provider. Simply purchasing an AED does not ensure appropriate usage during real-life events. Training by knowledgeable, skilled instructors is needed to minimize confusion and inappropriate AED use. Remove the AED and explain to them that AEDs are meant to be used only when a person is not breathing and has no pulse. Emphasize that it is appropriate to have the AED nearby in the event that a person goes into cardiorespiratory

arrest, but that it is not to be applied until then. After the patient has been transported to the hospital, tell the friends and family that you appreciate their willingness to be prepared for emergencies, and that you would like to see them be successful in their usage of their AED. If you or your department offers CPR/AED courses, offer to train them and/or point them in the right direction to receive the appropriate training.

3. Given the scene, you must assume that there is the likelihood for trauma. This means that you must assess and maintain his airway without manipulating his spine. Use the jaw-thrust maneuver and apply full c-spine precautions. Also, consider possible causes of his unconscious state, including any scene hazards and potential medical conditions.

Skills

Skill Drills

Skill Drill 11-1: Positioning the Patient

1. Kneel beside the patient, leaving room to roll the patient toward you.
2. Grasp the patient, stabilizing the cervical spine if needed.
3. Move the head and neck as a unit with the torso as your partner pulls on the distant shoulder and hip.
4. Move the patient to a supine position with legs straight and arms at the sides. (page 418)

Skill Drill 11-2: Performing Chest Compressions

1. Place the **heel** of one hand on the **sternum**, between the nipples.
2. Place the **heel** of your other **hand** over the first hand.
3. With your arms straight, lock your **elbows**, and position your shoulders directly over your **hands**. Depress the sternum **1.5″** to **2″** using a direct downward movement. Allow the chest to return to its normal position. **Compression** and relaxation should be of equal duration. (page 424)

Skill Drill 11-3: Performing One-Rescuer Adult CPR

1. Determine unresponsiveness and breathlessness, and call for help.
2. Check for a carotid pulse for no more than 10 seconds.
3. If there is no pulse, begin CPR until an AED is available. Give 30 chest compressions at a rate of at least 100 per minute.

4. Open the airway according to your suspicion of spinal injury.
5. Give two ventilations of 1 second each and observe for visible chest rise. Continue cycles of 30 chest compressions and two ventilations until additional personnel arrive or the patient starts to move.

Skill Drill 11-4: Performing Two-rescuer Adult CPR

1. Determine **unresponsiveness** and breathlessness and take positions.
2. Check for a(n) **carotid** pulse. If there is no pulse but a(n) **AED** is available, apply it now.
3. Begin CPR, starting with **chest compressions**. Give 30 chest compressions at a rate of **at least 100** per minute.
4. **Open** the airway according to your suspicion of spinal injury.
5. Give **two ventilations** of 1 second each and observe for **visible chest rise**. Continue cycles of 30 chest compressions and two ventilations (switch roles every 2 minutes) until ALS personnel take over or the patient starts to move.

Chapter 12: Medical Overview

General Knowledge

Matching

1. A (page 454)
2. G (page 454)
3. B (page 454)
4. I (page 454)
5. A (page 454)
6. F (page 454)
7. K (page 454)
8. C (page 454)
9. J (page 454)
10. E (page 454)
11. A (page 454)
12. D (page 454)
13. H (page 454)
14. B (page 454)
15. G (page 454)
16. D (page 454)
17. K (page 454)
18. D (page 454)
19. I (page 454)
20. C (page 454)

Multiple Choice

1. C (page 454)
2. B (page 454)
3. C (page 456)
4. A (page 456)
5. C (page 457)
6. B (page 457)
7. D (page 459)
8. C (page 460)
9. B (page 461)
10. B (page 462)
11. C (page 462)
12. C (page 464)
13. C (page 464)
14. A (page 465)
15. D (page 465)

True/False

1. T (page 454)
2. T (page 456)
3. F (page 455)
4. T (page 456)
5. F (page 457)
6. T (page 459)
7. T (page 461)
8. F (page 461)
9. F (page 462)
10. T (page 462)
11. F (page 463)
12. T (page 465)
13. T (page 465)
14. F (page 465)
15. T (page 466)
16. F (page 466)
17. T (page 457)
18. F (page 456)
19. T (page 460)
20. T (page 459)

Fill In-the-Blank

1. Hematologic emergencies (page 453)
2. Tunnel vision (page 454)
3. AVPU (page 455)
4. 5; 15 (page 458)
5. medical control (page 459)
6. AED (page 459)
7. Critical (page 459)
8. ground; air (page 459)
9. infectious disease (page 461)
10. Hepatitis (page 462)
11. Hepatitis A (page 463)
12. track marks (page 458)
13. Virulence (page 463)
14. Tuberculosis (page 463)
15. meningitis (page 463)

Fill-in-the-Table (page 461)

Causes of Infectious Disease		
Type of Organism	**Description**	**Example**
Bacteria	**Grow and reproduce outside the human cell in the appropriate temperature and with the appropriate nutrients**	*Salmonella*
Viruses	Smaller than bacteria; multiply only inside a host and die when exposed to the environment	**Human immunodeficiency virus**
Fungi	**Similar to bacteria in that they require the appropriate nutrients and organic material to grow**	**Mold**
Protozoa (parasites)	**One-celled microscopic organisms, some of which cause disease**	Amoebas
Helminths (parasites)	Invertebrates with long, flexible, rounded, or flattened bodies	**Worms**

Crossword Puzzle

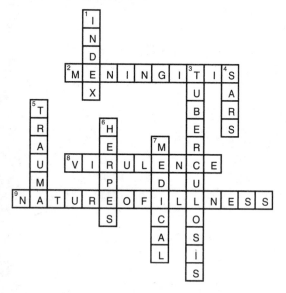

Critical Thinking

Short Answer

1.
 1. The patient's blood is splashed or sprayed into your eyes, nose, or mouth or into an open sore or cut; even microscopic openings in the skin are a possible source.
 2. You have blood from an infected patient on your hands and then touch your own eyes, nose, mouth, or an open sore or cut.
 3. A needle used to inject the patient breaks your skin.
 4. Broken glass at a motor vehicle collision or other incident may penetrate your glove (and skin), which may have already been covered with blood from an infected patient. (page 461)

2.
 1. Scene size-up
 2. Primary assessment
 3. History taking
 4. Secondary assessment
 5. Reassessment (pages 454–459)

3. **T** Tobacco
 A Alcohol
 C Caffeine
 O Over-the-counter medications/herbal supplements
 S Sexual and street drugs (page 457)

4. Unresponsive/altered mental status
 Airway/breathing problems
 Circulatory problems such as severe bleeding or signs of shock (page 459)

Ambulance Calls

1. It seems likely that this patient could be suffering from tuberculosis. You and your crew should apply protection immediately. You should place a HEPA respirator/mask on yourself and other crew members and a surgical mask on the patient. Although a surgical mask on the patient provides minimal protection, it provides a visual reminder to all who are involved in the patient's care of the possibility of an airborne communicable disease. The surgical mask should still allow for the placement of a nasal cannula for oxygen. Proper notification to the receiving hospital should be made so that isolation precautions can be in place when the patient arrives. Although the risk of contracting the illness is minimal to you and the crew, everyone should alert their management and follow their exposure-control plan. All crew members potentially exposed should receive a PPD skin test and follow up with a designated health care facility.

2. You should begin by verifying the chief complaint of chest pain. Ask the patient what she was doing when the pain began and whether anything potentially caused it. Does anything make the pain better or worse? Inquire as to the quality of the pain. Ask the patient to describe the pain, and determine if the pain is constant or intermittent. Where in her chest is the pain? Have the patient point to the painful area and determine whether the pain is localized to that area or if it radiates to other areas. Ask the patient to rate her pain on a scale from 1 to 10. Explain to her that 0 means no pain and that 10 means the worst pain. This will give you a baseline for reassessment after you begin treatment. Inquire as to how long she's had the pain. Is it just this incident or has she had previous episodes?

Chapter 13: Respiratory Emergencies

General Knowledge

Matching

1. N (page 475)
2. D (page 482)
3. H (page 508)
4. J (page 483)
5. L (page 487)
6. O (page 490)
7. G (page 475)
8. E (page 510)
9. M (page 479)
10. A (page 480)
11. K (page 489)
12. F (page 484)
13. I (page 488)
14. B (page 485)
15. C (page 487)

Multiple Choice

1. C (page 488)
2. C (page 476)
3. B (page 496)
4. C (page 476)
5. B (page 476)
6. C (page 508)
7. C (page 476)
8. A (page 479)
9. B (page 480)
10. A (page 482)
11. C (page 482)
12. A (page 483)
13. B (page 511)
14. B (page 495)
15. A (page 487)
16. C (page 485)
17. B (page 485)
18. D (pages 486–487)
19. C (page 487)
20. A (page 488)
21. B (page 489)
22. C (page 498)
23. D (page 491)
24. A (page 476)
25. A (page 500)
26. B (page 478)
27. D (page 499)
28. D (page 496)
29. C (page 500)
30. B (page 501)
31. D (page 512)
32. C (page 506)
33. B (page 507)
34. C (page 499)
35. A (page 485)

True/False

1. F (page 480)
2. T (page 487)
3. F (page 486)
4. F (page 485)
5. T (page 490)
6. T (pages 497, 512)
7. F (page 489)
8. T (page 483)
9. F (pages 483–484)
10. T (page 490)
11. T (pages 491–492)
12. T (pages 492–495)
13. F (page 479)
14. T (page 502)
15. F (page 507)
16. F (page 508)
17. T (page 510)
18. F (page 504)
19. T (page 492)
20. T (page 489)

Fill-in-the-Blank

1. carbon dioxide (page 476)
2. oxygen (page 478)
3. Oxygen (page 477)
4. alveoli (page 476)
5. HEPA respirator (page 491)
6. 12; 20 (page 478)
7. Carbon monoxide (page 489)
8. stridor (page 493)
9. Rales or crackles (page 493)
10. SAMPLE; OPQRST (page 496)
11. voice (page 508)
12. status epilepticus (page 488)
13. Pertussis (whooping cough) (page 511)
14. Rhonchi (page 493)
15. emphysema (page 498)

Labeling

1. Obstruction, Scarring, and Dilation of the Alveolar Sac (page 483)
   A. Bronchiole
   B. Inflammation or infection
   C. Obstruction
   D. Mucus
   E. Infection
   F. Alveolus
   G. Trapped air
   H. Dilated alveolus

Crossword Puzzle

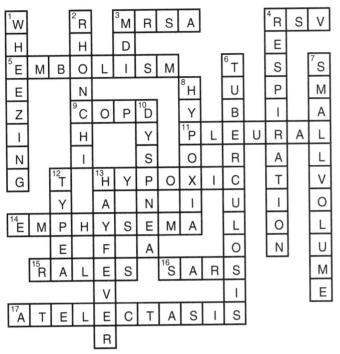

Critical Thinking

Short Answer

1. 1. Normal rate
    2. Regular pattern of inhalation and exhalation
    3. Clear and equal lung sounds on both sides of the chest
    4. Regular and equal chest rise and fall
    5. Adequate depth (page 478)

2. 1. Asthma
    2. Chronic obstructive pulmonary disease
    3. Congestive heart failure/pulmonary edema
    4. Pneumonia
    5. Bronchitis
    6. Anaphylaxis (page 493)

3. 1. Patient is unable to coordinate administration and inhalation.
    2. Inhaler is not prescribed for patient.
    3. You did not obtain permission from medical control or local protocol.
    4. Patient has already met maximum prescribed dose before your arrival.
    5. Medication is expired.
    6. There are other contraindications specific to the medication. (page 501)

4. An ongoing irritation of the respiratory tract; excess mucus production obstructs small airways and alveoli.

Protective mechanisms are impaired. Repeated episodes of irritation and pneumonia can cause scarring and alveolar damage, leading to COPD. (page 483)

5. Obstruction with secretions, mucus, foreign bodies, and/or airway swelling

    Bleeding

    Leaking

    Dislodgement

    Infection (page 508)

6. A condition characterized by a chronically high blood level of carbon dioxide in which the respiratory center no longer responds to high blood levels of carbon dioxide. In these patients, low blood oxygen causes the respiratory center to respond and stimulate respiration. If the arterial level of oxygen is then raised, as happens when the patient is given additional oxygen, there is no longer any stimulus to breathe; both the high carbon dioxide and low oxygen drives are lost. (page 478)

7. 1. Is the air going in?
    2. Does the chest expand with each breath?
    3. Does the chest fall after each breath?
    4. Is the rate adequate for the age of your patient? (page 492)

Ambulance Calls

1. This child has all the classics signs of epiglottitis. You should do nothing to excite or frighten the child, because doing so will likely cause his airway to spasm and close. Remember to use nonthreatening body language (place yourself below his eye level), give the child distance (until you establish trust), and perform any exam using the toe-to-head method. This is a true emergency that requires immediate transport to the hospital, but you must do so tactfully. Use parents to assist with patient care efforts such as applying humidified oxygen (blow-by or mask).

2. This patient's chief complaint, age, weight, smoking, and birth control use all place her at risk of pulmonary embolism (PE). PE patients most often experience a sudden onset of shortness of breath that they describe as sharp and worsening with inspiration. You should provide high-flow oxygen, obtain vital signs, and perform a secondary assessment en route to the hospital (including auscultation of lung sounds). Provide prompt transport to the nearest appropriate facility.

3. Place the patient in a position of comfort. Provide high-flow oxygen via nonrebreathing mask and monitor his vital signs. This patient requires rapid transport to the nearest appropriate facility.

4. This patient is likely experiencing pulmonary edema associated with his cardiac history. Place the patient in a sitting-up position and administer 100% oxygen through a nonrebreathing mask. Suction the frothy secretions from the patient's airway, as necessary. Consider CPAP for this patient and be prepared to provide full ventilatory support for this patient should he deteriorate. This patient requires prompt transport to the nearest appropriate facility.

Skills

Skill Drills

Skill Drill 13-1: Assisting a Patient With a Metered-Dose Inhaler

1. Check to make sure you have the correct medication for the correct patient. Check the expiration date. Ensure inhaler is at room temperature or **warmer**.

2. Remove oxygen mask. Hand inhaler to patient. Instruct about breathing and **lip seal**.

3. Instruct patient to press inhaler and inhale one puff. Instruct about **breath holding**.

4. Reapply **oxygen**. After a few **breaths**, have patient repeat **dose** if order or protocol allows. (pages 503–504)

Skill Drill 13-2: Assisting a Patient With a Small-Volume Nebulizer

1. Check to make sure you have the correct medication for the correct patient. Check the expiration date. Confirm you have the correct patient.

2. Insert the medication into the container on the nebulizer. In some cases, sterile saline may be added (about 3 mL) to achieve the optimum volume of fluid for the nebulized application.

3. Attach the medication container to the nebulizer, mouthpiece, and tubing. Attach oxygen tubing to the oxygen tank. Set the flowmeter at 6 L/min.

4. Instruct the patient on how to breathe. (pages 504–505)

Assessment Review

1. D (page 499)
2. B (page 489)
3. A (page 495)
4. B (page 499)
5. D (page 499)

Emergency Care Summary (page 517–519)

General Management of Respiratory Emergencies

Managing life threats to the patient's **ABCs** and ensuring the delivery of high-flow oxygen are the primary concerns with any respiratory emergency. Patients breathing at a rate of less than **8** breaths/min or greater than **30** breaths/min should have ventilations assisted with a **bag-mask device**. Continually assess the patient's mental status, and provide emotional support as needed. Transport in the position of comfort. For all respiratory emergencies, make sure you have taken the appropriate standard precautions, including the use of a **HEPA respirator**.

Upper or Lower Airway Infection

Dyspnea from an upper airway infection may be from **croup** or **epiglottitis**. Patients should receive **humidified** oxygen if available. Patients who are sitting forward, seem lethargic, or are drooling may have **epiglottitis**. Do not force the patient to lie down or attempt to suction or insert an **oropharyngeal** airway because this may cause a spasm and a complete airway **obstruction**. Transport should be rapid.

Lower airway infections may be from the common cold, bronchitis, or **pneumonia**. Patients need supplemental oxygen, monitoring of vital signs, and transport to the hospital.

Asthma, Hay Fever, and Anaphylaxis

Not all wheezing is the result of asthma! Obtain a thorough **history** from the patient or family. If the patient is wheezing and has asthma, assist with the patient's prescribed **inhaler** or administer a small-volume nebulizer containing **albuterol**. Provide supplemental oxygen and provide ventilatory support as needed. Patients whose asthma progresses to **status asthmaticus** require immediate transportation. Be prepared to assist their ventilations because they may become too exhausted to breathe.

Hay fever usually requires only support and transport, but if the condition has worsened from generalized cold symptoms, the patient may require supplemental oxygen and **airway** support.

Anaphylaxis is a true emergency that requires rapid intervention and **transport**. Airway, oxygen, and ventilatory support are paramount. Determine if the patient has a prescribed **EpiPen autoinjector** and assist with administration by placing it in the patient's hand. Guide the **EpiPen autoinjector** to the patient's thigh (lateral aspect) at a **90°** angle and administer the medication. Hold the **autoinjector** in place for **10** seconds. Transport promptly. Reassess the patient's condition en route to the hospital.

Pneumothorax

A pneumothorax may occur spontaneously or may be the result of a **traumatic event**. Place the patient in a position of comfort, and support the **ABCs**. Provide prompt transport, monitor the patient carefully, and be prepared to assist ventilations and provide **cardiopulmonary resuscitation** if necessary.

Obstruction of the Airway

Managing an airway obstruction is a priority. Use age-appropriate **basic** life support foreign body airway obstruction **maneuvers** to clear the airway. Administer supplemental oxygen, and transport the patient to the closest hospital. Some patients do not want to go to a hospital after the obstruction is cleared. Encourage them to be transported for evaluation of possible **injury** to the airway.

Hyperventilation

Gather a thorough **history**, and attempt to determine the **underlying cause** because the hyperventilation may be the result of a serious problem. Do not have the patient breathe into a **paper bag**; this maneuver could make things worse. Instead, **reassure** the patient, administer supplemental oxygen, and provide prompt transport to the hospital.

Chapter 14: Cardiovascular Emergencies

General Knowledge

Matching

1. L (page 525)	**6.** K (page 526)	**11.** F (page 531)	**16.** P (page 531)	**21.** A (page 536)
2. C (page 527)	**7.** H (page 525)	**12.** I (page 531)	**17.** G (page 531)	**22.** D (page 537)
3. O (page 526)	**8.** M (page 525)	**13.** J (page 534)	**18.** E (page 531)	**23.** B (page 537)
4. G (page 527)	**9.** B (page 531)	**14.** A (page 534)	**19.** F (page 532)	
5. N (page 526)	**10.** D (page 533)	**15.** E (page 534)	**20.** C (page 535)	

Multiple Choice

1. C (page 526)	**10.** A (page 531)	**19.** C (page 532)	**28.** C (page 538)	**37.** C (page 547)
2. D (page 526)	**11.** B (page 531)	**20.** A (pages 535–536)	**29.** B (page 540)	**38.** B (page 547)
3. A (page 526)	**12.** B (page 531)	**21.** B (page 535)	**30.** C (page 541)	**39.** C (page 548)
4. B (page 526)	**13.** D (page 532)	**22.** D (page 533)	**31.** A (page 536)	**40.** A (page 548)
5. A (page 526)	**14.** B (page 532)	**23.** A (page 534)	**32.** B (page 542)	**41.** D (page 538)
6. B (page 527)	**15.** A (page 532)	**24.** A (page 535)	**33.** C (page 543)	**42.** A (page 538)
7. C (page 529)	**16.** B (page 537)	**25.** D (page 536)	**34.** B (page 545)	**43.** D (page 551)
8. A (page 529)	**17.** C (page 532)	**26.** B (page 536)	**35.** A (page 545)	**44.** C (page 552)
9. C (page 529)	**18.** C (page 532)	**27.** C (page 533)	**36.** C (page 547)	**45.** C (page 554)

True/False

1. F (page 526)	**4.** F (page 531)	**7.** F (page 533)	**10.** F (page 529)	**13.** F (page 537)
2. F (page 527)	**5.** T (page 532)	**8.** F (pages 548, 550)	**11.** T (page 546)	**14.** T (page 533)
3. T (page 531)	**6.** F (page 532)	**9.** T (page 532)	**12.** T (page 546)	**15.** T (page 540)

Fill-in-the-Blank

1. septum (page 525)	**6.** Red blood (page 529)	**11.** dependent edema (page 537)
2. aorta (page 525)	**7.** Diastolic (page 529)	**12.** 160 mm Hg (page 537)
3. right (page 526)	**8.** four (page 525)	**13.** pulmonary veins (page 536)
4. atrioventricular (page 526)	**9.** left (page 526)	**14.** 90 mm Hg (page 536)
5. dilation (page 527)	**10.** CPAP (page 538)	**15.** inferior (page 533)

Labeling

1. **Right and Left Sides of the Heart**

   A. Superior vena cava (oxygen-poor blood from head and upper body)

   B. Left pulmonary artery (blood to left lung)

   C. Right pulmonary artery (blood to right lung)

   D. Right atrium

   E. Inferior vena cava (oxygen-poor blood from lower body)

   F. Right ventricle

   G. Oxygen-rich blood to head and upper body

   H. Right pulmonary veins (oxygen-rich blood from right lung)

   I. Left pulmonary veins (oxygen-rich blood from left lung)

   J. Left atrium

   K. Left ventricle

   L. Oxygen-rich blood to lower body (page 526)

2. Electrical Conduction System

  A. Atrioventricular (AV) node

  B. Bundle of His

  C. SA node

  D. Left bundle branch

  E. Internodal pathways

  F. Left posterior fascicle

  G. Right bundle branch

  H. Purkinje fibers

  I. Left anterior fascicle (page 526)

3. Pulse Points

  A. Carotid

  B. Femoral

  C. Brachial

  D. Radial

  E. Posterior tibial

  F. Dorsalis pedis (page 530)

Crossword Puzzle

Critical Thinking

Short Answer

1. In an AMI, the onset of pain is gradual, with additional symptoms. The pain is typically described as a tightness or pressure. The severity of pain increases with time and may wax and wane. The pain is usually substernal and very rarely radiates to the back. Peripheral pulses are equal.

With a dissecting aneurysm, the onset of pain is abrupt, without additional symptoms. The pain is typically described as sharp or tearing. The severity of pain is at its maximum from the onset and does not abate once started. The pain can be located in the chest with radiation to the back, between the shoulder blades. There can be a blood pressure discrepancy between the arms or a decrease in a femoral or carotid pulse. (pages 537–538)

2. **1.** Not having a charged battery

  2. Applying the AED to a patient who is moving

  3. Applying the AED to a responsive patient with a rapid heart rate (page 547)

3. **1.** If the patient regains a pulse

  2. After six to nine shocks have been delivered

  3. If the machine gives three consecutive "no shock" messages (page 554)

4. **1.** Be aware of the surface the patient is lying on. Wet and metal surfaces may conduct electricity, making defibrillation of the patient dangerous to EMTs.

  2. What is the age of the patient? Use pediatric AED pads when appropriate.

  3. Does the patient have a medication patch in the area where the AED pads will be placed? If so, remove the medication patch, wipe the area clean, and then attach the AED pad.

  4. Does the patient have an implantable pacemaker or internal defibrillator in the same area where the AED pads will be located? If so, place the AED pad below the pacemaker or defibrillator, or place the pads in anterior and posterior positions. (page 555)

5. Stable angina is characterized by pain in the chest of coronary origin that is relieved by the things that normally relieve it in a given patient, such as resting or taking nitroglycerin. Unstable angina is characterized by pain in the chest of coronary origin that occurs in response to progressively less exercise or fewer stimuli than ordinarily required to produce angina. If untreated, it can lead to AMI. (page 532)

6. 1. It may or may not be caused by exertion, but can occur at any time.

   2. It does not resolve in a few minutes.

   3. It may or may not be relieved by rest or nitroglycerin. (page 533)

7. 1. Sudden death

   2. Cardiogenic shock

   3. Congestive heart failure (CHF) (page 533)

8. 1. Sudden onset of weakness, nausea, or sweating without an obvious cause

   2. Chest pain/discomfort that does not change with each breath

   3. Pain, discomfort, or pressure in lower jaw, arms, back, abdomen, or neck

   4. Irregular heartbeat with syncope

   5. Shortness of breath, or dyspnea

   6. Pink, frothy sputum

   7. Sudden death (pages 532–533)

9. 1. Take vital signs, and give oxygen by nonrebreathing mask with an oxygen flow of 10 to 15 L/min.

   2. Allow the patient to remain sitting in an upright position with the legs down.

   3. Be reassuring; many patients with CHF are quite anxious because they cannot breathe.

   4. Patients who have had problems with CHF before will usually have specific medications for its treatment. Gather these medications and take them along to the hospital.

   5. Nitroglycerin may be of value if the patient's systolic blood pressure is greater than 100 mm Hg. If the patient has been prescribed nitroglycerin, and medical control or standing orders advises you to do so, you can administer it sublingually.

   6. Prompt transport to the emergency department is essential. (page 536)

Ambulance Calls

1. The patient is feeling better, so it is likely that he was experiencing an episode of angina; however, because you cannot rule out an AMI, this patient should be strongly encouraged to go to the hospital for evaluation. Place the patient in a position of comfort. Provide high-flow oxygen via nonrebreathing mask. Monitor his vital signs and provide normal transport. If the patient continues to have chest pain, reassess and consider administering an additional nitroglycerin tablet, if local protocol permits. In addition to BLS care, this patient will also benefit from ALS care; therefore, an attempt to rendezvous with an ALS unit should be made.

2. Denial is one of the biggest indicators of heart attack. Although this patient is considered "younger" and otherwise healthy, he is having signs and symptoms of a myocardial infarction. It may take some convincing of the need for treatment and transport, but you must be clear on the potential consequences of his refusal of care (informed refusal). If he initially refuses, explain what physical signs you see that lead you to believe he is likely having a heart attack, express genuine concern for his well-being, and allow him to speak directly with medical control. More often than not, when patients hear the same or similar information from a physician, it makes a different impact. If he allows you to examine, treat, and transport him, apply high-flow oxygen, transport promptly, and follow local protocols.

3. This patient could be having a heart attack. A common symptom that women (especially postmenopausal women) experience when having a heart attack is the sudden onset of generalized weakness. Although chest pain is a common indicator of heart attack, if a patient is not experiencing pain or pressure it does not necessarily mean they are not experiencing a cardiac event. It is important to note that heart disease is the number one killer of women in the United States, taking more lives than cancer and killing more women than men every year. If your patient exhibits any combination of the "associated symptoms" of heart attack such as nausea; vomiting; shortness of breath; pain or numbness in the neck, jaw, back, or arm(s); or cool, pale, sweaty skin, you should suspect the possibility of a heart attack. You should apply high-flow oxygen, obtain vital signs, allow the patient to maintain a position of comfort, and provide immediate transport to the nearest appropriate facility.

Fill-in-the-Patient Care Report

EMS Patient Care Report (PCR)				
Date: Today's Date	**Incident No.:** 011543	**Nature of Call:** Chest Pain		**Location:** 1574 S. Main St
Dispatched: 1901	**En Route:** 1901	**At Scene:** 1909	**Transport:** 1921	**At Hospital:** 1926 **In Service:** 1935

Patient Information	
Age: 58 Years	**Allergies:** Aspirin
Sex: Male	**Medications:** lisinopril, nitroglycerin, metformin, and metoprolol
Weight (in kg [lb]): Unknown	**Past Medical History:** hypertension, angina, and diabetes
	Chief Complaint: Chest tightness

Vital Signs				
Time: 1914	**BP:** 136/88	**Pulse:** 88	**Respirations:** 22	**Sao2:** 99%
Time: 1921	**BP:** 122/74	**Pulse:** 84	**Respirations:** 18	**Sao2:** 98%

EMS Treatment				
(circle all that apply)				
Oxygen @ 15 L/min via (circle one): NC **(NRM)** Bag-Mask Device		**Assisted Ventilation**	**Airway Adjunct**	**CPR**
Defibrillation	**Bleeding Control**	**Bandaging**	**Splinting**	**Other Shock Treatment**

Narrative
9-1-1 dispatch for 58-year-old man complaining of chest pain. Arrived on scene and was met by patient's wife at the front door who stated that patient has been experiencing chest pain for approximately 30 minutes with no relief from two nitroglycerin tablets. We were directed to the living room, where we found our patient sitting up on the couch with some obvious shortness of breath. Patient stated that he was sitting on the couch when he began to feel "incredible constant pressure" in his chest. Stated that he initially thought it was his angina, but reported that "this feels different." Patient currently rates pain as a 5/10. Oxygen was applied at 15 L/min via nonrebreathing mask. Primary and secondary assessment performed, along with vital signs. Per local protocol, because the patient's systolic blood pressure was above 100 mm Hg, one tablet of nitroglycerin was administered sublingually to the patient. The patient was secured to stretcher and taken to unit. Patient was transported to local facility. Reassessment of patient indicated his pain was now a 4/10. Upon arrival at facility, patient was stable. Care was transferred to ED staff. Verbal report was given to staff. No further incidents. Unit cleaned and restocked. Crew went available and returned to station. **End of Report**

Skills

Skill Drills

Skill Drill 14-1: Administration of Nitroglycerin

1. Obtain an order from **medical control**. Take the patient's blood pressure. Administer **nitroglycerin** only if the **systolic** blood pressure is greater than 100 mm Hg.

2. Check the medication and expiration date. Ask the patient about the last dose and its **effects**. Make sure that the patient understands the route of **administration**. Prepare to have the patient lie down to prevent **fainting**.

3. Ask the patient to lift his or her **tongue**. Place the tablet or spray the dose under the **tongue** (while wearing gloves), or have the patient do so. Have the patient keep his or her mouth **closed** with the tablet or spray under the tongue until it is dissolved and absorbed. Caution the patient against **chewing** or swallowing the tablet.

4. Recheck the blood pressure within 5 minutes. Record each medication and the time of administration. Reevaluate the **chest pain** and blood pressure, and repeat treatment, if necessary. (page 544)

Skill Drill 14-2: AED and CPR

1. Assess compression effectiveness if CPR is already in progress. If the patient is unresponsive and CPR has not been started yet, begin providing chest compressions and rescue breaths as a ratio of 30 compressions to two breaths, continuing until an AED arrives and is ready for use.

2. Turn on the AED. Apply the AED pads to the chest and attach the pads to the AED. Stop CPR.

3. Verbally and visually clear the patient. Push the Analyze button, if there is one. Wait for the AED to analyze the cardiac rhythm. If no shock is advised, perform five cycles (about 2 minutes) of CPR and then reanalyze the cardiac rhythm. If a shock is advised, recheck that all are clear, and push the Shock button. After the shock is delivered, immediately resume CPR, beginning with chest compressions.

4. After five cycles (about 2 minutes) of CPR, reanalyze the cardiac rhythm. Do not interrupt chest compressions for more than 10 seconds.

5. If a shock is advised, clear the patient, push the Shock button, and immediately resume CPR compressions. If no shock is advised, immediately resume CPR compressions. After five cycles (2 minutes) of CPR, reanalyze the cardiac rhythm. Repeat the cycle of five cycles (2 minutes) of CPR, one shock (if indicated), and 2 minutes of CPR. Transport, and contact medical control as needed.

Assessment Review

1. B (page 537)
2. A (page 540)
3. D (page 558)
4. C (page 540)
5. B (page 545)

Emergency Care Summary (page 560)

General Management of Cardiovascular Emergencies

Managing life threats to the patient's ABCs and ensuring the delivery of high-flow oxygen are primary concerns with any cardiovascular emergency. If the patient is unconscious, determine whether CPR is needed. In conscious patients, obtain a thorough history. "Time is **muscle**," so rapid transport will be needed to a **cardiac care** facility for patients presenting with signs and symptoms of a **myocardial** infarction. If local protocols allow, administer aspirin and assist the patient in taking his or her prescribed nitroglycerin. Be prepared to **defibrillate** if the patient becomes pulseless.

Cardiogenic Shock

Shock is a state of hypoperfusion. The hypoperfusion from cardiogenic shock is due to failure of the pump (heart). The container (blood vessels) is intact, and the fluid (blood) is still present within the container. EMTs need to be able to recognize cardiogenic shock over other types of shock because the management is different. The first clue is that there is no **mechanism of injury**. **Chest pain** is usually the chief complaint. The pulse may be irregular. The patient may have respiratory distress due to fluid buildup in the lungs (**pulmonary edema**) due to poor cardiac output. As with other shocks, the blood pressure is low. *Do not* place this patient in the shock or **Trendelenburg's** position because it will increase the workload of the heart and cause increased fluid collection in the lungs. Place the patient in a position of comfort. Administer high-concentration oxygen. Request ALS support if transport is delayed. *Do not* give **nitroglycerin**; the blood pressure is already low. If a specialty center is close by, transport there; if not, transport to the nearest hospital.

Congestive Heart Failure

Fluid in the lungs is called pulmonary edema. Pulmonary edema can be caused by cardiac failure after an AMI (CHF) or a noncardiogenic cause such as a toxic inhalation. In either case, the outcome is the same, fluid in the lungs prevents the efficient exchange of oxygen and carbon dioxide. The patient will present with respiratory distress, usually severe, and appear very anxious. The skin will be cool, pale, and **moist**. The patient's blood pressure is often high unless the AMI is so severe as to cause **cardiogenic shock**. Patients with a history of CHF will often sleep with multiple pillows or upright in a recliner. Jugular vein distention is common. The patient needs high-flow oxygen. Assisted ventilation or CPAP is often helpful. Assist the patient in taking his or her prescribed nitroglycerin if medical control or protocol allows, ensuring the systolic blood pressure is more than **100** mm Hg before giving the nitroglycerin. Patients experiencing pulmonary edema may require positive-pressure ventilation with a bag-mask device or CPAP. **CPAP** is the most effective way to assist a person with CHF to breathe effectively and prevent an invasive airway management technique. Transport promptly to the closest emergency department.

Chapter 15: Neurologic Emergencies

General Knowledge

Matching

1. M (page 571)
2. N (page 572)
3. D (page 574)
4. O (page 567)
5. K (page 567)
6. E (page 567)
7. H (page 576)
8. B (page 575)
9. F (page 575)
10. L (page 570)
11. A (page 572)
12. C (page 573)
13. I (page 574)
14. J (page 570)
15. G (page 571)

Multiple Choice

1. D (page 573)
2. A (page 567)
3. A (page 568)
4. C (page 567)
5. C (page 570)
6. A (page 571)
7. B (page 571)
8. B (page 570)
9. D (page 571)
10. A (page 576)
11. D (page 576)
12. A (page 580)
13. D (page 585)
14. C (page 576)
15. B (page 576)
16. C (page 576)
17. C (page 569)
18. A (page 570)
19. B (page 571)
20. D (page 569)
21. A (page 572)
22. B (page 578)
23. C (page 572)
24. C (page 579)
25. B (page 581)
26. D (page 580)
27. B (page 572)
28. A (page 570)
29. D (page 584)

True/False

1. F (page 572)
2. T (page 568)
3. T (page 575)
4. F (page 576)
5. T (page 569)
6. F (page 572)
7. T (page 569)
8. T (page 571)
9. F (page 571)
10. T (page 572)
11. F (page 572)
12. F (page 573)
13. T (page 575)
14. T (page 584)
15. F (page 577)
16. T (page 577)
17. T (page 583)
18. F (page 584)
19. F (page 584)
20. T (page 584)

Fill-in-the-Blank

1. 12 (page 567)
2. cerebellum (page 567)
3. ischemic; hemorrhagic (pages 570–571)
4. oxygen; glucose; temperature (page 568)
5. carbon monoxide poisoning (page 569)
6. simple partial (page 573)
7. opposite (page 567)
8. temporal (page 573)
9. Incontinence (page 575)
10. epileptic seizures (pages 574–575)
11. postictal state (page 574)
12. hemiparesis (page 576)
13. foreign body obstruction (page 579)
14. Glasgow Coma Scale (page 582)
15. Thrombolytic therapy (page 585)

Labeling

1. Brain (page 568)
   A. Cerebrum
   B. Skull
   C. Brain stem
   D. Cerebellum
   E. Spinal cord

2. Spinal Cord (page 568)
   A. Cerebrum
   B. Cerebellum
   C. Brain stem
   D. Foramen magnum
   E. Spinal cord
   F. Spinal nerves

Crossword Puzzle

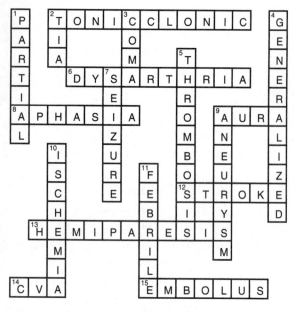

Critical Thinking

Short Answer

1. **1.** Facial droop—Ask patient to show teeth or smile.

   Normal: Both sides of the face move equally well.

   Abnormal: One side of the face does not move as well as the other.

   2. Arm drift—Ask patient to close eyes and hold arms out with palms up.

   Normal: Both arms move the same, or both arms do not move.

   Abnormal: One arm does not move, or one arm drifts down compared to the other side.

   3. Speech—Ask patient to say, "The sky is blue in Cincinnati."

   Normal: Patient uses correct words with no slurring.

   Abnormal: Patient slurs words, uses inappropriate words, or is unable to speak. (page 582)

2. Newer thrombolytic therapies may be helpful in reversing damage in certain kinds of strokes, but treatment must be started within 3 hours after onset of the event. (pages 585–586)

3. A period of time after a seizure, generally lasting from 5 to 30 minutes, that is characterized by some degree of altered mental status and labored respirations. The patient's muscles relax, becoming almost flaccid, or floppy. In some situations, the postictal state may be characterized by hemiparesis, resembling a stroke. However, unlike a stroke, these symptoms will resolve. (page 572)

4. A partial seizure begins in one part of the brain and is classified as simple or complex. In a simple partial seizure, there is no change in mental status. Patients may complain of numbness, weakness, or dizziness. A simple partial seizure may also cause twitching of the muscles and the extremities that may spread slowly from one part of the body to another, but it is not characterized by the dramatic severe twitching and muscle movements seen in a generalized seizure.

   In a complex partial seizure, the patient has an altered mental status and does not interact normally with his or her environment. This type of seizure results from abnormal discharges from the temporal lobe of the brain. Other characteristics may be lip smacking, eye blinking, and isolated convulsions or jerking of the body or one part of the body, such as an arm. (page 573)

5. **1.** Hypoglycemia

   2. Postictal state

   3. Subdural or epidural bleeding (page 572)

6. **A.** Eye Opening—4—Patient is looking at you.

Verbal—4—Patient is confused about the date/year.

Motor—5—Patient does not respond to commands, localized to pain.

Total: 13

B. Eye Opening—2—Patient opens eyes to painful stimulus.

Verbal—2—Patient uses incomprehensible sounds.

Motor—4—Patient withdraws to pain.

Total: 8

C. Eye Opening—1—Patient does not open eyes to any stimuli.

Verbal—1—Patient has no verbal response.

Motor—1—Patient does not move extremities to any stimuli.

Total: 3

D. Eye Opening—4—Patient is looking at you.

Verbal—5—Patient is able to have an oriented conversation.

Motor—6—Patient is able to follow commands.

Total: 15 (page 583)

Ambulance Calls

1. Given these signs, your patient is likely experiencing a left hemispheric stroke. Any problems related to his ability to understand or use language will be frustrating for both you and the patient. After performing your primary assessment, the Cincinnati Prehospital Stroke Scale can provide valuable information regarding the presence of a stroke. This assessment measures abnormalities in speech and the presence of facial droop and arm drift. Stroke is a true emergency that requires prompt transport. You should apply high-flow oxygen and take care during transport to prevent injury of affected body parts, because the patient will not be able to protect them on his own. It is helpful to place the patient on the affected side and elevate his head approximately 6″ (15 cm) to facilitate swallowing. Be sure to relate your positive findings of stroke to the hospital to avoid any unnecessary delays in patient care upon arrival to the emergency department.

2. Maintain the airway—high-flow oxygen

   Suction, if necessary, or position lateral recumbent to clear secretions

   Check glucose level

   Provide rapid transport.

3. This patient's signs and symptoms cause you to suspect the presence of a hemorrhagic stroke. You should apply high-flow oxygen and provide immediate transport. This patient will be more likely to experience seizure activity than patients suffering from ischemic stroke. There is no way for you to determine the type or extent of her stroke, because this can be accomplished only in the hospital. Your job is to recognize the seriousness of the situation, provide supportive measures within your scope of practice, and provide prompt transport and notification to the receiving facility.

4. When a patient who experienced a seizure wants to refuse EMS care, the following questions need to be discussed and/or considered:

   1. Is the patient awake and completely oriented after the seizure (GCS score of 15)?

   2. Does your assessment show no evidence of trauma or complications from the seizure?

   3. Has the patient ever had a seizure before?

   4. Was this seizure the "usual" seizure in every way (length, activity, recovery)?

   5. Is the patient currently being treated with medications and receiving regular evaluations by a physician?

   If the answer to all these questions is "yes," you may consider agreeing to the patient's refusal for transport if the patient can be released to a responsible person and monitored. However, if the answer is "no" to any of the questions, you should strongly encourage the patient to be transported and evaluated.

Skills

Assessment Review

1. C (page 582)   2. B (page 572)   3. A (page 585)   4. C (page 571)

Chapter 16: Gastrointestinal and Urologic Emergencies

General Knowledge

Matching

1. I (page 607)	**6.** A (page 602)	**11.** G (page 602)	**16.** F (page 603)	**21.** A (page 603)
2. D (page 603)	**7.** C (page 610)	**12.** N (page 606)	**17.** B (page 603)	**22.** D (page 603)
3. E (page 599)	**8.** J (page 606)	**13.** L (page 607)	**18.** J (page 603)	**23.** H (page 603)
4. M (page 603)	**9.** F (page 602)	**14.** O (page 602)	**19.** I (page 603)	**24.** C (page 603)
5. K (page 607)	**10.** B (page 602)	**15.** H (page 601)	**20.** E (page 603)	**25.** G (page 603)

Multiple Choice

1. B (page 602)	**7.** B (page 599)	**13.** D (page 606)	**19.** C (page 605)	**25.** D (page 612)
2. A (page 602)	**8.** C (page 603)	**14.** A (page 606)	**20.** A (page 605)	**26.** C (page 600)
3. A (page 607)	**9.** B (page 603)	**15.** A (page 612)	**21.** C (page 605)	**27.** B (page 601)
4. B (page 605)	**10.** D (pages 603–605)	**16.** C (page 600)	**22.** B (page 604)	**28.** C (page 600)
5. D (page 611)	**11.** B (page 604)	**17.** B (page 606)	**23.** C (page 604)	**29.** D (page 600)
6. A (page 607)	**12.** C (page 609)	**18.** D (page 605)	**24.** A (page 610)	**30.** C (page 600)

True/False

1. F (page 602)	**3.** F (page 609)	**5.** T (page 602)	**7.** F (page 610)	**9.** T (page 603)
2. T (page 613)	**4.** T (page 609)	**6.** F (page 602)	**8.** T (page 607)	**10.** F (page 612)

Labeling

1. **Solid Organs**
   - **A.** Liver
   - **B.** Spleen
   - **C.** Pancreas
   - **D.** Kidney
   - **E.** Kidney
   - **F.** Ovaries (page 599)

2. **Hollow Organs**
   - **A.** Gallbladder
   - **B.** Stomach
   - **C.** Ureter
   - **D.** Small intestine
   - **E.** Large intestine
   - **F.** Fallopian tubes
   - **G.** Urinary bladder
   - **H.** Uterus (page 599)

3. **Urinary System**
   - **A.** Kidney
   - **B.** Ureter
   - **C.** Bladder
   - **D.** Prostate gland
   - **E.** Ureter opening
   - **F.** Urethra
   - **G.** Penis
   - **H.** External urethral opening (page 600)

Crossword Puzzle

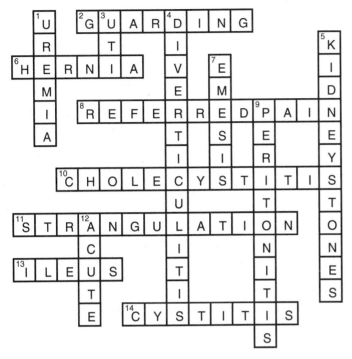

Critical Thinking

Short Answer

1. Occurs because of connections between the body's two nervous systems. The abdominal organs are supplied by autonomic nerves, which, when irritated, stimulate close-lying sensory (somatic) nerves. (page 602)

2. **1.** Has the patient's level of consciousness changed?
   2. Has the patient become more anxious?
   3. Have the skin signs started to change?
   4. Has the pain gotten better or worse?
   5. Has the bleeding become worse or better?
   6. Is current treatment improving the patient's condition?
   7. Has an already identified problem gotten better?
   8. Has an already identified problem gotten worse?
   9. What is the nature of any newly identified problems? (page 611)

3. Paralysis of muscular contractions in the bowel results in retained gas and feces. Nothing can pass through. (page 602)

4. **1.** Explain to the patient what you are going to do in terms of assessing the abdomen.
   2. Place the patient in a supine position with the legs drawn up and flexed at the knees to relax the abdominal muscles, unless there is any trauma, in which case the patient will remain supine and stabilized. Determine whether the patient is restless or quiet, and whether motion causes pain.
   3. Expose the abdomen and visually assess it. Does the abdomen appear distended (enlarged)? Do you see any pulsating masses? Is there bruising to the abdominal wall?
   4. Ask the patient where the pain is most intense. Palpate in a clockwise direction beginning with the quadrant after the one the patient indicates is tender or painful; end with the quadrant that the patient indicates is tender and painful. If the most painful area is palpated first, the patient may guard against further examination, making your assessment more difficult and less reliable.

5. Remember to be very gentle when palpating the abdomen.

6. Palpate the four quadrants of the abdomen gently to determine whether each quadrant is tense (guarded) or soft when palpated.

7. Note whether the pain is localized to a particular quadrant or diffuse (widespread).

8. Palpate and wait for the patient to respond, looking for a facial grimace or a verbal "ouch." Do not ask the patient, "Does it hurt here?" as you palpate.

9. Determine whether the patient exhibits rebound tenderness.

10. Determine whether the patient can relax the abdominal wall on command.

11. Guarding and rigidity may be detected. (pages 610–611)

Ambulance Calls

1. Appendicitis is a possibility. Place the patient in the position of comfort. Apply high-flow oxygen. Keep the patient warm. Provide rapid transport. Obtain a SAMPLE history. Document OPQRST. Monitor patient closely.

2. This patient is likely experiencing a bowel obstruction, secondary to an ileus, that is causing his pain and tenderness. If left untreated, his condition will deteriorate. When assessing his abdomen, explain what you will do, place him with knees slightly toward his abdomen, and gently palpate all four quadrants to determine the presence of rigidity or masses. If a patient points to a specific location of pain, palpate that area last. You must take great care in moving and transporting the patient, because it will be particularly painful if he is bumped or jostled. Apply high-flow oxygen, allow him to find his position of comfort, and move him gently. Do not delay transport to attempt to determine the cause of abdominal pain.

3. Individuals who have experienced a kidney stone(s) will tell you that it is an extremely painful experience. Provide prompt, gentle transport. Monitor his airway, breathing, and circulation. Be prepared for continued vomiting. Apply oxygen (which can ease nausea), obtain vital signs, do not give anything by mouth, and keep the patient as comfortable as possible. Be sure to thoroughly document all information regarding the patient's signs and symptoms as well as any treatment you provide. Always follow local protocols.

Skills

Assessment Review

1. D (page 608)

2. A (page 609)

3. B (page 609)

4. C (page602)

5. D (page 611)

Emergency Care Summary (page 617)

General Management of Gastrointestinal and Urologic Emergencies

1. Explain to the patient what you are going to do in terms of assessing the abdomen.

2. Establish and maintain a patent airway. Provide oxygen (**low**-flow reduces nausea). Monitor for vomiting and protect the airway against **aspiration**.

3. Allow the patient to assume a position of comfort. You will find that most patients want to be **supine** with their **legs** drawn up to relax the abdominal muscles, unless there is any trauma, in which case the patient will remain supine and stabilized.

4. Obtain SAMPLE history and vital signs.

5. Palpate the **four** quadrants of the abdomen gently to determine whether each quadrant is tense (**guarded**) or soft when palpated.

6. Determine whether the patient can relax the **abdominal wall** on command.

7. Request ALS support when intravenous fluids or pain management is necessary.

Chapter 17: Endocrine and Hematologic Emergencies

General Knowledge

Matching

1. J (page 621)
2. A (page 633)
3. C (page 622)
4. M (page 623)

5. O (page 622)
6. Q (page 625)
7. F (page 622)
8. G (page 634)

9. D (page 622)
10. B (page 625)
11. P (page 621)
12. E (page 623)

13. L (page 624)
14. K (page 621)
15. H (page 622)

16. N (page 635)
17. I (page 622)

Multiple Choice

1. A (page 622)
2. A (page 622)
3. A (page 634)
4. C (page 622)
5. C (page 635)
6. A (page 623)
7. C (page 622)
8. D (page 622)

9. D (page 625)
10. B (page 622)
11. B (page 623)
12. D (page 634)
13. D (page 622)
14. A (page 621)
15. A (page 622)
16. A (page 622)

17. C (page 623)
18. A (page 633)
19. B (page 626)
20. D (page 626)
21. C (page 626)
22. B (page 628)
23. A (page 625)
24. B (page 625)

25. C (page 627)
26. D (page 628)
27. B (page 636)
28. A (page 630)
29. D (page 632)
30. D (page 625)
31. B (page 625)
32. C (page 625)

33. D (page 636)
34. D (page 626)
35. A (page 626)
36. C (page 626)
37. C (page 632)

True/False

1. T (page 623)
2. F (page 622)
3. F (page 633)

4. T (page 625)
5. T (page 626)
6. T (page 635)

7. T (page 624)
8. T (page 622)
9. F (page 622)

10. F (page 634)
11. T (page 621)
12. T (page 622)

13. F (page 633)
14. T (page 622)

Fill-in-the-Blank

1. diabetes mellitus (page 622)
2. hemolytic; drop (page 634)
3. autoimmune (page 622)
4. Mediterranean; sickle cell (page 635)

5. ineffective (page 622)
6. diabetic coma (page 625)
7. Hematology; related (page 633)
8. sugar; insulin (page 629)

Fill-in-the-Table

	Hyperglycemia	Hypoglycemia
History		
Food intake	Excessive	Insufficient
Insulin dosage	Insufficient	Excessive
Onset	Gradual (hours to days)	Rapid, within minutes
Skin	Warm and dry	Pale, cool, and moist
Infection	Common	Uncommo
Gastrointestinal Tract		
Thirst	Intense	Absent
Hunger	Absent	Intense
Vomiting	Commo	Uncommon
Respiratory System		
Breathing	Rapid, deep (Kussmaul respirations)	Normal or rapid
Odor of breath	Sweet, fruity	Normal
Cardiovascular System		
Blood pressure	Normal to low	Low
Pulse	Rapid, weak, and thready	Rapid, weak
Nervous System		
Consciousness	Restlessness, possibly progressing to coma; abnormal or slurred speech; unsteady gait	Irritability, confusion, seizure, or coma; unsteady gait
Urine		
Sugar	Present	Absent
Acetone	Present	Absent
Treatment		
Response	Gradual, within 6 to 12 hours following medical treatment	Immediate after administration of glucose

Crossword Puzzle

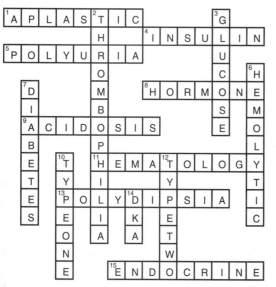

Critical Thinking

Multiple Choice

1. D (page 622)   **2.** C (page 624)   **3.** D (page 627)   **4.** A (page 626)   **5.** D (page 629)

Short Answer

1. Insulin is a hormone that enables glucose to enter the cells, which is essential for cellular metabolism. (page 623)

2. **1.** Glutose
   2. Insta-Glucose (page 630)

3. Due to the oblong shape of the red blood cells, they are poor oxygen carriers and can become lodged in blood vessels and organs. (page 633)

4. A patient who is unconscious or not able to swallow should not be given oral glucose. (page 630)

5. A patient with thrombophilia has a tendency to develop clots in the blood vessels. These clots can travel through the circulatory system and become lodged in the lungs, obstructing blood flow and oxygen exchange. (page 634)

6. **1.** Ketoacidosis
   2. Dehydration
   3. Hyperglycemia (page 625)

7. **1.** Kussmaul respirations
   2. Dehydration
   3. Fruity odor on breath
   4. Rapid, weak pulse
   5. Normal or slightly low blood pressure
   6. Varying degrees of unresponsiveness
   7. Polyuria, polydipsia, polyphagia (page 625)

8. Insulin shock; it develops rapidly as opposed to diabetic coma, which takes longer to develop. (page 626)

9. Spontaneous intracranial bleeding. (page 635)

Ambulance Calls

1. **1.** Turn the patient on her side immediately or use suction to clear the airway.
   2. Insert an oral or nasal airway and apply high-flow oxygen.
   3. Attempt to obtain a blood glucose level.
   4. Transport the patient rapidly because you should never give anything by mouth to an unresponsive patient.
   5. Monitor the patient closely.

2. The prehospital management of patients suffering from sickle cell crises will commonly include only comfort care and rapid transportation. You may also treat individual symptoms as they arise as per standard protocol. For example, a sickle cell patient presenting with difficulty breathing should receive oxygen therapy or ventilatory assistance if required.

3. You cannot give this patient anything by mouth because he is unconscious and therefore unable to protect his own airway. If available, you should request ALS providers, because they can administer intravenous dextrose (glucose). If you have no emergency providers available with this scope of practice within your system, you must transport this patient immediately. You may encounter family members who do not understand why you cannot "just give him some sugar." Hopefully, there will be no delays in explaining his need for transport or the seriousness of his condition. Perform a thorough assessment (including blood glucose testing, if permitted), provide high-flow oxygen, monitor his ABCs (using airway adjuncts, positive pressure ventilations, and suctioning, as needed), and provide prompt transport.

Fill-in-the-Patient Care Report

EMS Patient Care Report (PCR)					
Date: Today's Date	**Incident No.:** 2011-1234	**Nature of Call:** Laceration		**Location:** 12556 Old Lakehouse Drive	
Dispatched: 1752	**En Route:** 1755	**At Scene:** 1803	**Transport:** 1813	**At Hospital:** 1819	**In Service:** 1839

Patient Information					
Age: 14 Years			**Allergies:** Unknown		
Sex: Male			**Medications:** Unknown		
Weight (in kg [lb]): 60 kg (132 lb)			**Past Medical History:** Hemophilia		
			Chief Complaint: Bleeding Laceration		

Vital Signs				
Time: 1813	**BP:** 108/60	**Pulse:** 98	**Respirations:** 16 / GTV	**Sao2:** 96%

EMS Treatment
(circle all that apply)

Oxygen @ 15 L/min via (circle one): NC **(NRM)** Bag-Mask Device	**Assisted Ventilation**	**Airway Adjunct:**	**CPR**
Defibrillation / **(Bleeding Control)**	**(Bandaging:** Tourniquet**)**	**Splinting**	**(Other Shock Treatment)**

Narrative

9-1-1 dispatch for an arm laceration with uncontrolled bleeding. Arrived on scene and was directed to a second-floor bedroom where the patient, a 14-year-old boy, was holding pressure on a left forearm laceration. Patient's mother advised that he had hemophilia. Observed steady bleeding and attempted to control with pressure. Initiated oxygen therapy at 15 L/min via nonrebreathing mask and used the stair chair to move the patient down to the gurney where he was covered with blankets to conserve body temperature and loaded into the ambulance. Obtained vitals, which indicated that the patient might be hypoperfusing. Because steady pressure didn't stop the bleeding, applied a tourniquet proximal to the laceration, which did stop the bleeding. Monitored the patient while en route to the hospital, continued oxygen therapy, and notified the facility of our impending arrival. Delivered the patient to the trauma department, gave a full report to the charge RN, transferred patient care, and returned to service after cleaning/decontaminating the ambulance. **End of Report**

Skills

Skill Drills

Skill Drill 17-1: Administering Glucose

1. Make sure that the tube of glucose is intact and has not **expired**.

2. Squeeze a generous amount of oral glucose onto the **bottom third** of a **bite stick** or tongue depressor.

3. Open the patient's **mouth**. Place the tongue depressor on the **mucous membranes** between the cheek and the gum with the **gel side** next to the cheek. Repeat until the entire tube has been used. (page 631)

Assessment Review

1. B (page 626) **2.** B (page 626) **3.** C (page 627) **4.** D (page 627) **5.** D (page 630)

Chapter 18: Immunologic Emergencies

General Knowledge

Matching

1. D (page 647)
2. A (page 647)
3. H (page 647)
4. E (page 647)
5. B (page 653)
6. G (page 647)
7. C (page 649)
8. F (page 648)

Multiple Choice

1. A (page 656)
2. D (page 647)
3. A (page 652)
4. D (page 649)
5. C (page 653)
6. C (page 649)
7. D (page 652)
8. C (page 655)
9. D (page 654)
10. C (page 649)
11. A (page 649)
12. D (pages 652–653)
13. C (page 648)
14. C (page 647)
15. A (page 653)

True/False

1. T (page 647)
2. T (page 647)
3. F (page 647)
4. F (page 651)

Fill-in-the-Blank

1. bronchial passages (page 653)
2. urticaria (page 647)
3. barbed (page 648)
4. anaphylaxis (page 647)
5. hypoperfusion (page 653)
6. blood vessels (page 654)
7. imminent death (page 647)

Crossword Puzzle

Critical Thinking

Multiple Choice

1. C (page 647)

2. B (page 647)

3. D (page 655)

4. C (page 656)

5. D (page 656)

Short Answer

1. Increased blood pressure, tachycardia, pallor, dizziness, chest pain, headache, nausea, vomiting (page 659)

2.   **1.** Insect bites and stings

   2. Medications

   3. Plants

   4. Food

   5. Chemicals (pages 647–648)

3.   **1.** Obtain an order from medical control (or follow protocol or standing orders).

   2. Follow standard precautions.

   3. Make sure the medication was prescribed for that patient.

   4. Check for discoloration or expiration of medication.

   5. Remove the cap.

   6. Wipe the thigh with alcohol, if possible.

   7. Place the tip against the lateral midthigh.

   8. Push firmly until activation.

   9. Hold the auto-injector in place until the medication is injected.

   10. Remove and dispose.

   11. Record the time and dose.

   12. Reassess and record the patient's vital signs. (pages 655–657)

4. Respiratory: Shortness of breath (dyspnea); sneezing or itchy, runny nose; chest or throat tightness; dry cough; hoarseness; rapid, noisy, or labored respirations; wheezing and/or stridor

Circulatory: Decreased blood pressure (hypotension); increased pulse (tachycardia); pale skin; loss of consciousness and coma (page 652)

Ambulance Calls

1. Based on the information you have, there is no way to determine if the child fell out of the tree or climbed down. You should assume that the child fell, which will require the use of full spinal precautions. You also have the issue of scene safety, because the damaged hive is now lying on the ground next to the patient. You must take care not to receive multiple stings yourself, so proceed with caution. If the child is having a severe allergic reaction, hopefully you will have access to an EpiPen Junior. Provide high-flow oxygen and prompt transport according to local protocols.

2. Obtain a physician's order to administer the EpiPen to the patient. Check the EpiPen for clarity, expiration date, etc. Administer the EpiPen and promptly dispose of the auto-injector. Apply high-flow oxygen and provide rapid transport. Monitor the patient and assess vital signs frequently.

Fill-in-the-Patient Care Report

EMS Patient Care Report (PCR)			
Date: Today's Date	**Incident Number:** 2011-0101	**Nature of Call:** Allergic reaction	**Location:** 231 Seaside Parkway
Dispatched: 1734	**En Route:** 1734	**At Scene:** 1742	**Transport:** 1748	**At Hospital:** 1801	**In Service:** 1814

Patient Information	
Age: 37 Years	**Allergies:** Possible seafood
Sex: Male	**Medications:** N/A
Weight (kg [lb]): 63 kg (138 lb)	**Past Medical History:** N/A
	Chief Complaint: Allergic reaction

Vital Signs				
Time: 1748	**BP:** 110/64	**Pulse:** 116	**Respirations:** 26 Labored	**Sao$_2$:** 92%
Time: 1755	**BP:** 140/94	**Pulse:** 128	**Respirations:** 18 Adequate Tidal Volume	**Sao$_2$:** 96%

EMS Treatment

(circle all that apply)

Oxygen @ 15 L/min via (circle one): NC (NRM) (Bag-Mask Device)	(Assisted Ventilation)	Airway Adjunct	CPR
Defibrillation	Bleeding Control	Bandaging	Splinting	(Other Shock Treatment)

Narrative

Requested for an emergency response to a seafood restaurant for anaphylactic reaction. Arrived and led to patient—37-year-old man—who presented with generalized swelling of the face, neck, and hands; hives; and difficulty breathing. It was immediately apparent that the patient was becoming hypoxic, so we initiated oxygen therapy and requested an ALS rendezvous. We then began transport of the patient, and initial vitals indicated that the patient was anaphylactic. Began to assist ventilations with bag-mask device until rendezvous with ALS crew. Paramedic Johnson boarded ambulance and administered epinephrine and patient responded to treatment quickly. Second set of vitals confirmed reversal of anaphylaxis. Provided verbal report and ETA to the receiving facility, and the rest of the transport was without incident. On arrival at the facility, patient was appropriately turned over to the receiving staff after we provided a complete verbal report to the charge nurse. **End of Report**

Skills

Skill Drill

Skill Drill 18-2: Using a Twinject Auto-Injector

1. Remove the **injector** from the container.
2. Clean the administration site with an **alcohol** preparation. Pull off **green** cap "1" to expose a round **red** tip. Do not cover the rounded tip with your **hand**. Pull off green cap "2."
3. Place the **round** red tip against the **lateral** part of the thigh. The injection can be administered outside of **clothing** if necessary. Once the needle has entered the skin, press hard for **10** seconds. Remove the Twinject. Check to make sure the **needle** is visible. If the **needle** is not visible, repeat the steps.
4. If symptoms recur or have not improved within **10** minutes, repeat the dose. Carefully unscrew and remove the **red** tip. Hold the **blue** plastic, pulling the syringe out of the barrel without touching the **needle**. Slide the yellow collar off the plunger without pulling on the **plunger**.
5. Insert the **needle** into the skin on the lateral part of the **thigh** and push the plunger down. (pages 658–659)

Assessment Review

1. A (page 651)
2. D (pages 656–657)
3. D (page 657)
4. C (page 652)
5. D (page 652)

Emergency Care Summary (page 664)

Using an Auto-injector

1. Remove the auto-injector's **safety cap**, and quickly wipe the **thigh** with antiseptic.
2. Place the tip of the auto-injector against the **lateral** part of the **thigh**.
3. Push the auto-injector firmly against the **thigh**, and hold it in place until all the medication is injected (about **10** seconds).

Using Twinject

1. Remove the injector from the container.
2. Clean the administration site with an **alcohol** preparation. Pull off **green cap** "1" to expose a **round red** tip. Do not cover the rounded tip with your hand.
3. Pull off green cap "2."
4. Place the round red tip against the lateral part of the thigh. The injection can be administered outside of clothing if necessary. Once the needle has entered the skin, press hard for 10 seconds.
5. Remove the Twinject. Check to see whether the needle is visible. If the needle is *not* visible, the dose was not administered and all the steps should be repeated.
6. If symptoms recur or have not improved within 10 minutes, repeat the dose. Carefully unscrew and remove the **red tip**. Hold the blue plastic, pulling the syringe out of the barrel without touching the **needle**. Slide the yellow collar off the plunger without pulling on the **plunger**.
7. Insert the needle into the skin on the lateral part of the thigh and push the plunger down.

Chapter 19: Toxicology

General Knowledge

Matching

1. F (page 669)
2. H (page 669)
3. G (page 671)
4. D (page 679)
5. J (page 685)
6. I (page 669)
7. K (page 680)
8. E (page 683)
9. B (page 669)
10. A (page 682)
11. C (page 684)

Multiple Choice

1. B (page 674)
2. B (page 669)
3. C (page 689)
4. C (page 685)
5. A (page 670)
6. C (page 671)
7. C (page 679)
8. B (page 680)
9. C (page 681)
10. D (page 682)
11. A (page 684)
12. C (page 683)
13. A (page 685)
14. B (page 687)
15. A (page 683)
16. D (page 683)
17. C (page 679)
18. A (page 684)
19. B (page 683)
20. D (page 672)
21. C (page 672)
22. B (page 673)
23. C (page 676)
24. D (page 674)
25. A (page 676)
26. B (page 680)
27. D (page 681)
28. A (page 672)
29. C (page672)
30. A (page 674)
31. D (page 675)
32. A (page 672)
33. D (page 674)
34. C (page 679)
35. C (page 679)
36. B (page 679)
37. C (page 679)
38. B (page 679)
39. D (page 685)
40. B (page 685)

True/False

1. T (page 679)
2. F (page 679)
3. F (page 679)
4. F (page 672)
5. F (page 679)
6. T (page 681)
7. T (page 685)
8. F (page 680)
9. T (page 681)
10. T (page 683)
11. T (page 686)
12. F (page 689)

Fill-in-the-Blank

1. ABCs (page 679)
2. alcohol (page 680)
3. adsorbing (page 679)
4. 5 to 10; 15 to 20 (page 673)
5. respiratory depression (page 681)
6. hypoglycemia (page 680)
7. recognize (page 669)
8. 1 gram; kilogram (page 679)
9. outward (page 673)
10. ingestion (page 674)
11. delirium tremens (page 681)
12. ignite (page 674)
13. addiction (page 679)
14. Hypovolemia (page 681)

Fill-in-the-Table (page 670)

Toxidromes: Typical Signs and Symptoms of Specific Overdoses	
Agent	**Signs and Symptoms**
Opioid (Examples: heroin, oxycodone)	• Hypoventilation or respiratory arrest • **Pinpoint pupils** • Sedation or coma • **Hypotension**
Sympathomimetics (Examples: epinephrine, albuterol, cocaine, methamphetamine)	• Hypertension • **Tachycardia** • Dilated pupils • Agitation or seizures • **Hyperthermia**
Sedative-hypnotics (Examples: diazepam [Valium], secobarbital [Seconal], flunitrazepam, [Rohypnol])	• **Slurred speech** • Sedation or coma • Hypoventilation • **Hypotension**
Anticholinergics (Examples: atropine, Jimson weed)	• **Tachycardia** • **Hyperthermia** • Hypertension • Dilated pupils • **Dry skin and mucous membranes** • Sedation, agitation, seizures, coma, or delirium • **Decreased bowel sounds**
Cholinergics (Examples: pilocarpine, nerve gas)	• **Excess defecation or urination** • **Muscle fasciculations** • Pinpoint pupils • Excess lacrimation (tearing) or salivation • **Airway compromise** • **Nausea or vomiting**

Crossword Puzzle

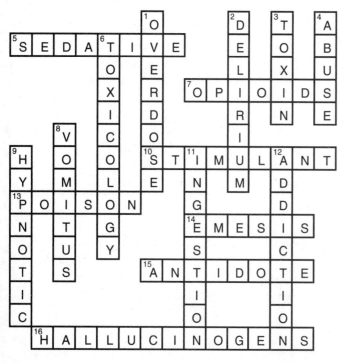

Critical Thinking

Short Answer

1. Activated charcoal adsorbs (binds to) the toxin and keeps it from being absorbed in the gastrointestinal tract. (page 679)

2. **1.** Ingestion
    2. Inhalation
    3. Injection
    4. Absorption (surface contact) (page 671)

3. Hypertension, tachycardia, paranoia, dilated pupils, along with irritability, agitation, anxiety, restlessness, or seizures (pages 683–684)

4. **1.** The organism itself causes the disease.
    2. The organism produces toxins that cause disease. (page 687)

5. Symptoms of acetaminophen overdose do not appear until the damage is irreversible, up to a week later. Finding evidence at the scene can save a patient's life. (page 686)

6. They describe patient presentation in cholinergic poisoning (ie, organophosphate insecticides, wild mushrooms).
    DUMBELS: Defecation, urination, miosis, bronchorrhea, emesis, lacrimation, salivation
    SLUDGE: Salivation, lacrimation, urination, defecation, gastrointestinal irritation, eye constriction/emesis (page 685)

7. **1.** Opioids
    2. Sedative-hypnotics
    3. Inhalants
    4. Sympathomimetics
    5. Hallucinogens
    6. Anticholinergic agents
    7. Cholinergic agents
    8. Miscellaneous drugs (pages 681–685)

8. **1.** What substance did you take?
    2. When did you take it or become exposed to it?
    3. How much did you ingest?
    4. What actions have been taken?
    5. How much do you weigh? (page 670)

9. Because they ignite when they come into contact with water (page 674)

Ambulance Calls

1. You should attempt to identify the substance. Some rat poisons are actually blood-thinning agents or anticoagulants, such as warfarin. You should collect the substance and call the poison control center and/or the hospital emergency department for patient care instructions. Some substances require the administration of activated charcoal, whereas others do not. Perform your initial assessment, start high-flow oxygen (blow-by), and provide prompt transport. Know your local protocols.

2. This patient obviously abuses alcohol and illegal substances. However, you cannot automatically assume that his decrease in mentation is directly related to alcohol intoxication or influence of other substances. He may have other medical conditions, which may mimic intoxication or even be obscured by it. You should perform a thorough assessment, take his vital signs, monitor his ABCs (because these could change at any time), and transport him to the nearest appropriate medical facility for evaluation. It is also important to be aware of the possibility of used needles when performing assessments and/or removing clothing when visualizing any potential injuries. Protect yourself.

3. Maintain the airway with an adjunct and high-flow oxygen via bag-mask device or nonrebreathing mask with 100% oxygen. Monitor vital signs and provide supportive measures and rapid transport. Take the pill bottle along to the emergency department. Be alert for possible vomiting, monitor the patient closely, and be prepared for the possible need for CPR.

Skills

Assessment Review

1. C (pages 677–678)
2. B (page 684)
3. B (page 687)
4. B (page 683)
5. A (page 679)

Emergency Care Summary (page 696)

General Management of Toxicologic Emergencies

1. Rescues from a toxic environment should only be performed by trained rescuers wearing appropriate **personal protective equipment**.
2. Establish and maintain a patent airway. Provide high-flow oxygen. Monitor for vomiting and protect against **aspiration**.
3. Obtain **SAMPLE** history and **vital signs**. Ascertain what toxin may be involved.
4. Request **ALS** when necessary.
5. Take all containers, bottles, and labels of poisons to the receiving hospital.
6. For patients who have taken alcohol, opioids, sedative-hypnotics, or abused inhalants, monitor the level of consciousness and airway patency because these drugs produce **central nervous system** depression and respiratory depression.
7. For abused inhalants, patients are prone to **seizures** and ventricular fibrillation.
8. For stimulants and anticholinergics, it is critical to monitor patients for hypertension and/or other **cardiovascular** effects.
9. For **cholinergic** agents, decontamination is a necessity. Monitor the patient for excessive **respiratory** secretions and seizures.
10. For patients who have plant poisoning, contact the regional poison center for assistance in identifying the plant.
11. For patients who have **food** poisoning, transport the food suspected to be responsible for the poisoning.

Administer **activated charcoal** for poisonous ingestions according to local protocol. Follow these steps:

1. Do not give activated charcoal if the patient exhibits an **altered mental status**, has ingested a substance for which charcoal is contraindicated, or is unable to **swallow**.
2. Obtain an order from medical direction or follow protocol.
3. Shake the activated charcoal container well.
4. Place the activated charcoal suspension in a covered cup with a straw and ask the patient to drink. The dose for infants and children is **12.5** to 25 g and the dose for adults is 25 to **50** g.

Chapter 20: Psychiatric Emergencies

General Knowledge

Matching

1. I (page 708)
2. F (page 705)
3. J (page 709)
4. D (page 702)
5. G (page 702)
6. A (page 702)
7. E (page 703)
8. H (page 702)
9. C (page 702)
10. B (page 703)

Multiple Choice

1. C (page 710)
2. B (page 701)
3. D (page 701)
4. B (page 702)
5. C (page 702)
6. B (page 702)
7. A (page 702)
8. D (page 702)
9. C (page 703)
10. B (page 703)
11. C (page 703)
12. B (pages 707–708)
13. D (page 703)
14. B (page 704)
15. A (page 709)
16. B (page 709)
17. A (page 709)
18. A (page 709)
19. C (pages 710–711)
20. C (page 712)
21. B (page 712)
22. D (page 712)
23. A (page 710)
24. A (pages 705–706)
25. D (page 712)
26. B (page 712)

True/False

1. F (page 701)
2. T (page 703)
3. F (page 702)
4. F (page 712)
5. F (page 710)
6. T (page 704)
7. F (page 708)
8. T (page 711)
9. F (page 701)
10. T (page 712)
11. T (page 712)
12. F (page 712)
13. T (page 707)
14. T (page 706)
15. T (page 705)

Fill-in-the-Blank

1. Behavior (page 702)
2. behavioral crisis (page 702)
3. depression (page 702)
4. Organic brain syndrome (page 703)
5. suicide (page 708)
6. schizophrenia (page 708)
7. law enforcement (page 711)
8. implied consent (page 711)
9. Alzheimer dementia (page 711)
10. minimum (page 712)

Crossword Puzzle

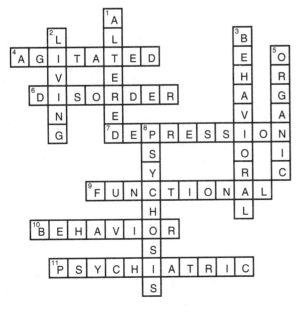

Critical Thinking

Short Answer

1. A behavioral crisis is a temporary change in behavior that interferes with activities of daily living or that is unacceptable to the patient or others. A psychiatric emergency involves a patient showing violence, agitation, or a threat to himself, herself, or others. (page 702)

2. 1. Improper functioning of the central nervous system.
    2. Drugs or alcohol
    3. Psychogenic circumstances (page 705)

3. 1. The degree of force necessary to keep the patient from injuring self or others
    2. Patient's gender, size, strength, and mental status
    3. The type of abnormal behavior the patient is exhibiting (page 712)

4. 1. Be prepared to spend extra time.
    2. Have a definite plan of action.
    3. Identify yourself calmly.
    4. Be direct.
    5. Assess the scene.
    6. Stay with the patient.
    7. Encourage purposeful movement.
    8. Express interest in the patient's story.
    9. Do not get too close to the patient.
    10. Avoid fighting with the patient.
    11. Be honest and reassuring.
    12. Do not judge. (page 704)

5. 1. Depression at any age
    2. Previous suicide attempt
    3. Current expression of wanting to commit suicide or sense of hopelessness
    4. Family history of suicide
    5. Age older than 40 years, particularly for single, widowed, divorced, alcoholic, or depressed individuals
    6. Recent loss of spouse, significant other, family member, or support system
    7. Chronic debilitating illness or recent diagnosis of serious illness
    8. Feeling anxious, agitated, angry, reckless, or aggressive
    9. Financial setback, loss of job, police arrest, imprisonment, or some sort of social embarrassment
    10. Substance abuse, particularly with increasing usage
    11. Children of an alcoholic or abusive parent
    12. Withdrawal from family and friends or a lack of social support, resulting in isolation
    13. Anniversary of death of loved one, job loss, marriage after the death of a spouse, etc.
    14. Unusual gathering or new acquisition of things that can cause death, such as purchase of a gun, a large volume of pills, or increased use of alcohol (page 709)

6. A technique used by mental health professionals to gain insight into a patient's thinking. It involves repeating, in question form, what the patient has said, encouraging the patient to expand on the thoughts. (pages 705–706)

7. 1. History
    2. Posture
    3. The scene
    4. Vocal activity
    5. Physical activity (pages 713–714)

Ambulance Calls

1. Removing restraints (especially when the patient has a known history of recent violence) is ill-advised and potentially against local protocols. Restraints, although uncomfortable, afford you and your patient a safe environment. You should continually monitor the restraints to ensure they are not too tight and that no manner of restraints (whether applied initially by you in the field or by hospital personnel for an interfacility transport) affects the patient's ability to breathe. Know your local laws regarding the use of restraints and your local protocols for appropriate use and discontinuation.

2. Although he tells you that he is fine, you cannot simply walk away. Those individuals who contemplate suicide often tell people they are "fine." With information passed along by his sister, you must take action. Because there is no evidence that the patient has tried to harm himself and he did not express directly to you that he intends to, you must use persuasive techniques to gain consent to treatment and transport.

3. Be understanding and listen. Explain to the patient that she needs medical care. Monitor vital signs and reassure patient en route.

Skills

Assessment Review

1. D (page 706)
2. A (page 713)
3. C (page 709)
4. B (page 714)
5. A (page 714)

Emergency Care Summary (page 720)

General Management of Psychiatric Emergencies

Managing life threats to the patient's **ABCs** and ensuring the delivery of high-flow oxygen are primary concerns with any psychiatric emergency. Without an underlying medical or trauma cause, there is usually little **hands-on** care for the EMT to perform. Competent adults have the right to refuse treatment and transport, but in the case of psychiatric emergencies, you may have a reasonable belief that the patient may harm himself, herself, or others. If this is the case, contact **law enforcement** to take the patient into custody. If **restraint** is required, consult with medical control, ensure law enforcement personnel are at the scene, and make sure that there are at least **four** people present. Use only approved restraint devices. Do not transport the patient in a **prone** position because the patient may experience severe respiratory distress or cardiac arrest, often called **positional asphyxia**.

Chapter 21: Gynecologic Emergencies

General Knowledge

Matching

1. G (page 725)	**4.** B (page 726)	**7.** D (page 726)	**10.** J (page 727)
2. E (page 725)	**5.** H (page 726)	**8.** C (page 727)	**11.** I (page 728)
3. K (page 725)	**6.** A (page 726)	**9.** F (page 726)	

Multiple Choice

1. D (page 728)	**5.** D (page 726)	**9.** C (page 732)	**13.** D (page 734)	**17.** C (pages 732–733)
2. B (page 728)	**6.** A (page 727)	**10.** A (page 732)	**14.** A (page 734)	**18.** D (page 734)
3. B (pages 732–733)	**7.** C (page 727)	**11.** A (page 732)	**15.** C (page 733)	
4. B (page 726)	**8.** B (page 729)	**12.** D (page 733)	**16.** A (page 732)	

True/False

1. T (page 727)	**4.** T (page 728)	**7.** T (page 730)	**10.** F (page 732)	**13.** F (page 732)
2. T (page 728)	**5.** T (page 730)	**8.** F (page 730)	**11.** T (page 730)	**14.** F (pages 733–734)
3. F (page 728)	**6.** F (page 730)	**9.** T (page 730)	**12.** T (page 731)	**15.** T (page 731)

Fill-in-the-Blank

1. ovaries (page 725)
2. puberty (page 726)
3. Pelvic inflammatory disease (page 727)
4. Gynecologic emergencies (page 728)
5. Ectopic pregnancy; spontaneous abortion (page 728)
6. external pads (page 732)
7. Vaginal bleeding (page 729)
8. law enforcement (page 732)
9. gonorrhea (page 728)
10. menopause (page 727)

Labeling

1. Female Reproductive System

A. Uterine (fallopian) tube
B. Uterus
C. Ovary
D. Cervix
E. Vagina (page 725)

2. External Genitalia

A. Labia minora
B. Labia majora
C. Urethra
D. Vaginal orifice
E. Perineum
F. Anus (page 726)

Crossword Puzzle

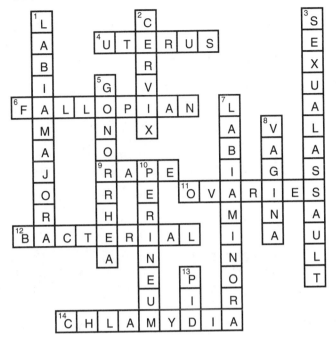

Critical Thinking

Short Answer

1. Where or in what position is the patient found?
   What is the condition of the residence? Clean, filthy, or wrecked?
   Is there evidence of a fight?
   Are alcohol, tobacco products, or drug paraphernalia present?
   Are there pictures of loved ones? Is there a noticeable absence of pictures?
   Does the patient live alone or with other people? (pages 728–729)

2. 1. Painful urination
    2. Burning or itching
    3. Yellowish or bloody discharge associated with a foul odor
    4. Blood associated with vaginal intercourse
    5. Cramping and abdominal pain
    6. Nausea and vomiting
    7. Bleeding between menstrual periods (page 728)

3. Use external pads to control bleeding. Keep the patient warm, place her in a supine position with her legs elevated, and provide her with supplemental oxygen even if she is not experiencing any difficulty breathing. Provide prompt transport to the hospital and reassess her vital signs every 5 minutes. (pages 728–732)

Ambulance Calls

1. The patient is most likely suffering from pelvic inflammatory disease (PID), one of the most common gynecologic reasons why women call for EMS. A patient with PID will complain of abdominal pain that generally starts during or after normal menstruation. The pain is typically described as "achy" and can be worse with walking. Other symptoms include vaginal discharge, fever and chills, and pain or burning on urination.

   Prehospital treatment is limited to supportive care, and nonemergency transport is usually recommended. Place the patient in a position of comfort and monitor vital signs. Consider oxygen. Keep in mind that although this condition is typically not an emergency, these patients require monitoring for any signs of deterioration.

2. The first issue is the medical treatment of the patient. You should assess and treat life threats and inquire about pain. The second issue focuses on the psychological care of the patient. Many women report feeling violated when subjected to interrogation, so do not cross-examine the patient or pass judgment on her during the assessment. Take the patient's history, and limit any physical examination to a brief survey for life-threatening injuries. Keep in mind that this patient has been through a traumatic experience, and your compassion for her will help to gain the patient's confidence. Limit the number of people involved in the assessment/examination process to protect the patient's privacy and dignity. Remember that you are at a crime scene. Do not cut through any clothing or throw away anything from the scene. Place bloodstained articles in a separate paper bag. You should gently persuade the patient to refrain from cleaning herself, urinating, changing clothes, moving her bowels, or rinsing her mouth, because this could potentially destroy evidence.

When documenting this incident, keep the report concise and record only what the patient stated in her own words. Use quotations marks to indicate that you are reporting the patient's version of the events. Refrain from inserting your own opinion into the documentation. Record all of your observations during the physical exam, including the patient's emotional state, the condition of her clothing, obvious injuries, and so forth.

Fill-in-the-Patient Care Report

EMS Patient Care Report (PCR)					
Date: Today's Date	**Incident No.:** 011689		**Nature of Call:** Assault		**Location:** 538 N. 10th Street, Apartment 4-C
Dispatched: 2101	**En Route:** 2103	**At Scene:** 2109	**Transport:** 2120	**At Hospital:** 2131	**In Service:** 2147

Patient Information					
Age: 32 Years			**Allergies:** None Known		
Sex: Female			**Medications:** lispro, Lantus, lisinopril		
Weight (in kg [lb]): Unknown			**Past Medical History:** Diabetes		
			Chief Complaint: Pain to the nose, face, and groin		

Vital Signs				
Time: 2114	**BP:** 144/98	**Pulse:** 102	**Respirations:** 22	**Sao$_2$:** 98%
Time: 2125	**BP:** 148/92	**Pulse:** 108	**Respirations:** 20	**Sao$_2$:** 97%

EMS Treatment (circle all that apply)				
Oxygen @ 2 L/min via (circle one): (NC) NRM Bag-Mask Device		**Assisted Ventilation**	**Airway Adjunct**	**CPR**
Defibrillation	**Bleeding Control**	**Bandaging**	**Splinting**	**Other Shock Treatment**

Narrative
9-1-1 dispatch for 32-year-old assault victim. Dispatcher advised that police were already on scene. No other information was provided. Upon arrival, crew was directed by PD through a well-kept apartment into a dark room where we found our patient. The patient had obvious multiple contusions to her face and appeared to be emotionally upset. When inquired about the incident, the patient blurted out that she was "raped by a maintenance worker here at the apartment complex." The patient initially stated that she was unsure if she wanted to go to the hospital. She stated that she did want to "change her clothes" and "take a shower." Both EMS and PD stated to patient that she could potentially disrupt any evidence, and that changing her clothes and showering were not advised. The patient complained of pain to the nose, face, and groin. She denied any bleeding. The patient appeared withdrawn and reluctant to speak with EMS. A female EMT was offered to the patient; however, the patient stated "No." No obvious life threats were noted on minimal exam. The patient was asked about the incident; however, she declined to comment. Due to the patient's status and limited injuries, no further examination performed at this time. Patient was continuously monitored for any signs of hemorrhaging or deterioration. The patient was loaded into the unit and transported to the local facility. Radio report was carried out by partner/driver. Upon arrival at facility, the patient was stable with no change in status noted. Care was transferred to the ED staff. A verbal report was given to the nurse with patient privacy precautions taken. No further incidents. Unit cleaned and restocked. Crew available. **End of Report**

Chapter 22: Trauma Overview

General Knowledge

Matching

1. H (page 758)
2. G (page 749)
3. F (page 748)
4. E (page 747)
5. C (page 749)
6. A (page 749)
7. D (page 749)
8. B (page 748)

Multiple Choice

1. B (page 747)
2. C (page 748)
3. C (page 749)
4. B (page 749)
5. D (page 757)
6. B (page 750)
7. C (pages 750–751)
8. D (page 765)
9. C (page 759)
10. A (page 751)
11. C (page 762)
12. B (page 751)
13. D (page 761)
14. A (page 752)
15. A (page 760)
16. B (page 752)
17. B (page 762)
18. B (page 754)
19. C (page 755)
20. B (page 757)
21. C (pages 750–751)
22. A (page 750)
23. B (page 751)
24. A (page 756)
25. C (page 748)
26. A (page 765)
27. B (page 757)
28. D (page 760)
29. D (pages 760–761)
30. C (page 763)

True/False

1. T (page 748)
2. F (page 749)
3. F (page 748)
4. T (page 753)
5. T (page 763)
6. T (page 757)
7. T (page 747)
8. F (page 762)
9. T (page 754)
10. F (page 753)
11. T (page 755)
12. F (page 756)
13. F (page 760)
14. T (page 763)
15. T (page 763)

Fill-in-the-Blank

1. doubles; quadruples (page 749)
2. Penetrating trauma (page 749)
3. coup-contrecoup (page 751)
4. KE = ½ MV^2 (page 749)
5. rear-end (page 753)
6. deceleration (page 752)
7. burns (page 749)
8. lateral (page 750)
9. ejection (page 755)
10. solid (pages 763–764)
11. Glasgow Coma (page 767)
12. pneumothorax (page 763)
13. Platinum 10 (page 764)
14. Newton's first law (page 748)
15. medical (page 747)

Fill-in-the-Table (page 759)

Recognizing Developing Problems in Trauma Patients		
Mechanism of Injury	**Signs and Symptoms**	**Index of Suspicion**
Blunt or penetrating trauma to the neck	• **Noisy or labored breathing** • **Swelling of the face or neck**	• Significant bleeding or foreign bodies in the upper or lower airway, causing obstruction • Be alert for airway compromise.
Significant chest wall trauma from motor vehicle crashes, car-versus-pedestrian, and other crashes; penetrating trauma to the chest wall	• **Significant chest pain** • **Shortness of breath** • **Asymmetrical chest wall movement**	• Cardiac or pulmonary contusion • Pneumothorax or hemothorax • Broken ribs, causing breathing compromise
Any significant blunt force trauma from motor vehicle crashes or penetrating injury	• **Blunt or penetrating trauma to the neck, chest, abdomen, or groin** • **Blows to the head sustained during motor vehicle crashes, falls, or other incidents, producing loss of consciousness, altered mental status, inability to recall events, combativeness, or changes in speech patterns** • **Difficulty moving extremities; headache, especially with nausea and vomiting**	• Injuries in these regions may tear and cause damage to the large blood vessels located in these body areas, resulting in significant internal and external bleeding. • Be alert to the possibility of bruising to the brain and bleeding in and around the brain tissue, which may cause the development of excess pressure inside the skull around the brain.
Any significant blunt force trauma, falls from a significant height, or penetrating trauma	• **Severe back and/or neck pain, history of difficulty moving extremities, loss of sensation or tingling in the extremities**	• Injuries to the bones of the spinal column or to the spinal cord

Crossword Puzzle

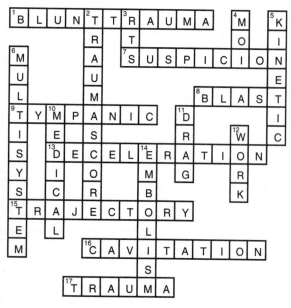

Critical Thinking

Short Answer

1. Potential energy is the product of mass (weight), force of gravity, and height and is mostly associated with the energy of falling objects. (page 749)

2. 1. Collision of the car against another car or other object
   2. Collision of the passenger against the interior of the car
   3. Collision of the passenger's internal organs against the solid structures of the body (pages 750–751)

3. 1. The height of the fall
   2. The surface struck
   3. The part of the body that hit first, followed by the path of energy displacement (page 758)

4. A bullet, because of its speed, creates pressure waves that emanate from its path, causing distant damage. (page 758)

5. The size (mass) and speed (velocity) of the projectile affect the potential damage. If the mass is doubled, the potential energy is doubled. If the velocity is doubled, the potential energy is quadrupled. (page 749)

6. Lateral chest and abdominal/internal organ injuries on the side of impact; fractures of the lower extremities, pelvis, and ribs; and injuries to the aorta (page 754)

7. Deformity of the motorcycle, the side of most damage, the distance of skid in the road, the deformity of stationary objects or other vehicles, and the extent and location of deformity in the helmet (page 756)

8. 1. Confirmed blood pressure of less than 90 mm Hg at any time in adults, and age-specific hypotension in children
   2. Respiratory compromise, obstruction, and/or intubation
   3. Receiving blood to maintain vital signs
   4. Emergency physician's discretion
   5. Glasgow Coma Scale score of less than or equal to 8 with mechanism attributed to trauma
   6. Gunshot wound to the abdomen, neck, or chest (page 767)

Ambulance Calls

1. Given the highway speeds and lack of a shoulder belt and airbag, along with his complaints of head and neck pain, your index of suspicion for head and spinal injuries is very high. It is a positive sign that he is awake and able to communicate; however, this should not encourage you to spend any more time on scene than is necessary to extricate this patient and place him in full spinal precautions. His condition could change at any time, and his inability to remember the details of the event likely indicate the presence of a closed head injury. Provide high-flow oxygen and prompt transport.

2. Each story is 10' (3 m), so this patient fell approximately 20' (6 m) from the ladder to the hard ground. He is now unconscious. Assume he has significant head and spinal injuries; determine if he is responsive and manage his airway, because he will be unable to protect it. Provide high-flow oxygen and prompt transport to the nearest appropriate facility, taking care not to waste time in determining other injuries.

3. 1. Apply high-flow oxygen.
   2. Stabilize the object in place with bulky dressings.
   3. Monitor his vital signs.
   4. Transport the patient in a supine position. Provide rapid transport due to abdominal penetration.

4. 1. Estimate the speed of the vehicle that struck the patient.
   2. Determine whether the patient was thrown through the air and at what distance.
   3. Determine if the patient was struck and pulled under the vehicle.
   4. Evaluate the vehicle for structural damage that might indicate contact points with the patient and alert you to potential injuries.

Chapter 23: Bleeding

General Knowledge

Matching

1. J (page 778) **4.** F (page 778) **7.** B (page 782) **10.** A (page 783) **13.** G (page 781)
2. E (page 778) **5.** C (page 778) **8.** I (page 783) **11.** D (page 782)
3. K (page 778) **6.** H (page 778) **9.** M (page 793) **12.** L (page 781)

Multiple Choice

1. B (page 778)   **8.** B (page 778)   **15.** D (page 780)   **22.** C (page 782)   **29.** B (page 783)
2. D (page 778)   **9.** D (page 779)   **16.** B (page 781)   **23.** D (page 782)   **30.** D (page 783)
3. C (page 778)   **10.** C (page 779)   **17.** B (page 781)   **24.** B (page 782)   **31.** D (page 783)
4. C (page 778)   **11.** B (page 780)   **18.** B (page 781)   **25.** C (page 781)   **32.** D (pages 783–784)
5. B (page 778)   **12.** C (page 780)   **19.** A (page 781)   **26.** A (page 788)   **33.** C (page 784)
6. A (page 778)   **13.** C (page 779)   **20.** B (page 782)   **27.** A (page 788)
7. D (page 778)   **14.** A (page 780)   **21.** C (page 782)   **28.** C (pages 792–793)

True/False

1. F (page 782)   **3.** F (page 788)   **5.** F (page 790)   **7.** F (page 785)   **9.** F (page 790)
2. F (page 781)   **4.** T (page 781)   **6.** T (page 793)   **8.** F (page 788)   **10.** T (page 794)

Fill-in-the-Blank

1. right (page 778)
2. Perfusion (page 780)
3. bruise (page 783)
4. Internal (page 783)
5. 100 (page 787)
6. Hematemesis (page 783)
7. Capillary (page 782)
8. autonomic nervous (page 779)
9. Capillaries (page 778)
10. involuntary (page 778)

Labeling

1. Left and Right Sides of the Heart
  A. Left pulmonary artery
  B. Superior vena cava
  C. Right pulmonary artery
  D. Right atrium
  E. Inferior vena cava
  F. Right ventricle
  G. Right pulmonary veins
  H. Oxygen-rich blood to head and upper body
  I. Left pulmonary veins
  J. Left atrium
  K. Left ventricle
  L. Oxygen-rich blood to lower body (page 778)

2. Perfusion
  A. Artery
  B. Arterioles
  C. Capillaries
  D. Organ or tissue
  E. Capillaries
  F. Venules
  G. Vein (page 780)

3. Arterial Pressure Points
  A. Superficial temporal
  B. External maxillary
  C. Carotid
  D. Brachial
  E. Ulnar
  F. Femoral
  G. Radial
  H. Posterior tibial
  I. Dorsalis pedis (page 790)

Crossword Puzzle

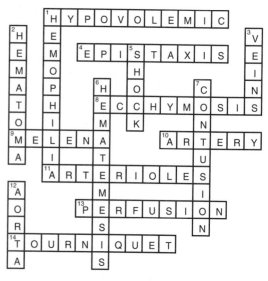

Critical Thinking

Multiple Choice

1. C (page 792) **2.** D (page 792) **3.** D (page 793) **4.** B (page 793) **5.** B (page 782)

Short Answer

1. It redirects blood away from nonessential organs to the heart, brain, lungs, and kidneys. (page 779)
2. **Artery:** Bright red, spurting
   Vein: Dark color with steady flow
   Capillary: Darker color, oozes (page 782)
3. 1. Direct pressure and elevation
   2. Pressure dressings
   3. Pressure points (for upper and lower extremities)
   4. Tourniquets
   5. Splints (page 788)
4. 1. Change in mental status (restlessness, anxiety, combativeness)
   2. Weakness, fainting, or dizziness on standing (early sign) or at rest (later sign)
   3. Tachycardia
   4. Thirst
   5. Nausea and vomiting
   6. Cold, moist (clammy) skin
   7. Shallow, rapid breathing
   8. Dull eyes
   9. Slightly dilated pupils, slow to respond to light
   10. Capillary refill in infants and children of more than 2 seconds
   11. Weak, rapid (thready) pulse
   12. Decreasing blood pressure
   13. Altered level of consciousness
   14. Cyanosis (pages 781, 784)
5. 1. Follow standard precautions.
   2. Maintain the airway.
   3. Administer high-flow oxygen.
   4. Control all obvious external bleeding.
   5. Apply splints to extremity, if a limb is involved.
   6. Monitor and record the patient's vital signs.
   7. Give the patient nothing by mouth.
   8. Elevate the legs 6″ to 12″ (15 to 31 cm) in nontrauma patients.
   9. Keep the patient warm.
   10. Provide immediate transport. (pages 795–796)

Ambulance Calls

1. Control bleeding with direct pressure, elevation, pressure point, and a tourniquet as a last resort. Apply high-flow oxygen and place the patient in a position of comfort. Monitor the patient's vital signs and provide rapid transport.
2. You must control bleeding through direct pressure, elevation, pressure dressings, and pressure points, as needed. You must also transport the amputated portion of the limb with the patient to the hospital. Quickly attempt to determine how much blood has been lost and assess his skin and vital signs, because these will provide accurate indicators of the significance of blood loss. Place the patient in Trendelenburg's position, as needed, apply high-flow oxygen; and provide prompt transport.
3. This is an isolated injury that, depending on the severity of the laceration to the antecubital vein, can result in significant blood loss. Attempt to control bleeding through direct pressure, elevation, pressure dressings, and pressure points, as needed. Something as benign as a pen can cause significant damage in the hands of a determined person.

Fill-in-the-Patient Care Report

EMS Patient Care Report (PCR)					
Date: Today's date	**Incident No.:** 2010-123	**Nature of Call:** Laceration		**Location:** 1467 Abner Lane	
Dispatched: 1653	**En Route:** 1653	**At Scene:** 1658	**Transport:** 1710	**At Hospital:** 1715	**In Service:** 1735

Patient Information	
Age: 42 Years **Sex:** Male **Weight (in kg [lb]):** 77 kg (170 lb)	**Allergies:** Amoxicillin **Medications:** Crestor **Past Medical History:** TIA—1 year ago **Chief Complaint:** Laceration to lower left leg

Vital Signs				
Time: 1704	**BP:** 136/86	**Pulse:** 88 strong/reg	**Respirations:** 16 GTV	**Sao₂:** 97%
Time: 1710	**BP:** 122/76	**Pulse:** 102 weak	**Respirations:** 20 shallow	**Sao₂:** 94%
Time: N/A	**BP:** N/A	**Pulse:** N/A	**Respirations:** N/A	**Sao₂:** N/A

EMS Treatment (circle all that apply)				
Oxygen @ 15 **L/min via (circle one):** NC (NRM) Bag-Mask Device	**Assisted Ventilation**	**Airway Adjunct**		**CPR**
Defibrillation	(Bleeding Control)	(Bandaging)	Splinting	(Other Shock Treatment)

Narrative

Dispatched for a leg laceration. Arrived on scene to find the patient, a 42-year-old man, on the back deck of his home. He was conscious and alert, had a patent airway, and was breathing with good tidal volume. The patient was holding a blood-soaked shirt on his lower leg and was sitting in a large pool of blood. Patient stated that he had been chopping wood when the axe blade had bounced off the wood and struck his leg. I immediately applied direct pressure using a large sterile dressing and manually elevated the patient's leg. I then applied a pressure dressing to maintain bleeding control. We initiated oxygen therapy via nonrebreathing mask at 15 L/min and obtained the patient's vitals. The patient's skin was found to be pale, cool, and diaphoretic. Patient's wife disclosed patient history of TIA (1 year ago), amoxicillin allergy, and current Crestor use. Placed patient onto gurney, covered with a blanket, elevated his legs, and moved him into the ambulance. I continued to monitor the patient's condition while en route. He remained conscious and alert but vital sign trending indicated possible hypoperfusion. Checked pressure dressing and found that bleeding was still controlled. Called in report to receiving facility and subsequently delivered patient without incident. Gave verbal report to the ED charge nurse. **End of Report**

Skills

Skill Drills

Skill Drill 23-1: Controlling External Bleeding
1. Apply **direct pressure** over the wound. Elevate the injury above the **level** of the **heart** if no **fracture** is suspected.
2. Apply a **pressure dressing**.
3. If direct pressure with a **pressure dressing** does not control the bleeding, apply a **tourniquet** above the level of the **bleeding**. (page 789)

Skill Drill 23-2: Applying a Commercial Tourniquet
1. Hold **pressure** over the bleeding site and place the tourniquet just **above** the injury.
2. Click the buckle into place, pull the strap tight, and turn the tightening dial **clockwise** until pulses are no longer palpable **distal** to the tourniquet or until bleeding has been **controlled**. (page 791)

Assessment Review

1. C (page 788)   2. A (page 785)   3. B (page 786)   4. D (page 787)   5. C (pages 787–788)

Emergency Care Summary

(pages 800-801)

External Bleeding

Steps to Caring for Patient With External Bleeding
1. Follow standard precautions—at least gloves and eye protection.   .
2. Maintain cervical stabilization if MOI suggests possible **spinal injury**.
3. Administer high-flow oxygen as necessary, once significant bleeding is controlled.
4. Control external bleeding using as many of the following means as necessary:
- **Direct pressure**, elevation, and pressure dressings
- Tourniquets
- **Splints**
5. Apply direct local pressure to bleeding site, elevate the bleeding extremity, and apply a **pressure** dressing.
6. If bleeding is not immediately controlled with the use of direct pressure, apply a **tourniquet**. Follow local protocol for approved methods of bleeding control.

Applying a Commercial Tourniquet
1. Follow standard precautions.
2. Hold direct pressure over the bleeding site.
3. Place the tourniquet around the extremity just **above** the bleeding site.
4. Click the **buckle** into place and pull the strap tight.
5. Turn the tightening dial **clockwise** until pulses are no longer palpable distal to the tourniquet or until bleeding is controlled.

Treating Epistaxis
1. Follow standard precautions.
2. Help the patient to sit, leaning forward.
3. Apply direct pressure for at least **15** minutes by pinching nostrils together.
4. Keep the patient calm and quiet.
5. Apply ice over the nose.
6. Maintain the pressure until bleeding is completely controlled.
7. Provide prompt transport.
8. If bleeding cannot be controlled, transport patient immediately. Treat for **shock** and administer oxygen via nonrebreathing mask if necessary.

Internal Bleeding

Steps to Caring for Patient with Internal Bleeding
1. Follow BSI precautions.
2. Maintain the airway with cervical immobilization if MOI suggests possible spinal injury.
3. Administer high-flow oxygen.
4. Control all obvious external bleeding.
5. Apply a **splint** to an extremity where internal bleeding is suspected.
6. Monitor and record vital signs at least every 5 minutes.
7. Give the patient **nothing** by mouth.
8. Elevate the legs 6" to 12" (15 to 31 cm) in significant trauma patients.
9. Keep the patient warm.
10. Provide immediate transport for patients with signs and symptoms of shock. Report changes in the patient's condition to hospital personnel.

Chapter 24: Soft-Tissue Injuries

General Knowledge

Matching

1. G (page 806)
2. B (page 806)
3. D (page 806)
4. F (page 806)
5. H (page 806)
6. J (page 809)
7. E (page 809)
8. A (page 805)
9. C (page 810)
10. I (page 819)

Multiple Choice

1. C (page 805)
2. B (page 806)
3. B (page 806)
4. A (page 806)
5. B (page 806)
6. C (page 808)
7. B (page 808)
8. B (page 808)
9. D (page 808)
10. C (page 808)
11. C (page 817)
12. B (page 809)
13. D (page 809)
14. D (page 811)
15. A (page 819)
16. D (pages 812–813)
17. D (page 817)
18. C (page 819)
19. C (page 821)
20. D (page 822)
21. D (page 823)
22. C (page 824)
23. B (page 824)
24. C (page 824)
25. D (page 825)
26. B (page 827)
27. D (page 828)
28. A (page 836)
29. D (page 837)
30. B (page 807)
31. B (page 821)

True/False

1. T (page 824)
2. F (page 824)
3. T (page 824)
4. T (page 825)
5. T (page 823)
6. T (page 834)
7. F (page 835)
8. T (page 828)
9. F (page 808)
10. T (page 836)
11. F (page 836)
12. F (page 837)
13. T (page 836)
14. F (page 808)
15. F (page 809)

Fill-in-the-Blank

1. alpha; beta; gamma (page 830)
2. cool (page 806)
3. dermis (page 806)
4. crush syndrome (page 808)
5. constrict (page 806)
6. cheek; chest (page 821)
7. Thermal; 111 (page 807)
8. amputation (page 810)
9. epidermis; dermis (page 806)
10. radiated (page 806)

Labeling

1. Skin
    A. Hair
    B. Pore
    C. Epidermis
    D. Germinal layer of epidermis
    E. Sebaceous gland
    F. Erector pillae muscle
    G. Dermis
    H. Nerve (sensory)
    I. Sweat gland
    J. Hair follicle
    K. Blood vessel
    L. Subcutaneous fat
    M. Fascia
    N. Subcutaneous tissue
    O. Muscle (page 806)

2. Rule of Nines
    A. 9
    B. 18
    C. 9
    D. 18
    E. 9
    F. 12
    G. 18
    H. 18
    I. 1
    J. 9
    K. 18
    L. 18
    M. 18
    N. 9
    O. 18
    P. 9
    Q. 9
    R. 1
    S. 1
    T. 16.5
    U. 16.5
    V. 13.5
    W. 13.5 (page 825)

Crossword Puzzle

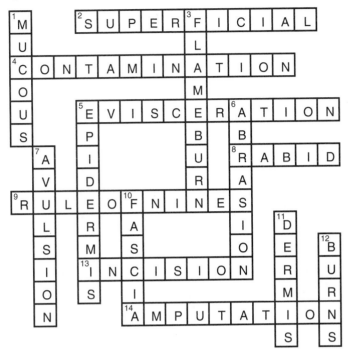

Critical Thinking

Multiple Choice

1. D (page 824)   **2.** D (page 811)   **3.** C (page 817)   **4.** A (page 809)   **5.** B (page 818)

Short Answer

1. **1.** Superficial (first degree)
   2. Partial thickness (second degree)
   3. Full thickness (third degree) (page 824)
2. **1.** Closed injuries
   2. Open injuries
   3. Burns (pages 806–807)
3. **R:** rest
   I: ice
   C: compression
   E: elevation
   S: splinting (page 817)
4. Any full-thickness burn
   Partial-thickness burns covering more than 20% of the body's total surface area
   Burns involving the hands, lower legs, feet, face, airway, buttocks, or genitalia (pages 825–826)
5. Brush off dry chemicals, and then remove the patient's clothing, (including shoes, stockings, gloves, jewelry, and glasses) because there may be small amounts of chemicals in the creases. (page 826)

6. First, there may be a deep tissue injury not visible on the outside. Second, there is a danger of cardiac arrest from the electrical shock. (page 827)
7. **1.** Primary
   2. Secondary
   3. Tertiary (page 811)
8. **1.** To control bleeding
   2. To protect the wound from further damage
   3. To prevent further contamination and infection (page 836)
9. **1.** Abrasions
   2. Lacerations
   3. Avulsions
   4. Penetrating wounds (page 809)
10. **1.** Depth of the burn
    2. Extent of the burn
    3. Involvement of critical areas (face, upper airway, hands, feet, genitalia)
    4. Preexisting medical conditions or other injuries
    5. Age younger than 5 years or older than 55 years (page 823)

Ambulance Calls

1. Take standard precautions and apply direct pressure. Elevate the extremity and apply a pressure dressing. If the bleeding is not controlled, move to the use of a tourniquet. Once the bleeding is controlled, splint the arm to decrease movement. Apply high-flow oxygen and transport the patient in a position of comfort. Monitor her vital signs en route to the hospital.

2. Unfortunately, this scenario has occurred in households throughout the country. This is why it is so important to "turn pot handles in" when cooking in the home of a small, inquisitive child. You must evaluate the child quickly to determine the extent and severity of the burns. Assess airway, breathing, and circulation, and quickly apply sterile dressings and high-flow oxygen. Promptly transport the patient according to local protocols.

3. Apply direct pressure to control any bleeding using sterile dressings. Have the patient lie down, because this injury will be quite painful. Even the toughest person can suddenly feel faint, especially if he or she looks at the injury. Find the piece of avulsed tissue, wrap it in sterile dressings, and transport it with you to the hospital. Oxygen via nasal cannula can assist with nausea that the patient may experience.

Fill-in-the-Patient Care Report

EMS Patient Care Report (PCR)				
Date: Today's Date	**Incident No:** 2011-2222	**Nature of Call:** GSW		**Location:** 14th and Berry
Dispatched: 1321	**En Route:** 1321	**At Scene:** 1329	**Transport:** 1334	**At Hospital:** 1341	**In Service:** 1411

Patient Information	
Age: 24 Years	**Allergies:** Unknown
Sex: Male	**Medications:** Unknown
Weight (kg [lb]): 73 kg (161 lb)	**Past Medical History:** Unknown
	Chief Complaint: GSW to neck

Vital Signs				
Time: 1334	**BP:** 92/60	**Pulse:** 120	**Respirations:** 20 Shallow	**Sao₂:** 92%
Time: 1337	**BP:** 92/58	**Pulse:** 124	**Respirations:** 20 Shallow	**Sao₂:** 94%

EMS Treatment

(circle all that apply)

Oxygen @ 15 L/min via (circle one): NC (NRM) Bag-Mask Device	Assisted Ventilation	Airway Adjunct	CPR
Defibrillation (Bleeding Control)	(Bandaging)	(Splinting)	(Other Shock Treatment)

Narrative

Medic 19 dispatched on emergency call for a police officer with a gunshot wound. Arrived on scene and was led to 24-year-old patient with GSW on left lateral neck. Bleeding was manually controlled, but evidence of severe blood loss was present. Patient was conscious and alert but subdued. Placed occlusive dressing and pressure dressing over wound and initiated high-flow oxygen therapy. Patient was secured to a long spine board due to MOI and immediate transport was initiated; no other wounds present. Baseline vital signs indicated that patient was hypoperfusing so we transported rapidly and covered the patient with blankets to retain body heat. Called report to the receiving trauma center and provided ETA. Subsequent vital signs showed no improvement of the shock condition but also no further deterioration. Remainder of transport was without incident, and we then delivered the patient to the emergency department and gave verbal report to the attending physician and charge nurse.

Medic 19 returned to service at 1411. **End of Report**

Skills

Skill Drills

Skill Drill 24-1: Controlling Bleeding From an Open Soft-Tissue Injury

1. Apply **direct pressure** with a sterile **dressing**.
2. Apply a **pressure** dressing.
3. If bleeding continues or recurs, apply a **tourniquet** above the level of **bleeding**. (page 818)

Skill Drill 24-3: Caring for Burns

1. Follow **standard** precautions to help prevent **infection**. If safe to do so, remove the **patient** from the burning area; extinguish or **remove** hot clothing and jewelry as necessary. If the wound(s) is (are) still burning or hot, **immerse** the hot area in **cool**, sterile **water**, or cover with a wet, cool **dressing**.
2. Provide high-flow **oxygen**, and continue to assess the **airway**.
3. Estimate the **severity** of the burn, and then cover the area with a **dry**, sterile dressing or clean **sheet**. Assess and treat the patient for any other **injuries**.
4. Prepare for transport. Treat for **shock**.
5. Cover the patient with **blankets** to prevent loss of **body heat**. Transport promptly. (pages 834–835)

Assessment Review

1. C (page 832)   **2.** B (page 833)   **3.** D (page 834)   **4.** A (page 834)   **5.** D (page 821)

Emergency Care Summary (pages 842, 845)

General Management of Closed Injuries

1. Ensure an open airway and adequate **ventilations**. Treat as required.
2. Be alert for and treat for shock (hypoperfusion) by raising the legs or backboard 6″ to 12″, maintain **body** temperature, and administer high-concentration oxygen.
3. Treat a closed soft-tissue injury by applying the mnemonic RICES:
   - Rest to keep patient quiet and comfortable
   - Ice to **constrict** blood vessels and reduce **pain**
   - Compression to compress blood vessels to slow **bleeding**
   - Elevation to raise injured part above level of the heart to decrease **swelling**
   - **Splinting** of extremity to decrease bleeding and pain

General Management of Open Injuries

1. Ensure you have followed standard precautions.
2. Ensure an open airway and adequate ventilations. Treat as required.
3. Apply an **occlusive** dressing to open chest injuries.
4. Apply direct pressure over the wound with a dry, **sterile** dressing.
5. Apply a **pressure** dressing.
6. If bleeding continues or recurs, apply a tourniquet to an extremity **above** the level of bleeding.
7. Be alert for and treat for **shock** (hypoperfusion) by raising legs or backboard 6″ to 12″, maintain body temperature, and administer high-concentration oxygen.

General Management of Burn Injuries

1. Stop the **burning** process.
2. Take appropriate standard precautions.
3. Treat life threats involving the ABCs.
4. Cool the burned area with sterile water or **saline**. Immerse or continuously irrigate the affected area, following local treatment protocols.
5. Cover the burned area with a **sterile** dressing. Dressing will be moist or dry depending on local protocol.
6. Maintain body temperature and treat for shock.

Chapter 25: Face and Throat Injuries

General Knowledge

Matching

1. G (page 854)	**4.** C (page 853)	**7.** I (page 852)	**10.** B (page 854)	**13.** A (page 870)
2. H (page 853)	**5.** J (page 853)	**8.** E (page 852)	**11.** F (page 853)	**14.** D (page 871)
3. L (page 871)	**6.** K (page 854)	**9.** O (pages 853–854)	**12.** M (page 852)	**15.** N (page 854)

Multiple Choice

1. D (page 851)	**5.** A (page 852)	**9.** A (page 860)	**13.** D (page 857)	**17.** A (page 853)
2. B (page 851)	**6.** D (page 852)	**10.** D (page 870)	**14.** C (page 872)	**18.** C (page 861)
3. C (page 851)	**7.** C (page 852)	**11.** B (page 870)	**15.** D (page 873)	**19.** B (pages 862–863)
4. D (page 852)	**8.** D (pages 854–855)	**12.** C (page 871)	**16.** A (page 874)	**20.** C (page 864)

True/False

1. T (page 856)	**5.** T (page 873)	**9.** T (page 856)	**13.** F (page 861)	**17.** F (page 869)
2. T (page 856)	**6.** T (page 851)	**10.** F (page 859)	**14.** F (page 865)	**18.** T (page 875)
3. F (page 859)	**7.** F (page 851)	**11.** T (page 859)	**15.** T (page 866)	**19.** F (page 859)
4. F (page 872)	**8.** F (page 852)	**12.** T (page 868)	**16.** F (page 867)	**20.** T (page 859)

Fill-in-the-Blank

1. carotid (page 852)	**5.** cartilage (page 852)	**9.** basilar skull fracture (page 870)
2. cervical (page 852)	**6.** men; women (page 852)	**10.** crown; root (pages 873)
3. temporal (page 851)	**7.** foramen magnum (page 851)	**11.** air embolism (page 875)
4. trachea (page 852)	**8.** blowout fracture (page 867)	

Labeling

1. **The Face**
   - **A.** Nasal bone
   - **B.** Zygoma
   - **C.** Maxilla
   - **D.** Mandible (page 851)

2. **The Larynx**
   - **A.** Laryngeal prominence (Adam's apple)
   - **B.** Thyroid cartilage
   - **C.** Cricothyroid membrane
   - **D.** Cricoid cartilage
   - **E.** Trachea (page 853)

3. **The Eye**
   - **A.** Anterior compartment filled with aqueous humor
   - **B.** Posterior compartment filled with vitreous humor
   - **C.** Anterior chamber
   - **D.** Posterior chamber
   - **E.** Vein
   - **F.** Iris
   - **G.** Cornea
   - **H.** Pupil
   - **I.** Artery
   - **J.** Lens
   - **K.** Optic nerve
   - **L.** Retina
   - **M.** Choroid
   - **N.** Sclera (page 853)

4. **The Ear**
   - **A.** Pinna
   - **B.** External auditory canal
   - **C.** Tympanic membrane
   - **D.** Cochlea
   - **E.** Hammer
   - **F.** Anvil
   - **G.** Stirrup (page 871)

Crossword Puzzle

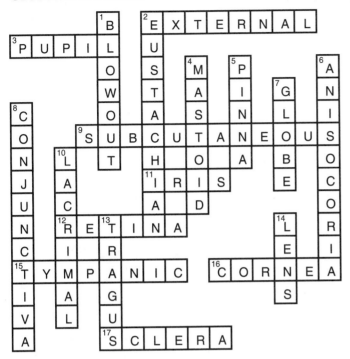

Critical Thinking

Short Answer

1. Apply direct manual pressure with a dry dressing. Use roller gauze around the circumference of the head to hold the pressure dressing in place. Make sure you do not apply excessive pressure if there is a possibility of an underlying skull fracture. (page 859)

2. **1.** Apply direct pressure to the bleeding site using a gloved fingertip if necessary to control bleeding.

   2. Apply a sterile occlusive dressing to ensure that air does not enter a vein or artery.

   3. Secure the dressing in place with roller gauze, adding more dressings if needed.

   4. Wrap the gauze around and under the patient's shoulder. To avoid possible airway and circulation problems, do not wrap the gauze around the neck. (page 874)

3. Start on the outer aspect of the eye and work your way in toward the pupil. Examine the eye for any obvious foreign matter. Observe for discoloration of the eye. Evaluate the clarity of the patient's vision. Assess for redness of or bleeding into the iris. Look for symmetry between the two eyes. Assess the pupils for equal size and reaction to light. Determine if unequal pupils are caused by physiologic or pathologic issues. Determine if the patient is able to follow your finger with their eyes. Assess visual acuity by having them read normal print. Question about blurry vision or sensitivity to light. (pages 857–858)

4. **1.** Never exert pressure on or manipulate the injured eye (globe) in any way.

   2. If part of the eyeball is exposed, gently apply a moist, sterile dressing to prevent drying.

   3. Cover the injured eye with a protective metal eye shield, cup, or sterile dressing. Apply soft dressings to both eyes, and provide prompt transport to the hospital. (page 866)

5. **1.** One pupil larger than the other

   2. The eyes not moving together or pointing in different directions

   3. Failure of the eyes to follow the movement of your finger as instructed

   4. Bleeding under the conjunctiva, which obscures the sclera of the eye

   5. Protrusion or bulging of one eye (pages 868–869)

Ambulance Calls

1. Depending on where the dog's teeth have punctured the skin, you may have a variety of soft-tissue injuries and swelling. If you notice the presence of subcutaneous emphysema, the dog punctured or perforated the child's trachea. You must also assume the presence of cervical spine injuries and take appropriate precautions. Assess his level of consciousness, airway, breathing, and circulation. Control any bleeding and apply other dressings, as needed, after airway management is accomplished and while en route to the hospital. Always follow local protocols.

2. Apply direct pressure to the bleeding site using gloved fingertips and a sterile occlusive dressing. Secure the dressing in place and apply pressure, if necessary. You may need to treat for shock. Provide prompt transport with the patient immobilized to a backboard and apply high-flow oxygen en route.

3. You should determine what objects were used to cause injury to this man's face. Baseball bats would be readily available and would increase your index of suspicion. You should determine the presence of head and neck pain. If the area of injury is limited to his nose, and the need for spinal precautions is not indicated, you can instruct the patient in controlling his bleeding by ensuring that he pushes on the cartilage of his nose and does not lean his head backwards. Swallowing blood will cause nausea. Do not allow the patient to blow his nose, and consider using ice, as needed, to reduce swelling and pain. Transport according to local protocols.

Skills

Skill Drills

Skill Drill 25-1: Removing a Foreign Object From Under the Upper Eyelid

1. Have the patient look **down**, grasp the upper **lashes**, and gently pull the **lid** away from the eye.
2. Place a cotton-tipped applicator on the **outer** surface of the **upper** lid.
3. Pull the lid **forward** and **up**, folding it back over the applicator.
4. Gently remove the foreign object from the eyelid with a moistened, **sterile**, cotton-tipped applicator. (page 862)

Skill Drill 25-2: Stabilizing a Foreign Object Impaled in the Eye

1. To prepare a doughnut ring, wrap a 2″ (5-cm) roll around your fingers and thumb seven or eight times. Adjust the diameter by spreading your fingers or squeezing them together.
2. Remove the gauze from you hand and wrap the remainder of the gauze roll radially around the ring that you have created.
3. Work around the entire ring to form a doughnut.
4. Place the dressing over the eye and impaled object to hold the impaled object in place, and then secure it with a roller bandage. (page 863)

Assessment Review

1. D (page 856)
2. B (page 858)
3. D (page 870)
4. A (page 873)
5. C (page 872)

Emergency Care Summary (page 882)

Ear Injuries

Place a soft, padded dressing between the ear and the scalp. If the ear is avulsed, wrap it in a(n) **moist**, sterile dressing and place in a plastic bag. Keep the avulsed tissue **cool** and transport to the hospital with the patient. Leave any foreign object within the ear for the physician to remove. Note any clear fluid coming from the ear.

Facial Fractures

Remove and save loose teeth or **bone** fragments from the mouth and transport them with you. Remove any loose dentures or dental bridges to protect against **airway** obstruction. Maintain an open airway.

Injuries to the Neck

1. Apply **direct** pressure to the bleeding site using a gloved fingertip if necessary to control bleeding.
2. Apply a sterile **occlusive dressing** to ensure that air does not enter a vein or artery.
3. Use **roller gauze** to secure a dressing in place.
4. Wrap the **bandage** around and under the patient's **shoulder**.

Chapter 26: Head and Spine Injuries

General Knowledge

Matching

1. D (page 897) **3.** H (page 895) **5.** A (page 896) **7.** B (page 894) **9.** J (page 891)
2. E (page 898) **4.** G (page 896) **6.** C (page 896) **8.** I (page 889) **10.** F (page 888)

Multiple Choice

1. D (page 887) **8.** D (page 888) **15.** B (page 909) **22.** D (page 895) **29.** C (page 907)
2. B (page 887) **9.** C (page 890) **16.** A (page 909) **23.** C (page 900) **30.** B (page 915)
3. C (page 887) **10.** A (page 891) **17.** A (page 906) **24.** B (page 899) **31.** D (page 916)
4. C (page 891) **11.** D (page 899) **18.** B (page 912) **25.** B (page 905) **32.** C (page 919)
5. A (page 888) **12.** D (page 898) **19.** D (pages 895–896) **26.** C (page 898) **33.** A (page 924)
6. B (page 890) **13.** B (page 891) **20.** B (page 896) **27.** C (page 899)
7. D (page 889) **14.** D (page 901) **21.** C (page 896) **28.** A (page 895)

True/False

1. T (page 897) **3.** F (page 889) **5.** F (page 890) **7.** F (page 898) **9.** T (page 912)
2. F (page 889) **4.** T (page 890) **6.** F (page 909) **8.** T (page 909) **10.** T (page 917)

Fill-in-the-Blank

1. motor (page 889)
2. meninges (page 888)
3. central (page 887)
4. 31 (page 889)
5. cranial (page 889)
6. intervertebral disks (page 891)
7. cranium; face (page 890)
8. arachnoid; pia mater (page 888)
9. sympathetic (page 890)
10. parasympathetic (page 890)
11. intracerebral hematoma (page 895)
12. contusion (page 897)
13. padding (page 923)
14. pulse; motor; sensory (page 911)
15. jaw-thrust (page 905)

Labeling

1. Brain
   A. Cerebrum
   B. Parietal lobe
   C. Frontal lobe
   D. Occipital lobe
   E. Temporal lobe
   F. Brain stem
   G. Cerebellum
   H. Spinal cord
   I. Foramen magnum (page 888)

2. Connecting Nerves in the Spinal Cord
   A. Motor nerve
   B. Sensory nerve
   C. Connecting nerve cell
   D. Spinal cord (page 889)

3. Spinal Column
   A. Cervical (7)
   B. Thoracic (12)
   C. Lumbar (5)
   D. Sacrum (5)
   E. Coccyx (4) (page 891)

Crossword Puzzle

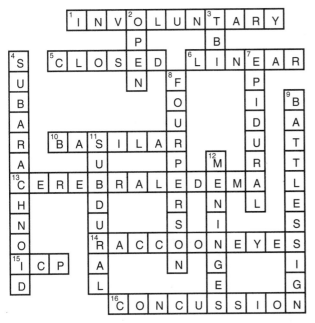

Critical Thinking

Short Answer

1. 1. Motor vehicle collision
   2. Pedestrian–motor vehicle collision
   3. Falls
   4. Blunt trauma
   5. Penetrating trauma to the head, neck, back, or torso
   6. Motorcycle crashes
   7. Rapid deceleration injuries
   8. Hangings
   9. Diving accidents
   10. Recreational accidents (page 898)

2. Muscle spasms in the neck
   Substantial increased pain
   Numbness, tingling, or weakness in the arms or legs
   Compromised airway or ventilations (page 909)

3. Primary brain injury is injury to the brain and its associated structures that results instantaneously from impact to the head. Secondary brain injury refers to a multitude of processes that increase the severity of a primary brain injury, and therefore negatively impact outcome. Secondary brain injuries result from cerebral edema, intracranial hemorrhage, increased intracranial pressure, cerebral ischemia, and infection. Hypoxia and hypotension are the two most common causes of secondary brain injuries. (page 893)

4. Lacerations, contusions, or hematomas to the scalp
   Soft area or depression on palpation
   Visible fractures or deformities of the skull
   Decreased mentation
   Irregular breathing pattern
   Widening pulse pressure
   Slow pulse rate
   Ecchymosis about the eyes or behind the ear over the mastoid process
   Clear or pink cerebrospinal fluid leakage from a scalp wound, the nose, or the ear
   Failure of the pupils to respond to light
   Unequal pupil size
   Loss of sensation and/or motor function
   A period of unconsciousness
   Amnesia
   Seizures
   Numbness or tingling in the extremities
   Irregular respirations
   Dizziness
   Visual complaints
   Combative or other abnormal behavior
   Nausea or vomiting
   Posturing (decorticate or decerebrate) (page 892)

5. **1.** Establish an adequate airway.

   2. Control bleeding.

   3. Assess the patient's baseline level of consciousness. (page 905)

6. **1.** Is the patient's airway clear?

   2. Is the patient breathing adequately?

   3. Can you maintain the airway and assist ventilations if the helmet remains in place?

   4. Can the face guard be easily removed to allow access to the airway without removing the helmet?

   5. How well does the helmet fit?

   6. Can the patient move within the helmet?

   7. Can the spine be immobilized in a neutral position with the helmet on? (page 919)

Ambulance Calls

1. This incident involves a significant mechanism of injury. The impact with the car, the lack of a helmet, the obvious head trauma, and the patient's decreased level of consciousness all indicate significant life-threatening injuries. You must quickly apply full spinal precautions and manage her airway. Provide prompt transport and high-flow oxygen, and perform ongoing assessments while en route to the nearest appropriate medical facility.

2. This child landed face down on a concrete surface with significant force. She is now unconscious with a partially obstructed airway. You must move her to a supine position to manage her airway. Take note of any apparent injuries to her back as you reposition her. Ideally, you will have the appropriate equipment and adequate staffing to quickly and safely move her to a long backboard immediately. However, do not delay appropriately moving her to a supine position, because you must do this to assess and manage her airway. This may be difficult, because she likely has facial fractures and possibly broken teeth, blood, and secretions in her airway. Be prepared to suction her airway and apply positive-pressure ventilations (this may be especially challenging in the presence of significant facial fractures). Use high-flow oxygen and promptly transport her to the nearest appropriate facility according to your local protocols.

3. Leave the patient in his car seat. Pad appropriately to immobilize the patient. Use blow-by oxygen if the patient will tolerate it. Monitor vital signs. Continue assessment. Provide rapid transport due to mechanism of injury and death in vehicle.

Skills

Skill Drills

Skill Drill 26-1: Performing Manual In-Line Stabilization

1. Kneel behind the patient and place your hands firmly around the **base** of the **skull** on either **side**.

2. Support the lower jaw with your **index** and **long** fingers, and the head with your **palms**. Gently lift the head into a **neutral**, **eyes-forward** position, aligned with the torso. Do not **move** the head or neck excessively, forcefully, or rapidly.

3. Continue to **support** the head manually while your partner places a rigid **cervical collar** around the neck. Maintain **manual support** until you have completely secured the patient to a backboard. (page 908)

Skill Drill 26-2: Immobilizing a Patient to a Long Backboard

1. Apply and maintain cervical motion restriction. Assess distal functions in all extremities.

2. Apply a cervical collar.

3. Rescuers kneel on one side of the patient and place hands on the far side of the patient.

4. On command, rescuers roll the patient toward themselves, quickly examine the back, slide the backboard under the patient, and roll the patient onto the board.

5. Center the patient on the board.

6. Secure the upper torso first.

7. Secure the pelvis and upper legs.

8. Begin to secure the patient's head using a commercial immobilization device or rolled towels.

9. Place tape across the patient's forehead to secure the immobolization device.

10. Check all straps and readjust as needed. Reassess distal functions in all extremities. (pages 910–911)

Skill Drill 26-4: Immobilizing a Patient found in a Standing Position

1. While **manually** stabilizing the head and neck, apply a **cervical collar**. Position the board **behind** the patient.
2. Position EMTs at **sides** and **behind** the patient. Side EMTs reach under the patient's **arms** and grasp **handholds** at or slightly above **shoulder** level.
3. Prepare to lower the patient to the **ground**.
4. On command, **lower** the backboard to the ground as a unit under the direction of the EMT at the **head**. (pages 915–916)

Skill Drill 26-5: Application of a Cervical Collar

1. Apply in-line **motion restriction**.
2. Measure the proper **collar size**.
3. Place the **chin support** first.
4. **Wrap** the collar around the neck and **secure** the collar.
5. Ensure proper **fit** and maintain **neutral, in-line** motion restriction until the patient is secured to a **backboard**.

Assessment Review

1. D (page 900)
2. C (page 916)
3. B (page 909)
4. C (pages 911–912)
5. A (page 920)

Emergency Care Summary (page 930)

General Management of Head Injuries

1. Establish and maintain a **patent** airway. Provide high-flow **supplemental** oxygen and provide **ventilatory** assistance, if needed.
2. Control **bleeding**. Do not apply pressure to an open or **depressed** skull injury. Begin **cardiopulmonary** resuscitation, if necessary.
3. Assess the patient's baseline level of **consciousness**, and continuously monitor it.
4. Assess and treat other injuries.
5. Anticipate and manage **vomiting** to prevent aspiration.
6. Be prepared for **convulsions** and changes in the patient's condition.
7. Transport the patient promptly and with extreme care.

General Management of Spine Injuries

1. Open and maintain a patent airway with the **jaw-thrust** maneuver.
2. Hold the head still in a **neutral**, in-line position.
3. Consider inserting an **oropharyngeal** airway.
4. Have a **suctioning** unit available.
5. Provide high-flow oxygen.
6. Continuously monitor the patient's airway.
7. Perform manual, in-line stabilization to protect the **cervical** spine.
8. Prepare the patient for transport according to patient's **position**.
9. Transport to the appropriate **trauma center**.

Chapter 27: Chest Injuries

General Knowledge

Matching

1. B (page 935)   **4.** A (page 937)   **7.** I (page 940)   **10.** G (page 940)
2. D (page 937)   **5.** E (page 936)   **8.** J (page 948)   **11.** C (page 936)
3. K (page 937)   **6.** H (page 938)   **9.** F (page 939)

Multiple Choice

1. B (page 936)   **6.** C (page 939)   **11.** D (pages 945–946)   **16.** A (page 949)
2. A (page 937)   **7.** A (page 951)   **12.** B (pages 948–949)   **17.** C (page 951)
3. C (page 937)   **8.** C (page 941)   **13.** C (page 947)   **18.** D (page 944)
4. D (pages 938–939)   **9.** D (page 945)   **14.** A (page 948)   **19.** A (page 943)
5. D (page 939)   **10.** C (page 945)   **15.** C (page 951)   **20.** B (page 936)

True/False

1. T (page 940)   **4.** F (page 949)   **7.** F (page 935)   **10.** T (page 939)   **13.** T (page 941)
2. F (page 940)   **5.** F (page 948)   **8.** T (page 937)   **11.** F (page 944)   **14.** T (page 940)
3. T (page 947)   **6.** F (page 952)   **9.** F (page 946)   **12.** F (page 943)   **15.** F (page 936)

Fill-in-the-Blank

1. back (page 936)   **6.** ribs (page 936)   **11.** Ventilation (page 935)
2. decreases (page 937)   **7.** diaphragm (page 937)   **12.** C6; C7 (page 935)
3. sternum (page 936)   **8.** Pleura (page 936)   **13.** Tidal volume (page 937)
4. bronchi (page 936)   **9.** aorta (page 953)   **14.** respiratory rate (page 944)
5. phrenic (page 937)   **10.** contracts (page 937)   **15.** immobilized (page 950)

Labeling

1. Anterior Aspect of the Chest
   A. Subclavian artery
   B. Superior vena cava
   C. Heart
   D. Aorta
   E. Pulmonary arteries
   F. Pleural lining
   G. Lungs
   H. Diaphragm (page 936)

2. Pneumothorax
   A. Parietal pleura
   B. Air in the pleural space
   C. Wound site
   D. Lung
   E. Collapsed lung
   F. Heart
   G. Visceral pleura
   H. Diaphragm (page 945)

Crossword Puzzle

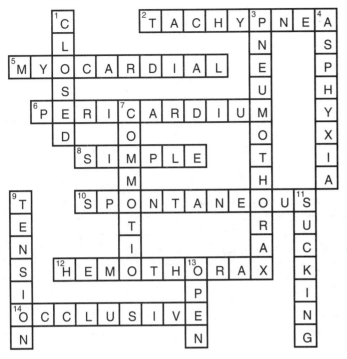

Critical Thinking

Short Answer

1. Pain at the site of injury
   Pain localized at the site of injury that is aggravated by or increased with breathing
   Bruising to the chest wall
   Crepitus with palpation of the chest
   Any penetrating injury to the chest
   Dyspnea (difficulty breathing, shortness of breath)
   Hemoptysis (coughing up blood)
   Failure of one or both sides of the chest to expand normally with inspiration
   Rapid, weak pulse and low blood pressure
   Cyanosis around the lips or fingernails (page 939)

2. **1.** Seal the wound with a large airtight dressing that seals all four sides.
   2. Seal the wound with a dressing that seals three sides with the fourth side as a flutter valve.
   Your local protocol will dictate the way you are to care for this injury. (pages 945–946)

3. Tape a bulky pad against the segment of the chest or use a pillow. (page 950)

4. Sudden severe compression of the chest, causing a rapid increase of pressure within the chest. Characteristic signs include distended neck veins, facial and neck cyanosis, and hemorrhage in the sclera of the eye. (page 951)

5. **1.** Airway obstruction
   2. Bronchial disruption
   3. Diaphragmatic tear
   4. Esophageal injury
   5. Open pneumothorax
   6. Tension pneuomothorax
   7. Massive hemothorax
   8. Flail chest

9. Cardiac tamponade
10. Thoracic aortic dissection
11. Myocardial contusion
12. Pulmonary contusion (page 942)

Ambulance Calls

1. You should be concerned with the presence of rib and sternal fractures as well as pulmonary contusions and pneumothoraces. This patient may require assistance in breathing, because it will be extremely painful for him to breathe in. If he requires assistance with a bag-mask device, you must be careful not to become too aggressive in your ventilations. Time your ventilations with the patient's respirations and be gentle. Provide high-flow oxygen and take spinal precautions according to your local protocols.

2. This patient's chest has been crushed with a significant amount of weight. This mechanism of injury indicates the high potential for rib, sternal, and thoracic fractures as well as other soft-tissue injuries. Patients who experience sternal fractures will find it difficult to be placed supine, because this will likely increase their pain. There will be little you can do to ease this pain, because they should be immobilized on a long backboard. Provide prompt transport, high-flow oxygen, and monitor the pulse, motor, and sensations particularly distal to the suspected spinal injury.

3. Apply high-flow oxygen via nonrebreathing mask or bag-mask device. Fully c-spine immobilize the patient. Provide rapid transport and monitor vital signs en route.

Skills

Assessment Review

1. B (page 945)
2. D (page 945)
3. C (page 946)
4. D (page 950)
5. A (page 958)

Emergency Care Summary (page 959)

General Management of Chest Injuries

Managing life threats to the patient's **ABCs** is the primary concern with any traumatic emergency. The MOI that caused the chest injury may also have caused a **spinal** injury or other fracture, and these must be managed at the appropriate time following local protocols. **Breathing** difficulties are often present with chest injuries, as are injuries involving bleeding. With all chest injuries, once crew safety has been established, management of airway, breathing, and circulatory problems is a priority. For all of the following specific chest injuries, begin with the following steps:

1. Ensure scene safety.
2. Determine the **MOI**.
3. Consider **spinal immobilization**.
4. Open, clear, and maintain the patient's airway.
5. Inspect, palpate, and **auscultate** the chest.
6. Administer high concentration oxygen via a nonrebreathing mask or bag-mask device, as appropriate.
7. Control bleeding and treat for **shock**.
8. Transport to the appropriate treatment facility.

Chapter 28: Abdominal and Genitourinary Injuries

General Knowledge

Matching

1. E (page 969)
2. I (page 971)
3. F (page 972)
4. A (page 970)
5. H (page 968)
6. C (page 973)
7. D (page 971)
8. G (page 968)
9. B (page 968)

Multiple Choice

1. D (page 967)
2. B (page 968)
3. C (page 968)
4. D (page 968)
5. B (page 968)
6. C (page 968)
7. A (page 968)
8. C (pages 969–970)
9. B (page 973)
10. A (page 967)
11. A (page 973)
12. C (page 971)
13. B (page 969)
14. A (page 971)
15. B (page 971)
16. B (page 972)
17. B (page 975)
18. B (page 973)
19. D (page 976)
20. D (page 970)
21. C (page 977)
22. A (page 971)
23. D (page 971)
24. D (page 978)
25. A (page 981)
26. C (page 981)
27. D (page 982)
28. C (page 987)
29. A (page 987)
30. B (page 987)
31. B (page 984)
32. B (page 988)

True/False

1. F (page 968)
2. T (pages 971–972)
3. F (page 977)
4. T (page 968)
5. F (page 978)
6. F (page 982)
7. T (page 968)
8. F (page 967)
9. T (pages 970–971)
10. T (page 980)

Fill-in-the-Blank

1. solid (page 968)
2. urinary (page 981)
3. retroperitoneal (page 969)
4. other organs (page 982)
5. peritonitis (page 968)
6. peritoneal cavity (pages 968–969)
7. blunt injuries (page 969)
8. penetrating injuries (page 971)
9. flank (page 972)
10. evisceration (page 971)

Labeling

1. Hollow Organs
   A. Stomach
   B. Gallbladder
   C. Bile duct
   D. Large intestine
   E. Ureter
   F. Small intestine
   G. Fallopian tubes
   H. Rectum
   I. Appendix
   J. Uterus
   K. Urinary bladder (page 968)

2. Solid Organs
   A. Liver
   B. Spleen
   C. Adrenal gland
   D. Adrenal gland
   E. Pancreas
   F. Kidney
   G. Kidney
   H. Ovaries (page 968)

Crossword Puzzle

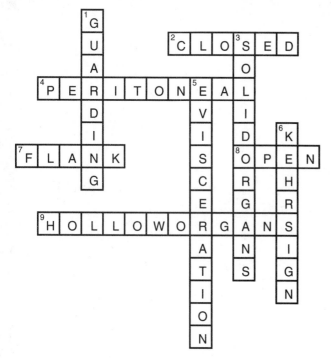

Critical Thinking

Short Answer

1. Stomach, intestines, ureters, bladder, gallbladder, bile duct, appendix, uterus, fallopian tubes, and rectum (page 968)

2. Liver, spleen, pancreas, adrenal glands, ovaries, and kidneys (page 968)

3. Pain

   Guarding

   Distention

   Tenderness

   Bruising and discoloration

   Abrasions

   Tachycardia

   Shock signs

   Lacerations

   Bleeding

   Difficulty with movement because of pain (pages 969–973)

4. 1. Log roll the patient to a supine position on a backboard.

    2. Inspect the patient's back and sides for exit wounds.

    3. Apply a dry, sterile dressing to all open wounds.

    4. If the penetrating object is still in place, apply a stabilizing bandage around it to control external bleeding and to minimize movement of the object.

    5. Monitor the patient's vital signs for indications of shock.

    6. Administer oxygen, if needed.

    7. Keep the patient warm with blankets.

    8. Provide prompt transport to the emergency department. (pages 979–980)

5. **1.** Cover the wound with sterile gauze compresses moistened with sterile saline solution.

   2. Secure the gauze with a sterile dressing.

   3. Treat the patient for shock.

   4. Provide high-flow oxygen.

   5. Transport the patient to the highest level trauma center available. (pages 980–981)

6. An abrasion, laceration, or contusion in the flank

A penetrating wound in the region of the lower rib cage (the flank) or the upper abdomen

Fractures on either side of the lower rib cage or of the lower thoracic or upper lumbar vertebrae

A hematoma in the flank region (page 982)

Ambulance Calls

1. Assess the patient's ABCs and apply high-flow oxygen. Control any bleeding. Stabilize the knife in place with bulky dressings—*do not remove it*. Keep movement of the patient to the bare minimum, so as not to create further injury. (Sliding the patient very carefully onto a backboard may help to minimize movement.) Monitor vital signs, and provide rapid transport. Bandage minor lacerations en route.

2. Quickly visualize the area to determine how badly he has cut himself and whether he has in fact amputated any portion of his penis. You will need to control bleeding, because blood loss in this area can be significant. Use pressure dressings and/or pressure points as needed to control bleeding. Provide high-flow oxygen and prompt transport. Also, request the presence of a police officer during transport, because this patient will likely need to be restrained and could be unpredictable during transport.

3. Cover the abdomen and the portion of the protruding bowel with a moistened, sterile dressing and/or an occlusive dressing. Secure these dressings with tape. Allow the patient to draw up his knees as needed for comfort. Apply high-flow oxygen, cover the patient to preserve warmth, and promptly transport to the hospital.

Skills

Assessment Review

  1. A (page 980)

  2. B (page 987)

  3. D (page 976)

  4. D (pages 987–988)

  5. C (page 988)

Emergency Care Summary (pages 994, 997)

Abdominal Trauma

Blunt Abdominal Injuries

Log roll the patient to a **supine** position on a backboard. If the patient vomits, turn him or her to one side and clear the mouth and throat of vomitus. Monitor the patient's vital signs for any indication of **shock**. If shock is present, administer high-flow supplemental oxygen via a nonrebreathing mask and treat for shock. Keep the patient **warm**. Provide prompt transport to the emergency department.

Penetrating Abdominal Injuries

The injuries from penetrating trauma may not be so obvious. Large amounts of **external bleeding** may not be present, yet there can be significant blood loss internally. Accurate assessment of a penetrating injury takes place in the **operating room**. Prehospital treatment consists of controlling any external bleeding, immobilizing the patient on a long spine board, treating for shock, and transporting the patient to the appropriate specialty center. If the penetrating object is still in place (impaled), stabilize the object in place.

Abdominal Evisceration

Never attempt to replace protruding organs. Cover the exposed organs with a **moist**, sterile dressing. If local protocol allows, cover the sterile dressing with an **occlusive** dressing. Maintain body temperature, treat for shock, and transport to the highest level trauma center available.

Genitourinary Trauma

Kidney Injuries

Damage to the kidneys may not be obvious on inspection of the patient. You may or may not see bruises or lacerations on the overlying skin. You will see signs of shock if the injury is associated with significant blood loss. Another sign of kidney damage is **blood** in the urine (hematuria). Treat shock and associated injuries in the appropriate manner. Provide prompt transport to the hospital, monitoring the patient's vital signs carefully en route.

Urinary Bladder Injuries

Suspect a possible injury of the urinary bladder if you see blood at the **urethral** opening or physical signs of trauma on the lower abdomen, pelvis, or **perineum**. There may be blood at the tip of the penis or a stain on the patient's underwear. The presence of associated injuries or of shock will dictate the urgency of transport. In most instances, provide prompt transport, and monitor the patient's vital signs en route.

Genitalia Injuries

Soft-tissue injuries to the external genitalia should be treated like any other soft-tissue injury once all life threats have been assessed and managed. Female patients with external genitalia trauma should be questioned about the possibility of **pregnancy**. Use only external dressings, never place anything into the **vagina**.

Trauma to the abdomen or genitourinary area may produce injury to the female patient's uterus, **fallopian tubes**, and ovaries. Treat for shock because injuries to these organs may be hidden.

Rectal Bleeding

Rectal bleeding can be significant and lead to shock. Place dressings in the crease between the **buttocks** to manage bleeding. Contact medical control to determine the need for transport.

Sexual Assault

Follow local protocol for crime scene management and **evidence** preservation. If available, an EMT of the same sex as the patient should perform the assessment and treatment. Advise the patient not to change clothes, **shower**, drink, or eat. Maintain patient privacy at all times. Sexual assault victims may have serious multisystem trauma. Assessment and treatment should consist of managing life-threatening injuries. Do not examine the genitalia unless obvious bleeding must be managed.

Chapter 29: Orthopaedic Injuries

General Knowledge

Matching

1. G (page 1001)
2. J (page 1001)
3. D (page 1002)
4. I (page 1004)
5. F (page 1005)
6. B (page 1007)
7. K (page 1008)
8. A (page 1007)
9. C (page 1005)
10. E (page 1007)
11. H (page 1021)

Multiple Choice

1. A (page 1041)
2. B (page 1002)
3. A (page 1002)
4. B (page 1004)
5. C (page 1005)
6. B (page 1005)
7. C (page 1005)
8. A (page 1006)
9. D (page 1006)
10. A (page 1006)
11. B (page 1006)
12. C (page 1006)
13. D (page 1007)
14. B (page 1007)
15. C (page 1007)
16. D (page 1007)
17. A (page 1007)
18. C (page 1008)
19. D (page 1008)
20. A (page 1008)
21. C (page 1008)
22. B (page 1008)
23. A (page 1008)
24. C (page 1008)
25. D (page 1010)
26. C (pages 1010–1011)
27. D (page 1015)
28. B (page 1011)
29. D (page 1015)
30. A (page 1020)
31. C (page 1021)
32. D (page 1021)
33. B (page 1026)
34. A (page 1031)
35. B (page 1031)
36. B (page 1033)
37. D (page 1042)
38. C (page 1043)
39. B (page 1043)
40. D (page 1043)
41. C (page 1044)
42. B (page 1044)
43. A (page 1046)
44. C (page 1046)
45. A (page 1047)

True/False

1. T (pages 1013, 1020)
2. T (page 1020)
3. F (page 1021)
4. T (page 1021)
5. T (page 1020)
6. F (page 1020)
7. T (page 1015)
8. T (page 1015)
9. T (page 1015)
10. F (page 1015)

Fill-in-the-Blank

1. calcaneus (page 1046)
2. blood cells (page 1002)
3. hinged (page 1003)
4. clavicle (page 1031)
5. mechanism of injury (page 1012)
6. open fracture (page 1014)
7. sciatic nerve (page 1042)
8. Pelvic binders (page 1028)
9. crepitus (page 1008)
10. reduce (page 1010)
11. neurovascular status (page 1047)

Labeling

1. **Pectoral Girdle**
   - **A.** Sternoclavicular joint
   - **B.** Clavicle
   - **C.** Acromioclavicular joint
   - **D.** Clavicle
   - **E.** Manubrium
   - **F.** Acromion process
   - **G.** Acromion process
   - **H.** Humerus
   - **I.** Glenoid fossa
   - **J.** Sternum
   - **K.** Humerus
   - **L.** Glenohumeral (shoulder) joint
   - **M.** Scapula (page 1003)

2. **Anatomy of the Wrist and Hand**
   - **A.** Index
   - **B.** Long
   - **C.** Ring
   - **D.** Small
   - **E.** Phalanges
   - **F.** Thumb
   - **G.** Metacarpals
   - **H.** Scaphoid
   - **I.** Carpals
   - **J.** Radius
   - **K.** Ulna (page 1004)

3. **Bones of the Thigh, Leg, and Foot**
   - **A.** Pelvis (hip bone)
   - **B.** Hip
   - **C.** Femur
   - **D.** Thigh
   - **E.** Patella (knee cap)
   - **F.** Knee
   - **G.** Fibula
   - **H.** Leg
   - **I.** Tibia (shin bone)
   - **J.** Ankle
   - **K.** Tarsals (ankle)
   - **L.** Foot
   - **M.** Metatarsals
   - **N.** Phalanges (page 1004)

Crossword Puzzle

Critical Thinking

Short Answer

1. 1. Direct blows
    2. Indirect forces
    3. Twisting force
    4. High-energy injury (page 1006)
2. Deformity
    Tenderness (point)
    Guarding
    Swelling
    Bruising
    Crepitus
    False motion
    Exposed fragments
    Pain
    Locked joint (pages 1008–1009)
3. 1. Pulse
    2. Capillary refill
    3. Sensation
    4. Motor function (page 1015)
4. 1. Remove clothing from the area.
    2. Note and record the patient's neurovascular status distal to the site of the injury.
    3. Cover all wounds with a dry, sterile dressing before splinting.
    4. Do not move the patient before splinting.
    5. For a suspected fracture of the shaft of any bone, immobilize the joints above and below the fracture.
    6. For a joint injury, immobilize the bones above and below the injured joint.
    7. Pad all rigid splints.
    8. Maintain manual immobilization to minimize movement of the limb and to support the injury site.
    9. If a fracture of a long-bone shaft has resulted in severe deformity, use a constant, gentle manual traction to align the limb.
    10. If you encounter resistance to limb alignment, splint the limb in its deformed position.
    11. Stabilize all suspected spinal injuries in a neutral in-line position on a backboard.
    12. If the patient has signs of shock, align the limb in the normal anatomic position, and provide transport.
    13. When in doubt, splint. (page 1020)
5. 1. Stabilize the fracture fragments to prevent excessive movement.
    2. Align the limb sufficiently to allow it to be placed in a splint.
    3. Avoid potential neurovascular compromise. (page 1021)

Ambulance Calls

1. This patient likely has a compression injury to his lumbar spine. The force exerted on his body from the landing will be transferred up from his feet through his legs to his pelvis and spine. You must take all spinal precautions, apply high-flow oxygen, and provide prompt transport to the nearest appropriate facility. Continue to monitor any changes in the pulse, motor, and sensation, specifically in his lower body.
2. Because circulation is intact, splint the arm in the position found. Use a board splint for support with a sling and swathe. Immobilize the hand in the position of function. Apply oxygen as needed and transport the patient in a position of comfort. Provide normal transport and monitor vital signs.
3. This man not only has probable injuries and swelling to his airway, but also significant likelihood for distraction injuries to his cervical spine. You must take c-spine precautions as you open his airway and determine the presence of breathing. The information provided does not include whether he has a pulse. Assess airway, breathing, and circulation; apply full spinal precautions, high-flow oxygen, positive-pressure ventilations, and CPR, as needed. Transport to an appropriate facility immediately. If ALS was not initially dispatched, request them during your scene size-up. Keep in mind that your patient is a prisoner and that special precautions may be necessary for transport regardless of the patient's condition. Communication with prison staff will be essential for a safe transport.

Skills

Skill Drills

Skill Drill 29-1: Assessing Neurovascular Status

1. Palpate the **radial** pulse in the upper extremity.
2. Palpate the **posterior tibial** and dorsalis pedis pulse in the lower extremity.
3. Assess capillary refill by blanching a fingernail or **toenail**.
4. Assess sensation on the flesh near the **tip** of the **index** finger and thumb, as well as the little finger.
5. On the foot, first check sensation on the flesh near the **tip** of the **big toe**.
6. Also check foot sensation on the **lateral side** of the foot.
7. For an upper extremity injury, evaluate motor function by asking the patient to **open** the hand. (Perform motor tests only if the hand or foot is not **injured. Stop** a test if it causes pain.)
8. Also ask the patient to **make** a **fist**.
9. For a lower extremity injury, ask the patient to **extend** the foot.
10. Also have the patient **flex** the foot and **wiggle** the toes. (pages 1016–1017)

Skill Drill 29-3: Applying a Rigid Splint

1. Provide gentle **support** and **in-line traction** for the limb.
2. Place the splint **alongside** or **under** the limb. **Pad** between the limb and the splint as needed to ensure even pressure and contact.
3. Secure the splint to the limb with **bindings**.
4. Assess and record **distal neurovascular** function. (page 1022)

Skill Drill 29-6: Applying a Vacuum Splint

1. Your partner **stabilizes** and **supports** the injury.
2. Place the splint, and **wrap** it around the limb.
3. **Draw** the air out of the splint through the **suction valve**, and then **seal** the valve. (page 1025)

Assessment Review

1. C (page 1013)
2. B (page 1017)
3. A (page 1015)
4. B (page 1040)
5. D (page 1028)

Skill Drill 29-7: Applying a Hare Traction Splint

1. Expose the injured limb and check pulse and motor and sensory function. Place the splint beside the uninjured limb, adjust the splint to proper length, and prepare the straps.
2. Support the injured limb as your partner fastens the ankle hitch about the foot and ankle.
3. Continue to support the limb as your partner applies gentle in-line traction to the ankle hitch and foot.
4. Slide the splint into position under the injured limb.
5. Pad the groin and fasten the ischial strap.
6. Connect the loops of the ankle hitch to the end of the splint as your partner continues to maintain traction. Carefully tighten the ratchet to the point that the splint holds adequate traction.
7. Secure and check support straps. Assess pulse and motor and sensory functions.
8. Secure the patient and splint to the backboard in a way that will prevent movement of the splint during patient movement and transport. (pages 1026-1027)

Skill Drill 29-10: Splinting the Hand and Wrist

1. Support the injured limb and move the hand into the **position** of **function**. Place a soft **roller bandage** in the palm.
2. Apply a **padded board** splint on the **palmar** side with fingers **exposed**.
3. Secure the splint with a **roller bandage**. (page 1039)

Chapter 30: Environmental Emergencies

General Knowledge

Matching

1. J (page 1062)
2. H (page 1080)
3. K (page 1062)
4. O (page 1070)
5. A (page 1079)
6. N (page 1063)
7. I (page 1062)
8. C (page 1076)
9. B (pages 1072–1073)
10. E (page 1062)
11. G (page 1062)
12. M (page 1070)
13. L (page 1070)
14. D (page 1076)
15. F (page 1087)

Multiple Choice

1. D (page 1062)
2. A (page 1062)
3. D (page 1062)
4. C (page 1063)
5. C (page 1064)
6. B (page 1063)
7. A (page 1063)
8. C (page 1064)
9. D (page 1068)
10. D (page 1065)
11. A (page 1070)
12. D (page 1070)
13. D (page 1070)
14. A (page 1070)
15. D (page 1071)
16. A (page 1077)
17. A (page 1071)
18. D (page 1071)
19. B (page 1076)
20. D (page 1081)
21. B (page 1080)
22. C (page 1083)
23. B (page 1079)
24. B (page 1080)
25. A (page 1080)
26. D (page 1080)
27. A (page 1080)
28. D (page 1086)
29. A (page 1090)
30. A (page 1091)
31. B (page 1089)
32. C (page 1091)
33. A (page 1086)
34. D (pages 1089–1090)
35. B (page 1071)
36. B (page 1063)
37. A (page 1062)
38. B (page 1063)
39. D (page 1067–1068)
40. C (page 1061)
41. A (page 1062)

True/False

1. T (page 1070)
2. T (page 1063)
3. F (page 1064)
4. T (page 1070)
5. T (page 1070)
6. F (page 1084)
7. T (page 1079)
8. F (page 1089)
9. F (page 1088)
10. T (pages 1087–1088)
11. F (page 1091)
12. F (page 1091)
13. F (page 1066)
14. T (page 1069)
15. T (page 1085)
16. F (page 1062)
17. F (page 1081)
18. T (page 1066)
19. F (page 1071)

Fill-in-the-Blank

1. moderate; severe (pages 1068–1069)
2. ascent (page 1080)
3. rewarming (page 1069)
4. high-altitude pulmonary edema (page 1084)
5. Shivering (page 1062)
6. diving reflex (page 1079)
7. Radiation (page 1062)
8. 90°F (32°C); 95°F (35°C) (page 1064)
9. cardiovascular; nervous (page 1085)
10. Lightning (page 1085)
11. Antivenin (page 1086)
12. Hymenoptera (page 1087)
13. April; October (page 1088)
14. rattlesnake (page 1088)
15. Scorpions (page 1090)
16. summer (page 1091)
17. bull's-eye (page 1091)
18. acetic acid (page 1091)
19. envenomations (page 1091)
20. heat sensitive (page 1092)

Crossword Puzzle

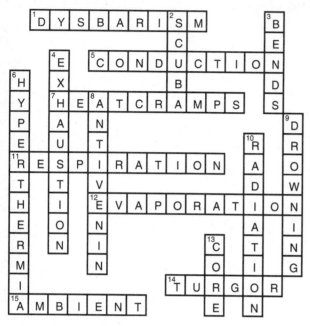

Critical Thinking

Short Answer

1. 1. Increase or decrease heat production: shiver, jump, walk around, etc.
   2. Move to an area where heat loss is decreased or increased: out of wind, into sun, etc.
   3. Wear insulated clothing, which helps decrease heat loss in several ways: layer with wool, down, synthetics, etc. (page 1062)

2. 1. Move the patient out of the hot environment and into the ambulance.
   2. Set the air conditioning to maximum cooling.
   3. Remove the patient's clothing.
   4. Administer high-flow oxygen. If needed, assist the patient's ventilations with a bag-mask device and appropriate airway adjuncts as per your protocol.
   5. Apply cool packs to patient's neck, groin, and armpits.
   6. Cover the patient with wet towels or sheets, or spray the patient with cool water and fan him or her.
   7. Aggressively and repeatedly fan the patient with or without dampening the skin.
   8. Transport immediately.
   9. Notify the hospital. (page 1075)

3. An air embolism is a bubble of air in the blood vessels caused by breath-holding during rapid ascent. The air pressure in the lungs remains at a high level while the external pressure on the chest decreases. As a result, the air inside the lungs expands rapidly, causing the alveoli in the lungs to rupture. (page 1080)

4. Treatment of air embolism and decompression sickness. The recompression treatment allows the bubbles of the gas to dissolve into the blood and equalize the pressures inside and outside the lungs. (page 1081)

5. 1. Remove the patient from the cold.
   2. Handle the injured part gently and protect it from further injury.
   3. Administer oxygen.
   4. Remove wet or restricting clothing.
   5. Consider active rewarming if there is no chance of reinjury.
   6. Splint the extremity and cover it loosely with a dry, sterile dressing.
   7. Be sure not to rub the injured tissue. (page 1069)

6. 1. Do not break blisters.
    2. Do not rub or massage area.
    3. Do not apply heat or rewarm unless instructed by medical control.
    4. Do not allow patient to stand or walk on a frostbitten foot.
    5. Do not reexpose the injury to cold. (page 1069)
7. 1. Have the patient lie flat and stay quiet.
    2. Wash the bite area with soapy water; consider a constricting band for hypotensive patients.
    3. Splint the extremity.
    4. Mark the skin with a pen to monitor advancing swelling. (pages 1089–1090)
8. **Black widow:** Bite has a systemic effect (venom is neurotoxic).
    Brown recluse: Bite destroys tissue locally (venom is cytotoxic). (pages 1086–1087)

Ambulance Calls

1. Provide BLS. Administer oxygen. Transport the patient in the left lateral recumbent position with the head down. Transport to a facility with hyperbaric chamber access.

2. Your main concern for this patient is hypothermia. Although this patient could also likely have localized cold injuries such as frostbite or frostnip, hypothermia can be fatal. You must handle this patient carefully, remove him from the cold environment, remove any wet clothing, and prevent further heat loss. Assessing the extent of the hypothermia through mentation will be difficult in this case, because your patient is likely confused. Take note of the presence of shivering (this protective mechanism stops at core temperatures > 90°F or 32°C), and, if possible, take his temperature (rectally). Assess airway, breathing, and circulation. Provide warm, humidified oxygen (if possible) and passive rewarming measures, such as increasing the heat in the patient compartment and prompt transport.

3. This patient has severe dehydration. Her use of diuretics and laxatives combined with strenuous exercise and a "body wrap," have depleted her body's volume. There is also the possibility that she is suffering from hyperthermia, because her lack of fluids will affect her body's thermoregulatory mechanisms. She needs fluid replacement therapy and assessment of her core temperature. You should remove excess layers of clothing (in this case, the body wrap), give high-flow oxygen, encourage oral fluid replacement if fully alert, and provide nonaggressive cooling measures.

Skills

Skill Drills

Skill Drill 30-1: Treating for Heat Exhaustion
  1. Move the patient to a **cooler environment**. Remove extra **clothing**.
  2. Give **oxygen**. Place the patient in a **supine** position, elevate the **legs**, and fan the patient.
  3. If the patient is fully alert, give **water** by mouth.
  4. If **nausea** develops, secure and transport on his or her side. (page 1074)

Skill Drill 30-2: Stabilizing a Suspected Spinal Injury in the Water
  1. Turn the patient to a supine position by rotating the entire upper half of the body as a single unit.
  2. As soon as the patient is turned, begin artificial ventilation using the mouth-to-mouth method or a pocket mask.
  3. Float a buoyant backboard under the patient.
  4. Secure the patient to the backboard.
  5. Remove the patient from the water.
  6. Cover the patient with a blanket and apply oxygen if breathing. Begin CPR if breathing and pulse are absent. (pages 1078–1079)

Assessment Review

1. B (page 1065)
2. A (page 1063)
3. B (page 1070)
4. B (page 1085)
5. C (page 1091)

Emergency Care Summary (pages 1097, 1099)

Cold Exposure Emergency

1. Establish and maintain a patent airway. Provide oxygen. Monitor for **vomiting** and protect against aspiration.
2. Carefully move the patient to a protected environment. Remove any **wet** clothing. Place dry **blankets** over and under the patient.
3. Handle the patient gently to avoid further injury. With severe **hypothermia**, careful handling of the patient is necessary to prevent cardiac arrest; rough handling can cause ventricular fibrillation.
4. If the hypothermia is mild, begin **active rewarming**.
5. If the hypothermia is moderate or severe, prevent further heat loss and follow local protocols.

Diving Injuries

1. Remove the patient from the water.
2. Begin CPR if pulse and breathing are absent.
3. If pulse and breathing are present, administer **oxygen**.
4. Place the patient in a **left lateral recumbent** position with the head **down**.
5. Provide prompt transport to the nearest **recompression** facility for treatment.

Spider Bites

1. Provide basic life support for respiratory distress.
2. Apply **ice** to the bite area and clean the wound with soap and water.
3. Transport the patient and, if possible, the spider to the hospital.

Snake Bites

1. Calm the patient and minimize movement.
2. Clean the bite area gently with soap and water or a mild **antiseptic**. Do not apply **ice**.
3. Transport the patient and, if possible, the snake to the emergency department.
4. Notify the emergency department that you are bringing in a snake bite victim.

Chapter 31: Obstetrics and Neonatal Care

General Knowledge

Matching

1. D (page 1108)
2. C (page 1111)
3. L (page 1108)
4. B (page 1108)
5. N (page 1107)
6. H (page 1108)
7. M (page 1110)
8. E (page 1108)
9. F (page 1111)
10. O (page 1128)
11. K (page 1128)
12. I (page 1110)
13. A (page 1122)
14. G (page 1128)
15. J (page 1112)

Multiple Choice

1. C (page 1122)
2. B (page 1122)
3. D (page 1123)
4. B (page 1124)
5. A (page 1127)
6. C (page 1127)
7. D (page 1127)
8. D (page 1126)
9. A (page 1128)
10. A (page 1129)
11. B (page 1130)
12. A (page 1110)
13. B (page 1110)
14. C (page 1111)
15. A (page 1111)
16. C (page 1111)
17. B (page 1111)
18. B (page 1112)
19. D (page 1109)
20. C (page 1109)
21. D (page 1112)
22. D (page 1129)
23. C (page 1112)
24. B (page 1112)
25. A (page 1111)
26. B (page 1129)
27. D (page 1111)
28. D (page 1122)
29. C (page 1111)
30. C (page 1123)
31. D (page 1124)
32. B (page 1107)
33. C (page 1107)
34. B (page 1112)
35. B (page 1126)
36. C (page 1130)
37. A (page 1131)
38. D (page 1131)
39. C (page 1132)
40. B (page 1124)

True/False

1. T (page 1108)
2. F (page 1111)
3. F (page 1110)
4. F (page 1110)
5. F (page 1118)
6. T (page 1128)
7. T (page 1124)
8. F (page 1124)
9. F (page 1124)
10. T (page 1128)
11. T (page 1130)
12. T (page 1115)
13. F (page 1123)
14. T (page 1130)
15. T (page 1131
16. F (page 1131)
17. T (page 1132)

Fill-in-the-Blank

1. placenta (page 1108)
2. arteries; vein (page 1108)
3. 500; 1,000 (page 1108)
4. 36; 40 (page 1131)
5. 20 (page 1109)
6. body fluids (page 1111)
7. ectopic pregnancy (page 1112)
8. resuscitate (page 1114)
9. fontanelles (page 1122)
10. Spina bifida (page 1129)
11. abortion (page 1129)
12. Braxton-Hicks (page 1110)
13. umbilical vein (page 1108)
14. perineum (page 1108)
15. falls (page 1113)

Fill-in-the-Table

Apgar Scoring System			
Area of Activity	Score		
	2	1	0
Appearance	Entire infant is pink.	Body is pink, but hands and feet remain blue.	Entire infant is blue or pale.
Pulse	More than 100 beats/min.	Fewer than 100 beats/min.	Absent pulse.
Grimace or irritability	Infant cries and tries to move foot away from finger snapped against sole of foot.	Infant gives a weak cry in response to stimulus.	Infant does not cry or react to stimulus.
Activity or muscle tone	Infant resists attempts to straighten hips and knees.	Infant makes weak attempts to resist straightening.	Infant is completely limp, with no muscle tone.
Respiration	Rapid respirations.	Slow respirations.	Absent respirations.

Labeling

1. Anatomic Structures of the Pregnant Woman
    A. Placenta
    B. Uterus
    C. Cervix
    D. Amniotic fluid
    E. Sacrum
    F. Rectum
    G. Bladder
    H. Vagina
    I. Pubic symphysis

Crossword Puzzle

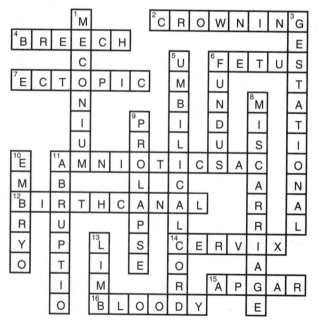

Critical Thinking

Multiple Choice

1. C (page 1127)
2. A (page 1127)
3. B (page 1127)

Short Answer

1. Early: spontaneous abortion (miscarriage) or ectopic pregnancy.
   Late: Placenta previa or abruptio placenta (page 1112)

2. On the left side, to prevent supine hypotensive syndrome (low blood pressure occurring from the weight of the fetus compressing the inferior vena cava) (page 1112)

3. 1. Uterine contractions
   2. Bloody show
   3. Rupture of amniotic sac (page 1110)

4. 1. How long have you been pregnant?
   2. When are you due?
   3. Is this your first baby?
   4. Are you having contractions? If so, how far apart are the contractions? How long do the contractions last?
   5. Do you feel as though you will have a bowel movement?
   6. Have you had any spotting or bleeding?
   7. Has your water broken?
   8. Were any of your previous children delivered by cesarean section?
   9. Did you have any problems in a previous pregnancy?
   10. Do you use drugs, drink alcohol, or take any medications?
   11. Do you know if there is a chance of a multiple birth?
   12. Does you doctor expect any complications? (pages 1117–1118)

5. Exert gentle pressure on the head as it emerges to prevent rapid expulsion with a strong contraction. (page 1120)

6. The brain is covered by only skin and membrane at the fontanelles. (page 1122)

7. Applying gentle pressure across the perineum with a sterile gauze pad and applying gentle pressure to the head while stretching the perineum. Always follow local protocol. (page 1120)

8. 1. During a breech delivery to protect the infant's airway
   2. When the umbilical cord is prolapsed (pages 1128–1129)

9. 1. Prematurity
   2. Low birth weight
   3. Severe respiratory depression (page 1130)

10. 1. Headache
    2. Seeing spots
    3. Swelling on the hands and feet (edema)
    4. Anxiety
    5. High blood pressure (page 1111)

Ambulance Calls

1. This patient has classic signs of preeclampsia. If she does not receive medical care soon to control her hypertension, she will likely experience a seizure. Provide high-flow oxygen, obtain a set of vital signs (especially blood pressure), and provide prompt transport with the patient on her left side. Consider ALS intercept, if available.

2. Recent laws have been enacted to provide protection for new mothers who do not wish to keep their babies. They can release their newborns and infants to fire stations and hospitals without fear of criminal charges (as the young woman in this scenario chose to do). You should notify other providers in your station as you begin measures to dry, warm, stimulate, and suction the baby's airway. These measures are very effective in improving a newborn's oxygenation and perfusion status. Blow-by oxygen will help immensely, but if those measures fail to quickly improve the newborn's status, bag-mask ventilations should be initiated. Provide chest compressions if the newborn's heart rate is less than 60 beats/min, and take note of the condition of the umbilical cord to ensure no blood loss occurs. Provide prompt transport and notify the hospital of the incoming patient.

3. Position the mother for delivery and apply high-flow oxygen. As crowning occurs, use a clamp to puncture the sac, away from the baby's face. Push the ruptured sac away from the infant's face as the head is delivered. Clear the baby's mouth and nose immediately. Continue with the delivery as normal.

Skills

Skill Drill

Skill Drill 31-1: Delivering the Baby

1. Support the bony parts of the head with your hands as it emerges. Suction fluid from the mouth, then nostrils.
2. As the upper shoulder appears, guide the head down slightly, if needed, to deliver the shoulder.
3. Support the head and upper body as the lower shoulder delivers, guiding the head up if needed.
4. Handle the infant firmly but gently, keeping the neck in neutral position to maintain the airway. Keep the infant approximately at the level of the vagina until the umbilical cord is cut.
5. Place the umbilical cord clamps 2″ to 4″ (5 to 10 cm) apart, and cut between them.
6. Allow the placenta to deliver itself. Do not pull on the cord to speed delivery. (pages 1121–1122)

Assessment Review

1. A (page 1120)
2. A (page 1126)
3. A (page 1117)
4. D (page 1123)
5. B (page 1123)

Emergency Care Summary (pages 1139–1141)

General Management of Obstetric Emergencies

Managing life threats to the patient's ABCs are primary concerns with any obstetric emergency. Avoid tunnel vision. Complete a **full-body** scan, remaining alert for signs and symptoms of **shock**. Manage as per local protocol. Request additional resources if delivery is imminent or has occurred. Provide high-concentration oxygen.

Delivery Complications

Nuchal Cord
When the **umbilical cord** is wrapped around the infant's neck, it is called a nuchal cord. If it is wound tightly it will strangle the infant, so it must be removed. Attempt to slip the cord over the infant's head or shoulder. If you are unable to slip the cord over the head or shoulder, you will need to clamp the cord in **two** places about 2″ (5 cm) apart, if possible, and cut the cord between the clamps. After cutting the cord, you can unwrap it and continue with the delivery as usual.

Spontaneous Abortion (Miscarriage)
If the delivery is occurring before the **20th** week of gestation, be prepared to treat the patient for bleeding and shock. Place a sterile pad/dressing on the **vagina**. Collect any expelled tissue to take to the hospital, but never pull tissue out of the vagina. Transport immediately, continually monitoring the patient's ABCs while assessing for signs of shock.

Multiple Gestation
The procedure for delivering multiple infants is the same as that for a single newborn. If you suspect more than one infant, **additional resources** should be called for immediately. Record the time of birth for each infant separately, making sure to label them for identification after the delivery process is over. At 1- and 5-minute intervals, assess and record the **Apgar** score for each infant.

Postterm Pregnancy
Pregnancies lasting more than 42 weeks can lead to problems with the mother and infant. Infants can be larger, leading to a more difficult delivery and injury to the infant. **Meconium** aspiration risk increases, as does infection and **stillborn** birth. Respiratory and **neurologic** functions may be affected, so be prepared to resuscitate the infant.

Chapter 32: Pediatric Emergencies

General Knowledge

Matching

1. C (page 1152)
2. I (page 1175)
3. F (page 1149)
4. A (page 1159)
5. D (page 1196)
6. G (page 1148)
7. J (page 1173)
8. H (page 1151)
9. B (page 1160)
10. E (page 1150)

Multiple Choice

1. B (page 1149)
2. C (page 1149)
3. D (page 1150)
4. C (page 1151)
5. A (page 1153)
6. A (page 1154)
7. D (page 1155)
8. B (page 1155)
9. C (page 1156)
10. C (page 1160)
11. A (page 1162)
12. B (page 1162)
13. A (page 1163)
14. D (page 1165)
15. C (page 1166)
16. C (page 1167)
17. C (pages 1168–1169)
18. B (pages 1169–1171)
19. D (page 1170)
20. B (page 1171)
21. A (page 1171)
22. A (page 1172)
23. A (page 1172)
24. D (page 1180)
25. C (page 1180)
26. D (page 1181)
27. D (page 1182)
28. B (page 1182)
29. C (page 1183)
30. A (page 1184)
31. D (page 1184)
32. A (page 1185)
33. B (page 1185)
34. D (page 1186)
35. C (page 1186)
36. D (page 1187)
37. B (page 1192)
38. B (page 1192)
39. B (page 1194)
40. C (page 1196)
41. D (page 1197)
42. A (page 1199)

True/False

1. F (page 1149)
2. T (page 1150)
3. F (page 1151)
4. T (page 1152)
5. T (page 1153)
6. F (page 1154)
7. T (page 1156)
8. T (page 1156)
9. F (page 1161)
10. F (page 1164)
11. F (page 1167)
12. T (page 1171)
13. T (page 1173)
14. F (page 1176)
15. T (page 1186)
16. T (page 1188)
17. F (page 1193)
18. T (page 1196)
19. T (page 1196)
20. F (page 1199)

Fill-in-the-Blank

1. oxygen demand (page 1154)
2. chest (page 1154)
3. Respiratory failure (page 1155)
4. fontanelles (page 1156)
5. pediatric assessment triangle (page 1158)
6. sniffing position (page 1160)
7. forward-facing, rear-facing (page 1164)
8. oxygen (page 1169)
9. Epiglottitis (pages 1169–1170)
10. Chest compressions (page 1171)
11. Asthma (page 1171)
12. oropharyngeal airway (page 1176)
13. Hemophilia (page 1181)
14. Appendicitis (page 1183)
15. Drowning (page1186)
16. blunt trauma (page 1190)
17. infection (page 1192)
18. Neglect (page 1196)

Crossword Puzzle

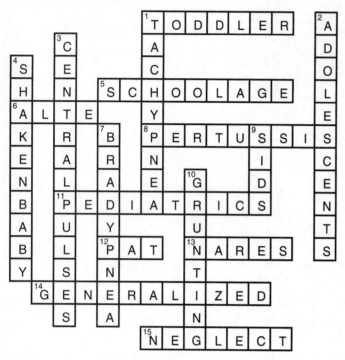

Critical Thinking

Short Answer

1. Tone

   Interactiveness

   Consolability

   Look or gaze

   Speech or cry (page 1158)

2. **Accessory muscle use:** Contractions of the muscles above the clavicles

   Retractions: Drawing in of the muscles between the ribs or of the sternum during inspiration

   Head-bobbing: The head lifts and tilts back during inspiration, then moves forward during expiration

   Nasal flaring: The nares widen; usually seen during inspiration

   Tachypnea: Increased respiratory rate (page 1161)

3. Unsafe scene

   Significant MOI

   History compatible with a serious illness

   Physiologic abnormality noted during the primary assessment

   Potentially serious anatomic abnormality

   Significant pain

   Altered mental status or signs and/or symptoms of shock (page 1164)

4. 70 + (2 × child's age in years) = systolic blood pressure (page 1167)

5. **Pulse:** Assess both the rate and quality of the pulse. A weak, "thready" pulse is a sign that there is a problem. The appropriate rate depends on the patient's age; anything over 160 beats/min suggests shock.

Skin signs: Assess the temperature and moisture of the hands and feet. How does this compare with the temperature of the skin on the trunk of the body? Is the skin dry and warm, or cold and clammy?

Capillary refill time: Squeeze a finger or toe for several seconds until the skin blanches, and then release it. Does the fingertip return to its normal color within 2 seconds, or is it delayed?

Color: Assess the patient's skin color. Is it pink, pale, ashen, or blue? (page 1180)

Ambulance Calls

1. Young children typically experience febrile seizures when their temperature rises rapidly. As with any call, you should assess airway, breathing, and circulation of this 2-year-old patient. Ensure that his airway is patent; assist him with breathing using a bag-mask device and airway adjunct, as necessary; apply high-flow oxygen; and remove excessive clothing. The child's level of consciousness should improve. If the child's level of consciousness doesn't improve or if the child experiences additional seizure activity, then this is a very serious sign that should be relayed to the receiving emergency department.

2. Immediately open and suction the airway. Assess breathing and apply high-flow oxygen via nonrebreathing mask or bag-mask device. Assess the patient further en route during rapid transport. Obtain the history from the grandmother en route. Reassess the patient's airway and vital signs en route as well.

3. Allow the child to remain in the mother's arms to decrease her anxiety. Offer oxygen via a nonrebreathing mask with the mother holding it. If she will not tolerate the nonrebreathing mask, use blow-by oxygen. Allow the mother to ride in the patient compartment of the ambulance to comfort the child. Provide rapid transport in a position of comfort with as much oxygen as she will tolerate. Continually assess the patient for signs of altered mental status and decreasing tidal volume; be prepared to assist ventilations. Obtain further history en route.

4. This infant is deceased, possibly as a result of SIDS. After you have quickly assessed the infant and made this determination, you must communicate the condition of the baby to the mother and family. This may be difficult, and they will possibly request resuscitation attempts regardless of your findings. This becomes a judgment call, which can be clarified by utilizing online medical direction and/or standing orders. You should survey the scene and document any history of recent illness, congenital conditions, and so forth. Be supportive of family members and assist them as appropriate. Calls involving infants and children can be traumatic experiences for emergency medical providers as well. Request debriefing as necessary and follow local protocols.

Skills

Skill Drills

Skill Drill 32-1: Positioning the Airway in a Pediatric Patient
1. Position the pediatric patient on a **firm** surface.
2. Place a **folded** towel about **1**-inch thick under the **shoulders** and **back**.
3. **Immobilize** the forehead to limit **movement** and use the head tilt–chin lift maneuver to open the airway. (page 1161)

Skill Drill 32-2: Inserting an Oropharyngeal Airway in a Pediatric Patient
1. Determine the appropriately **sized** airway. Confirm the correct size **visually**, by placing it next to the patient's **face**.
2. Position the pediatric patient's **airway** with the appropriate method.
3. Open the mouth. Insert the airway until the **flange** rests against the **lips**. **Reassess** the airway. (page 1174)

Skill Drill 32-3: Inserting a Nasopharyngeal Airway in a Pediatric Patient
1. Determine the correct airway size by comparing its **diameter** to the opening of the **nostril** (naris). Place the airway next to the pediatric patient's **face** to confirm correct **length**. **Position** the airway.
2. Lubricate the airway. Insert the **tip** into the right naris with the bevel pointing toward the **septum**.
3. Carefully move the tip forward until the **flange** rests against the **outside** of the nostril. Reassess the **airway**. (page 1175)

Skill Drill 32-4: One-Rescuer Bag-Mask Device Ventilation on a Pediatric Patient

1. Open the airway and insert the appropriate airway adjunct.

2. Hold the mask on the patient's face with a one-handed head tilt–chin lift technique (E-C grip). Ensure a good mask–face seal while maintaining the airway.

3. Squeeze the bag using the correct ventilation rate of 12 to 20 breaths/min. Allow adequate time for exhalation.

4. Assess effectiveness of ventilation by watching bilateral rise and fall of the chest. (page 1179)

Skill Drill 32-6: Immobilizing a Patient in a Car Seat

1. Carefully **stabilize** the patient's head in a **neutral** position.

2. Place an appropriately sized **cervical** collar on the patient if available. Otherwise, place rolled **towels** or padding alongside the patient.

3. Carefully secure the **padding**, using tape to keep it in place.

4. Secure the car seat to the **stretcher**. (page 1190)

Skill Drill 32-7: Immobilizing a Patient Out of a Car Seat

1. Stabilize the head in neutral position.

2. Place an immobilization device between the patient and the surface he or she is resting on.

3. Slide the patient onto the board.

4. Place a towel under the back, from the shoulders to the hips, to ensure neutral head position.

5. Secure the torso first; pad any voids.

6. Secure the head to the board. (page 1191)

Chapter 33: Geriatric Emergencies

General Knowledge

Matching

1. E (page 1225)   **3.** G (page 1229)   **5.** J (page 1230)   **7.** D (page 1234)   **9.** A (page 1234)
2. C (page 1228)   **4.** I (page 1229)   **6.** F (page 1227)   **8.** H (page 1235)   **10.** B (page 1227)

Multiple Choice

1. C (page 1217)   **13.** C (page 1220)   **25.** A (page 1228)   **37.** B (page 1236)
2. A (page 1215)   **14.** A (page 1221)   **26.** D (page 1229)   **38.** D (page 1237)
3. D (page 1215)   **15.** D (page 1223)   **27.** B (page 1231)   **39.** B (page 1244)
4. C (pages 1215–1216) **16.** B (page 1223)   **28.** A (page 1231)   **40.** D (page 1240)
5. A (page 1216)   **17.** A (page 1224)   **29.** C (page 1232)   **41.** C (page 1241)
6. C (page 1217)   **18.** C (page 1225)   **30.** C (page 1233)   **42.** D (page 1242)
7. D (page 1218)   **19.** A (page 1226)   **31.** D (page 1233)   **43.** A (page 1243)
8. C (page 1218)   **20.** D (pages 1226–1227) **32.** A (page 1234)   **44.** D (page 1245)
9. A (page 1218)   **21.** C (page 1229)   **33.** C (page 1234)   **45.** B (pages 1244–1245)
10. A (page 1219)   **22.** B (page 1227)   **34.** B (page 1235)
11. D (page 1220)   **23.** D (page 1228)   **35.** D (page 1236)
12. B (page 1220)   **24.** D (page 1228)   **36.** C (page 1236)

True/False

1. T (page 1215)   **6.** T (page 1219)   **11.** T (page 1227)   **16.** F (page 1232)   **21.** F (page 1237)
2. T (page 1216)   **7.** T (page 1221)   **12.** T (page 1228)   **17.** T (page 1233)   **22.** F (page 1238)
3. F (page 1217)   **8.** F (page 1223)   **13.** T (page 1229)   **18.** T (page 1234)   **23.** T (page 1239)
4. T (page 1218)   **9.** F (page 1225)   **14.** F (page 1230)   **19.** F (page 1235)   **24.** T (page 1241)
5. F (page 1219)   **10.** F (page 1226) **15.** T (page 1231)   **20.** T (page 1236)   **25.** T (page 1243)

Fill-in-the-Blank

1. name (page 1216)
2. osteoporosis (page 1217)
3. Oxygen (page 1221)
4. Pneumonia (page 1223)
5. fever (page 1224)
6. Arteriosclerosis (page 1225)
7. aneurysm (page 1225)
8. left-sided (page 1227)
9. Presbycusis (page 1228)
10. touch, pain (page 1229)
11. Diverticulosis (page 1231)
12. Pressure ulcers (page 1234)
13. cerebral bleeding (page 1237)
14. Bystander information (page 1238)
15. airway obstruction (page 1238)
16. flaccid abdominal wall (page 1239)
17. kyphosis (page 1240)
18. pelvic (page 1240)
19. Nursing homes (page 1241)
20. Advance directives (page 1242)

Fill-in-the-Table (page 1244)

Categories of Elder Abuse	
Physical	• **Assault** • **Neglect** • **Dietary** • **Poor maintenance of home** • **Poor personal hygiene**
Psychological	• **Benign neglect** • **Verbal** • **Treating the person as an infant** • **Deprivation of sensory stimulation**
Financial	• **Theft of valuables** • **Embezzlement**

Crossword Puzzle

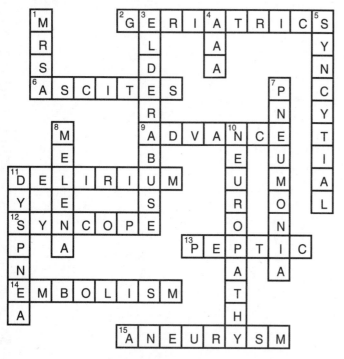

Critical Thinking

Short Answer

1. **1.** Hypertension
   2. Diagnosed arthritis
   3. Heart disease
   4. Cancer
   5. Diabetes
   6. Sinusitis (page 1217)

2. Motor nerves: muscle weakness, cramps, spasms, loss of balance, and loss of coordination.

Sensory nerves: tingling, numbness, itching, and pain; burning, freezing, or extreme sensitivity to touch

Autonomic nerves: affected involuntary functions that could include changes in blood pressure and heart rate, constipation, bladder and sexual dysfunction. (pages 1230–1231)

3. HHNC is a type 2 diabetic complication. It does not cause ketosis; instead, it leads to osmotic diuresis and a shift of fluid to the intravascular space that results in dehydration. The blood glucose level in HHNC is greater than 300 mg/dL. HHNC does not present with Kussmaul respirations.

DKA is a type 1 diabetic complication. It causes ketosis as a result of the hyperglycemia. The blood glucose is typically over 500 mg/dL in DKA, and patients tend to present with Kussmaul respirations. (page 1233)

4. Repeated visits to the emergency department or clinic

A history of being "accident prone"

Soft-tissue injuries

Unbelievable or vague explanations of injuries

Psychosomatic complaints

Chronic pain without medical explanation

Self-destructive behavior

Eating and sleep disorders

Depression or lack of energy

Substance and/or sexual abuse (page 1244)

5. **1.** Arrhythmias and heart attack: The heart is beating too fast or too slowly, the cardiac output drops, and blood flow to the brain is interrupted. A heart attack can also cause syncope.

2. Vascular and volume changes: Medication interactions can cause venous pooling and vasodilation, which results in a drop in blood pressure and inadequate blood flow to the brain. Another cause of syncope is a drop in blood volume because of hidden bleeding from a condition such as an aneurysm.

3. Neurologic cause: A transient ischemic attack or stroke can sometimes mimic syncope. (page 1231)

Ambulance Calls

1. This situation appears to be one of neglect and possible elder abuse. Perform a thorough assessment, especially if the patient is confused or is otherwise unable to express how or why she ended up on the floor. Ask for the patient's medical chart to obtain accurate information regarding her medical condition(s) and current medications. Immobilize her affected leg (and spine if needed) using the most comfortable methods possible. Geriatric patients need gentle care and many cannot tolerate conventional methods of splinting and immobilizing. Mechanisms of injury not viewed as significant in young, healthy patients can prove quite devastating or result in serious injury in older patients with frail skin and brittle bones.

2. Osteoporosis can be quite insidious in its onset. Individuals who were once relatively strong and healthy can suddenly find themselves with a fracture from something they may have done many times in the past. Postmenopausal, thin, Caucasian women are at higher risk of developing osteoporosis, and a spinal fracture in this scenario should be suspected. Perform an assessment to determine the presence of other injuries, provide full spinal immobilization, apply oxygen, and promptly transport this patient to the nearest appropriate facility. Always follow local protocols.

3. Hip fractures are a misnomer because true "hip fractures" are in fact fractures of the femur. You should determine if the mechanism of injury or suspicion exists for possible spinal fractures. Survey the scene to determine if there was a reason for the fall or if the break was spontaneous, giving the patient the impression of "tripping" on an object. If you believe that it was a spontaneous fracture, this patient suffers from extreme osteoporosis and likely suffered other fractures during the fall. If no spinal immobilization is deemed necessary, isolated hip fracture care requires an assessment of the patient's pulse, motor, and sensation of both lower extremities. You should also determine if the affected extremity is the same length or shorter than the uninjured side. It is also helpful to note if the leg is rotated inward, outward, or not at all. Immobilize the injured leg using blankets, pillows, and cravats or straps after placing the patient on a long spine board or scoop stretcher. After immobilization has occurred, reassess the pulse and motor and sensory functions of the injured extremity. Provide reassurance for the patient, because many feel that hip fractures signal the loss of their independence. Always follow local protocols.

4. Patients with kyphosis are extremely uncomfortable when immobilized on long spine boards. You should pad all voids using pillows, blankets, towels, or other appropriate forms of padding. Failure to adequately pad a patient's spine can result in increased pain and the inability of the patient to remain still. This can result in exacerbated injuries as well as a very unhappy patient. Thoracic spine injuries and injuries to the ribs can make it difficult for patients to breathe without pain. Determine whether her shortness of breath is related to pain during inspiration and/or whether she has a history of respiratory disease such as emphysema, chronic bronchitis, or asthma. Local weather conditions have probably contributed to her fall. Depending on the length of exposure to the elements, she could be suffering from hypothermia as well. Geriatric patients generally do not tolerate extremes in weather; avoiding extended periods of time in cold temperatures will minimize the likelihood for hypothermia.

Fill-in-the-Patient Care Report

EMS Patient Care Report (PCR)				
Date: Today's Date	**Incident No.:** 011727	**Nature of Call:** Unknown Medical Emergency		**Location:** 222 Orchid Lane
Dispatched: 0843	**En Route:** 0843	**At Scene:** 0849	**Transport:** 0902	**At Hospital:** 0908	**In Service:** 0915

Patient Information	
Age: 78 Years **Sex:** Male **Weight (in kg [lb]):** Unknown	**Allergies:** Aspirin
	Medications: metoprolol, Lisinopril, Actos, metformin, Zocor, Celebrex, allopurinol, Lasix, K-dur, Plavix, and multivitamin
	Past Medical History: MI, CHF, Hypertension, Diabetes, Arthritis, Gout, High Cholesterol
	Chief Complaint: "My head hurts."

Vital Signs				
Time: 0853	**BP:** 110/68	**Pulse:** 86	**Respirations:** 20	**Sao$_2$:** 98%
Time: 0902	**BP:** 116/76	**Pulse:** 84	**Respirations:** 18	**Sao$_2$:** 100%

EMS Treatment (circle all that apply)				
Oxygen @ 15 **L/min via (circle one):** NC (NRM) Bag-Mask Device		**Assisted Ventilation**	**Airway Adjunct**	**CPR**
Defibrillation	(**Bleeding Control**)	(**Bandaging**)	(**Splinting:** Full Body/ Cervical Immobilization)	**Other Shock Treatment**

Narrative
9-1-1 dispatch for 78-year-old man with an unknown medical problem. Local fire department was also dispatched for an assist per the dispatcher. Arrived on scene and was met by patient's wife at the front door who stated that patient was lying on the bathroom floor and she was unable to help him up. We were directed to the bathroom, where we found our patient lying supine on the floor in no obvious distress with a hematoma and laceration noted to his right forehead. Patient stated that he was on the toilet and must have fallen, but cannot completely remember the incident. The patient denied any chest pain, SOB, N/V, dizziness, or sweating. The patient complained of "head pain," which he rated as a 4/10. The patient denied radiation of pain or neck pain. Cervical immobilization was manually maintained while immobilization supplies were gathered. The patient was fully immobilized onto a backboard to include cervical collar, longboard, and head immobilization device. Immobilization was assisted by fire personnel. Oxygen was applied at 15 L/min via nonrebreathing mask. Primary and secondary assessment performed, along with vital signs. The patient was secured to litter and taken to unit. Patient was transported to Mercy Hospital per his request. Reassessment of patient indicated his pain continued to be a 4/10. Upon arrival at facility, patient was stable. Care was transferred to ED staff. Verbal report was given to staff. Room 4. No further incidents. Unit cleaned and restocked. Crew went available and returned to station. **End of Report**

Chapter 34: Patients With Special Challenges

General Knowledge

Matching

1. C (page 1266)
2. H (page 1273)
3. F (page 1261)
4. J (page 1262)
5. A (page 1273)
6. D (page 1268)
7. G (page 1265)
8. I (page 1272)
9. B (page 1268)
10. E (page 1269)

Multiple Choice

1. C (page 1261)
2. B (page 1262)
3. D (pages 1262–1263)
4. A (page 1263)
5. A (page 1263)
6. C (page 1264)
7. D (page 1264)
8. B (page 1264)
9. D (page 1265)
10. A (page 1265)
11. A (page 1266)
12. B (page 1266)
13. C (page 1267)
14. A (page 1268)
15. B (page 1270)
16. C (page 1270)
17. D (page 1271)
18. C (page 1272)
19. B (page 1272)
20. B (page 1272)
21. A (page 1273)
22. C (page 1273)
23. D (page 1274)
24. A (page 1275)
25. B (page 1268)

True/False

1. T (page 1264)
2. F (page 1264)
3. T (page 1268)
4. F (page 1268)
5. F (page 1269)
6. T (pages 1269–1270)
7. F (page 1269)
8. T (page 1271)
9. T (page 1272)
10. T (page 1273)

Fill-in-the-Blank

1. Autism (page 1262)
2. shoulder (page 1264)
3. Hearing aids (page 1265)
4. sensorineural; conductive (page 1265)
5. Cerebral palsy (page 1266)
6. vitamin B (folic acid) (page 1268)
7. left ventricular assist device (page 1271)
8. Shunts (page 1272)
9. dehydration (page 1273)
10. palliative care (page 1274)

Fill-in-the-Table (page 1269)

DOPE Mnemonic	
D	Displaced, dislodged, or damaged tube
O	Obstruction of the tube (secretions, blood, mucus, vomitus)
P	Pneumothorax, pulmonary problems
E	Equipment failure (kinked tubing, ventilator malfunction, empty oxygen supply)

Crossword Puzzle

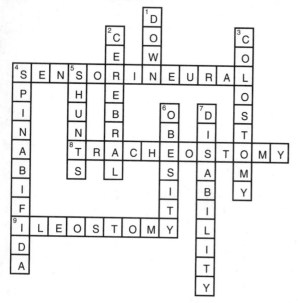

Critical Thinking

Short Answer

1. **1.** Speak slowly and distinctly into a less-impaired ear, or position yourself on that side.
   2. Change speakers. Look for a team member with a low-pitched voice if you think pitch is the issue.
   3. Provide paper and a pencil so that you may write your questions and the patient may write responses.
   4. Only one person should ask interview questions, to avoid confusing the patient.
   5. Try the "reverse stethoscope" technique: Put the earpieces of your stethoscope in the patient's ears and speak softly into the diaphragm of the stethoscope. (pages 1265–1266)

2. Make sure the hearing aid is turned on.
   Try a fresh battery, and check the tubing to make sure it is not twisted or bent.
   Ensure the switch is set on M (microphone), not T (telephone).
   Try a spare cord for a conventional body type aid; the old one may be broken or shorted.
   Make sure the ear mold is not plugged with wax. (page 1266)

3. **1.** Behind-the-ear type
   2. Conventional body type
   3. In-the-canal and completely in-the-canal type
   4. In-the-ear type (page 1266)

4. **1.** Treat the patient with dignity and respect.
   2. Ask your patient how it is the best to move him or her before attempting to do so.
   3. Avoid trying to lift the patient by only one limb, which would risk injury to overtaxed joints.
   4. Coordinate and communicate all moves to all team members prior to starting to lift.
   5. If the move becomes uncontrolled at any point, stop, reposition, and resume.
   6. Look for pinch or pressure points from equipment because they could cause a deep venous thrombosis.
   7. Very large patients may have difficulty breathing if you lay the patient in a supine position.
   8. Many manufacturers make specialized equipment for morbidly obese patients, and some areas have specially equipped bariatric ambulances for such patients.
   9. Plan egress routes to accommodate large patients, equipment, and the lifting crew members.
   10. Notify the receiving facility early to allow special arrangements to be made prior to your arrival to accommodate the patient's needs. (page 1269)

5. **1.** What type of heart disorder does the patient have?

   2. How long has this device been implanted?

   3. What is the patient's normal baseline rhythm and pulse rate?

   4. Is the patient's heart completely dependent on the pacemaker device?

   5. At what pulse rate will the defibrillator fire?

   6. How many times has the defibrillator shocked the patient? (page 1271)

Ambulance Calls

1. An internal cardiac pacemaker is implanted under the patient's skin to regulate the pulse rate and rhythm. You should provide oxygen and airway management for this patient. Because the automated implanted cardioverter defibrillator is firing, it is likely that the patient has an underlying arrhythmia. ALS should be contacted for a rendezvous. In addition, you should be prepared for this patient to go into cardiac arrest. Remember not to place AED pads directly over the implanted device. Transport immediately, maintain ABCs, and rendezvous with ALS.

2. Many patients with Down syndrome have epilepsy. Most of the seizures are tonic-clonic. Patient management is the same as with other patients with seizures. Because the patient has had two witnessed seizures, consider requesting ALS. It is likely the patient will seize again. In addition, use the parents and family as a resource for information. These people are likely to be very familiar with the patient's medical history and complications. Maintain ABCs, apply oxygen, and assess for any potential injuries that may have occurred during the seizure. Be aware of the potential airway complications faced in patients with Down syndrome, such as a large tongue and smaller oral and nasal cavities.

Skills

Assessment Review

1. C (page 1262)

2. D (page 1264)

3. D (page 1270)

4. B (page 1273)

Chapter 35: Lifting and Moving Patients

General Knowledge

Matching

1. C (page 1306)   **3.** H (page 1293)   **5.** A (page 1319)   **7.** F (page 1306)   **9.** D (page 1293)
2. J (page 1318)   **4.** E (page 1319)   **6.** I (page 1294)   **8.** B (page 1317)   **10.** G (page 1313)

Multiple Choice

1. D (page 1285)   **9.** D (page 1294)   **17.** A (page 1300)   **25.** B (page 1312)
2. B (pages 1300–1301) **10.** A (page 1295)   **18.** B (page 1300)   **26.** B (page 1313)
3. D (page 1287)   **11.** D (page 1295)   **19.** C (page 1300)   **27.** D (page 1294)
4. C (pages 1287–1288) **12.** B (page 1296)   **20.** B (page 1286)   **28.** B (page 1300)
5. B (page1287)   **13.** A (page 1296)   **21.** A (page 1303)   **29.** A (page 1290)
6. A (page 1289)   **14.** C (pages 1296–1297) **22.** C (page 1310)   **30.** D (page 1309)
7. B (page 1293)   **15.** C (page 1298)   **23.** A (page 1319)
8. A (page 1295)   **16.** B (page 1299)   **24.** D (page 1295)

True/False

1. T (page 1318)   **4.** F (page 1298)   **7.** F (page 1293)   **10.** T (page 1313)   **13.** F (page 1318)
2. T (page 1287)   **5.** T (page 1300)   **8.** F (page 1302)   **11.** T (page 1321)   **14.** F (page 1315)
3. F (page 1295)   **6.** F (page 1320)   **9.** F (page 1295)   **12.** T (page 1321)   **15.** T (page 1315)

Fill-in-the-Blank

1. body mechanics (page 1285)   **6.** 250 (page 1295)   **11.** spine movement (page 1302)
2. upright (page 1287)   **7.** sideways (page 1298)   **12.** direct ground lift (page 1306)
3. power lift (page 1287)   **8.** locked (page 1299)   **13.** extremity lift (page 1306)
4. palm (page 1289)   **9.** overhead (page 1299)   **14.** fluid resistant (page 1314)
5. locked-in (page 1292)   **10.** less strain (page 1300) **15.** scoop stretcher (page 1320)

Crossword Puzzle

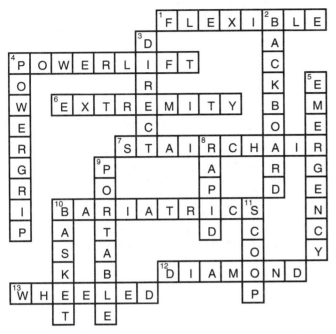

Critical Thinking

Short Answer

1. 1. Body drag
   2. Fire fighter's drag
   3. Front cradle
   4. One-person walking assist
   5. Fire fighter's carry
   6. Pack strap (pages 1300–1302)
2. 1. The vehicle or scene is unsafe.
   2. Explosives or other hazardous materials are on the scene.
   3. There is a fire or a danger of fire.
   4. The patient cannot be properly assessed before being removed from the car.
   5. The patient needs immediate intervention that requires a supine position.
   6. The patient has a life-threatening condition that requires immediate transport to the hospital.
   7. The patient blocks the EMT's access to another seriously injured patient. (page 1303)
3. 1. Make sure there is sufficient lifting power.
   2. Follow the manufacturer's directions for safe and proper use of the stretcher.
   3. Make sure that all stretchers and patients are fully secured before you move the ambulance. (page 1318)
4. 1. Be sure that you know or can find out the weight, both of the patient and the associated equipment, to be lifted and the limitations of the team's abilities.
   2. Coordinate your movements with those of the other team members while constantly communicating with them.
   3. Do not twist your body as you are carrying the patient.
   4. Keep the weight that you are carrying as close to your body as possible while keeping your back in a locked-in position.
   5. Be sure to flex at the hips, not at the waist, and bend at the knees, while making sure that you do not hyperextend your back by leaning back from your waist. (page 1290)
5. Always keep your back in a straight, upright position and lift without twisting. (page 1287)

Ambulance Calls

1. Immobilize the patient on a long spine board, apply high-flow oxygen, and consider the use of a basket stretcher. Use four people to carry the patient back up the ledge. Plan the route, and brief your helpers before moving the patient. Clarify whether you will move on "three" or count to three, then move. Coordinate the move until the patient is loaded into the ambulance.

2. It is highly unlikely that you will be able to move this patient, especially without significantly hurting yourself or your partner. You should immediately request additional personnel. You can attempt to move the patient, but if you cannot successfully do so, you will have to open his airway, etc., in his current position. Do the best you can until the patient can be moved.

3. Patients whose conditions will be exacerbated by physical activity should not walk to the stretcher or ambulance. If a patient's condition is such that it is not medically necessary that you carry him or her, it is safer for the patient to walk on his or her own power to the ambulance. However, this patient should not/cannot walk. This produces a safety issue for you and your partner, especially given the fact that there is no elevator. Fortunately, this patient can sit upright; thus, the use of a stair chair would be appropriate in this situation. Regardless, you should ask for more personnel given the patient's large size. Back injuries are very common in EMS. For providers to avoid these injuries, correct lifting techniques should be used and assistance should be requested whenever the patient is large or in a position not conducive to correct lifting procedures.

Skills

Skill Drills

Skill Drill 35-1: Performing the Power Lift

1. Lock your back into a(n) **upright** curve. **Spread** and bend your legs. Grasp the backboard, palms up and just in front of you. **Balance** and **center** the weight between your arms.
2. Position your feet, **straddle** the object, and **distribute** weight.
3. Lift by **straightening** your legs, keeping your back locked in. (page 1288)

Skill Drill 35-2: Performing the Diamond Carry

1. Position yourselves facing the patient.
2. The EMTs at the sides each turn the head-end hand palm down and release the other hand.
3. The EMTs at the side turn toward the foot end. The EMT at the foot turns to face forward. (page 1291)

Skill Drill 35-3: Performing the One-Handed Carrying Technique

1. **Face** each other and use both **hands**.
2. Lift the backboard to **carrying height**.
3. **Turn** in the direction you will walk and **switch** to using one hand. (page 1292)

Skill Drill 35-6: Performing the Rapid Extrication Technique

1. The first EMT provides in-line manual support of the head and cervical spine.
2. The second EMT gives commands, applies a cervical collar, and performs the primary assessment.
3. The second EMT supports the torso. The third EMT frees the patient's legs from the pedals and moves the legs together, without moving the pelvis or spine.
4. The second EMT and the third EMT rotate the patient as a unit in several short, coordinated moves. The first EMT (relieved by the fourth EMT or a bystander as needed) supports the patient's head and neck during rotation (and later steps).
5. The first (or fourth) EMT places the backboard on the seat against patient's buttocks.
6. The third EMT moves to an effective position for sliding the patient. The second and third EMTs slide the patient along the backboard in coordinated, 8″ to 12″ (20- to 30-cm) moves until the patient's hips rest on the backboard.
7. The third EMT exits the vehicle, moves to the backboard opposite the second EMT, and they continue to slide the patient until the patient is fully on the board.
8. The first (or fourth) EMT continues to stabilize the head and neck while the second EMT and the third EMT carry the patient away from the vehicle and onto the prepared stretcher. (pages 1304–1305)

Skill Drill 35-8: Extremity Lift

1. The patient's hands are **crossed** over the chest. The first EMT grasps the patient's wrists or **forearms** and pulls the patient to a **sitting** position.

2. The second EMT moves to a position between the patient's **legs**, facing in the **same** direction as the patient, and places his or her hands under the **knees**.

3. Both EMTs rise to a **crouching** position. On **command**, both lift and begin to move. (page 1308)

Skill Drill 35-9: Direct Carry

1. Place the stretcher **parallel** to the bed with the patient's **feet** facing the head of the stretcher. Secure the **stretcher** to prevent movement. Face the patient while standing between the **bed** and the **stretcher**. Slide one arm under the patient's **neck** and cup the patient's **shoulder**. Your partner should slide his or her hand under the patient's **hip** and lift slightly. You should then slide your other arm under the patient's **back**, and your partner should place both arms underneath the patient's **hips** and **calves**.

2. Lift the patient in a smooth, **coordinated** fashion. Slowly walk the patient around, and position him or her over the **stretcher**.

3. Slowly and **gently** lower the patient onto the stretcher. (page 1309)

Skill Drill 35-10: Using a Scoop Stretcher

1. Adjust the **length** of the **stretcher**.

2. **Lift** the patient slightly and **slide** the stretcher into place, one side at a time.

3. **Lock** the stretcher ends together, avoiding **pinching** the patient.

4. **Secure** the patient to the scoop stretcher, and **transfer** it to the stretcher. (page 1311)

Chapter 36: Transport Operations

General Knowledge

Matching

1. D (page 1354)   **3.** E (page 1349)   **5.** F (page 1331)   **7.** B (page 1345)
2. A (page 1347)   **4.** G (page 1346)   **6.** C (page 1345)

Multiple Choice

1. C (page 1331)   **9.** B (page 1337)   **17.** B (page 1342)   **25.** C (page 1352)
2. A (page 1332)   **10.** D (page 1338)   **18.** D (page 1347)   **26.** B (page 1352)
3. A (page 1332)   **11.** A (page 1338)   **19.** B (page 1348)   **27.** D (page 1342)
4. B (page 1332)   **12.** D (page 1341)   **20.** A (page 1350)   **28.** D (page 1344)
5. D (page 1333)   **13.** D (page 1341)   **21.** C (page 1350)   **29.** C (page 1345)
6. D (page 1336)   **14.** C (page 1341)   **22.** D (page 1352)   **30.** D (pages 1345–1346)
7. A (page 1336)   **15.** C (page 1342)   **23.** B (page 1352)   **31.** D (page 1355)
8. D (page 1336)   **16.** D (page 1347)   **24.** C (page 1352)

True/False

1. T (page 1333)   **3.** T (page 1333)   **5.** F (page 1350)   **7.** T (page 1356)   **9.** F (page 1355)
2. F (page 1337)   **4.** F (page 1342)   **6.** T (page 1349)   **8.** F (page 1353)

Fill-in-the-Blank

1. jump kit (page 1338)   **4.** First-responder vehicles (page 1331)   **7.** airway (page 1336)
2. Star of Life® (page 1332)   **5.** nine (page 1332)   **8.** CPR board (page 1337)
3. hearse (page 1331)   **6.** decontaminate (page 1336)

Labeling

1. Helicopter Hand Signals

A. Move right
B. Move forward
C. Move rearward
D. Move upward
E. Move downward
F. Move left (page 1357)

Crossword Puzzle

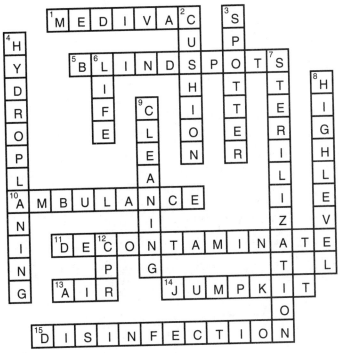

Critical Thinking

Multiple Choice

1. A (page 1342)
2. B (page 1332)
3. D (page 1337)
4. C (page 1344)
5. A (page 1344)

Short Answer

1. **Type I:** Conventional, truck cab-chassis with modular ambulance body that can be transferred to a newer chassis as needed

   Type II: Standard van, forward-control integral cab-body ambulance

   Type III: Specialty van, forward-control integral cab-body ambulance (page 1332)

2. 1. Preparation for the call
   2. Dispatch
   3. En route to scene
   4. Arrival at scene
   5. Transfer of patient to the ambulance
   6. En route to the receiving facility (transport)
   7. At the receiving facility (delivery)
   8. En route to station
   9. Postrun (page 1332)

3. *Siren syndrome* is the term for the increase in anxiety of other drivers that commonly causes them to drive faster in the presence of sirens. (page 1350)

4. **1.** To the best of your knowledge, the unit must be on a true emergency call.

   2. Both audible and visual warning devices must be used simultaneously.

   3. The unit must be operated with due regard for the safety of all others, on and off the roadway. (page 1352)

5. **1.** At the time of dispatch, select the shortest and least congested route to the scene.

   2. Avoid routes with heavy traffic congestion; know alternative routes to each hospital during rush hours.

   3. Avoid one-way streets. Do not go against the flow of traffic on a one-way street, unless absolutely necessary.

   4. Watch carefully for bystanders as you approach the scene.

   5. Once you arrive at the scene, park the ambulance in a safe place. If you park facing into traffic, turn off your headlights so that they do not blind oncoming drivers unless they are needed to illuminate the scene. If the vehicle is blocking part of the road, keep your warning lights on to alert oncoming motorists; otherwise, turn them off.

   6. Drive within the speed limit while transporting patients, except in the rare extreme emergency.

   7. Go with the flow of the traffic.

   8. Always drive defensively.

   9. Always maintain a safe following distance. Use the "4-second rule."

   10. Try to maintain an open space or cushion in the lane next to you as an escape route in case the vehicle in front of you stops suddenly.

   12. Use your siren if you turn on the emergency lights, except when you are on a freeway.

   13. Always assume that other drivers will not hear the siren or see your emergency lights. (page 1348)

6. A hard, level surface a minimum of 100′ by 100′ (30 m by 30 m).

   A clear site that is free of loose debris, electric or telephone poles and wires, or any other hazards that might interfere with the safe operation of the helicopter. (page 1355)

Ambulance Calls

1. Fire departments have a distinct chain of command. You should obtain permission to place yourself en route to this medical emergency from your shift captain or appropriate fire officer. Just because a call is dispatched does not mean you should automatically place yourself en route to that location. The incident commander of the confirmed structure fire may need your immediate assistance on the scene. Because you do not know the nature of the medical emergency at this point, it would be prudent to place that decision in appropriate hands. Always follow local protocols and chain of command.

2. Ideally, you should be very familiar with your response area, and you should take time every shift to study local roads. This can be done individually or as a group shift activity. Obviously, the larger your coverage area the more difficult it becomes to memorize addresses, especially if you are not native to the area. Regardless, you should be able to read maps quickly, and you should not rely on your memory to assist in locating a new address. To attempt to memorize all local streets is a good goal, but failing to consult with a map before leaving the station for reasons of pride is downright foolish. Ensure that each and every agency vehicle used in response to emergencies is equipped with local maps and other resources to ensure that you arrive promptly at emergency scenes. Utilize your local dispatch center for directions, if necessary.

3. Park your ambulance in a safe area and ensure your personal safety. Either you or your partner should handle traffic control until the police arrive. The person not handling traffic control should assess the patient. Provide patient care while ensuring personal safety and patient safety.

Fill-in-the-Patient Care Report

EMS Patient Care Report (PCR)			
Date: Today's Date	**Incident No.:** 2011-8999	**Nature of Call:** MVC	**Location:** Hwy 12 and Nest Creek Rd
Dispatched: 0512	**En Route:** 0513	**At Scene:** 0523 **Transport:** 0532	**At Hospital:** 0546 **In Service:** 0557

Patient Information	
Age: 41 Years	**Allergies:** None
Sex: Female	**Medications:** Lisinopril
Weight (in kg [lb]): 90 kg (198 lb)	**Past Medical History:** TIA at age 36
	Chief Complaint: Facial pain following MVC

Vital Signs				
Time: 0532	**BP:** 142/100	**Pulse:** 100	**Respirations:** 16 Unlabored	**Sao₂:** 98%
Time: 0543	**BP:** 142/100	**Pulse:** 100	**Respirations:** 14 Unlabored	**Sao₂:** 98%

EMS Treatment

(circle all that apply)

Oxygen @ 15 L/min via (circle one): NC (NRM) Bag-Mask Device	Assisted Ventilation	Airway Adjunct	CPR
Defibrillation	**Bleeding Control**	**Bandaging** (Splinting)	**Other Shock Treatment**

Narrative

Dispatched on an emergency call to a motor vehicle collision on Hwy 12. Arrived on scene to find two vehicles involved and one injured driver (other driver denied any injury). Patient, 41-year-old woman with a swollen and bleeding nose, was contacted while still belted into the driver's seat of her damaged car. She was conscious and alert and followed directions appropriately. C-spine precautions were taken. The patient was properly secured to a long spine board, removed from the vehicle, and given high-concentration oxygen via nonrebreathing mask. Patient was loaded into the ambulance and was found to have no other obvious or stated injuries. Initial vital signs indicated elevated blood pressure, which the patient stated was normal; all other observations indicated that the patient was stable. While en route, I contacted the receiving facility to provide report and completed a second set of vital signs to compare to the first and found no change other than a slightly lower respiratory rate. Transport was completed without incident. Once at the County Medical Center, the patient was transferred appropriately to the staff's care. I provided a full verbal report to the accepting nurse. Ambulance was then cleaned and restocked, and we returned to service without delay. **End of Report**

Chapter 37: Vehicle Extrication and Special Rescue

General Knowledge

Matching

1. E (page 1368)	**4.** F (page 1370)	**7.** D (page 1373)	**10.** G (page 1379)
2. A (page 1372)	**5.** B (page 1376)	**8.** H (page 1374)	**11.** K (page 1379)
3. L (page 1380)	**6.** J (page 1378)	**9.** I (page 1376)	**12.** C (page 1371)

Multiple Choice

1. B (page 1368)	**4.** B (page 1370)	**7.** D (page 1370)	**10.** C (page 1371)	**13.** C (page 1376)
2. D (page 1368)	**5.** D (page 1370)	**8.** B (page 1370)	**11.** A (page 1372)	**14.** D (page 1378)
3. A (page 1369)	**6.** C (page 1370)	**9.** B (page 1371)	**12.** B (page 1372)	**15.** B (page 1379)

True/False

1. T (page 1379)	**5.** T (page 1376)	**9.** F (page 1370)	**13.** F (page 1372)	**17.** F (page 1368)
2. F (page 1379)	**6.** F (page 1369)	**10.** T (page 1374)	**14.** T (page 1372)	
3. T (page 1377)	**7.** T (page 1374)	**11.** F (page 1374)	**15.** F (page 1371)	
4. T (page 1376)	**8.** T (page 1374)	**12.** T (page 1373)	**16.** T (page 1368)	

Fill-in-the-Blank

1. hazardous materials (page 1380)	**10.** battery (page 1371)	**18.** air medical unit (page 1377)
2. mentally; physically (page 1367)	**11.** stabilized (page 1371)	**19.** incident commander (page 1378)
3. Entrapment (page 1368)	**12.** protective gear (page 1372)	**20.** Vibration (page 1378)
4. safe (page 1368)	**13.** rescue team (page 1370)	**21.** four feet (page 1378)
5. Size-up (page 1369)	**14.** Communication (page 1374)	**22.** structure fire (page 1379)
6. emergency lights (page 1368)	**15.** leadership (page 1374)	
7. EMS personnel (page 1370)	**16.** fire-resistant canvas; blanket (page 1375)	
8. fire fighters (page 1370)	**17.** specialized rescue (page 1376)	
9. danger zone (page 1371)		

Crossword Puzzle

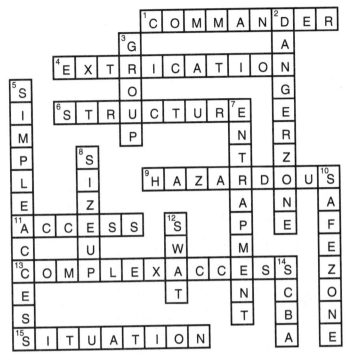

Critical Thinking

Short Answer

1. **EMS personnel:** Responsible for assessing and providing immediate medical care, performing triage and assigning priority to patients, packaging the patient, providing additional assessment and care as needed once the patient has been removed, and providing transport to the emergency department.

   Fire fighters: Responsible for extinguishing any fire, preventing additional ignition, ensuring that the scene is safe, and washing down spilled fuel.

   Law enforcement: Responsible for traffic control and direction, maintaining order at the scene, investigating the crash or crime scene, and establishing and maintaining lines so bystanders are kept at a safe distance and out of the way of rescuers.

   Rescue team: Responsible for properly securing and stabilizing the vehicle, providing safe entrance and access to patients, extricating any patients, ensuring that patients are properly protected during extrication or other rescue activities, and providing adequate room so that patients can be removed properly. (page 1370)

2. 1. Is the patient in a vehicle or in some other structure?
   2. Is the vehicle or structure severely damaged?
   3. What hazards exist that pose risk to the patient and rescuers?
   4. In what position is the vehicle? On what type of surface? Is the vehicle stable or is it apt to roll or tip? (page 1372)

3. 1. Provide manual stabilization to protect the c-spine, as needed.
   2. Open the airway.
   3. Provide high-flow oxygen
   4. Assist or provide for adequate ventilation.
   5. Control any significant external bleeding.
   6. Treat all critical injuries. (pages 1373–1374)

4. **1.** Preparation

   2. En route to the scene

   3. Arrival and scene size-up

   4. Hazard control

   5. Support operations

   6. Gaining access

   7. Emergency care

   8. Removal of the patient

   9. Transfer of the patient

   10. Termination (page 1368)

5. Ensure that each EMT can be positioned so that he or she can lift and carry at all times. Move the patient in a series of smooth, slow, controlled steps, with stops designed between steps to allow for repositioning and adjustments. Plan the exact steps and pathway that you will follow. Choose a path that requires the least manipulation of the patient or equipment. Make sure that sufficient personnel are available. Make sure that you move the patient as a unit. While moving the patient, continue to protect him or her from any hazards. (pages 1375–1376)

Ambulance Calls

1. You cannot assume that the man has left the premises, and you must act in the best interest of the patient. If the man is unconscious or otherwise incapacitated, time is of the essence. You should look inside the residence to see if the patient (in whole or part) is visible. Law enforcement should be summoned to the scene immediately for legal purposes if you feel that forced entry is justified. Always "try before you pry," checking open windows and doors to gain access; if this is not possible, choose a small window to break rather than a door. It is less expensive to repair. Sometimes windows adjacent to doors can be broken and access to the interior lock can be gained. You must be careful when entering, because there is a family dog that will most likely protect the property. Animal control should be requested if you feel the dog presents a safety hazard. It is prudent to err on the side that the patient needs immediate assistance rather than waiting for the third-party caller to arrive with keys. Always follow local protocols.

2. Entering the water could be a death sentence for you both. If you have a cellular phone and/or department radio with you, your best course of action would be to inform incoming units of the boy's location and situation. It would be advisable to direct some responding units downstream so that if the boy should lose his grasp on the log, other responders will be available to retrieve him. If your department has areas that contain the possibility of swift water rescue (even if only seasonal), training should be conducted and appropriate helmets, throw bags, and life jackets should be made available for safe response. You must assess the scene before trying to effect immediate rescue operations. Many responders have been killed by "jumping into" all types of rescues without performing a scene size-up or using the proper gear. Don't become a victim. Doing so will only make you part of the problem.

3. Try to learn as much about the chemical as possible by having the dispatcher contact CHEMTREC or another agency to find out about possible effects to the patient. Prepare necessary equipment to manage the airway and ventilation. Be prepared to do CPR, if necessary. Have all equipment within reach. Once the patient is brought to you, rapidly begin to manage the ABCs and prepare for rapid transport.

Chapter 38: Incident Management

General Knowledge

Matching

1. H (page 1404)
2. N (page 1411)
3. B (page 1409)
4. J (page 1409)
5. E (page 1410)
6. O (page 1389)
7. L (page 1400)
8. I (page 1410)
9. A (page 1403)
10. G (page 1404)
11. C (page 1396)
12. F (page 1403)
13. D (page 1396)
14. M (page 1388)
15. K (page 1410)

Multiple Choice

1. B (page 1387)
2. D (page 1387)
3. A (page 1388)
4. D (page 1389)
5. A (page 1390)
6. C (page 1392)
7. B (page 1392)
8. C (page 1392)
9. D (page 1393)
10. B (page 1393)
11. B (page 1394)
12. A (page 1394)
13. B (page 1396)
14. C (page 1396)
15. B (page 1396)
16. D (page 1396)
17. A (page 1397)
18. C (page 1390)
19. A (page 1398)
20. C (page 1398)
21. A (page 1398)
22. A (page 1399)
23. B (page 1401)
24. D (page 1402)
25. C (page 1403)
26. C (page 1404)
27. B (page 1405)
28. A (page 1406)
29. D (page 1410)
30. B (pages 1413–1414)

True/False

1. T (page 1387)
2. T (page 1388)
3. F (page 1389)
4. F (page 1392)
5. T (page 1393)
6. F (pages 1393–1394)
7. T (page 1394)
8. T (page 1397)
9. F (page 1398)
10. F (page 1401)
11. T (page 1402)
12. T (page 1403)
13. F (page 1405)
14. T (page 1408)
15. F (pages 1412–1413)

Fill-in-the-Blank

1. flexibility; standardization (page 1387)
2. span of control (page 1388)
3. single (page 1389)
4. planning (page 1390)
5. Preparedness (page 1391)
6. triage supervisor (page 1393)
7. Treatment supervisors (page 1393)
8. number; category (page 1396)
9. location; building (pages 1401–1402)
10. bulk; nonbulk (page 1402)
11. Storage bags (page 1403)
12. Control zones (page 1409)
13. warm zone (page 1410)
14. decontamination (page 1410)
15. intermodal tank (page 1403)

Fill-in-the-Table (page 1397)

Triage Priorities	
Triage Category	**Typical Injuries**
Red tag: first priority (immediate) Patients who need immediate care and transport Treat these patients first, and transport as soon as possible	• **Airway and breathing difficulties** • **Uncontrolled or severe bleeding** • **Severe medical problems** • **Signs of shock (hypoperfusion)** • **Severe burns** • **Open chest or abdominal injuries**
Yellow tag: second priority (delayed) Patients whose treatment and transport can be temporarily delayed	• **Burns without airway problems** • **Major or multiple bone or joint injuries** • **Back injuries with or without spinal cord damage**
Green tag: third priority, minimal (walking wounded) Patients who require minimal or no treatment and transport can be delayed until last	• **Minor fractures** • **Minor soft-tissue injuries**
Black tag: fourth priority (expectant) Patients who are already dead or have little chance for survival; treat salvageable patients before treating these patients	• **Obvious death** • **Obviously nonsurvivable injury, such as major open brain trauma** • **Respiratory arrest (if limited resources)** • **Cardiac arrest**

Crossword Puzzle

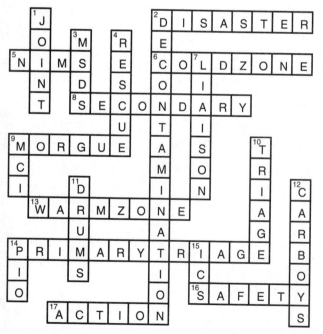

Critical Thinking

Short Answer

1. Command and management

   Preparedness

   Resource management

   Communications and information management

   Supporting technologies

   Ongoing management and maintenance (pages 1387–1388)

2. 1. Check-in at the incident

    2. Initial incident briefing

    3. Incident record keeping

    4. Accountability

    5. Incident demobilization (page 1391)

3. The total number of patients

   The number of patients in each of the triage categories

   Recommendations for extrication and movement of patients to the treatment area

   Resources needed to complete triage and begin movement of patients (page 1396)

4. An understanding of what hazardous substances are and the risks associated with them

   An understanding of the potential outcomes of an incident

   The ability to recognize the presence of hazardous substances

   The ability to identify the hazardous substances, if possible

   An understanding of the role of the first responder awareness individual in the emergency response plan

   The ability to determine the need for additional resources and to notify the communication center (pages 1400–1401)

5. The name of the chemical, including any synonyms for it

   Physical and chemical characteristics of the material

   Physical hazards of the material

   Health hazards of the material

   Signs and symptoms of exposure

   Routes of entry

   Permissible exposure limits

   Response-party contact

   Precautions for safe handling (including hygiene practices, protective measures, and procedures for cleaning up spills or leaks)

   Applicable control measures, including personal protective equipment

   Emergency and first-aid procedures

   Appropriate waste disposal (page 1407)

Ambulance Calls

1. The 4-year-old should be triaged as first priority (red). The 27-year-old should be triaged as third priority (green). The 42-year-old should be triaged as fourth priority (black).

2. It is fortunate that this is occurring on shift change, because members from two shifts are available to respond to this mass casualty incident. Because this is a remote area, implying response times are extended, you should use this time to gather information from the crop-duster pilot/responsible parties regarding the substance and to notify all local hospitals. Area HazMat team members should be requested, and once the chemicals have been identified appropriate first aid and other instructions should be relayed to the affected patients on-scene through the dispatch center. Law enforcement should be requested to cordon off the area to prevent more individuals, such as coworkers and family members, from entering the contaminated area. Consult HazMat team members and/or CHEMTREC for appropriate information, including medical treatment, PPE, and minimum distances that are required to avoid exposure to the identified substance. Obviously, do not enter the area unless you have been trained and have the proper equipment to do so.

3. The good news is that you are uphill from the possible hazardous materials. You should be uphill and upwind from contaminated areas (especially when dealing with an unidentified substance). Each chemical reacts differently to outside air, temperature, and other ambient conditions. You should immediately instruct all civilians along the road to move out of the immediate area and/or instruct them to wait in a specific location if you feel that they have already been contaminated by the substance. Do not allow the driver to contaminate the passersby. Immediately notify law enforcement as well as the local HazMat team. Attempt to gain information regarding the shipment, keeping a safe distance (using binoculars, PA system to relay instructions, etc.). Prevent exposure to yourself and your crew and the members of the public. Always follow local protocols.

Skills

Assessment Review

1. C (page 1398)
2. B (page 1398)
3. A (page 1398)
4. B (pages 1398–1399)

Chapter 39: Terrorism Response and Disaster Management

General Knowledge

Matching

1. L (page 1433)
2. O (page 1433)
3. E (page 1439)
4. N (page 1434)
5. J (page 1442)
6. K (page 1440)
7. B (page 1432)
8. F (page 1437)
9. D (page 1433)
10. M (page 1441)
11. C (page 1439)
12. I (page 1442)
13. H (page 1439)
14. A (page 1445)
15. G (page 1439)

Multiple Choice

1. D (pages 1427–1428)
2. A (page 1428)
3. B (page 1429)
4. B (page 1430)
5. A (page 1430)
6. A (page 1432)
7. B (page 1432)
8. C (page 1433)
9. A (page 1434)
10. A (page 1435)
11. A (page 1436)
12. B (page 1434)
13. A (page 1437)
14. B (page 1439)
15. D (page 1440)
16. D (page 1441)
17. C (page 1441)
18. A (page 1442)
19. A (page 1443)
20. B (page 1444)
21. B (page 1445)
22. D (page 1447)
23. B (page 1448)

True/False

1. F (page 1427)
2. T (page 1428)
3. F (page 1429)
4. T (page 1429)
5. T (page 1430)
6. F (page 1432)
7. F (page 1433)
8. F (page 1433)
9. T (page 1434)
10. F (page 1435)
11. F (page 1436)
12. T (page 1434)
13. T (page 1438)
14. F (page 1439)
15. F (page 1440)
16. T (page 1441)
17. T (page 1442)
18. F (page 1442)
19. F (page 1443)
20. F (page 1444)
21. T (page 1445)
22. T (page 1447)
23. T (page 1448)

Fill-in-the-Blank

1. domestic terrorism (page 1427)
2. weapon of mass destruction/casualty (page 1428)
3. State-sponsored terrorism (page 1429)
4. orange (page 1430)
5. Cross-contamination (page 1431)
6. Route of exposure (page 1433)
7. contact hazard (page 1433)
8. Nerve agents (page 1434)
9. Off-gassing (page 1435)
10. Dissemination (page 1439)
11. Virus (page 1439)
12. viral hemorrhagic fevers (page 1440)
13. Anthrax (page 1441)
14. lymph nodes (page 1441)
15. botulinum (page 1442)
16. Points of distribution (page 1444)
17. radiologic dispersal device (page 1445)
18. secondary blast injury (page 1447)

Crossword Puzzle

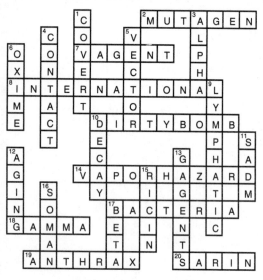

Critical Thinking

Short Answer

1. 1. What are your initial actions?
   2. Whom should you notify, and what should you tell them?
   3. What type of additional resources might you require?
   4. How should you proceed to address the needs of the victims?
   5. How do you ensure your own and your partner's safety, as well as the safety of the victims?
   6. What is the clinical presentation of a victim exposed to a WMD?
   7. How are WMD patients to be assessed and treated?
   8. How do you avoid becoming contaminated or cross-contaminated with a WMD agent? (page 1427)

2. 1. Vesicants (blister agents)
   2. Respiratory agents (choking agents)
   3. Nerve agents
   4. Metabolic agents (cyanides) (page 1429)

3. 1. Type of location
   2. Type of call
   3. Number of patients
   4. Victims' statements
   5. Pre-incident indicators (page 1430)

4. 1. Skin irritation, burning, and reddening
   2. Immediate intense skin pain
   3. Formation of large blisters
   4. Gray discoloration of skin
   5. Swollen and closed or irritated eyes
   6. Permanent eye injury
   7. If vapors inhaled:
      a. Hoarseness and stridor
      b. Severe cough
      c. Hemoptysis
      d. Severe dyspnea (page 1433)

5. **1.** Shortness of breath

   2. Chest tightness

   3. Hoarseness and stridor due to upper airway constriction

   4. Gasping and coughing (page 1434)

6. **1.** Salivation, sweating

   2. Lacrimation

   3. Urination

   4. Defecation, drooling, diarrhea

   5. Gastric upset and cramps

   6. Emesis

   7. Muscle twitching, miosis (page 1436)

7. **1.** Shortness of breath and gasping respirations

   2. Tachypnea

   3. Flushed skin

   4. Tachycardia

   5. Altered mental status

   6. Seizures

   7. Coma

   8. Apnea

   9. Cardiac arrest (page 1437)

8. **1.** Fever

   2. Chills

   3. Headache

   4. Muscle aches

   5. Nausea

   6. Vomiting

   7. Diarrhea

   8. Severe abdominal cramping

   9. Dehydration

   10. Gastrointestinal bleeding

   11. Necrosis of liver, spleen, kidneys, and gastrointestinal tract (page 1443)

9. **1.** Hospitals

   2. Colleges and universities

   3. Chemical and industrial sites (page 1445)

10. **1.** Time

   2. Distance

   3. Shielding (page 1447)

Ambulance Calls

1. There is no confirmation regarding the nature of the explosion. It could have been caused by a number of hazards, but precautions should be taken any time there is the chance for a terrorist attack. No one should rush into the scene, because terrorists have been known to deliberately target first responders by placing secondary explosive devices. Request all available resources, including local, state, and federal specialized HazMat and law enforcement agencies, to assist in this call. Notify all local and regional hospitals of the situation; assess the scene from a distance. Establish command and designate a staging area for incoming units. Enter the scene only when it has been determined to be safe. Regularly scheduled mock drills to include expected agencies to respond in this type of situation can greatly improve communications and the overall effectiveness and efficiency of response.

2. The presence of numerous people with the same signs and symptoms, who were in the same location at the same time, should immediately send up red flags. These patients were exposed to contaminated food, air, or water in which they ingested some sort of toxin. Ingestion of ricin can produce these signs and symptoms within 4 to 8 hours after exposure. It can be difficult to initially determine what substances caused these signs and symptoms, but through careful history taking and investigation of the patients' commonalities the exposure can be found. Unfortunately, there is no vaccination or other specific treatment available for exposure to ricin. Only supportive measures for airway, breathing, and circulation can be applied.

3. Cyanide is colorless and has an odor similar to bitter almonds. It interferes with the body's ability to utilize oxygen and can result in headache, shortness of breath, tachypnea, altered levels of consciousness, apnea, seizures, and even death. Antidotes can be given, but are rarely carried on ambulances. Patients' clothing must be removed to avoid exposure to the cyanide because it is released as a gas from the clothing fibers. For most patients, simply removing them from the source of cyanide and providing supportive therapy for their ABCs will be all that is needed. However, those with significant exposure may require aggressive airway intervention.

Assessment Review

1. C (page 1439)
2. B (page 1441)
3. D (page 1441)
4. A (page 1440)

Chapter 40: ALS Assist

General Knowledge

Matching

1. H (page 1474)
2. F (page 1488)
3. K (page 1480)
4. G (page 1482)
5. B (page 1488)
6. A (page 1468)
7. I (page 1466)
8. M (page 1493)
9. D (page 1482)
10. C (page 1496)
11. E (page 1476)
12. N (page 1477)
13. O (page 1476)
14. J (page 1465)
15. L (page 1480)

Multiple Choice

1. B (page 1463)
2. C (page 1463)
3. C (page 1463)
4. C (page 1464)
5. D (page 1465)
6. B (pages 1469–1470)
7. A (page 1466)
8. C (page 1467)
9. B (page 1468)
10. A (page 1468)
11. C (page 1470)
12. B (page 1473)
13. C (page 1473)
14. A (pages 1474–1475)
15. B (pages 1476)
16. C (page 1476)
17. B (page 1476)
18. D (page 1476)
19. B (page 1479)
20. D (page 1480)
21. C (page 1482)
22. B (page 1482)
23. D (page 1487)
24. B (page 1488)
25. C (page 1489)
26. D (page 1490)
27. B (page 1491)
28. A (page 1492)
29. B (page 1491)
30. C (page 1496)

True/False

1. T (page 1495)
2. F (page 1492)
3. F (page 1493)
4. T (page 1492)
5. T (page 1497)
6. T (page 1497)
7. F (page 1473)
8. F (page 1468)
9. F (page 1466)
10. F (page 1482)
11. T (page 1488)
12. F (page 1490)
13. T (page 1488)
14. T (page 1482)
15. F (page 1488)

Fill-in-the-Blank

1. inhalation (page 1464)
2. Cuffed (page 1467)
3. 15/22-mm (page 1468)
4. electrical conduction system (page 1491)
5. Sinus rhythm (page 1492)
6. Ventricular fibrillation (page 1495)
7. Asystole (page 1495)
8. Chest leads (page 1496)
9. gastric tube (page 1477)
10. CPAP (page 1478)
11. Saline locks (page 1481)
12. phlebitis (page 1488)
13. Macrodrip sets (page 1481)
14. Catheter shear (page 1489)
15. administration set (page 1480)

Labeling

1. ECG Rhythms

   A. Sinus tachycardia

   B. Asystole

   C. Ventricular fibrillation

   D. Normal sinus rhythm

   E. Sinus bradycardia

   F. Ventricular tachycardia (pages 1493, 1495–1496)

Crossword Puzzle

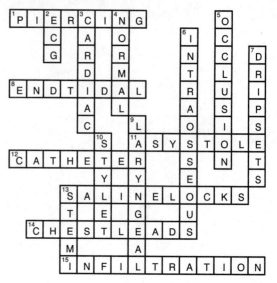

Critical Thinking

Short Answer

1. The sinoatrial node

Internodal pathways

Atrioventricular node

The bundle of His

The left bundle

The right bundle

The Purkinje system (page 1491)

2. Baseline period

SA node produces impulse

P wave forms

Impulse passes through AV node (PR interval)

QRS begins to form as impulse passes through ventricles

T wave forms during muscle repolarization

The final phase occurs when the impulse returns to baseline (page 1493)

3. **1.** Intubating the right mainstem bronchus

   2. Intubating the esophagus

   3. Aggravating a spinal injury

   4. Taking too long to intubate

   5. Patient vomiting

   6. Laryngospasm

   7. Trauma

   8. Mechanical failure

   9. Patient intolerance of ETT

   10. Decrease in heart rate (pages 1474–1476)

4. Infiltration

   Phlebitis

   Occlusion

   Vein irritation

   Hematoma (page 1488)

5. Allergic reactions

   Air embolus

   Catheter shear

   Circulatory overload

   Vasovagal reactions (page 1489)

Ambulance Calls

1. Do not be afraid to inform the paramedic that the leads have not been appropriately attached. You can save valuable time by simply relaying what you have seen. Sometimes EMTs can feel intimidated by the presence of paramedics and become afraid to speak out when they see something that doesn't appear right. Do not underestimate your ability to help, because sometimes you may notice things that the paramedic does not.

2. If successful intubation has occurred, you will hear equal, bilateral breath sounds and no sounds over the epigastrium. This endotracheal tube should be removed, and the patient should be ventilated with high-flow oxygen via bag-mask device and the placement of an oral airway. Secondary placement devices should be utilized when assessing placement of the ET tube. Direct visualization of the ET tube passing through the cords along with the use of esophageal detector devices and/or end-tidal carbon dioxide detectors can ensure successful placement has been accomplished. If endotracheal intubation is not possible, consider the use of multilumen airways such as the Esophageal Tracheal Combitube (ETC), King LT airway, or Laryngeal Mask Airway (LMA). Always follow local protocols.

3. You should immediately slow the IV to a TKO rate, raise the patient's head, and apply high-flow oxygen (or increase the current L/min). Notify the receiving facility of the error. Healthy adults can handle the sudden influx of intravenous fluids without detrimental effects, but individuals who have diseased or otherwise weakened hearts, lungs, or kidneys do not possess the ability to cope with the fluid overload. To avoid this occurrence, check and double-check the drip chamber/flow rate to prevent accidental fluid boluses.

Skills

Skill Drills

Skill Drill 40-1: Performing Orotracheal Intubation

1. Open and clear the airway. Insert an oral airway, and oxygenate with a bag-mask device.
2. Assemble and test the intubation equipment.
3. Position the patient's head, perform the Sellick maneuver, and remove the oral airway.
4. For trauma patients, maintain the cervical spine in-line and neutral.
5. Visualize the vocal cords and watch the ET tube pass between them. Remove the laryngoscope and stylet. Hold the tube carefully.
6. Inflate the balloon cuff, and remove the syringe as your partner prepares to ventilate.
7. Ventilate and confirm placement.
8. Secure the tube. Note the depth of insertion. Reconfirm placement with every move. (pages 1472–1473)

Skill Drill 40-2: Spiking the Bag

1. Remove the pigtail from the port on the IV bag and the cover from the spike on the administration set.
2. Slide the spike into the IV bag port.
3. Prime the chamber.
4. Prime the line to remove air.
5. Check the drip chamber. It should only be half filled. If the fluid level is too low, squeeze the chamber until it fills. If the drip chamber fills completely, invert the IV bag and squeeze the excess back into the bag. (page 1482)

Skill Drill 40-3: Starting an IV

1. Prepare the solution and tubing to be used. Fill the drip chamber halfway by squeezing it.
2. Flush or "bleed" the tubing to remove any air bubbles by opening the roller clamp.
3. Tear the tape before venipuncture, or have a commercial device available.
4. Apply gloves before making contact with the patient. Palpate a suitable vein.
5. Apply the constricting band above the intended IV site.
6. Clean the area using aseptic technique.
7. Choose the appropriately sized catheter, and examine it for any imperfections.
8. Insert the catheter at an angle of approximately 45° with the bevel up while applying distal traction with the other hand.
9. Observe for "flashback" as blood enters the catheter.
10. Occlude the catheter to prevent blood leaking while removing the stylet.
11. Dispose of all sharps in the proper container.
12. Attach the prepared IV line.
13. Remove the constricting band.
14. Open the IV line to ensure fluid is flowing and the IV is patent. Observe for swelling and infiltration around the IV site.
15. Secure the catheter with tape or a commercial device. Secure IV tubing and adjust the flow rate. (pages 1484–1486)

Notes

Notes

Notes

Notes